# Statistical Methods in Epilepsy

Epilepsy research promises new treatments and insights into brain function, but statistics and machine learning are paramount for extracting meaning from data and enabling discovery. **Statistical Methods in Epilepsy** provides a comprehensive introduction to statistical methods used in epilepsy research. Written in a clear, accessible style by leading authorities, this textbook demystifies introductory and advanced statistical methods, providing a practical roadmap that will be invaluable for learners and experts alike.

Topics include a primer on version control and coding, pre-processing of imaging and electrophysiological data, hypothesis testing, generalized linear models, survival analysis, network analysis, time-series analysis, spectral analysis, spatial statistics, unsupervised and supervised learning, natural language processing, prospective trial design, pharmacokinetic and pharmacodynamic modeling, and randomized clinical trials.

**Features:**

- Provides a comprehensive introduction to statistical methods employed in epilepsy research
- Divided into four parts: Basic Processing Methods for Data Analysis; Statistical Models for Epilepsy Data Types; Machine Learning Methods; and Clinical Studies
- Covers methodological and practical aspects, as well as worked-out examples with R and Python code provided in the online supplement
- Includes contributions by experts in the field

This handbook targets clinicians, graduate students, medical students, and researchers who seek to conduct quantitative epilepsy research. The topics covered extend broadly to quantitative research in other neurological specialties and provide a valuable reference for the field of neurology.

**Sharon Chiang** is a fellow in the Department of Physiology and the Epilepsy Division in the Department of Neurology at the University of California, San Francisco, USA. Her research focuses on state-space models, network models, and the cellular circuit mechanisms of memory impairment in epilepsy.

**Vikram R. Rao** is an Associate Professor of Clinical Neurology, Ernest Gallo Distinguished Professor, and Chief of the Epilepsy Division in the Department of Neurology at the University of California, San Francisco, USA. His clinical and research interests involve applications of neurostimulation devices for drug-resistant epilepsy, neuropsychiatric disorders, and seizure forecasting.

**Marina Vannucci** is Noah Harding Professor of Statistics at Rice University, Houston, TX, USA, and also holds an Adjunct Professor appointment at the MD Anderson Cancer Center, Houston, TX, USA. Her research is focused on the development of Bayesian statistical methodologies for application in genomics, neuroscience, and neuroimaging.

**CHAPMAN & HALL/CRC Interdisciplinary Statistics Series**
Series editors: B.J.T. Morgan, C.K. Wikle, P.G.M. van der Heijden

**Recently Published Titles**

**Correspondence Analysis in Practice, Third Edition**
M. Greenacre

**Capture-Recapture Methods for the Socialand Medical Sciences**
D. Böhning, P. G. M. van der Heijden, and J. Bunge (editors)

**The Data Book: Collection and Management of Research Data**
M. Zozus

**Modern Directional Statistics**
C. Ley and T. Verdebout

**Survival Analysis with Interval-Censored Data: A Practical Approach with Examples in R, Sas, and Bugs**
K. Bogaerts, A. Komarek, and E. Lesaffre

**Statistical Methods in Psychiatry and Related Field: Longitudinal, Clustered and Other Repeat Measures Data**
R. Gueorguieva

**Bayesian Disease Mapping: Hierarchical Modeling in Spatial Epidemiology, Third Edition**
A.B. Lawson

**Flexbile Imputation of Missing Data, Second Edition**
S. van Buuren

**Compositional Data Analysis in Practice**
M. Greenacre

**Applied Directional Statistics: Modern Methods and Case Studies**
C. Ley and T. Verdebout

**Design of Experiments for Generalized Linear Models**
K.G. Russell

**Model-Based Geostatistics for Global Public Health: Methods and Applications**
P.J. Diggle and E. Giorgi

**Statistical and Econometric Methods for Transportation Data Analysis, Third Edition**
S. Washington, M.G. Karlaftis, F. Mannering and P. Anastasopoulos

**Parameter Redundancy and Identifiability**
D. Cole

**Mendelian Randomization: Methods for Causal Inference Using Genetic Variants, Second Edition**
S. Burgess, S. G. Thompson

**Bayesian Modelling of Spatio-Temporal Data with R**
Sujit Kumar Sahu

**Statistical Methods in Epilepsy**
Sharon Chiang, Vikram R. Rao, and Marina Vannucci

For more information about this series, please visit: https://www.crcpress.com/Chapman--HallCRC-Interdisciplinary-Statistics/book-series/CHINTSTASER

# Statistical Methods in Epilepsy

Edited by
Sharon Chiang, Vikram R. Rao, and Marina Vannucci

CRC Press
Taylor & Francis Group
Boca Raton London New York

CRC Press is an imprint of the
Taylor & Francis Group, an **informa** business
A CHAPMAN & HALL BOOK

First edition published 2024
by CRC Press
62385 Executive Center Drive, Suite 320, Boca Raton, FL 33431, U.S.A.

and by CRC Press
4 Park Square, Milton Park, Abingdon, Oxon, OX14 4RN

*CRC Press is an imprint of Taylor & Francis Group, LLC*



ISBN: 978-1-032-18435-7 (hbk)
ISBN: 978-1-032-18436-4 (pbk)
ISBN: 978-1-003-25451-5 (ebk)

DOI: 10.1201/9781003254515

Typeset in Latin Modern font
by KnowledgeWorks Global Ltd.

*Publisher's note:* This book has been prepared from camera-ready copy provided by the authors.

Access the support material: www.routledge.com/9781032184357

*To our families,*
*and to our patients and friends living with epilepsy*

# Contents

# Preface

Epilepsy is a common neurological disorder characterized by recurrent seizures, paroxysmal attacks associated with high morbidity and mortality. Seizures have myriad manifestations and seem to occur at random, features that have engendered fascination and fear since antiquity. The earliest accounts of epilepsy come from the Babylonians, whose diagnostic manuals written in cuneiform script over 3000 years ago describe different seizure types associated with different outcomes as well as treatments that involved spiritual intervention. Hippocrates was among the first to attribute seizures to organic brain dysfunction, but belief in a supernatural etiology of epilepsy was widespread and proved tenacious. The scientific foundation for epileptology was laid by John Hughlings Jackson in the late nineteenth century, and the development of electroencephalography (EEG) by Hans Berger soon thereafter enabled the study of brain electrical activity in relation to seizures. In 1912, Alfred Hauptmann discovered the anticonvulsant properties of phenobarbital, and the ensuing century saw exponential growth in the number of anti-seizure medications. Milestones in epilepsy along the way have included effective surgical therapies, improved EEG systems, sophisticated neuroimaging modalities, genetic diagnostics, implanted neurostimulation devices, seizure prediction strategies, and wearable sensors. With these advances, modern clinicians have an unprecedented array of tools to care for people living with epilepsy.

These advances have also introduced new challenges. For researchers in this age of 'Big Data', multimodal epilepsy data are often collected in the petabytes but still require careful curation and pre-processing before analysis. Measurements of human brain activity now span a wide spatial range (single-cell to whole-brain) over long timescales (months to years), and these data demand analytical methods that account for spatially organized and temporally ordered processes. Seizures are typically infrequent events and studying longitudinal zero-inflated count data necessitates certain mathematical approaches. Similarly, investigation of cyclical phenomenon in epilepsy requires application of circular statistics. For clinicians, the expanding armamentarium of therapeutic options makes rigorous evaluation of clinical trial data essential, though this requires background in the relevant statistics. With electronic health records now ubiquitous, clinicians would also benefit from background in natural language processing methods that can distill valuable information from a sea of unstructured free text. Artificial intelligence and deep learning methods have permeated epilepsy, and some clinicians may feel inadequately prepared to appreciate the promises and perils of this technology. Indeed, medical education is criticized for not including enough statistical training, and this knowledge gap will only be more exposed in the years ahead.

This textbook was written with an aim to bridge this gap. The intended audience is diverse, including epilepsy clinicians and researchers, applied statisticians, neural engineers, and data scientists. Each chapter focuses on teaching the reader how to conduct statistical analysis pertinent to the chapter topic.

The first four chapters provide foundational material for data analysis. The first chapter covers basic coding practices in two common programming languages, `R` and Python. Two chapters are dedicated to pre-processing data from electroencephalography, magnetoencephalography, and neuroimaging, including data acquisition principles and artifact rejection methods. A separate chapter reviews fundamental principles of hypothesis generation, validity assessment, and correction for multiple testing.

The next six chapters review common types of data encountered in epilepsy, including spatial imaging data, with an emphasis on Bayesian methodologies; time-series data, including inference and prediction methods from data such as chronic EEG; spectral analysis to model oscillatory phenomena in brain electrical activity; and network estimation and graph theoretic metrics that describe relationships between interconnected components in complex systems. One chapter focuses on generalized linear models that relate clinical covariates to outcomes, and a separate chapter is dedicated to non-parametric and semi-parametric survival analyses that model time to an event.

The next three chapters focus on machine learning methods. One chapter reviews unsupervised learning methods that can reveal meaningful structure in large, complex datasets without requiring response variables or labels. Another chapter covers supervised learning methods in the context of seizure detection and seizure classification. Natural language processing, large language models, and deep learning are reviewed in a chapter focused methods that generate rich numeric representations of sequences of words.

The last three chapters are dedicated to clinical studies. A chapter on prospective cohort design reviews study design, data collection, and analysis issues encountered in observational studies that follow a group of patients over time. Given that anti-seizure medications are the mainstay of epilepsy treatment, one chapter is dedicated to pharmacokinetic parameters (e.g., absorption, distribution, metabolism, and elimination) and study design methods that depend on the intensity of data sampling. The final chapter discusses epilepsy-specific considerations in randomized controlled trials.

This textbook can serve as curriculum material for undergraduate, graduate, or medical school courses; for clinical neurophysiology or epilepsy fellowships; and for continuing education programs for neurologists and advanced practice providers. Although focused on epilepsy, the statistical principles described here are broadly applicable in many areas of medicine and biomedical research.

We thank our families for their enduring support during this project. We are also immensely grateful to the chapter authors, who generously dedicated their time, energy, and expertise to creating a resource that is practical and accessible for all. Just as a supernatural etiology for epilepsy was eventually debunked, we hope this textbook may help demystify statistical methods in epilepsy.

Sharon Chiang, M.D., Ph.D. – University of California, San Francisco, USA

Vikram R. Rao, M.D., Ph.D. – University of California, San Francisco, USA

Marina Vannucci, Ph.D. – Rice University, USA

June 2023

# *Foreword*

A thorough understanding of statistics is required for a successful career in medical research. Unfortunately, training in statistical methods can be difficult to obtain for many in academic medicine due to barriers involving other time commitments and the lack of clear, concise resources that are tailored to those in medicine. In neurology, the challenge is even greater, with few dedicated statistical trainings focused on neuroscience in general, let alone those that are dedicated to specific areas of study within the field.

The pace of advances in epilepsy research over the last decade has been nothing short of spectacular. New approaches for dataset interpretation as well as clinical trial execution seem to arise monthly as the field catches up not only with other areas of neurology such as stroke, but other specialties of medicine including oncology which historically have utilized advanced research approaches to answer key epidemiologic questions while allowing for innovation and rapid adoption of new therapies for patients. It is in this context that this book edited by Drs. Sharon Chiang, Vikram R. Rao, and Marina Vannucci meets an important unmet gap. For those interested in any research in neurology, but particularly those studying epilepsy, this incredible *tour de force* can be useful for teaching both basic and advanced statistical methods ranging from coding and modeling to machine learning and clinical trial design. The more novel techniques described here are particularly essential in an era when reproducible research and ethical issues surrounding artificial intelligence are so important to the field and to society at large. Unlike many books on statistical methods, the chapters in this text are well written, accessible, and easy to understand, even for those with only modest statistical backgrounds.

The Editors have performed a remarkable job of carefully selecting authors who not only are experts in the field, but who demonstrate a communication style that readers will immediately recognize as not typical of similar texts. The varied topics contained and amazing diversity of approaches outlined, from classic to cutting-edge, will serve as a tremendous resource for years to come, encapsulating the future of epilepsy research as well as the most recent past. It can be imagined that some readers will choose to digest this book from cover to cover, like taking an inspiring statistical course in college or professional school. In this manner, the book's educational potential for trainees and even senior researchers cannot be overstated; contained herein is a true masterclass in statistics for those dedicated to a career in research. For others, this book can be used more sporadically, serving as an important resource for the bookshelf (or electronic bookshelf), to function as a key reference work whenever exploring new and exciting avenues of epilepsy investigation.

It is rare in 2023 to see a book published that is truly unique and fills an important need, given the large number of texts that are produced each and every year – this is a rare and delightfully exciting exception. *Statistical Methods in Epilepsy* stands as an incredibly important addition to the field, and I hope that readers enjoy it as much as I have.

S. Andrew Josephson, M.D. – University of California, San Francisco, USA

June 2023

# Part I

# Basic Processing Methods for Data Analysis

# 1

# *Coding Basics*

**Emilian R. Vankov**
*Wayfair (USA)*

**Rob M. Sylvester**
*Reltio (USA)*

**Christfried H. Focke**
*AppFolio (USA)*

## CONTENTS



This chapter provides a primer to version control and programming when carrying out statistical analysis for epilepsy studies. Introductions are made to version control, an aspect of coding practice employed in industry and academia to increase reproducibility and collaboration, and programming in two common software languages employed in applied statistical research, `R` and Python. We focus primarily on illustrating the basic coding principles in `R`, which is the preferred software of most statisticians, and provide a brief introduction to object-oriented programming in Python, another popular programming language among data scientists, machine learning engineers, and software engineers. Concepts are illustrated using a simulated dataset of interictal epileptiform discharges and electrographic seizure counts motivated by chronic ambulatory electrocorticography data from the Responsive Neurostimulation System (RNS® System) (NeuroPace, Inc., Mountain View, CA).

DOI: 10.1201/9781003254515-1

## 1.1 Introduction

This chapter presents a basic primer to programming and version control in reproducible collaborative research. Whether the reader is new to these concepts or an experienced researcher, this chapter is intended to serve as an overview of basic concepts when working with Github, version control systems, and two widely used programming languages for statistical analysis and machine learning – R and Python. Following a primer on Github and software versioning, we cover the essential programming concepts for getting started in the R programming language, including topics such as data structures, importing data and basic operations, data wrangling, and exploratory data analysis. Concepts are illustrated using a simulated example bivariate time-series dataset of interictal epileptiform discharges (IEDs) and long episodes (LEs), a proxy for electrographic seizures, motivated by data collected from the RNS System. Last, we provide a brief introduction to object-oriented programming in Python.

## 1.2 Version Control

Oftentimes, both in academia and industry, scripts are written that may or may not run on other computers. Results may be difficult to reproduce, and time is often spent writing code for something that someone has already written. Version control through software version management and collaborative platforms offers a solution to these issues by allowing users to track and manage their projects and software versions with ease, a practice that is necessary for increasing reproducibility in epilepsy research.

A version control system (VCS) is essentially a bookkeeping device for software development. While humans can theoretically achieve this collaboration manually, manual management generally impedes collaborative and reproducible research, leading to non-standardized naming conventions, generation of multiple duplicative copies of work, logistical challenges resulting from simultaneous editing or distributing changes, and generation of conflicts from multiple edits to the same file. Many of these headaches can be solved using a VCS. One popular VCS used in the industry and increasingly in academic research collaborations is Git. It is a free and open-source distributed VCS. Commonly partnered with Git is GitHub, a cloud-based repository, or location where code is stored and organized, that enables developers to store and manage their code easily. Using GitHub allows teams to have a single source of truth (SSOT) for the codebase used in a research collaboration. In this section, we walk the reader through an introduction to using the GitHub to setup and manage code repositories for research practice.

### 1.2.1 Getting Started with Git

In this section, we walk the reader through how to create a Github account, create a new repository, make local changes to the repository, and push the changes back to Github. These practices are necessary for using Github to manage a code repository in collaborative research.

### Installing Github and creating an account

On Mac, as well as some Linux distributions, Git is included with the operating system (OS). If it is not already installed on the system, it should be first downloaded and installed. On a Mac or Linux OS, open a program called *Terminal* that allows the user to run commands. From the terminal, type `git --version` to verify the installation and print your Git version. To install Git on Windows, follow the installation instructions for GitHub Desktop. After the installation on your OS is complete, create a GitHub account (`www.github.com`).

### Creating a repository

After installing Git and creating a Github account, create a new repository in GitHub called `test_repository`. Generally, it is advisable to create a new repository for each self-contained project. You should now have a reference URL for this new repository at https://github.com/<your_username>/test_repository.git. We will use this repository as a running example in this section.

### Committing changes

Before making modifications to the repository, you should create a local copy, called a *clone*, of the repository. This allows you and any collaborators to make modifications to the files, including descriptions of what changed, that you can later sync back to the source of truth (the original repository). To clone the repository from the terminal, run the command git clone <your_git_url>. You will now have a folder named `test_repository` on your machine.

To make changes to this repository and push the changes back to GitHub, follow the below steps:

1. Navigate to the local directory for `test_repository`.
2. Create and save a new text file called `test.txt`. Optionally include contents in this text file.
3. *Stage* your new changes by running `git add test.txt`.
4. *Commit* your new changes by running `git commit -m ``added new file ''`.
5. *Push* your new changes to GitHub (your source of truth) by running `git push`.

Steps 3–5 (*staging*, *committing*, and *pushing* changes) are the common sequence of actions that authors use to create historical records of change in the repository. The *commit* itself is the atomic unit of change that takes the repository from one stable state to another. Ideally, it contains a commit message, "*added new file*" that allows authors to describe what is changed in the new state. It is advisable to package your semantically related changes together in commits so that your development history is easy to maintain, trace, and recover across time. The commits are full snapshots of the code in your repository, which are stored efficiently without the need for multiple copies of your file.

Although a full walkthrough of Git is beyond the scope of this text, the above steps will enable the reader to get started creating a repository and committing changes for research projects. Tutorials for how to perform other steps, such as proposing changes to other researchers' projects or creating branches, are available at `docs.github.com`. It is recommended, for example, that the reader becomes familiar with branching logic in Git for any projects with multiple collaborators. There are also other best practices that researchers should be aware of; for example, it is generally best to only commit source code files to Github repositories. Specifically, it is not recommended to commit files such as full datasets, generated files (such as PDFs, executable files, spreadsheets), or binary files to a repository. This is because, once committed to Github, files remain part of the repository's history, forever bloating its size for all collaborators.

While the setup for VCS has an initial learning curve, it is critical to the development of quality software according to industry standards. Within medical and academic research, which has a potential impact on patient care and scientific knowledge, it is likely even more critical. Maintaining a SSOT in coding practice is critical to facilitating reproducible and transparent research, avoiding mistakes attributable to outdated or conflicting versions of code, and helping researchers to efficiently streamline large-scale collaborative research.

### 1.2.2 R and Python Versioning

Keeping up-to-date with software programming languages such as `R` and Python is crucial for compatibility, stability, and access to the latest features and bug fixes. While both languages have multiple versions that are actively maintained, using the latest versions ensures not only the best performance but also access to these newest features and improved security. Both `R` and Python can be downloaded for free from their official websites (`https://cran.r-project.org/` and `https://www.python.org/`).

RStudio is an integrated development environment (IDE) according to that provides a user-friendly interface to simplify, installation and version management in `R`. It provides an interface for switching between R versions and includes a package manager to manage dependencies in `R` projects.

For Python, `pip` is the default package manager used to maintain versions of different Python packages. Python projects are often developed in a virtual environment, which is a self-contained directory that manages not only the user's version of Python but the version of software packages. The authors recommend `pyenv` as a tool for managing Python versions and `virtualenv` as part of the standard Python library to create virtual environments, or the software package `poetry` for a simplified solution that takes care of it all.

Visual Studio Code (VS Code) is a powerful IDE that supports both `R` and Python development. It offers a wide range of extensions and includes rich support for Git, debugging tools, virtual environments, and other everyday development tasks that make this a highly recommended IDE of choice.

## 1.3 Programming in R

In this section, we provide an introduction to data analysis and visualization with `R`.

### 1.3.1 Why R?

`R` is one of the most popular open-source programming languages used for data analysis, visualization, and statistics. It was specifically designed for statistical computing and data analysis and is widely used throughout academia by statisticians, which allows new statistical inference and machine learning algorithms to be made freely available for users. There is a vast repository of libraries and functions created for data manipulation, data visualization, statistical inference, and machine learning through the Comprehensive R Archive Network (CRAN), which makes `R` a great choice for the development of new algorithms as well as statistical analysis. Given a data set, it is very easy to get started with `R` and to be up and running with data analysis within a matter of minutes. Moreover, it is very well-suited for the development of new algorithms and statistical methodology, the overhead associated with data structures and initial setup common for other languages is abstracted away.

### 1.3.2 Data Structures

First, let us review the most common data structures used in `R` along with some of their benefits.

Like most programming languages that deal with numerical operations, `R` provides the users with *vector* and *matrix* structures. Atomic vectors in `R` can be one of the four types: integer, double, Boolean/logical and character. Each atomic vector can contain only a homogeneous type of data, i.e., at most one of the four types. The homogeneous structure of the vectors and matrices allows for a trade-off between computational efficiency and flexibility in storing data.

In contrast, *lists* are similar to atomic vectors, but they can contain more than one data type, including other lists, vectors, matrices, data frames, or functions. Lists are one of the most flexible data structures, with elements of lists able to contain multidimensional data types.

While lists offer great flexibility in handling heterogeneous or nested data, some datasets involve tabular structured data. To handle this sort of data, `R` uses *data frames*. A data frame is a two-dimensional tabular structure composed of rows and columns and is designed so that each row represents an observation and each column represents a variable. Unlike other data structures, data frames have row names and column names that allow for convenient subsetting and aggregation of data. Moreover, unlike matrices and vectors, data frames can store *factors*, a data type used for handling categorical data in `R`, and *strings*, a data type used to handle text. More recently, an enhanced version of data frames, called *tibbles*, was introduced to `R` through the `tibble` library. Some of the benefits that tibbles provide are that they have stricter rules of column types and enforce consistent types within each column in the dataset, which prevents accidental coercion of data. Tibbles can also be more memory efficient when working with large datasets, as they use a lazy evaluation approach, which means that they do not load the entire dataset into memory until necessary. For a more extensive treatment of the different data structures within `R`, we refer the readers to [7].

### 1.3.3 Basic Operations

Next, we demonstrate how to carry out several basic coding operations required for data analysis in `R`. The dataset that we explore in this and subsequent sections is a simulated dataset of electrographic seizures and IEDs. The dataset and code are available in the repository accompanying the book.

#### Importing Libraries

In `R`, *libraries* (also known as *packages*) are collections of R functions that extend the capabilities of the base `R` system. Libraries allow the user to access specialized algorithms that have been developed by the `R` community.

For example, in one of the upcoming sections, we demonstrate how to load data stored in JavaScript Object Notation (JSON) files into `R`. This capability is not present in the base

R system, but is available through the jsonlite library. To use a library in R, it must first be installed onto the system using the install.packages() function. Once the library is installed, it can then be loaded into the current R session using the library() function. For example, to install and load the jsonlite library, we would run:

```
# Install library
install.packages("jsonlite")
# Load library
library(jsonlite)
```

### Loading CSV Files

Next, we show how to load data from three file formats commonly encountered in research: CSV (comma-separated values) files, JSON files, and MATLAB data files.

The data provided in the repository for this chapter consists of 20 folders, each with data on IED counts from an individual simulated patient with epilepsy, motivated by data from the RNS system [4]. Within each patient's folder there are three files: (1) metadata.csv, which is a CSV file containing metadata on the patient, including the patient's ID (first column), age in years (second column), gender (third column), suspected seizure focus (fourth column), first clinic visit after RNS implantation (fifth column), and a column with only missing values (sixth column); (2) sdata.json, which is a JSON file containing 2000 hourly observations of IED counts from each of two RNS leads, hourly long episode counts (a proxy for electrographic seizures), and the patient ID; and (3) timedata.mat, which is a MATLAB file containing timestamps corresponding to each of the 2000 hourly observations from sdata.json.

We will start by loading the metadata for a single patient from the CSV file into our R session. To load a CSV file in R, we use the built-in function read.csv(), which takes the file location and filename as input arguments. Another optional argument to this function is a specification of whether the header of the CSV file should be used as column names, by setting the header argument to either TRUE or FALSE. To look up the documentation for read.csv() (or, for that matter, any function in R), we can type ? in front of the function name (i.e., ?read.csv) or call help on the function name (i.e., help(read.csv)).

To load the metadata.csv file from a single patient, we would run:

```
# Initialize required paths
data_path <- "<your_path>"
single_patient_folder <- "Patient_1"
filename <- "metadata.csv"

# Concatenate all directories (as strings)
file_path <- paste(data_path, '/', single_patient_folder ,'/', filename, sep="")

# Read in the CSV file for a single patient
metadata_patient1 <- read.csv(file_path, header = TRUE, sep = ",")
```

To run the above code, replace data_path <- "<your_path>" with the local directory where you have saved the individual patient folders.

This code results in the CSV file containing the metadata for Patient 1 being loaded into an object called metadata_patient1. The object is a data frame with a single row, and six columns, with each column corresponding to a different patient attribute. (Hint: To check the structure of an object in R, call str() on the object.)

### Loading JSON Files

Another common standard data format encountered in research is the JSON file format. Many machine learning and software applications rely on JSON files for storing data. JSON files can be read into R using the `read_json()` function. Specifically, to load a JSON file, we would run:

```
# Load jsonlite library
library(jsonlite)

# Set the working directory to data_path
setwd(data_path)

# Load JSON data
rdata <- read_json(paste('Patient_1/', 'sdata.json', sep=""), simplifyVector =
    TRUE)

# Convert the large JSON character into a dataframe
seizures_patient1 <- fromJSON(rdata)
```

This code results in the JSON file containing hourly IED and LE counts being loaded and converted into a data frame called `seizure_data`. The dimensions of this object are $2000 \times 4$, corresponding to 2000 hourly observations and 4 variables.

### Loading MATLAB Files

Ability to load MATLAB files into R is another useful skill, as MATLAB is a common programming language used in research, particularly in signal processing. For example, it may be the case that you may have processed EEG data in MATLAB (see, for example, Chapter 2), and saved the output as a MATLAB file, and you may wish to read this file into R for analysis. To read and write MATLAB files with file extension .mat into R, we first install and then load the `R.matlab` library. We will then use the `readMat()` function to read the MATLAB file (in our case, `timedata.mat`) into our R session:

```
# Install and load the required packages
install.packages("R.matlab")
library(R.matlab)

# Load MATLAB data
timedata_patient1 <- readMat(paste('Patient_1/','timedata.mat', sep=""))
```

### For Loops

In many applications, data is stored across multiple files. For example, in data collected from $T$ successive time points across $p$ variables for each of $N$ patients, the data may be stored as a $T \times p$ matrix, with a different file saved in each of $N$ folders.

Suppose, for example, that rather than loading the CSV file from only a single patient, we now wish to load the CSV metadata files from all 20 patients into a single data frame. One way to load data from multiple files is to repeat the same code for each file. This could be done by repeating the same code 20 times, or, more concisely, with a For Loop, where we tell R to iteratively loop through and load each patient's data as a new row.

To accomplish this, we create a character vector with all the patients' directory names and execute the desired code within a For Loop. First, we initialize a character vector with the names of the 20 patient directories:

```
# Initialize a character vector with all patient directory names
patients_list <- c()
# Populate vector with patient names
patient_size <- 20
for (i in 1:patient_size){
  patients_list[i] <- paste('Patient_', i, sep="")
```

```
}
```

Next, we loop through each directory, load the CSV file from each individual patient folder into memory, and concatenate the data frames into a single data frame called `df_metadata`:

```
# Initialize the vector where the patient's metadata will be stored
df_metadata <- data.frame()

for (i in 1:length(patients_list)){
  # Get the filepath for each patient
  file_path <- paste(data_path, patients_list[i], '/', filename, sep="")

  # Load the patient's metadata
  metadata_current_patient <- read.csv(file_path, header = TRUE, sep = ",")

  # Store the patient's metadata into a new data frame to avoid overwriting
  df_metadata <- rbind(df_metadata, metadata_current_patient)
}
```

The resulting data frame `df_metadata` contains the metadata from all 20 patients. Syntactically, when writing a For Loop in `R`, the conditions for start and termination of the loop are specified within the parentheses, and the code that should be executed within each loop is specified within the curly braces.

### List Apply

For Loops are well-suited for certain applications in `R`, such as those involving iterative operations that depend on the order of elements, or non-vectorized operations where elements either must be accessed based on a condition or involving operations that cannot be applied element-wise. However, For Loops in `R` can be improved upon, particularly for operations that could be vectorized or where a single function is being applied to each element.

In these applications, the `lapply()` function, which stands for "list apply," offers a more efficient alternative. To use the `lapply()` function to apply `read.csv()` to multiple files, we would run:

```
# Initialize the directory containing the files and provide the filenames within
    each folder
files <- dir(data_path, recursive = TRUE, full.names = TRUE, pattern = "metadata.
    csv$")

# Iteratively load all CSV files
metadata_list <- lapply(files, read.csv)
```

In the code above, `lapply()` is used to apply `read.csv` to each element of the object `files`. Syntactically, `lapply()` applies the function specified in its second input argument, to each element of a list or vector specified in the first input argument. In this example, the built-in function `dir()` is used to retrieve the names of all files in the directory `data_path`. More generally, `dir()` is used to retrieve a list of filenames or directory names in a specified directory. It can be particularly useful as it does not require specification or pre-existing knowledge of the number of files or names of the files in the directory.

Last, we combine the list of data frames in `metadata_list` into a single data frame using `unlist`:

```
# Convert the metadata to a data frame
metadata <- data.frame(matrix(unlist(metadata_list), nrow=length(metadata_list),
    byrow=TRUE), stringsAsFactors=FALSE)
```

```
# Assign the appropriate column names
names(metadata) <- names(unlist(metadata_list[1]))
```

Let us do the same to use `lapply()` to load the timestamps from all patients into a single data frame:

```
files <- dir(data_path, recursive = TRUE, full.names = TRUE, pattern = "timedata.
    mat$")
timedata <- lapply(files, readMat)
timedata <- unlist(timedata)
```

## Functions

Thus far, we have used various predefined functions in R, such as `read.csv()`, `read_json()`, and `readMat()`. However, it is also possible to to define your own functions in R. A function is defined as a reusable block of code that takes inputs, performs computations on the inputs, and returns an output. The basic syntax of a function in R is:

```
my_function <- function(arg1, arg2, ...) {
  # Perform computations
  # Return value using 'return' function
}
```

For example, suppose we wish to define a function `my_function()` that takes a single input (the name of a JSON file that we wish to import), performs internal computations to load the JSON file and convert it to a data frame, and then returns a single output (the data frame containing the loaded JSON file). We can define such a function as:

```
my_function <- function(file_list){

  # Load JSON file
  rdata <- read_json(file_list, simplifyVector = TRUE)

  # Convert the large JSON file into a data frame
  seizure_data <- fromJSON(rdata)

  # Return
  return(seizure_data)
}
```

Here, the input argument to `my_function()` is `file_list`. The code body reads in `file_list` and converts it to a data frame, and the `return` statement returns the data frame to the user.

We can use our newly defined function, `my_function()`, to iteratively load the JSON files for all patients:

```
install.packages("dplyr")
library(dplyr)

# Read in all json files
files <- dir(data_path, recursive = TRUE, full.names = TRUE, pattern = "sdata.
    json$")
data <- lapply(files, my_function)

# Convert the list of dataframes to a dataframe
seizure_data <- bind_rows(data)
```

### Date and Time Data

There are several libraries available for working with date and time data in R. The two most commonly used are base (using the base R system) and lubridate. These two libraries handle dates and date/times slightly differently. The base library allows you to create a Date object to handle dates (hint: ?as.Date), and POSIXct or POSIXlt objects to handle date/times (hint: ?as.POSIXct). The lubridate package contains a number of additional convenient functions for handling dates and date/times that are not present in the base library, including functions to perform arithmetic operations on date/time objects, handle time zones, and handle time intervals. To create date/time objects, lubridate provides functions including ymd() (year-month-day), ymd_hms() (year-month-day hour-minute-second), and dmy() (day-month-year). For example, if we wish to turn timedata into a date/time object using lubridate, we would run:

```
install.packages("lubridate")
library(lubridate)
timedata <- ymd_hms(timedata, tz="UTC")
```

This code converts the string structure currently stored in timedata to a date/time object. The date/time object can then undergo any of the various functions available for manipulation of dates and times through lubridate.

## 1.3.4 Data Wrangling

Once data have been imported into R, the next step is *data wrangling*, or the process of exploring, cleaning, and organizing the data into a format usable for statistical analysis.

The scenario we consider in this example demonstrates several of the issues commonly encountered in data wrangling in a real-life data analysis project. Oftentimes, for example, one might need to work with data from multiple files or databases, all of which may be in different formats (e.g., CSV, JSON, MATLAB, Excel). The data sources are usually related by some common identifier (such as patient ID), but each usually also contains unique information that is not available in the other files. There may also be data that is missing from the dataset, or incorrectly named variables or entries. The task at hand, then, is to first identify the structure of each dataset and then to join the datasets by the common identifier.

The values that the data sources share in common are referred to in relational databases as *keys*. Typically, there are two types of keys - primary and foreign keys. A *primary key* refer to the column that uniquely identifies each row in the table. A *foreign key* refers to the column or columns in the table that refers to the primary key of another table. Defining a foreign key creates a link between the tables. To make these concepts more concrete, we will make use of the metadata, seizure_data, and timedata data frames imported into our R session in Section 1.3.3.

### Initial Data Structure Exploration

A quick way to investigate the structure of an object in R is via str(), which provides a concise summary of the internal structure of the object, such as its type, dimensions, and the content of each of its components. For example, str(metadata) yields:

```
str(metadata)
'data.frame': 20 obs. of  6 variables:
 $ ID          : chr  "Patient_1" "Patient_10" "Patient_11" "Patient_12" ...
 $ Age         : chr  "30.5" "20.9" "27.7" "26.3" ...
 $ Gender      : chr  "M" "M" "FALSE" "FALSE" ...
```

```
 $ Seizure_Foci: chr  "left frontal" "supplementary motor cortex" "right
    hippocampus" "left parietal" ...
 $ NA.         : chr  "2017-07-03" "2018-09-27" "2018-01-03" "2018-02-26" ...
 $ NA..1       : chr  NA NA NA NA ...
```

This means that `metadata` is a data frame with 20 rows (observations) and 6 columns (variables), with column names 'ID', 'Age', 'Gender,', 'Seizure_Foci', 'NA.', and 'NA..1', all of which are characters (`chr`). In this case, the variable `ID` is the primary key for the data frame as it uniquely identifies the rows.

We can similarly explore the structure `str(seizure_data)`, which yields:

```
str(seizure_data)
'data.frame': 40000 obs. of  5 variables:
 $ iea_lead1     : int  0 0 0 0 0 0 0 0 0 0 ...
 $ iea_lead2     : int  0 0 0 0 1 2 0 3 0 2 ...
 $ LE            : int  0 0 0 0 0 0 1 0 0 0 ...
 $ patient_id    : int  1 1 1 1 1 1 1 1 1 1 ...
```

This means that `seizure_data` is a data frame with 40,000 observations and 4 variables, all of which are integers (`int`). Here, the variables `iea_lead1` and `iea_lead2` are the hourly IED counts at each time bin from leads 1 and 2 of the device, and `LE` is the hourly LE counts , with the starting date/time of each time bin defined in `timedata`. The primary key in this case is `patient_id`, which has an `int` structure.

### Joining Data Frames

In general, a simple way of adding a single variable to a data frame in `R`, such as adding the variable `timedata` to the `seizure_data` data frame, is:

```
seizure_data$hourly_markers <- timedata
```

If, however, the interest is in joining two or more data frames into a single data frame based on common variables, we can use the `merge()` function. In our example, the primary keys from `metadata` and `seizure_data` (`ID` and `patient_id`) are stored as different structures (a character and an integer). In addition, although they both represent patient ID number, the variables have different content; namely, notice that the `ID` variable in `metadata` is stored as the patient ID, preceded by the string 'Patient_'.

Before joining the two data frames, it is necessary to convert both primary keys to the same data structure and representation of the ID variable in order to avoid a faulty join. If we wish to add the string 'Patient_' to the ID variable in `metadata`, we can use `paste0()`:

```
seizure_data$patient_id <- paste0("Patient_", seizure_data$patient_id)
```

Then, to join the two data frames, we can use `merge()`:

```
seizure_data <- merge(seizure_data, metadata, by.x = 'patient_id', by.y = 'ID',
    all.x = TRUE, all.y = FALSE)
```

In this example, the `merge()` function is used to merge `seizure_data` and `metadata` based on the `patient_id` variable in the left data frame (`seizure_data`) and by the `ID` variable in the right data frame (`metadata`). We also specify that we want to include all rows from the left data frame in the merged result, even if there are no matching rows in the right data frame, but that we only want to include rows from the right data frame if there are matching rows in the left data frame. The merge function also allows you to control the type of merge (inner, left, right, or full) and more (see `?merge`).

The merged data frame has 40,000 rows and 10 columns, and contains all the data that is available in both the original `seizure_data` and `metadata`. Of note, an alternative way to join these data frames would have been to perform an inner join. In an inner join, only the rows that have matches in both data frames are returned. Using `merge()` in R, an inner join can be performed by setting `all.x=TRUE` and `all.y = TRUE`.

### Data Cleaning

After joining all data frames into a single data frame, we would like to clean the data into an organized format that can be then input into one of the statistical models in the subsequent chapters of this book. Running `str(seizure_data)` quickly reveals a few issues with our data:

1. *Some variables have incorrect data types.* For example, `str(seizure_data)` reveals that `Age` was read in as a character rather than as a numeric. To convert the age variable into a float, we would run:

```
seizure_data$Age <- as.numeric(seizure_data$Age)
```

   Alternatively, if we wished to convert age into an integer, we would run `as.integer(seizure_data$Age)`.

2. *Some column names are capitalized, while others are lower case letters.* For consistency, one can change all column names to lower case by `tolower()`:

```
names(seizure_data) <- tolower(names(seizure_data))
```

3. *For the gender variable,* `R` *incorrectly read in the value 'female' as 'FALSE'; we need to replace all instances of 'FALSE' with the string 'female'.* There are several ways to convert `FALSE` to `F` to match more standard representations. As an example, we can use `gsub("FALSE", "F", seizure_data$gender)`. The function will find all occurrences of the first string, replace it with the second and insert it into the `gender` column in the data frame `seizure_data`. The same outcome can be accomplished the same way using:

```
install.packages("stringi")
library(stringi)
stri_replace_all_fixed(seizure_data$gender, "FALSE", "F")
```

   from the `stringi` package [2]. Since both functions accomplish the same outcome, a natural question is which one should be used. One way to answer this question is to compare the execution time of each function applied to the data frame:

```
install.packages('microbenchmark')
library(microbenchmark)
microbenchmark(gsub("FALSE", "F", seizure_data$gender),
    stri_replace_all_fixed(seizure_data$gender, "FALSE", "F"))
```

   The output is shown in Table 1.1.

**TABLE 1.1**
Comparison of execution time in milliseconds over 100 trials of `gsub()` and `stringi()`.

| | Minimum | Q1 | Mean | Median | Q3 | Maximum | # trials |
|---|---|---|---|---|---|---|---|
| gsub | 15.02 | 15.64 | 16.19 | 16.12 | 16.41 | 21.44 | 100 |
| stringi | 5.29 | 5.60 | 5.96 | 5.74 | 5.92 | 19.15 | 100 |

As we see, `stri_replace_all_fixed()` via `stringi` is about three times faster than `gsub()`. Generally, this advantage is further increased for larger datasets.

Using `stringi` to replace `"FALSE"` to `"F"` within `gender`, then, we would run:

```
# Replace "FALSE" with "F"
seizure_data$gender <- stri_replace_all_fixed(seizure_data$gender, "FALSE
    ", "F")
```

4. *There is a column named* `na.`*, which contains content on the date of the patient's first clinic visit after RNS implantation; this column should be renamed.* To rename the variable, we can run:

```
# Change column names
col_names <- colnames(seizure_data)
colnames(seizure_data)[col_names == "na."] <- 'first_visit_date'
```

   This replaces the original column name `na.` with `first_visit_date`, which is much more informative.

5. *There is a column named* `na..1`*, which contains only* NA *values; this column should be dropped.* One way to drop a column from a data frame in `R` is to use the subset operator:

```
# Drop the column using the subset operator
seizure_data <- seizure_data[, -which(names(seizure_data) == 'na..1')]
```

   Here, `which()` returns the index/indices of the columns satisfying the condition `names(seizure_data == 'na..1')`.

### Missing data

When dealing with data, there are often observations that contain missing values. Sometimes, as in the instance of `na..1`, there are variables which are completely missing. In the majority of instances, however, missing values constitute only a percentage of observations. Understanding the percentage and distribution of missingness is important to appropriate missing data treatment. There are a number of built-in functions in `R` for imputing missing data, including the `mice` library, which provides multiple imputation by chained equations; `missForest`, which imputes missing data using random forests; `VIM`, which provides functions for visualizing and analyzing missing data, as well as offering various imputation methods; `Hmisc`, which provides various other functions for imputation; and `imputeTS`, which provides methods for time-series imputation.

There are different ways to treat missing values, which depend on the mechanism of missingness (see Chapter 14). The simplest way to treat missing data is *complete-case analysis*, which drops the entire row if any of the columns contain missing data. This can be implemented via `na.omit()`:

```
# If NA is present in any row of the data frame, drop that row
any_na_drop = na.omit(seizure_data)
```

This code yields a new data frame, `any_na_drop`, which contains only observations for which there was no missing data. Alternatively, we could carry out complete-case analysis using the `complete.cases()` function to return which observations are complete, i.e., have no missing values, and take the subset of `seizure_data` with those observations.

Of note, complete-case analysis is a straightforward method for handling missing data, but leads to reduction in sample size as well as introduction of potential bias if the missingness mechanism is not missing completely at random (MCAR) or at least unrelated to the variables being analyzed. An alternative method for handling missing data includes imputation, which uses available information to fill in missing values. Imputation-based methods can be broadly divided into two categories: single imputation methods and model-based imputation. Single imputation methods replace each missing value with a single value, such as the mean (*mean imputation*), median (*median imputation*), randomly selected values from similar observations for which data is non-missing (*hot-deck imputation*), or $k$-nearest neighbors imputation (see Chapter 11). Another common class of methods are multiple imputation approaches; rather than imputing a single value for a missing value, multiple plausible values for each missing value are imputed using statistical models, and the average is treated as the final imputed value. Model-based imputation methods, on the other hand, use statistical models or machine learning methods to estimate missing values, and include methods such as regression-based imputation, decision tree-based imputation, Bayesian imputation, and deep learning-based imputation. Low-rank matrix completion is discussed in Chapter 11. Although methods for handling missing data are beyond the scope of this chapter, we refer the reader to several external resources for further reading [1, 3, 5].

For illustrative purposes about coding in R, we demonstrate how one can write a function to carry out median imputation. Median imputation proceeds as follows:

1. Calculate the median of each variable using the non-missing data.
2. Replace missing values of each variable with the median calculated from the non-missing data in that variable.

If we wish to code our own functions to carry out median imputation in R, we can define the following two functions:

```
# Create a function for filling NAs with median
median_noNA <- function(vec){
  # Return the median value of x removing NA
  return(replace(vec, is.na(vec), median(vec, na.rm = TRUE)))
}

# Execute the function on each row in the data frame
replace_na <- function(df, impute_function){

  # Get only the numeric columns
  is_numeric <- sapply(df, is.numeric)

  # Replace missing values  with the median
  clean_df <- replace(df, is_numeric, lapply(df[is_numeric], impute_function))
  return(clean_df)
}
```

The first function takes a vector of values and replaces all missing values in the vector with the median. The second function takes in a data frame and a general imputation function as inputs, and returns the data frame with the imputed missing values.

The missing values in `seizure_data` can then be imputed via:

```
# Impute missing values in place
seizure_data = replace_na(seizure_data, median_noNA)
```

The modular structure of the functions we have defined allows for easy substitution with other user-defined functions that can be used to impute the missing values. For example, if one would like to impute the missing values with the mean instead of median, we can instead write a function to replace missing values with the mean:

```
mean_noNA <- function(df){
  # Return the mean value of x removing NA
  return(replace(df, is.na(df), mean(df, na.rm = TRUE)))
}
```

and then run `replace_na(seizure_data, mean_noNA)`. Note that, since we have already performed median imputation at the previous step, we would need to reinitialize `seizure_data` in order to perform mean imputation.

**Arithmetic operations and transformations of columns**

Data must sometimes undergo transformations or arithmetic operations prior to usage in statistical models. Examples include standardization/normalization prior to use in many supervised and unsupervised machine learning algorithms, log transformations of count or skewed data, or performing arithmetic operations on multiple columns. In our example, each of the individual lead columns represents the hourly IED counts detected by each lead. If, however, the *total* hourly IED counts between the two leads is of interest, then it may be useful to instead to add the values in the two columns to create a new column, and then to drop the original individual variables. We can add the values in the two variables `iea_lead1` and `iea_lead2` and then use the `subset()` function to drop the original variables as follows:

```
# Add IED counts from the two leads into a new variable
seizure_data$iea_lead_agg = seizure_data$iea_lead1 + seizure_data$iea_lead2
# Drop the original variables
seizure_data <- subset(seizure_data, select = -c(iea_lead1,iea_lead2) )
```

### 1.3.5 Exploratory Data Analysis

Typically, once data cleaning and preparation are complete, exploratory data analysis can begin to uncover the underlying data structure, formulate hypotheses, or identify data quality issues that may require further data cleaning and transformations. In this section, we walk the reader through an example exploratory data analysis of our simulated RNS dataset.

A good starting practice in exploratory data analysis is to always start first with examination of visual representations of the data to obtain a high-level understanding of patterns, prior to proceeding to more specific exploratory data analysis techniques. Histograms are a commonly used plotting approach which allows for evaluation of the distribution of continuous variables and can be generated in `R` using the `hist()` function. In our running example, let us construct histograms of the two variables of interest: hourly long episodes (`le`) and the total hourly IED counts observed from both leads (`iea_lead_agg`):

```
# Plot histograms for LE and IED counts
hist(seizure_data$le, main = "", xlab = "Seizures", ylab = "Density", freq = FALSE
    )
hist(seizure_data$iea_lead_agg, main = "", xlab = "Seizure Spikes", ylab = "
    Density", freq=FALSE)
```

Examination of the histograms in Figure 1.1 reveals that, the majority of the time, there are zero LEs in any given hour. Moreover, the greatest number of LEs experienced by any of the patients in the sample is one. Similarly, the majority of the time, the number of IEDs per hour is zero. However, there are more IEDs per hour than seizures; specifically, the density of IEDs is right-skewed and tapers off after about 100 IEDs per hour, with very

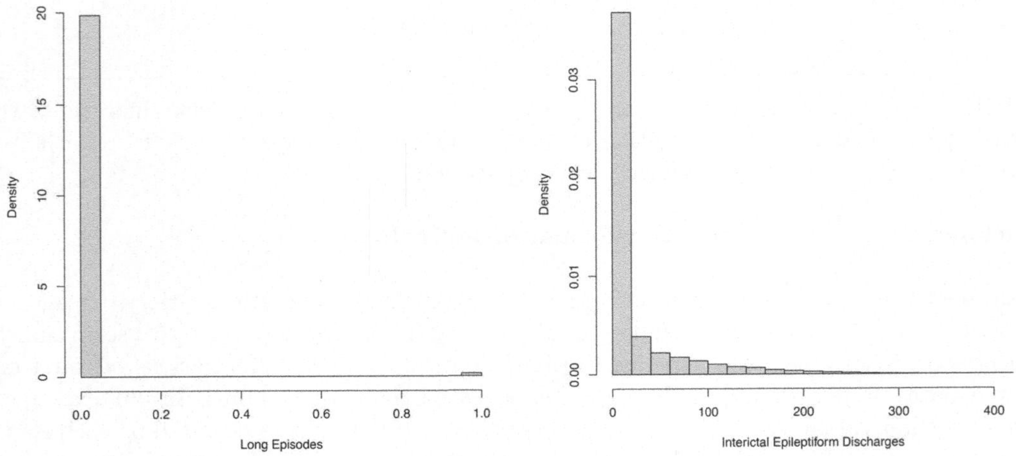


**FIGURE 1.1**
Histograms of (left panel) the number of long episodes per hour across all patients, and (right panel) the number of interictal epileptiform discharges per hour across all patients.

few instances involving more than 200 IEDs per hour. This may be seen, for example, in devices with a maximum hourly bin capacity for recording.

Another common evaluation technique in exploratory data analysis is in the computation of summary statistics for each variable, including measures such as the mean, median, mode, standard deviation, range, and quantiles of the distribution. Summary statistics can be calculated through the `summary()` function. For our data, this yields:

```
summary(seizure_data$iea_lead_agg)

> Min. 1st Qu.  Median    Mean 3rd Qu.    Max.
0.00    1.00    6.00   26.05   22.00  406.00
```

These summary statistics quantitatively confirm our observation of right skewness from Figure 1.1, as the mean exceeds the median. We also see that the maximum number of IEDs per hour is 406, with 75% of the data involving fewer than 22 IEDs per hour.

What if we wish instead to explore the distribution of seizures and IEDs on a daily rather than hourly basis? This can be accomplished by summing across the timestamps within each hour:

```
# Extract the dates from the time stamps as Date objects
seizure_data$seizure_date <- as.Date(seizure_data$hourly_markers)

# Aggregate seizures and IEDs on daily level into a new data frame
daily_seizures_iea <- seizure_data %>%
  group_by(patient_id, seizure_date) %>%
  summarise(total_le = sum(le), total_iea_lead_agg = sum(iea_lead_agg))

# Plot the histograms
hist(daily_seizures_iea$total_le, main = "", xlab = "Seizures", ylab = "Density",
    freq = FALSE)
hist(daily_seizures_iea$total_iea_lead_agg, main = "", xlab = "Seizure Spikes",
    ylab = "Density", freq = FALSE)
```

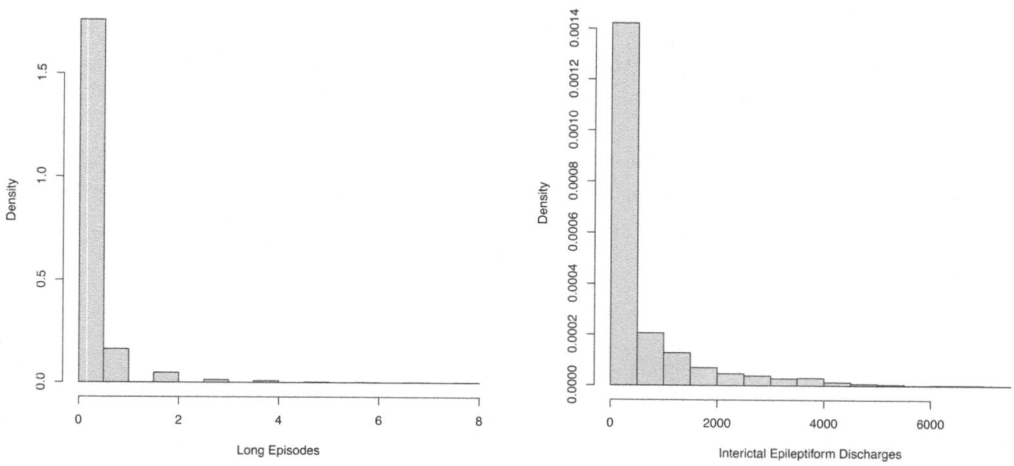


**FIGURE 1.2**
Histograms of (left panel) the number of long episodes per day across all patients, and (right panel) the number of interictal epileptiform discharges per day across all patients.

In the first block of code, `as.Date()` extracts the date from the timestamp as a date object and assigns it to `seizure_date`. The second block of code uses the `dplyr` convention to group the data frame by patient ID and the seizure occurrence date (`group_by`), and then calculates the total number of seizures and IEDs per day by summing across all seizures and all IEDs for each group. The result is a new data frame, `daily_seizures_iea`, which contains 1,686 observations and 4 variables (patient ID, the date of the seizure, the total number of seizures per day (`total_le`), and the total number of IEDs per day (`total_iea_lead_agg`). Histograms of the total number of seizures and IEDs after daily aggregation are shown in Figure 1.2. The distribution of daily IEDs in Figure 1.2 is similar to the distribution in Figure 1.1, which is expected, given that one value is a monotonic transformation of the other. The distribution of daily seizures shows that the maximum number of seizures that a patient had in a day was eight seizures, with the vast majority involving zero or one seizures per day.

Next, let us look at the demographic characteristics of our study sample, including the age, gender, and distribution of suspected seizure foci among these 20 patients. To find the unique values of the distribution of seizure foci, let us use the `unique()` function to check `unique(seizure_data$seizure_foci)`. The output indicates that there are eight unique values - left hippocampus, right hippocampus, left insula, left frontal, right frontal, supplementary motor cortex, left parietal, and left postcentral gyrus. To check how many suspected seizure foci each patient has, we can run:

```
seizure_data %>%
  group_by(patient_id) %>%
  summarise(count = n_distinct(seizure_foci))
```

The result is a tibble outputting the number of distinct seizure foci per patient. It seems that each patient was suspected to have a single focus. To find specifically which patients had, for example, left hippocampal and right hippocampal foci, we can run:

```
aggregate(patient_id ~ seizure_foci, seizure_data, function(x) paste(unique(x),
    collapse = ", "))
```

Here, the `aggregate()` function allows to specify how the data should be subset and what function should be applied to each group. In this case, the code specifies that for each patient ID, the unique value of the suspected seizure focus should be returned. Notice that the way we define a function inside `aggregate()` is to incorporate an existing function within the grouping. In this case, `unique()` is used. For more information, see `?aggregate`.

Table 1.2 shows the results of the aggregation. We see that the majority of the patients in this sample have a suspected right hippocampal focus, followed by the left hippocampus and supplementary motor cortex.

**TABLE 1.2**
Distribution of seizure foci in data example.

| Seizure focus | Patient ID |
|---|---|
| Left frontal | Patient 1 |
| Left hippocampus | Patient 2, Patient 6, Patient 9 |
| Left insula | Patient 20 |
| Left parietal | Patient 12 |
| Left postcentral gyrus | Patient 19, Patient 8 |
| Right frontal | Patient 5 |
| Right hippocampus | Patient 11, Patient 13, Patient 14, Patient 15, Patient 18, Patient 3, Patient 4, Patient 7 |
| Supplementary motor cortex | Patient 10, Patient 16, Patient 17 |

We can also check the distribution of gender for the study sample. Running `str(seizure_data$gender)` shows that `gender` is currently a string-valued variable. If, instead, we wish to analyze `gender` as a categorical variable, we can convert it to a factor. Let us also convert `seizure_foci` to a factor:

```
# Convert the gender and seizure foci columns to factors
factor_cols <- c('gender', 'seizure_foci')
seizure_data[factor_cols] <- lapply(seizure_data[factor_cols], factor)
```

Inspecting the data frame confirms that the `gender` and `seizure_foci` variables have been converted to factors with two and eight levels, respectively.

Last, as `seizure_data` is time-series data, let us look at the distribution of seizures and IEDs over time.

First, let us see the range of dates that the sample of recordings is taken from. To extract the minimum and maximum dates for the time-series, we can check `min(seizure_data$hourly_markers)` and `max(seizure_data$hourly_markers)`. The timestamps range from January 5, 2017, to April 4, 2019.

Next, let us see how long the recording was for each patient. We can do this by grouping all unique time stamps for each patient:

```
seizure_data %>%
  group_by(patient_id) %>%
  summarise(count = n_distinct(hourly_markers))
```

The results indicate that all patients have around 2000 hours of recording. However, Patient 2 and Patient 5 have 1999 distinct observations each, indicating duplicate timestamps in the data. To drop the duplicate observations, we would run:

```
seizure_data <- seizure_data[!duplicated(seizure_data), ]
```

Oftentimes, clinical interest lies in seizure prediction to reduce morbidity, mortality, and impacts on quality of life from unexpected seizures. Prior to applying prediction models, a good first step in understanding which time-series or sequence models may be useful (see Chapters 8 and 13) is to visualize and gain better understanding the time structure of seizures. Let us visualize the time-series of seizures and IEDs for a single patient, Patient 6, during a time period of interest of February 1, 2017 to March 20, 2017. To extract the subset of data corresponding only to Patient 6, we would run:

```
seizure_data_2017_patient_6 <- seizure_data[seizure_data$patient_id == 'Patient_6'
    , ]
```

If we specifically wish to focus on the time period of February 1, 2017 to March 20, 2017, for Patient 6, we would run:

```
seizure_data_subset_2017_patient_6 <- seizure_data_2017_patient_6[(seizure_data_
    2017_patient_6$hourly_markers > '2017-02-01 00:00:00 UTC') & (seizure_data_
    2017_patient_6$hourly_markers <= '2017-03-20 00:00:00 UTC'),]
```

In this code, there are two conditions to subset on: we want timestamps that are later than February 1, 2017, AND earlier than March 20, 2017. The logical 'AND' operator is represented by the symbol '&'.

Figure 1.3 shows a line plot of the number of IEDs per hour for Patient 6 between February 1, 2017, and March 20, 2017, with the grey line indicating the number of IEDs per hour and the black circles indicating the timing of the seizures.

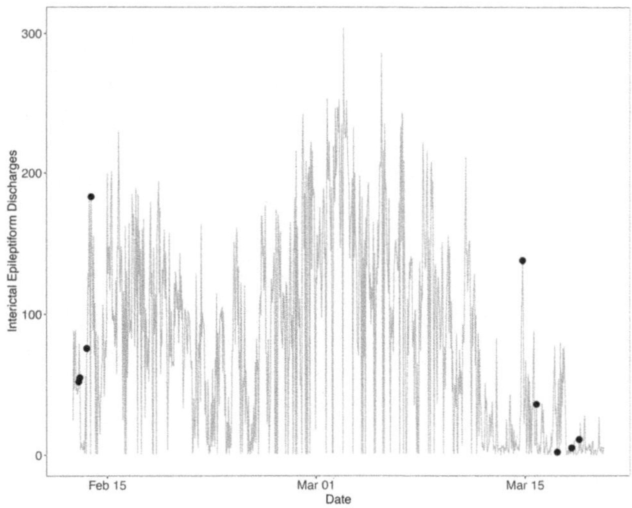


**FIGURE 1.3**
Hourly IEDs (grey line) and seizures (black circles) for a sample patient.

To produce the line chart and superimposed seizures, we use ggplot2 [6]:

```
install.packages("ggplot2")
library(ggplot2)
# Plot IEDs
spikes <- ggplot() + geom_line(data = seizure_data_subset_2017_patient_6, aes(x =
    hourly_markers, y = iea_lead_agg)) + xlab("Date") + ylab("Spikes")

# Add seizures
spikes + geom_point(data = seizure_data_subset_2017_patient_6[
    seizure_data_subset_2017_patient_6$le > 0, ], aes(x = hourly_markers, y =
    iea_lead_agg), color='black')
```

From this plot, we make a few observations: (1) the IEDs vary quite a bit over time, ranging from 0 to about 300 IEDs per hour and a mean of 82; (2) there appears to be periodicity in the IED rate with a length of about two weeks, with IEDs increasing until mid February, decreasing until late February, increasing until early March, and then decreasing until late March; and (3) seizures appear to cluster at certain times relative to the IEDs, with four of the nine seizures in this period occurring between Feb 1 and Feb 15, and the other five seizures occurring between March 15 and March 20. These observations from exploratory data analysis may suggest the appropriateness of further exploration using circular data analysis, discussed in Chapter 8.

## 1.4 Python

Python is another popular and powerful programming language used widely among software engineers, web developers, machine learning engineers, and data scientists. While R's libraries and community are generally more focused on statistical analysis, algorithm development, and data visualization, Python's libraries and community have a broader focus that ranges from front- or back-end web application development to machine learning, and more. Because of these libraries and suite of tools built around Python development, Python is a good choice for developers tasked with going from writing scripts and functions to writing full-blown applications hosted across different servers. Similar to the repository of libraries available in R through CRAN, Python hosts an extensive repository of libraries in the Python Package Index (PyPI) such as NumPy, SciPy, scikit-learn, and PyTorch.

In general, principles of code-writing and syntax differ between R and Python. We will illustrate only a brief example of a few differences; as this book primarily is written in R, we refer the reader interested in learning Python to the numerous resources available from both Python.org and the various other courses available online. A Python version of code to replicate the analyses in Section 1.3 is available in the repository accompanying the book.

The following 'Hello World!' example helps to illustrate the syntax of importing a Python module, accessing methods belonging to the module, and defining functions. To see the example, run the following code in your Python console:

```
import random

def main():
    print("Hello World!")
    a = random.random()
    return a

if __name__ == "__main__":
    result = main()
    print(result)
}
```

You should see the output `Hello World` on one line, and on the second line you should see a randomly generated number between 0 and 1. Let us break down what is going on here under the hood:

- The first thing that happens in the 'Hello World!' code is that we import a *module* called `random`. This module houses a library of code related to random number generation. When you install Python, it comes packaged with the standard library, which is a catalog of modules providing useful functionality. Other modules can be imported to use other functionalities.

- The next thing that happens in this file is that we define a function called `main()`. Similar to `R`, functions in Python have zero or more inputs and zero or more outputs. This specific function has no inputs, and one output.
  - Here, the first line of `main()` prints `Hello World!` to the console.
  - The second line of `main()` uses the `random()` method from the `random` library to generate a pseudo-random number between 0 and 1. This value is assigned to the variable `a`.
  - If a function has an output, its execution finishes with a `return` statement. Functions can also print output directly to the console by using the `print` function.
- The line `if __name__ == "__main__":` is a common way of defining the execution point of a piece of code. It tells your machine where to begin when you run the command `python hello_world.py`. In this case we call our function, receive its returned value, and print it to the console. The other critical piece of this statement is that it prevents your code from being executed if it is imported somewhere else.

### 1.4.1 Defining Classes in Object-Oriented Programming

One core difference between programming in `R` and Python is that `R` is a functional programming language while Python is an object-oriented language. Whereas functional programming treats computation as the evaluation of mathematical functions, object-oriented programming focuses on creating objects that contain both data and functions, within units called classes.

Using Python classes is one of the most efficient ways to organize code into reusable components. An *object* is a entity that combines functions (called *methods*) and data (called *attributes*). The purpose of an object is to bundle together related code to simplify composition and reuse, in order to make the code overall more readable and digestible. Objects are created by initializing (*instantiating*) *classes*. Classes have an `__init__` method that is called upon initialization.

To see how to define a class called `Patient`, run the following:

```
class Patient:
    def __init__(self, name: str, age: int):
        self.name = name
        self.age = age

    def get_age_difference(
        self, other: "Patient"
    ) -> int:
        return abs(self.age - other.age)

def main():
    p1 = Patient("Rob", 100)
    p2 = Patient("Chris", 75)

    age_difference = p1.get_age_difference(p2)
    print(age_difference)

if __name__ == "__main__":
    main()
```

Let us break down this code as well.

- In the first code block, a class called `Patient` is defined with a name as well as an `__init__` method. Notice this `__init__` method takes '`self`' as a first argument. All methods in Python classes begin with the 'self' argument; it stores a reference to the object itself, which means that at any time you can access other attributes and methods by referencing 'self'. In the `__init__` method, we store two argument values to the object, the *name* and *age*.

- Next, the `get_age_difference` method in class `Patient` accesses the stored *age* attribute for the current object, as well as another *Patient* object passed in as the first argument, and computes the absolute difference.

- The reusability of classes is most obvious when they are instantiated many times. Classes tend to be nouns, and their methods tend to be verbs associated with their behavior. In the defined `main()` function, for example, we instantiate two Patient classes. In large software systems, it is common to design the high-level classes need before writing too much code.

## 1.5 Summary

In this chapter, we provide a brief primer to version control and programming in R and Python. It is our hope that this sets a basic foundation for the reader's journey through programming and data analysis in epilepsy, and that the principles discussed here will prove useful for equipping readers with the ability to independently implement statistical methods both in the remainder of this book and in research practice.

## Bibliography

[1] Amanda N Baraldi and Craig K Enders. An introduction to modern missing data analyses. *Journal of School Psychology*, 48(1):5–37, 2010.

[2] Marek Gagolewski. stringi: Character string processing facilities. *R Journal*, 9(2):439–461, 2021.

[3] Roderick JA Little and Donald B Rubin. *Statistical Analysis with Missing Data*, volume 793. John Wiley & Sons, 2019.

[4] Vikram R Rao. Chronic electroencephalography in epilepsy with a responsive neurostimulation device: current status and future prospects. *Expert Review of Medical Devices*, 18(11):1093–1105, 2021.

[5] Stef van Buuren. *Flexible Imputation of Missing Data.* CRC Press, Boca Raton, FL, 2018.

[6] Hadley Wickham. ggplot2: Elegant graphics for data analysis. *Journal of Statistical Software*, 77(9):1–3, 2016.

[7] Hadley Wickham. *Advanced R.* Chapman and Hall/CRC, Boca Raton, FL, 2nd edition, 2019.

# 2

# *Preprocessing Electrophysiological Data: EEG, iEEG, and MEG Data*

**Kristin K. Sellers**

*Department of Neurological Surgery, University of California, San Francisco (USA)*

**Joline M. Fan**

*Department of Neurology, University of California, San Francisco (USA)*

**Leighton B.N. Hinkley**

*Department of Radiology, University of California, San Francisco (USA)*

**Heidi E. Kirsch**

*Department of Neurology, University of California, San Francisco (USA)*

## CONTENTS



The measurement and understanding of brain activity time series is integral to epilepsy care and research. Brain signals may be acquired using external sensors, as with scalp electroencephalography (EEG) and magnetoencephalography (MEG), or using implanted internal sensors, as with intracranial EEG (iEEG). These techniques can provide high temporal resolution recordings of electrical or electromagnetic activity relevant to epilepsy, cognitive processing, and many other functions, but require data processing and cleaning

DOI: 10.1201/9781003254515-2

ahead of analysis. We first describe how EEG and iEEG are acquired, discuss similarities and differences, and elaborate on fundamental data preprocessing steps. We next provide example MATLAB functions for the most common preprocessing steps. Subsequently, we provide an overview of why MEG recordings may be beneficial, discuss acquisition considerations, and review preprocessing steps. Finally, we comment on popular software toolboxes.

## 2.1 Introduction

Preprocessing of electrophysiology recordings is an essential step to using brain electrical activity for clinical and research applications. Preprocessing steps allow for the extraction of the most relevant physiologic information within noisy time-series data and the preparation of data for source-localization and/or time or frequency domain analyses. Here, we introduce key principles and basic preprocessing building blocks for scalp EEG, iEEG, and MEG recordings. Although some aspects of signal processing are used across these recording modalities, specific considerations are also given to the processing of each recording modality.

In this chapter, we first review basic principles of EEG and iEEG recording and the utility of these recording modalities. We subsequently discuss materials and methods required for the acquisition of EEG and iEEG. We describe key preprocessing steps for EEG and iEEG analysis, providing examples and explanations of their uses. We then introduce MEG as an additional non-invasive method and touch on specific differences in preprocessing. Preprocessing steps for MEG mirror those for EEG and may also include advanced denoising procedures and source reconstruction. Finally, we close the chapter with a list of important preprocessing software tools that are commonly leveraged for the preprocessing of electrophysiology data.

## 2.2 Preprocessing for EEG and iEEG

The extracellular voltage measured using EEG and iEEG (which includes electrocorticography (ECoG), stereotactic-EEG (sEEG), and chronic iEEG) arises from a combination of synaptic activity, action potentials, calcium spikes, intrinsic currents, afterhyperpolarizations, and gap junctions [7]. Each of these tools measures changes in extracellular voltage, with various degrees of spatial filtering. In using these methods, we are interested in changes in voltage over time. This can provide a wealth of information, for example about the physiological (or pathological, as in the case of seizures) synchrony between brain regions during rest or cognitive processing. Substantial prior research has examined correlative and causal relationships between extracellular voltage measurements and behavior, sensory perception, cognition, and alterations in disease [10, 13, 18, 48, 51].

### 2.2.1 Key Principles

In general, the most common dataset in epilepsy is recorded from scalp EEG, which can be obtained from short-duration routine studies in the outpatient setting or from days-long evaluations in the epilepsy monitoring unit (EMU). For patients undergoing surgical intervention, iEEG may be acquired through three paradigms: brief intraoperative recordings using portable equipment, sub-chronic implants in the EMU typically lasting one to two weeks, or chronic years-long recordings using implanted devices such as the Responsive Neurostimulation System (RNS® System) (NeuroPace, Inc., Mountain View, CA). We will discuss equipment and acquisition considerations for each of these paradigms, as they influence downstream preprocessing and limitations of the data for subsequent analyses. As a preface to this discussion, we remind the reader of a few principles and properties that are highly relevant:

- Brain signals follow a $1/f$ to $1/f^4$ relationship, meaning there is power-law scaling of neural power as frequency increases [29].
- The Nyquist Theorem states that an analog signal must be sampled at least twice as fast as the bandwidth of the signal to accurately reconstruct the waveform. Following directly from this, frequencies can be measured up to $F_s/2$ ($F_s$ = sampling rate), and thus, the sampling rate determines the maximum frequency content resolvable in a signal.
- All acquisition systems have a noise floor, or lower bound, below which any signal of interest cannot be detected.

### 2.2.2 Why Multiple EEG Methods?

In this section, we discuss EEG and iEEG. These methods have similarities and differences that are important for selecting appropriate data processing steps and for downstream interpretation (Table 2.1). Scalp EEG is a non-invasive recording modality, whereas iEEG is an invasive recording modality and includes ECoG, stereo EEG (sEEG), hybrid approaches, and chronically implanted iEEG. ECoG requires a craniotomy to place electrodes on the surface of the brain (typically but not always subdurally), while sEEG requires burr holes to insert depth electrodes into the brain parenchyma. Some institutions also combine subdural and depth electrodes for intracranial monitoring to achieve a hybrid approach [12]. Chronically implanted iEEG can include a combination of subdural or depth electrodes, depending on the target location.

In both EEG and iEEG, the activity of interest (electric fields generated in the brain) is the same, but the biophysical properties that are relevant based on the location of the sensing electrode differ for each method. In the case of EEG, the electrical field must travel through the layers of connective tissue around the brain, cerebrospinal fluid, skull, subcutaneous tissue, and scalp to reach the sensing electrode. This results in substantial volume conduction and signal attenuation. A single scalp EEG electrode records a signal that is integrated over an area of 10 $cm^2$ or more [7]. While the electrical potentials generated by populations of neurons are on the order of 0.5–1 mV when measured extracellularly by invasive electrodes capable of detecting single units, this amplitude drops to the $\mu$V range for EEG. Because of the $1/f$ property of neural signals, lower amplitude of activity recorded at the scalp, and the layers of tissue acting as a low pass filter, activity recorded using most conventional EEG acquisition systems is analyzed up to $\tilde{8}0$ Hz [4, 5]. Signals above this frequency are often below the noise floor and no longer resolvable. Thus, EEG sampling rates are typically 256 or 512 Hz. However, the non-invasive nature of EEG does allow for electrodes to be placed on the full scalp. Thus, a spatially non-specific but full-brain picture of cortical electrical potentials is possible.

ECoG arrays are placed on the brain surface. Configuration is highly individualized but typically includes strip and grid arrays. Standard electrode sizes used for clinical care are 2–4 mm in diameter, with center-to-center pitch of 8–15 mm. Many research applications use higher density grids with smaller contact sizes and denser spacing [24, 44, 45]. Activity measured from a single ECoG electrode has a spatial resolution of $< 5$ mm$^2$ [7].

sEEG employs depth electrodes, which are penetrative probes with multiple recording contacts along the z-axis. Typical electrode sizes for clinical use are 2–2.5 mm in length with center-to-center pitch of 5–10 mm. These electrodes are used when deep brain structures (e.g. amygdala, hippocampus) are implicated and recording of localized activity from these structures is needed.

Both ECoG and sEEG are typically acquired at sampling rates between 1 kHz and 25 kHz. Most commonly, activity is only analyzed up to about 300 Hz, although there is some evidence for meaningful information in higher frequency ranges [35]. Higher frequency activity can be accessed using these methods because direct recordings provide higher amplitude signals, which allow for more frequency content to be above the noise floor of amplifiers. In addition to allowing for higher frequency signals to be acquired, high sampling rates can also be advantageous when recording concurrently with electrical stimulation, as the stimulation waveform can more accurately be recorded and offline artifact rejection techniques can be applied to clean the data [43].

**TABLE 2.1**
Similarities and differences between EEG and intracranial EEG (iEEG).

| | EEG | iEEG |
|---|---|---|
| Invasiveness | Non-invasive | Invasive |
| Coverage | Full brain | Cortical surface portion (ECoG) or local deep brain structure (sEEG) |
| Signal amplitude | 1–10s $\mu$V | 10s–100s $\mu$V |
| Frequencies of interest | 1–80 Hz | 1–300 Hz |
| Sampling rate | 256 Hz or 512 Hz | 1 kHz–25 kHz |

Lastly, the types of artifacts which most commonly contaminate signals vary somewhat based on the modality. Artifact is a catch-all term for physiological or non-physiological contributions to the signal that are not generated by the brain and thus contaminate the signal. See Table 2.2 for common artifacts for each recording modality.

### 2.2.3 Amplification, Digitization, and Filtering in the EMU

Due to the small amplitude of activity sensed by EEG and iEEG electrodes, specialized equipment is necessary to successfully acquire these signals. When acquisition is conducted in the EMU, electrodes (EEG, ECoG, or sEEG) are physically connected using specialized cables to a differential amplifier, analog-to-digital converter (ADC), and acquisition computer. The amplifier conditions and multiplies the signal to prevent loss below the noise floor; the ADC then converts the analog signal into a digital signal that can be processed and saved by the acquisition computer. Sampling rate, measured in Hz, determines the number of samples per second for the creation of the digital signal. As mentioned above, following the Nyquist principle, frequency content can be resolved up to a frequency of $F_s/2$, although if equipment permits it is preferable to acquire at a rate that is 3–5x higher than the max frequency of interest. Acquisition systems may impose filtering at multiple steps to ensure signal integrity. Analog filters (e.g. high pass filters) may be applied to remove DC-offset, thereby keeping the signal within the input range of the amplifier. If this is not done, the amplifier may saturate, at which point no usable signal is recorded. Additional analog filtering (e.g. low pass filters) must also be used to prevent aliasing – if there is

**TABLE 2.2**
Common artifacts in EEG and intracranial EEG (iEEG).

| Source of artifact | Presentation | Modality affected | Methods for mitigation |
|---|---|---|---|
| Line noise | 50/60 Hz sinewave | EEG, iEEG | Physical separation of power lines from recording cables; battery-powering equipment; specialized wearable Faraday cage* |
| Eyeblink and eye movement | Large amplitude rolling activity, more concentrated in frontal electrodes | EEG | Eye fixation during recordings; post-processing to remove artifact |
| Cardiac | Repetitive and regular EKG waveform | EEG, iEEG | Re-position electrodes away from major blood vessels; post-processing to remove artifact |
| Muscle activity | Intermittent prominent wideband activity, often correlated with tensing jaw muscles | EEG, iEEG | Have participant relax jaw muscles; no eating or drinking during recordings |
| Cable handling | Sharp cuts in the signal | EEG, iEEG | Do not move cables during recordings |
| Interictal epileptiform discharges† | Spike and slow wave complex, spikes, sharp waves | EEG, iEEG | Post-processing to remove artifact |

* Wearable Sensing, San Diego, CA.
† Whether this is considered an artifact may depend on the specific scientific question.

frequency content above $F_s/2$ in the analog signal, it can contaminate the signal at lower frequencies; after digitization, it is impossible to disentangle the true low frequency content from aliased signal.

A few key technical specifications of the equipment influence the resulting signal. Amplifier input impedance should be at least 100x larger than the electrode impedances. EEG and ECoG electrodes typically have impedances in the range of 0.1–20 $k\Omega$ (measured at 1 kHz) [53]. If this is not met, there will be significant signal attenuation. Bit resolution and input range influence the granularity of the analog to digital conversion. There is typically a trade-off between the smallest step between voltages being too large (and thus losing information) versus having very fine voltage steps but being limited to a smaller total range of amplitudes covered. What settings to choose can be influenced by the specific experiment and scientific question. For example, when using electrical stimulation which creates an artifact, having a larger input range to prevent saturation of the amplifiers is typically preferable over the most fine-grained voltage resolution.

Prior to digitization, the EEG or iEEG signal is extremely susceptible to external artifacts. We will discuss more about artifacts and mitigation strategies in a following section.

### 2.2.4 Ground and Reference

By definition, electrical potentials must be measured as the difference between two points. In the case of EEG and iEEG, we often use 3 electrodes for each measurement. Measurements between parts of the human body will reveal variable, non-zero potential. Therefore, we need a signal baseline, or ground (GND) (not to be confused with true earth ground, which is typically not relevant in the context of EEG and iEEG). The potential measured at the ground electrode is assigned 0V (when measured against itself it is zero) to provide a baseline. The signal of interest, site, is recorded from the site relative to this ground electrode (Site – GND). While this is the bare bones required for acquisition, it is typically advantageous to add a bit of complexity to improve signal interpretability and quality. The differential recording between site and ground is susceptible to electrical noise from the amplifier and other sources. Therefore, a reference electrode is also measured relative to the ground electrode (REF – GND). The (REF – GND) signal also picks up electrical noise from the amplifier and other sources but should not have the same signal-of-interest as the site. Thus, when the two differential signals are subtracted, this common mode noise is removed from the final signal:

$$[E_{site} - E_{ground} + noise] - [E_{reference} - E_{ground} + noise] = E_{site} - E_{reference}. \quad (2.1)$$

Differential amplifiers, discussed above, are designed to perform acquisition in this manner. The benefit of this approach requires choosing appropriate locations for the ground and reference electrodes. The ground electrode should have very little physiological activity. This provides a 'stable' zero point, with little positive or negative overall shift in the resulting voltage values. An effective reference electrode is the same material as the recording electrodes but may be a larger in size with lower impedance, which allows for sensing of the same noise but not the same signal of interest. Together, this provides an acquisition setup in which the input range of the amplifiers is centered around zero, as defined by the ground electrode. Separate ground and reference electrodes (as described above) allow for common-mode noise to be removed. Shorting the ground and reference electrodes results in single-ended amplification, in which the common-mode noise gets amplified along with the physiological activity signal.

Optimal grounding and referencing are not always possible in practice, and preprocessing techniques conducted on the digital signal such as common average referencing (CAR), bipolar referencing, and surface Laplacian will be discussed which can combat resulting noise. However, thoughtful selection and placement of ground and reference electrodes can greatly improve signal quality and resulting interpretation. For EEG, commonly used ground location(s) include Cz or linked mastoids (M1 + M2) and common reference locations include FCz or Cz (if not used for ground). For iEEG, ground and reference options include a separate electrical contact placed in the dura, a contact in white matter, or a contact that is outside the brain (in the case of sEEG). The same contact is sometimes used for both reference and ground – this can be done for experimental ease, although it does not allow for the rejection of common mode noise as described above.

### 2.2.5 Sensor versus Source Spaces

Regardless of the ground and reference chosen, all raw signals recorded using these modalities reflect sensor space – or activity based on the physical location of the placed electrodes. Particularly in the case of EEG, these signals are subject to volume conduction, in which there is propagation of the electric field through tissue to the sensor. Volume conduction may complicate interpretation of the signals, particularly in localizing the brain region responsible for a particular activity pattern. Inverse modeling can be conducted, in which assumptions are applied to estimate where sources are located in the brain which generated activity measured by the scalp electrodes [21]. However, analyzing source-estimated signals is accompanied by its own set of challenges.

### 2.2.6 The NeuroPace RNS® System

The RNS® System is an FDA-approved implantable device for treatment of seizures in adults with certain forms of drug-resistant focal epilepsy. Two four-contact leads are implanted and connected to an implantable neurostimulator that is contained within the skull. The device is capable of both delivering electrical stimulation and recording chronic iEEG from up to four channels simultaneously. The implanted device contains all the hardware required for amplification and digitization. Channels are recorded in a bipolar montage, where the differential recording is between two electrodes of the four-contact lead. Thus, this system does not have dedicated ground or reference electrodes. The device samples at 250 Hz, with default analog bandpass filters at [5 70] Hz and widest possible bandwidth of [1 90] Hz. In contrast to iEEG recordings conducted in the EMU, the RNS System allows for short recordings while a patient is in a variety of environments, without any bulky cabling or externalized electronics. RNS-specific preprocessing considerations are described in subsequent sections.

Equipped with this basic understanding of how EEG and iEEG signals are acquired, we will now dive into how to preprocess these data following acquisition.

### 2.2.7 Preprocessing Building Blocks

In the context of EEG and iEEG, preprocessing refers to a pipeline of mathematical computations that is deployed on the raw data in order to prepare them for subsequent analyses. The specific order and parameters of preprocessing steps varies depending upon application. Some preprocessing steps are conducted per channel while others incorporate data across channels. Here, we first describe separate building blocks of preprocessing pipelines and subsequently give an example of a full preprocessing pipeline with example traces (Figure 2.1).

- *Bandpass filters*: Bandpass filters are applied per channel to reject data with frequency activity below a high-pass cutoff and above a low-pass cutoff. Bandpass filtering can be used to remove artifacts that commonly occur in very low frequencies (perspiration of the scalp, movement of head and cables) and high frequencies (muscle activity). The low-pass portion is also critical to prevent aliasing of data when downsampling. If there are large transients in the data, filtering can temporally blur this activity, causing more artifact to be introduced. The MATLAB function `butterworthBPFilter` applies a zero-phase digital filter to the input data:

```
function [filtData] = butterworthBPFilter(data,passBand,order,Fs)
%
% Input parameters:
% data = channels x samples
% passBand = vector with passband frequencies, in Hz
% order = filter order
% Fs = data sampling rate, in Hz
%%

% If only 1 channel, want channel x samples
if iscolumn(data)
   data = data';
```

```
end

runOrder = order/2; % For bandpass designs, runOrder represents one-half the
    filter order

% Define filter parameters
Fc = passBand;
Fn = Fs/2;
Wn = Fc/Fn;
[b1, a1] = butter(runOrder, Wn, 'bandpass');

% Run notch filter
for iChan = 1:size(data,1)
    filtData(iChan,:) = filtfilt(b1,a1,data(iChan,:));
end

end
```

- *Notch filters*: Notch filters reject a narrow frequency range of activity, typically centered around the line noise frequency (or harmonics), 50 Hz or 60 Hz, depending on the country where recording was conducted. While best to minimize line noise interference during acquisition, in human experiments, it is often not possible to completely remove this artifact. Narrow notch filters can also be used to remove noise at the frequency of electrical stimulation. In the function `butterworthNotchFilter`, we reject data within +/- 2Hz of the specified `notchFreq`:

```
function [filtData] = butterworthNotchFilter(data,notchFreq,order,Fs)
%
% Input parameters:
% data = channels x samples
% notchFreq = frequency for centering notch filter, in Hz
% order = filter order
% Fs = data sampling rate, in Hz

%%
% If only 1 channel, want channel x samples
if iscolumn(data)
   data = data';
end

runOrder = order/2; % because implementing bandpass filter for notch

% Define filter parameters
Fc = [notchFreq-2 notchFreq+2];
Fn = Fs/2;
Wn = Fc/Fn;
[b1, a1] = butter(runOrder, Wn, 'stop');

% Run notch filter
for iChan = 1:size(data,1)
    filtData(iChan,:) = filtfilt(b1,a1,data(iChan,:));
end

end
```

- *Channel rejection*: Manual inspection of channels can be done to look for "bad" channels, which should be excluded from all subsequent calculations and analyses. Bad channels may result from physically broken connections in cabling, poor impedances, or electrodes that have fallen off (for EEG) or that have poor contact with the cortical surface (for ECoG).

- *Time period rejection*: Rejection of data across all channels for selected time periods may be needed. Bad time periods of data may result from movement of cables or other artifacts. While artifacts may only affect a subset of channels, it is typically preferable to reject data for that time segment across all channels for ease of data and time management. A key decision is what to put in place of the rejected data. Replacing the rejected samples with NaN values preserves the original timing of the recording, but may complicate subsequent analyses (e.g. frequency decomposition, which is sensitive to NaNs). We suggest replacement with NaNs during preprocessing, with the option to handle these samples differently later in analysis (e.g. remove those values, thus collapsing time; replace with interpolated values). The function `manuallyRejectTimeSegments` facilitates manual identification of time periods for rejection by plotting the data and prompting the user to highlight bad time periods, using functionality from EEGLAB. See the example pipeline for how to reject the identified bad time periods of data:

```
function manuallyRejectTimeSegments(data,Fs)
%
% Highlight data segments with bad data and return the indices of these periods
%
% Input parameters:
% data = channels x samples
% Fs = data sampling rate, in Hz
%
% Note: This function requires EEGLAB functions. 'tempMarkedRejection' in main
    workspace
% will have rejected data segment information
%%

% If only 1 channel, want channel x samples
if iscolumn(data)
   data = data';
end

rejCommand = [...
    'tempMarkedRejection = [];'...
    'if ~isempty(TMPREJ),'...
    'tempMarkedRejection  = eegplot2event(TMPREJ, -1);'...
    'end;'...
    ];

TMPREJ = [];
tempMarkedRejection = [];
eegplot(data,'srate',Fs,'winlength',15,'wincolor',[1 0 0],'command',rejCommand
    ,...
    'title','Select data segments to remove');
uiwait

end
```

- *Epoching*: Often used in trial-based experimental designs, epoching refers to segmenting the continuous data in time. Epochs are often defined by experimental triggers that are concurrently recorded with the EEG or iEEG data. Individual epochs can be rejected if artifact is present. Amplitude thresholding can be applied, and any epoch with activity exceeding the threshold (e.g. $\pm 75\mu V$ for EEG) is rejected from further analysis.

- *Re-referencing*: Re-referencing refers to looking across a subset (e.g. one grid array) or all signals recorded and recalculating the signal for each channel based on taking differences. This may be beneficial to look for more local signal and to remove noise shared across channels. However, it can also remove physiological activity such as an event-related potential (ERP) that is present on most channels. Re-referencing should be done after removing bad channels and bad time periods, as this procedure can also introduce artifacts to channels. There are different types of re-referencing:

- *Common average reference (CAR)*: Common average reference refers to subtracting the average of all the signals from each signal of interest in order to remove shared noise. If there are a small number of channels with large amplitude artifact, CAR mean will introduce this artifact to other channels (typically affecting lower frequencies). CAR median can introduce high frequency noise by jumping between the median value taken from different channels.

```
% CAR mean
reref = nanmean(filtData,1);
CAR_ECOG = bsxfun(@minus,filtData,reref);
```

- *Bipolar reference*: In bipolar referencing, the signals from adjacent electrodes are subtracted in order to obtain a more local signal.

- *Surface Laplacian*: In surface Laplacian, the signal of the four nearest neighbors is averaged and subtracted from the site of interest for each electrode. This serves to estimate the radial current flow at the scalp. This approach can be advantageous because it estimates a sharper topography, reducing the effect of volume conduction [8, 27].

• *Independent Component Analysis (ICA)*: ICA is a signal processing computation that seeks to separate independent sources of signals that are linearly mixed in several sensors. ICA can be run on an arbitrary number of dimensions. If 64 channels of data are input into ICA, 64 components will be returned, which represent a projection of the original data into a new space with maximal independence. The components can then be examined and those which represent artifacts (e.g. eye blink, cardiac signal, muscle artifact, etc.) can be removed and the data can be projected back into sensor space. This technique is strong at removing stereotyped artifacts but one limitation of the ICA approach is it can lead to removal of desired physiological activity that is included in the (mostly) artifactual components.

• *Downsampling*: Downsampling reduces the sampling rate of the data to preserve disk space and subsequent computational resources. This must be done in such a way as to avoid introducing aliasing; the MATLAB `resample` function applies a finite impulse response antialiasing low-pass filter. As a reminder, sampling rate determines the highest frequency activity that can be resolved, so downsampling should be done to an appropriate frequency depending on the analysis of interest. To downsample in MATLAB:

```
function [outputData] = changeFs(data,newFs,originalFs)
%
% Downsample data to desired sampling rate. Can accommodate fractional
   originalFs
%
% Input parameters:
% data = channels x samples
% newFs = desired sampling rate, in Hz
% originalFs = desired sampling rate, in Hz

%%
% If only 1 channel, want channel x samples
if iscolumn(data)
   data = data';
end
```

```
  [N,D] = rat(originalFs/newFs);
  temp = resample(data',D,N);

  outputData = temp';
  end
```

Following preprocessing, many analyses will include frequency decomposition using a method such as fast Fourier transform, wavelets, multi-taper, or filter/Hilbert (see Chapter 9 for more discussion). Prior preprocessing can influence the results of frequency decomposition and other event-related metrics such as ERPs [40].

Below is an example pipeline for iEEG preprocessing:

```
close all
clear all
clc

% Load raw data from .edf file
[header, rawData] = edfread(fileName);

% Extract sampling rate from file header
Fs = header.frequency(1);

% Bandpass filtering [1 500] -- should remove large transient from stim onset and
% offset
filterOrder = 4;
passBand = [1 500];
disp('Bandpass filtering data: [1-500]Hz')
filtData = butterworthBPFilter(rawData,passBand,filterOrder,Fs);

% Notch filter
notchFreq = 60;
filterOrder = 4;
disp('60Hz (and harmonics) notch filtering')
while notchFreq < 500
    filtData = butterworthNotchFilter(filtData,notchFreq,filterOrder,Fs);
    notchFreq = notchFreq + 60; % get harmonics
end

% CAR across all channels
disp('CAR rereferencing')
reref = nanmean(filtData,1);
CAR_ECOG = bsxfun(@minus,filtData,reref);

% Manually select bad periods of data
removeOrReplace = 1; % 1 = replace bad data with NaNs; 2 = remove bad data
manuallyRejectTimeSegments(CAR_ECOG,Fs);
cleanedECOG = CAR_ECOG;

if ~exist('tempMarkedRejection','var')
    tempMarkedRejection = [];
end
if removeOrReplace == 1 % Replacing bad data with NaNs
  if ~isempty(tempMarkedRejection)
    for iRejection = 1:size(tempMarkedRejection,1)
     cleanedECOG(:,tempMarkedRejection(iRejection,3):tempMarkedRejection(
    iRejection,4)) = NaN;
    end
      rejectionTimes = sortrows(tempMarkedRejection);
  end
```

```
elseif removeOrReplace == 2 % Removing bad data -- time is no longer accurate
    % Need to sort rejectionTimes so they are early to late
    rejectionTimes = sortrows(tempMarkedRejection);

    if ~isempty(tempMarkedRejection)
        for iRejection = size(rejectionTimes,1):-1:1
            cleanedECOG(:,rejectionTimes(iRejection,3):rejectionTimes(iRejection
    ,4)) = [];
        end
    end
end

% Downsample to 1000Hz
dsFs = 1000;
preprocessedECOG = changeFs(cleanedECOG,dsFs,Fs);
```

### 2.2.8 Preprocessing Considerations for RNS® Data

There are some differences in the acquisition and equipment employed by the NeuroPace RNS® System that affect how data should be preprocessed. Because the device is powered by a battery, there is no line noise (50/60Hz) added from a power source. However, there have been reports of line noise found in the signal, likely due to the use of the device wand during real-time in-clinic recordings. Therefore, it remains a decision for each user if notch filtering is appropriate. If needed, channel rejection of RNS data would occur at the level of the bipolar signal. With a maximum of four channels of data acquired at any given time, channel rejection should only be done if the signal is highly compromised. Time period rejection becomes critical if stimulation is enabled on the device. When stimulation is delivered on the RNS, the acquired iEEG may either be highly contaminated by stimulation artifact or blanked so the amplifier does not saturate. Either way, the data do not represent physiological activity and therefore must be pruned before spectral analysis of the full data segment can be interpreted. Re-referencing and ICA are inappropriate for RNS data as there are too few channels of simultaneously recorded data. Lastly, downsampling can be conducted on RNS data, although given the native sampling rate of 250 Hz, this is often not necessary.

The optimal preprocessing pipeline for RNS data depends upon the purpose of the analysis. Specifically, RNS data may be analyzed to inform programming of device detectors for triggering responsive stimulation. In these cases, it may make sense to analyze the raw data, without any preprocessing steps, as this most closely represents what the on-device algorithm will use as input. Most other analyses which use RNS data to make observations about neural activity, but do not inform stimulation programming, do benefit from preprocessing. A fundamental strength of RNS data stems from the more naturalistic settings during acquisition afforded by the chronically implanted device. However, precise synchronization of iEEG with external tasks and peripherals can be a challenge. Specialized setups may be required to achieve high levels of temporal accuracy [47]. To our knowledge, there are no published software toolboxes for analyzing RNS data. Research groups which work with these data typically develop code in-house, some of which has been made available via GitHub (`https://github.com/penn-cnt/RNS_processing_toolbox`).

### 2.2.9 Practical Considerations

There are a number of practical considerations when designing preprocessing pipelines for EEG and iEEG. As electrode counts increase with high density EEG and larger, more densely implanted arrays, computational requirements for preprocessing must be

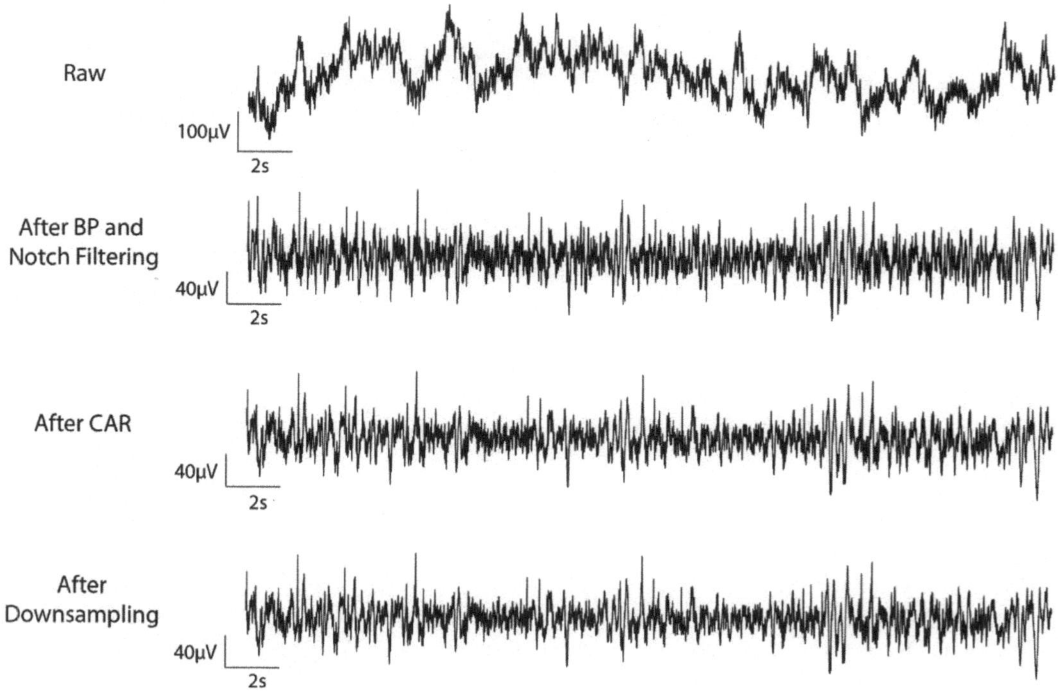


**FIGURE 2.1**
Intracranial EEG (iEEG) of 160 channels recorded for 210 seconds, originally acquired at 10 kHz, was preprocessed according to the steps in the example pipeline in Section 2.2.7. Here, we plot the same 30 seconds of data following subsequent preprocessing steps. All traces show data from one channel on the iEEG depth lead targeting right orbitofrontal cortex. Note the different y-scale for the raw trace.

considered. In addition, some pipelines which require manual checking or categorization may be tractable for 32 channels but much less feasible for 512 channels. Many of the above-mentioned toolboxes seek to fully automate ICA component categorization for precisely this reason. However, this is a difficult problem given the heterogeneity of artifacts and disruptions which can occur during electrophysiological recordings in humans.

As mentioned above, artifact rejection may lead to non-continuous recordings. This can result in a number of problems, including edge effects at the junctions, lack of stationarity, and missing values (which are incompatible with many types of downstream analyses). Depending on the experimental or clinical question, missing values can be interpolated from remaining data, or the edge effects introduced may be negligible (e.g. if averaging over a longer time period).

In addition, there are both clinical and research indications for electrical stimulation, which can be performed through either the same contacts used for sensing or different dedicated stimulation electrodes. This electrical stimulation produces artifacts that contaminate the recorded signal. There are numerous methods for removing the stimulation artifact from the signal, which are sensitive to recording sampling rate, stimulation frequency, and proximity of the stimulation electrode(s) to the sensing electrode(s).

With a plethora of acquisition systems available, there is an ever-increasing number of file formats used for human electrophysiological data. Some acquisition systems use proprietary file formats but allow for export into more open formats. There are numerous efforts underway to create data standards for human electrophysiological data to both

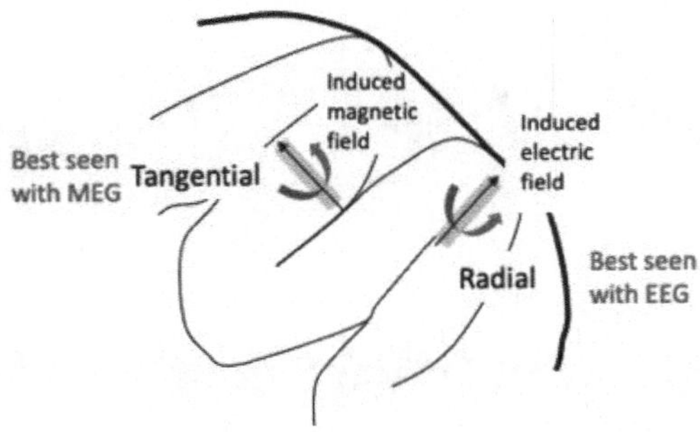


**FIGURE 2.2**
Illustration of cortical surface with tangentially versus radially oriented neural sources. While EEG captures radial sources most effectively, MEG can detect tangential sources. (Color version available in electronic supplement.)

ensure sufficient meta-data are included to allow for interpretation (e.g. channel labels and locations) and to facilitate data sharing / future meta analyses. For example, Neurodata Without Borders (NWB) [41, 46] has standard schema for common human neurophysiological data and metadata but also allows for customized extensions for special use cases. Databasing has also been created around the NWB standard [39]. iEEG-BIDS [26] also represents an extension to the common Brain Imaging Data Structure (BIDS), discussed in Chapter 3, specifically for iEEG data.

## 2.3 Preprocessing for MEG

MEG is a non-invasive neurophysiologic technique that is complementary to EEG and that measures changes in magnetic fields generated from underlying neural activity. Magnetic fields recorded by MEG capture the net contributions of excitatory and inhibitory postsynaptic potentials of dendrites [38]. As magnetic fields are generated orthogonally to electric currents, MEG improves the detection of tangentially oriented neural activity as compared to EEG, which best captures radial activity (Figure 2.2). Given the sensitivity to different components of neural activity, the combination of MEG and EEG has been demonstrated to improve the accuracy of source localization of epileptiform activity [1, 37].

In addition to being used as a complementary tool to capture orthogonally oriented neural activity, there are several advantages to consider for MEG recordings, as compared to EEG:

- Magnetic fields are not attenuated or distorted by changes in electric conductance, such as through the skull, subcutaneous tissue, and scalp. Therefore, there is reduced signal attenuation when measuring intracranial neural signals at the level of the scalp using MEG as compared to EEG. Considering the reduced signal attenuation and the sensitivity of the signal, MEG sensors can record a signal integrated over a cortical area of 3–4 $cm^2$ [3, 20].

- Given that MEG signals are not distorted by changes in electric conductance, MEG recordings and subsequent source localization may be particularly helpful in patients who have had prior surgeries that may alter such conductance (such as skull defects leading to breach rhythms on EEG or brain resections altering expected EEG surface topology).

- Due to the reduced signal attenuation and lack of other obstacles seen in EEG (such as electrode impedance), MEG can achieve high sampling rates (up to 12 kHz, with a typical sampling of 1 kHz), which enables the modeling of fast neurophysiological processes in the cortex.

- Finally, unlike the measurement of electric potentials by EEG (i.e. characterized by the difference across two points), MEG directly measures fluctuations in the magnetic field (i.e. calculated by the force exerted by a dipole). Therefore, MEG recordings do not require placement of a separate ground or reference electrode as a baseline for interpretation of the signal of interest; in this sense, MEG is commonly referred to as a "reference-free" modality. As such, common noise from a single ground or reference electrode, as potentially introduced in EEG, does not need to be considered. This is not to be confused with the presence of a reference sensor array, which is located away from the MEG helmet and is employed to capture external magnetic interference for isolating signals originating from the brain.

As compared to EEG, relative disadvantages of MEG include the inability to perform long-term monitoring or intentionally capture ictal recordings, given the required stationarity of the head within the MEG helmet. In addition, while EEG recordings can be performed in typical clinical environments or even in ambulatory settings, the specialized shielding required for MEG scanning limits its more general use. Finally, MEG scanning is more costly due to the underlying equipment and maintenance.

### 2.3.1 MEG Instrumentation and Acquisition

MEG recordings capture the synchronous activity of tens of thousands of neurons, which culminate in weak fluctuations of the magnetic field on the order of femtoteslas ($10^{-15}$ Tesla). To detect small changes in the magnetic fields produced by neural activity, MEG scanners are contained within a magnetically shielded room to isolate the scanner from environmental noise. In addition, measurements of these small fluctuations in the magnetic field are enabled by super-conducting quantum interference devices (SQUIDs) embedded within the helmet of the scanner. Current generation SQUIDs require cooling to sufficiently low temperature to enable superconducting properties. For this reason, MEG scanning can incur high costs related to cooling, which is typically done with liquid helium, a limited resource. Hardware development in MEG (including helium recyclers, optically pumped magnetometers (OPMs), and "room temperature" SQUIDs) is focused on overcoming these challenges in order to increase accessibility to this technology.

Flux transformers detect changes in the magnetic flux across a specified area and are coupled with the SQUIDs. Flux transformers are usually arrayed in one of two conformations: magnetometers or gradiometers. A magnetometer, the simpler setup, consists of a single superconducting coil that has high sensitivity but also picks up environmental noise. Gradiometers (either axial or planar orientations) comprise two oppositely configured coils, which are arranged to limit environmental noise from distant sources. To achieve high spatial sensitivity, MEG machines typically have from 256 to over 300 sensors to achieve whole brain coverage.

Clinical MEG recordings are typically acquired simultaneously with EEG to enable correlation of MEG and EEG signals for more accurate waveform identification and clinical correlation. All sources of magnetic noise, such as due to ferromagnetic materials including in clothes, jewelry, or make-up, should be removed prior to recording. When sources of magnetic noise cannot be physically removed, i.e. dental implants or surgical devices such as a cerebrospinal fluid (CSF) shunt or vagus nerve stimulator (VNS, which should be turned off for noise reduction), subsequent advanced denoising is necessary to reconstruct the MEG sensor data; however, even then, the signal may be unsalvageable. Additionally, because of the fixed head space within the helmet for MEG recording, head movements can lead to particularly large artifact; therefore, subjects are instructed to remain still for recording sessions. For epilepsy studies, recordings are recommended to be at least an hour long and to include both wake and sleep stages for characterizing epileptiform discharges. Although high sampling rates (in the kilohertz range) can be achieved using MEG, hardware filters for routine epilepsy assessments are typically set using a high-pass filter in the range of 1–4 Hz and a low pass filter in the range of 40–70 Hz. Review of the most up to date American Clinical MEG Society practice guidelines is recommended for further details on clinical data acquisition [2].

### 2.3.2 Experimental Design Considerations

For both clinical and research purposes, data are collected during both resting-state and behavioral task paradigms (i.e. motor, auditory, or language tasks). Resting-state recordings enable the detection of spontaneous neural activity, which includes non-task related state changes (e.g. wake and sleep state) and interictal epileptiform discharges. Because state-dependent network properties alter the morphology, localization, and field of epileptiform discharges [16, 17, 28], the acquisition of discharges across sleep-wake states is important for complete evaluation. The temporal fidelity of the resting-state MEG also provides an opportunity to examine whole-brain functional connectivity, as is performed with resting-state hemodynamic measures (e.g. functional MRI, positron emission tomography). Correlations/coherence and more advanced functional connectivity metrics (e.g. phase lag, entropy) using MEG sensor and source space reconstructions have demonstrated clinical significance in presurgical mapping and planning [14, 15, 50]. Two types of task-related experimental designs are considered: phase-locked (e.g. evoked) and non-phase locked (e.g. task-induced) designs.

- *Phase-locked trial designs* rely on precise temporal correlation of the task with an evoked response (e.g. auditory, visual, or sensory evoked responses). These trial designs are analogous to the single-trial averaging of datasets commonly done in EEG to look at event-related potentials and are most amenable to capturing the earliest stimulus response with the shortest latency. At the magnetometer level, evoked fields (e.g. auditory evoked field = AEF; visual evoked field = VEF) are averaged across multiple trials to improve the signal-to-noise ratio [22]. Longer-latency responses tend to exhibit more jitter and lower signal-to-noise when averaged across trials.

- *Non-phase locked trial designs* rely on the examination of activity within a window of time, and the analysis is most often performed in the frequency domain (i.e. spectral power within a frequency band of interest). As such, non-phase locked designs are effective when a response is expected to be consistent across trials but is less stringently time-locked to a stimulus.

Determination of the experimental design is essential prior to the acquisition of data to ensure accurate data collection with stimulus timing, the appropriate trial structure, and the adequate number of trials for subsequent statistical testing.

### 2.3.3 Preprocessing for MEG Signal Analysis

All preprocessing steps for EEG described in Section 2.2 are also considered for MEG signal analysis, except for re-referencing. As such, many toolboxes used for EEG are also used for the preprocessing of MEG data. Preprocessing is typically performed on the MEG

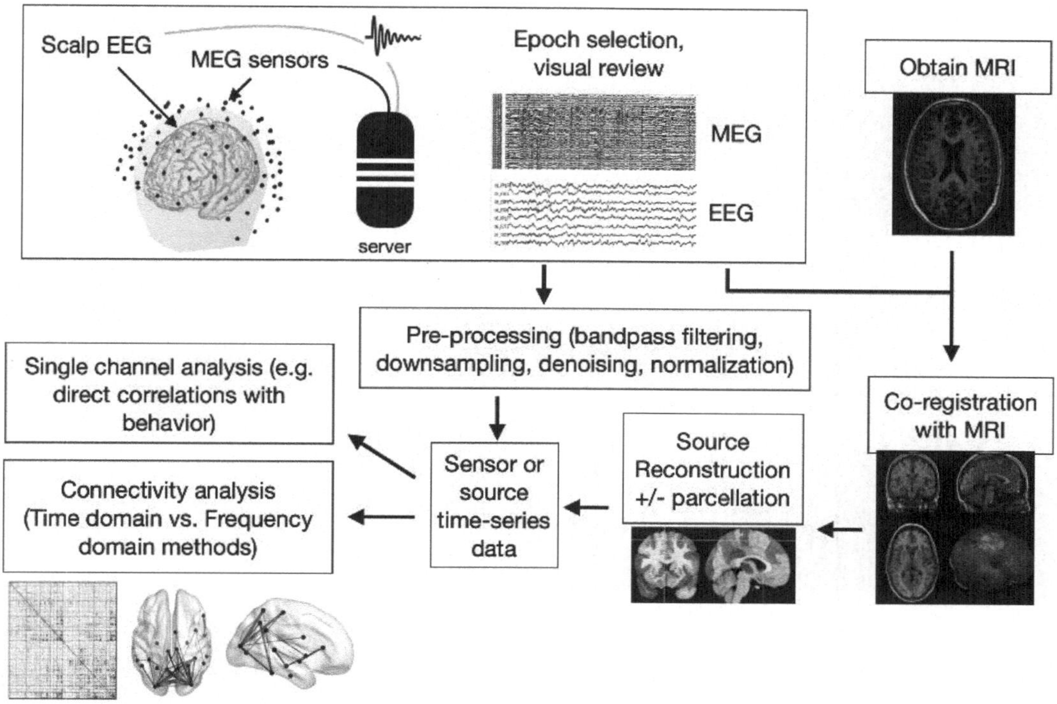


**FIGURE 2.3**
Workflow of MEG and EEG recording to analysis. Following MEG and EEG recording and epoch selection, raw signals undergo preprocessing prior to statistical analysis; time-series analysis can be performed on sensor or source time series data. (Color version available in electronic supplement.)

sensor data, although it can also be performed on source-reconstructed time series (Figure 2.3). MEG-specific considerations, including data sources, artifact reduction/denoising, and source reconstruction, are highlighted below.

- *Data sources*: MEG raw data formats differ from EEG and depend on a proprietary format designated by the machine manufacturer. Common raw formats include CTF, 4D/BTi, KIT/Yokogawa/RICOH, and Elekta/Neuromag data formats. Most manufacturers provide a stock series of data preprocessing tools (e.g. CTF DataEditor) built to handle data in the formats coming off the machine. These tools permit visualization of the raw data for cleaning, selection of high-quality data epochs, or rejection of epochs with movement artifact. Most toolboxes have import functions that work across datatypes and allow for data manipulation.

- *Artifact reduction*: To ensure high quality electrophysiology data, artifact reduction is typically performed in multiple steps. The first step often involves the visual review of the raw data to reject channels/trials/epochs with significant artifact (typically related to sensor noise or head movement) and can be performed within the manufacturer visualization tool (e.g. CTF DataEditor) or following data import into the MATLAB/Python environment. Channel selection typically refers to the rejection of channels with excessive artifact by manual inspection or using an automated technique requiring an independent evaluation criterion (i.e. distance measure or noise-threshold). Alternatively, channel selection may refer to the selection of a subset of channels if

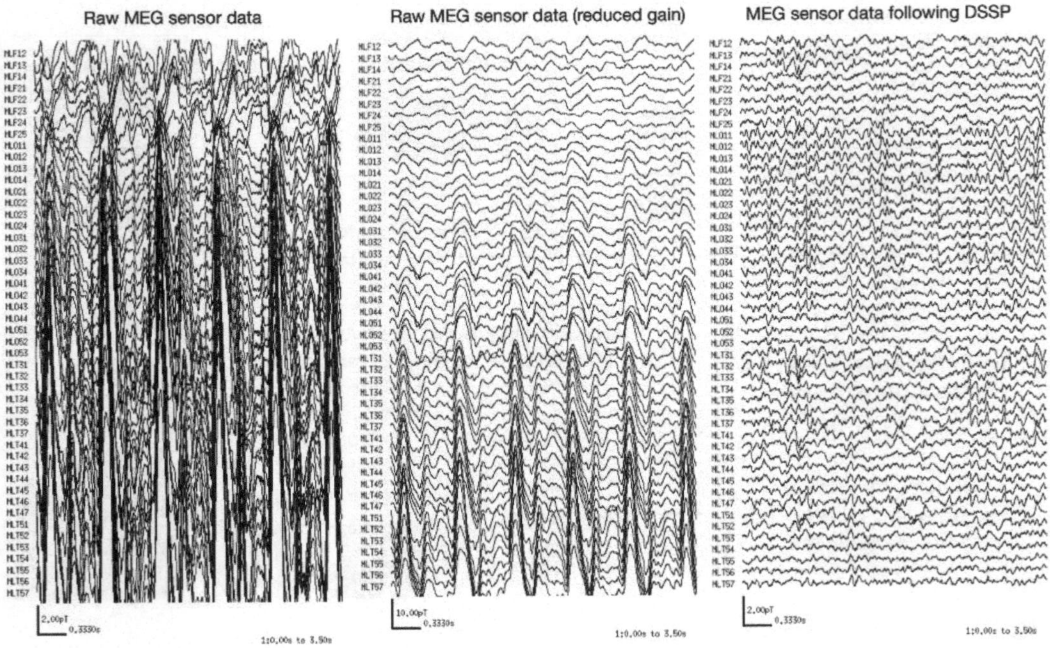


**FIGURE 2.4**
(Left and Middle) Example of MEG sensor background data that is heavily contaminated by VNS artifact. (Right) Dual SSP (DSSP) is performed as a denoising step, resulting in more interpretable signal.

the desired analysis is to be performed in sensor space of a specific region. Likewise, in multi-trial recordings (AEF, etc.) or continuous recordings, trial/epoch selection or rejection refers to the selection of high-quality segments or to the removal of segments where substantial noise is present across channels. Manual review is the gold standard; however, automated methods to detect trials or segments of time with overlying artifact are again often performed, such as with noise thresholding methods (e.g. root mean square thresholding). Subsequent preprocessing steps to remove systematic noise that may be shared across channels (e.g. eye blinks, cardiac artifact, or other movement) include techniques such as ICA or factor analysis [32].

- *Advanced denoising methods*: In MEG, unique noise that is not seen in EEG include metallic artifact from ferromagnetic hardware attached to the patient, e.g. dental hardware, pacemakers, CSF shunts, or a VNS. Advanced denoising procedures such as signal space separation (SSS) or signal-space projection (SSP), both spatial filtering algorithms that suppress external interference, can be performed on these recordings. In addition, there are even more advanced techniques for denoising of external interference, such as temporal SSS or dual SSP (DSSP), in which the denoising methods are performed in the spatio-temporal domain [42] (Figure 2.4).

As with EEG, standard preprocessing steps include frequency filtering, down-sampling, ICA, and epoching. Filtering is performed to limit the upper range (low-pass filter), bottom range (high-pass filter), and/or remove a specific band (e.g. notch filter) of frequency activity to resolve a neurophysiologic range of interest. Filters are designed with characteristic roll-off rates, which describe the steepness of the transition from the pass band to the stop band (or vice-versa), and variations in ripples at the transition, which represent amplitude errors of the filter within the pass or stop band. Commonly used filters in signal processing include Butterworth, Chebyshev, or Bessel filters, which differ in the roll-off rates and presence/absence of ripples.

Additional preprocessing steps includes normalization and averaging of the data, which depend on the experimental paradigm. For resting-state paradigms, normalization is often performed across the whole-trial, while in task-based paradigms, normalization may be performed relative to the pre-stimulus baseline. Normalization is also typically performed on a per-channel basis. To increase signal-to-noise, averaging across multiple trials is often performed for evoked or triggered events. Epileptiform waveforms captured during resting-state periods are overlayed and averaged based on peak detection of the waveforms. Task-related events may be averaged in the time-domain in the phase-locked trial design or based on maximal spectral changes within an explicit window in non-phase locked trial design, as described previously. If non-phase locked trial design is performed, the time-window (length, duration, and sliding/overlap parameters) and frequency band must be defined.

### 2.3.4 Brief Introduction to Source Reconstruction

As with EEG, signal analysis of MEG signals can be performed on the sensor or source reconstructed data. Given that MEG signal analysis is frequently performed in source space, we will briefly review the high-level steps for source reconstruction here. First, reconstruction of the source data requires generation of a lead field/gain matrix, often obtained by co-registering the MEG data with a high-resolution anatomical MRI (Figure 2.3). Co-registration requires a head coordinate system, which is based on landmarks identifiable on MRI (generally a T1-weighted image), usually defined by the anatomic landmarks of the nasion, inion, and bilateral pre-auricular points and are aligned with the MEG sensor array. A head model, such as a spherical head model, multisphere model, or boundary element method (BEM) head model, is then selected to approximate the properties of conductivity, and associated with the MEG acquisition for lead field/gain matrix generation of the forward model.

Source analysis can subsequently be performed on evoked potentials using a variety of inverse methods, which include beamformer (LCMV, SAM), minimum norm (sLORETA [36], dSPM), and Bayesian (Champagne [34], SAKETINI [54]) methods. Alternatively, source reconstruction can be performed to provide estimates for neural activity of each regional voxel. Using a voxel-to-regional anatomical atlas, such as the Automated Anatomical Labeling atlas [49], regional-times series data can be obtained and analyzed for whole brain functional connectivity estimates and other statistical analyses.

With the preprocessing steps applied to sensor or source-reconstructed time series recordings, subsequent analyses can be performed on individual channels/regions or the whole-brain, including correlations to behavior and connectivity analyses. In the next section, we will discuss specific toolboxes that can aid in the preprocessing pipeline.

## 2.4 Preprocessing Software Tools

There are numerous open-source and licensed software toolboxes available for EEG, iEEG, and MEG data. Here, we provide a brief overview of some popular programs:

- EEGLAB (`https://sccn.ucsd.edu/eeglab/index.php`) is an open-source toolbox for MATLAB with comprehensive analysis for EEG, which can also be largely applied to

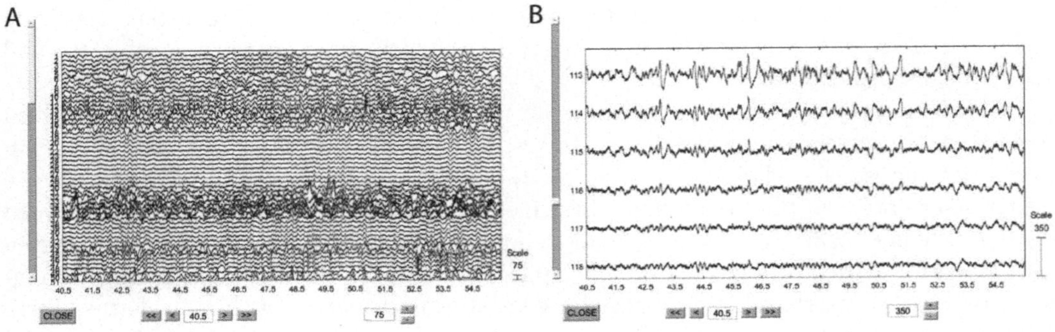

**FIGURE 2.5**
(A) Interactive EEGLAB plot displaying 15 seconds of data from 51 of 160 concurrently recorded sEEG traces. The user can scroll through time and across channels using the interactive plot and easily select to plot a different number of channels or amount of time. (B) Resized display showing 6 sEEG traces, illustrating an amplitude gradient across contacts of a single depth electrode. (Color version available in electronic supplement.)

iEEG data. EEGLAB can be used via a graphic user interface (GUI), or source code can be generated for further customization or incorporation of aspects of the processing pipeline with other analyses (as demonstrated in the functions above). EEGLAB is quite accessible to the beginning user, with default standard preprocessing routines, including ICA. The plotting functionality of EEGLAB is particularly useful for scrolling through large quantities of simultaneously recorded data (Figure 2.5).

- Fieldtrip (`https://www.fieldtriptoolbox.org/`) is another open-source toolbox for MATLAB with comprehensive analysis for EEG, MEG, and intracranial data. It does not include a GUI but provides functions which can be incorporated into a MATLAB script for analysis. Fieldtrip contains data read functions for common recording system data formats, along with more advanced analyses such as source reconstruction, connectivity analyses, and incorporating concurrent recording with some peripherals (e.g. eye tracking).
- MNE (`https://mne.tools/stable/index.html`) is an open-source Python package for the analysis and visualization of human neurophysiological data (EEG, iEEG, MEG, NIRS, etc). MNE is organized into modules, classes, and functions according to analysis step. MNE contains functionality for all part of analysis: data import, preprocessing, segmenting data, estimating evoked responses, time-frequency analysis, forward modeling, and source localization.
- Brainstorm (`https://neuroimage.usc.edu/brainstorm/`) is a package for analyzing EEG, iEEG, and MEG data through a powerful GUI interface that does not require programming knowledge. Brainstorm emphasizes practical aspects of data analysis, reproducibility, and productivity in electrophysiological datasets.
- SPM12 (`www.fil.ion.ucl.ac.uk/spm/`) is a MATLAB-based toolbox that has benefited from high popularity in the analysis of fMRI/PET data for well over two decades. SPM12 has expanded its capabilities to include analyses of EEG and MEG datasets, providing users a platform for analyzing separate EEG, MEG, and fMRI datasets in the same pipeline.
- NUTMEG (`https://www.nitrc.org/projects/nutmeg/`), the "Neurodynamic Utility Toolbox for Magnetoencephalographic Data" [11], is a MATLAB-based workbench

developed at UCSF that offers both GUI interfaces and command line scripting for its "sensor-to-statistics pipeline" for EEG and MEG datasets [25]. Strengths of the toolkit include a wide variety of inverse solutions and visualization of source solutions at both the single subject and group level.

Other stand-alone pipelines or plugins for the aforementioned comprehensive platforms address a particular challenge in the analysis pipeline. For example, substantial effort has been invested in automating high-quality artifact rejection:

- HAPPE [19], the "Harvard Automated Processing Pipeline for Electroencephalography," is a standardized, automated pipeline compatible with EEG recordings of variable lengths and artifact contamination levels, including high-artifact and short EEG recordings from young children or those with neurodevelopmental disorders.
- PREP pipeline [6] is a MATLAB library containing a standardized and completely automated early stage preprocessing pipeline for EEG data. The deployed steps try to preserve as much of the original signal as possible while also standardizing preprocessing steps across experiments. The authors provide explanations for each processing step and how they may affect resulting output data.
- FASTER [33], "Fully Automated Statistical Thresholding for EEG artifact Rejection," is a fully automated, unsupervised approach which takes raw EEG data as the input and outputs epoched, artifact-attenuated data. The pipeline includes automated ICA for artifact rejection.
- ADJUST [30], "Automatic EEG artifact Detection based on the Joint Use of Spatial and Temporal features," is a fully automated routine to identify ocular artifacts (blinks, vertical and horizontal eye movements) and discontinuities (anomalous events at a single electrode, typically due to high impedance or electrical instability).
- TAPEEG [23], "Tool for Automated Processing of EEG data," is a fully automated toolbox for preprocessing resting state EEG.
- ASR [31], "Artifact Subspace Reconstruction," is an approach to remove short-time, high-amplitude artifacts in continuous EEG data in real time. This real-time processing is particularly relevant for brain-computer interface applications.
- MARA [52], "Multiple Artifact Rejection Algorithm," is an EEGLAB plugin which uses supervised ICA to identify artifacts of multiple origins.
- SASICA [9], "Semi-Automated Selection of Independent Components of the electroencephalogram for Artifact correction," is a plugin for EEGLAB to facilitate user selection of physiological and artifactual ICA components by providing more quantitative information.

## 2.5 Summary

In this chapter, we have introduced EEG, iEEG, and MEG acquisition principles as they apply to data quality, interpretability, and preprocessing. We have outlined common artifacts encountered in these types of neurophysiological recordings and mitigation strategies. We have described popular software packages for preprocessing and provided building blocks for creating custom preprocessing pipelines. These preprocessing concepts and tools are critical to preparing neurophysiologic data for subsequent time series analysis and statistical testing, which will be described in subsequent chapters.

## Bibliography

[1] Ümit Aydin, Johannes Vorwerk, Matthias Dümpelmann, Philipp Küpper, Harald Kugel, Marcel Heers, and Jörg Wellmer. Combined EEG/MEG can outperform single modality EEG or MEG source reconstruction in presurgical epilepsy diagnosis. *PloS One*, 10(3):0118753, 2015.

[2] Anto I. Bagi, Robert C. Knowlton, Douglas F. Rose, and John S. Ebersole. American clinical magnetoencephalography society clinical practice guideline 1: Recording and analysis of spontaneous cerebral activity. *Journal of Clinical Neurophysiology*, 28:348–54, 2011.

[3] C. Baumgartner, E. Pataraia, G. Lindinger, and L. Deecke. Neuromagnetic recordings in temporal lobe epilepsy. *Journal of Clinical Neurophysiology: Official Publication of the American Electroencephalographic Society*, 17(2):177–89, 2000.

[4] Claude Bedard, H. Kröger, and Alain Destexhe. Model of low-pass filtering of local field potentials in brain tissue. *Physical Review. E*, 2006. *Statistical, Nonlinear, and Soft Matter Physics* 73 (June): 051911.

[5] Sándor Beniczky and Donald L. Schomer. Electroencephalography: Basic biophysical and technological aspects important for clinical applications. *Epileptic Disorders*, 22(6):697–715, 2020.

[6] Nima Bigdely-Shamlo, Tim Mullen, Christian Kothe, Kyung-Min Su, and Kay A. Robbins. The PREP pipeline: Standardized preprocessing for large-scale EEG analysis. *Frontiers in Neuroinformatics*, 9, 2015.

[7] György Buzsáki, Costas A. Anastassiou, and Christof Koch. The origin of extracellular fields and currents — EEG, ECoG, LFP and spikes. *Nature Reviews. Neuroscience*, 13(6):407–20, 2012.

[8] Claudio Carvalhaes and J.Acacio Barros. The surface Laplacian technique in EEG: Theory and methods. *International Journal of Psychophysiology*, 97(3):174–88, 2015.

[9] Maximilien Chaumon, Dorothy V.M. Bishop, and Niko A. Busch. A practical guide to the selection of independent components of the electroencephalogram for artifact correction. *Journal of Neuroscience Methods, Cutting-edge EEG Methods*, 250(July):47–63, 2015.

[10] Michael S. Clayton, Nick Yeung, and Roi Cohen Kadosh. The roles of cortical oscillations in sustained attention. *Trends in Cognitive Sciences*, 19(4):188–95, 2015.

[11] S.S. Dalal, J.M. Zumer, V. Agrawal, K.E. Hild, K. Sekihara, and S.S. Nagarajan. NUTMEG: A neuromagnetic source reconstruction toolbox. *Neurology*, 2004. *Clinical Neurophysiology*: NCN 2004 (November): 52.

[12] Rei Enatsu, Juan Bulacio, Imad Najm, Elaine Wyllie, Norman K. So, Dileep R. Nair, Nancy Foldvary-Schaefer, William Bingaman, and Jorge Gonzalez-Martinez. Combining stereo-electroencephalography and subdural electrodes in the diagnosis and treatment of medically intractable epilepsy. *Journal of Clinical Neuroscience*, 21(8):1441–5, 2014.

[13] Andreas K. Engel, Christian K.E. Moll, Itzhak Fried, and George A. Ojemann. Invasive recordings from the human brain: Clinical insights and beyond. *Nature Reviews Neuroscience*, 6(1):35–47, 2005.

[14] Dario J. Englot, Srikantan S. Nagarajan, Brandon S. Imber, Kunal P. Raygor, Susanne M. Honma, Danielle Mizuiri, Mary Mantle, Robert C. Knowlton, Heidi E. Kirsch, and Edward F. Chang. Epileptogenic zone localization using magnetoencephalography predicts seizure freedom in epilepsy surgery. *Epilepsia*, 56(6):949–58, 2015.

[15] Joline M. Fan, Anthony T. Lee, Kiwamu Kudo, Kamalini G. Ranasinghe, Hirofumi Morise, Anne M. Findlay, Heidi E. Kirsch, Edward F. Chang, Srikantan S. Nagarajan, and Vikram R. Rao. Network connectivity predicts effectiveness of responsive neurostimulation in focal epilepsy. *Brain Communications*, 4(3):104, 2022.

[16] Birgit Frauscher, Nicolás Ellenrieder, Franccois Dubeau, and Jean Gotman. EEG desynchronization during phasic REM sleep suppresses interictal epileptic activity in humans. *Epilepsia*, 57(6):879–88, 2016.

[17] Birgit Frauscher, Nicolás Ellenrieder, Taissa Ferrari-Marinho, Massimo Avoli, Franccois Dubeau, and Jean Gotman. Facilitation of epileptic activity during sleep is mediated by high amplitude slow waves. *Brain: A Journal of Neurology*, 138(Pt 6):1629–41, 2015.

[18] Karl J. Friston, André M. Bastos, Dimitris Pinotsis, and Vladimir Litvak. LFP and oscillations—what do they tell us? *Current Opinion in Neurobiology, SI: Brain Rhythms and Dynamic Coordination*, 31(April):1–6, 2015.

[19] Laurel J. Gabard-Durnam, Adriana S.Mendez Leal, Carol L. Wilkinson, and April R. Levin. The Harvard automated processing pipeline for electroencephalography (HAPPE): Standardized processing software for developmental and high-artifact data. *Frontiers in Neuroscience*, 12, 2018.

[20] Daniel M. Goldenholz, Seppo P. Ahlfors, Matti S. Hämäläinen, Dahlia Sharon, Mamiko Ishitobi, Lucia M. Vaina, and Steven M. Stufflebeam. Mapping the signal-to-noise-ratios of cortical sources in magnetoencephalography and electroencephalography. *Human Brain Mapping*, 30(4):1077–86, 2009.

[21] Roberta Grech, Tracey Cassar, Joseph Muscat, Kenneth P. Camilleri, Simon G. Fabri, Michalis Zervakis, Petros Xanthopoulos, Vangelis Sakkalis, and Bart Vanrumste. Review on solving the inverse problem in EEG source analysis. *Journal of NeuroEngineering and Rehabilitation*, 5(1):25, 2008.

[22] Peter Hansen, Morten Kringelbach, and Riitta Salmelin, editors. *MEG: An Introduction to Methods.* Oxford University Press, New York, 2010.

[23] F. Hatz, M. Hardmeier, H. Bousleiman, S. Rüegg, C. Schindler, and P. Fuhr. Reliability of fully automated versus visually controlled pre- and post-processing of resting-state EEG. *Clinical Neurophysiology*, 126(2):268–74, 2015.

[24] John Hermiz, Nicholas Rogers, Erik Kaestner, Mehran Ganji, Daniel R. Cleary, Bob S. Carter, David Barba, Shadi A. Dayeh, Eric Halgren, and Vikash Gilja. Sub-millimeter ECoG pitch in human enables higher fidelity cognitive neural state estimation. *NeuroImage*, 176(August):454–64, 2018.

[25] Leighton B.N. Hinkley, Corby L. Dale, Chang Cai, Johanna Zumer, Sarang Dalal, Anne Findlay, Kensuke Sekihara, and Srikantan S. Nagarajan. NUTMEG: Open source software for M/EEG source reconstruction. *Frontiers in Neuroscience* 14 (August): 710, 2020.

[26] Christopher Holdgraf, Stefan Appelhoff, Stephan Bickel, Kristofer Bouchard, Sasha D'Ambrosio, Olivier David, and Orrin Devinsky. IEEG-BIDS, extending the brain imaging data structure specification to human intracranial electrophysiology. *Scientific Data*, 6(1):102, 2019.

[27] Jürgen Kayser and Craig E. Tenke. On the benefits of using surface laplacian (current source density) methodology in electrophysiology. *International Journal of Psychophysiology : Official Journal of the International Organization of Psychophysiology*, 97(3):171–3, 2015.

[28] Graham A. McLeod, Parandoush Abbasian, Darion Toutant, Amirhossein Ghassemi, Tyler Duke, Conrad Rycyk, Demitre Serletis, Zahra Moussavi, and Marcus C. Ng. Sleep–wake states change the interictal localization of candidate epileptic source generators. *Sleep*, 45(6):062, 2022.

[29] Kai J. Miller, Larry B. Sorensen, Jeffrey G. Ojemann, and Marcel Nijs. Power-law scaling in the brain surface electric potential. *PLoS Computational Biology*, 5(12):1000609, 2009.

[30] Andrea Mognon, Jorge Jovicich, Lorenzo Bruzzone, and Marco Buiatti. ADJUST: An automatic EEG artifact detector based on the joint use of spatial and temporal features. *Psychophysiology*, 48(2):229–40, 2011.

[31] Tim Mullen, Christian Kothe, Yu Mike Chi, Alejandro Ojeda, Trevor Kerth, Scott Makeig, Gert Cauwenberghs, and Tzyy-Ping Jung. Real-time modeling and 3D visualization of source dynamics and connectivity using wearable EEG. In *2013 35th Annual International Conference of the IEEE Engineering in Medicine and Biology Society (EMBC)*, pages 2184–87, 2013.

[32] Srikantan S. Nagarajan, Hagai T. Attias, Kenneth E. Hild, and Kensuke Sekihara. A probabilistic algorithm for robust interference suppression in bioelectromagnetic sensor data. *Statistics in Medicine*, 26(21):3886–3910, 2007.

[33] H. Nolan, R. Whelan, and R.B. Reilly. FASTER: Fully automated statistical thresholding for EEG artifact rejection. *Journal of Neuroscience Methods*, 192(1):152–62, 2010.

[34] Julia P. Owen, David P. Wipf, Hagai T. Attias, Kensuke Sekihara, and Srikantan S. Nagarajan. Performance evaluation of the champagne source reconstruction algorithm on simulated and real M/EEG data. *NeuroImage*, 60(1):305–23, 2012.

[35] Martin Pail, Jan Cimbálník, Robert Roman, Pavel Daniel, Daniel J. Shaw, Jan Chrastina, and Milan Brázdil. High frequency oscillations in epileptic and non-epileptic human hippocampus during a cognitive task. *Scientific Reports*, 10(1):18147, 2020.

[36] Roberto D. Pascual-Marqui, Dietrich Lehmann, Martha Koukkou, Kieko Kochi, Peter Anderer, Bernd Saletu, and Hideaki Tanaka. Assessing interactions in the brain with exact low-resolution electromagnetic tomography. *Philosophical Transactions of the Royal Society A: Mathematical, Physical and Engineering Sciences*, 369:3768–84, 2011.

[37] Chris Plummer, Simon J. Vogrin, William P. Woods, Michael A. Murphy, Mark J. Cook, and David T.J. Liley. Interictal and ictal source localization for epilepsy surgery using high-density EEG with MEG: A prospective long-term study. *Brain: A Journal of Neurology*, 142(4):932–51, 2019.

[38] Malcolm Proudfoot, Mark W. Woolrich, Anna C. Nobre, and Martin R. Turner. Magnetoencephalography. *Practical Neurology*, 14(5):336–43, 2014.

[39] Marike L. Reimer, Lakshmi Bangalore, Stephen G. Waxman, and Andrew M. Tan. Core principles for the implementation of the Neurodata Without Borders data standard. *Journal of Neuroscience Methods*, 348(January):108972, 2021.

[40] Kay A. Robbins, Jonathan Touryan, Tim Mullen, Christian Kothe, and Nima Bigdely-Shamlo. How sensitive are EEG results to preprocessing methods: A benchmarking study. *IEEE Transactions on Neural Systems and Rehabilitation Engineering: A Publication of the IEEE Engineering in Medicine and Biology Society*, 28(5):1081–90, 2020.

[41] Oliver Rübel, Andrew Tritt, Ryan Ly, Benjamin K. Dichter, Satrajit Ghosh, Lawrence Niu, Ivan Soltesz, Karel Svoboda, Loren Frank, and Kristofer E. Bouchard. The Neurodata Without Borders ecosystem for neurophysiological data science. *BioRxiv*, 2021.

[42] Kensuke Sekihara, Yuya Kawabata, Shuta Ushio, Satoshi Sumiya, Shigenori Kawabata, Yoshiaki Adachi, and Srikantan S. Nagarajan. Dual signal subspace projection (DSSP): A novel algorithm for removing large interference in biomagnetic measurements. *Journal of Neural Engineering*, 13(3):036007, 2016.

[43] K.K. Sellers, W.L. Schuerman, H.E. Dawes, E.F. Chang, and M.K. Leonard. Comparison of common artifact rejection methods applied to direct cortical and peripheral stimulation in human ECoG. In *2019 9th International IEEE/EMBS Conference on Neural Engineering (NER)*, pages 77–80, 2019.

[44] Kristin K. Sellers, Jason E. Chung, Jenny Zhou, Michael G. Triplett, Heather E. Dawes, Razi Haque, and Edward F. Chang. Thin-film microfabrication and intraoperative testing of $\mu$ECoG and IEEE depth arrays for sense and stimulation. *Journal of Neural Engineering*, 18(4):045014, 2021.

[45] Mehdi Shokoueinejad, Dong-Wook Park, Yei Hwan Jung, Sarah K. Brodnick, Joseph Novello, Aaron Dingle, and Kyle I. Swanson. Progress in the field of micro-electrocorticography. *Micromachines*, 10(1), 2019.

[46] Jeffery L. Teeters, Keith Godfrey, Rob Young, Chinh Dang, Claudia Friedsam, Barry Wark, and Hiroki Asari. Neurodata Without Borders: Creating a common data format for neurophysiology. *Neuron*, 88(4):629–34, 2015.

[47] Uros Topalovic, Zahra M. Aghajan, Diane Villaroman, Sonja Hiller, Leonardo Christov-Moore, Tyler J. Wishard, and Matthias Stangl. Wireless programmable recording and stimulation of deep brain activity in freely moving humans. *Neuron*, 108(2):322–34 9, 2020.

[48] Roger D. Traub and Miles A. Whittington. *Cortical Oscillations in Health and Disease.* Oxford University Press, 2010.

[49] N. Tzourio-Mazoyer, B. Landeau, D. Papathanassiou, F. Crivello, O. Etard, N. Delcroix, B. Mazoyer, and M. Joliot. Automated anatomical labeling of activations in SPM using a macroscopic anatomical parcellation of the MNI MRI single-subject brain. *NeuroImage*, 15(1):273–89, 2002.

[50] Jayabal Velmurugan, Srikantan S. Nagarajan, Narayanan Mariyappa, Ravindranadh C. Mundlamuri, Kenchaiah Raghavendra, Rose Dawn Bharath, and Jitender Saini. Magnetoencephalography imaging of high frequency oscillations strengthens presurgical localization and outcome prediction. *Brain: A Journal of Neurology*, 142(11):3514–29, 2019.

[51] Xiao-Jing Wang. Neurophysiological and computational principles of cortical rhythms in cognition. *Physiological Reviews*, 90(3):1195–1268, 2010.

[52] Irene Winkler, Stephanie Brandl, Franziska Horn, Eric Waldburger, Carsten Allefeld, and Michael Tangermann. Robust artifactual independent component classification for BCI practitioners. *Journal of Neural Engineering*, 11(3):035013, 2014.

[53] Jonathan Wolpaw and Elizabeth Winter Wolpaw. *Brain-Computer Interfaces: Principles and Practice.* Oxford University Press, 2012.

[54] Johanna M. Zumer, Hagai T. Attias, Kensuke Sekihara, and Srikantan S. Nagarajan. A probabilistic algorithm integrating source localization and noise suppression for MEG and EEG data. *NeuroImage*, 37(1):102–15, 2007.

# 3

# *Acquisition and Preprocessing of Neuroimaging MRI Data*

**Hsiang J. Yeh**

*Department of Neurology, University of California, Los Angeles (USA)*

## CONTENTS



Analysis of functional neuroimaging data for epilepsy research hinges on the quality of the recorded imaging data and methods used in preprocessing. In this chapter, we describe practical methods to record high quality imaging data, and provide an example preprocessing pipeline for MRI. We discuss best practices for scanning, with the goal of obtaining imaging scans with high quality signal and avoiding artifact. We highlight common steps to follow for maintaining quality, consistency, and reducing artifacts during imaging data acquisition. Examples of preprocessing for several common neuroimaging modalities are provided using custom Bash scripts.

DOI: 10.1201/9781003254515-3

## 3.1 Introduction

Neuroimaging research in epilepsy demands careful and rigorous collection of data to ensure high-quality downstream analyses. This chapter presents practical methods and an example preprocessing pipeline for working with brain imaging data in an epilepsy research context. We first review best practices for scanning and discuss MRI physics, scanner upkeep, communication with the radiology team, and scanner software settings. Next, we demonstrate an example preprocessing pipeline using Bash scripting to automate the process. Example scripts provided in this chapter demonstrate conversion of DICOM to NifTI format, organizing into Brain Imaging Data Structure (BIDS), evaluating data quality, independent components analysis (ICA) denoising, nuisance regression, frequency filtering, time-series extraction, and a positron emission tomography (PET) preprocessing example. The methods and scripts presented in this chapter are intended to help facilitate collection and preprocessing of neuroimaging data in epilepsy research.

## 3.2 Data Acquisition

In this section, we provide a brief overview of best practices for imaging data acquisition, including MRI physics, scanner preparation, scanner software settings, and considerations in obtaining high-quality imaging.

### 3.2.1 Brief Overview of MRI

MRI and its derivatives, functional magnetic resonance imaging (fMRI), and diffusion tensor imaging (DTI), are commonly used modalities in epilepsy research. The key difference between MRI and computed tomography (CT) and positron emission tomography (PET) is the lack of exposure to ionizing radiation, since CT involves X-rays, while PET involves injecting a radioactive tracer into the body. Another noteworthy difference lies in how MRI signals are recorded and then transformed into the familiar 3D or 4D image. While CT and PET directly detect radioactive signals, MRI uses carefully crafted radio frequency pulses and magnetic field shifts to encode the signal, which is detected by receiver coils. As the physics behind an MRI scanner is vastly complicated, an exhaustive explanation of how MRI works is not within the scope of this section. Instead, we will provide a brief overview on MRI physics, with focus rather on how data quality may be impacted by the sensitive machinery involved.

Magnetic resonance imaging works on the principle that protons within a strong magnetic field will become aligned in the same precession direction. A radiofrequency (RF) pulse applied at the Larmor frequency will cause protons precessing at the exact frequency to resonate and go into a higher energy state. When the RF pulse is removed, the protons will return to the lower energy state, and release the energy back at the same exact frequency. This resonant RF signal can then be picked up by receiving RF coils. The Larmor frequency is defined by the particle and the magnetic field strength it lies in. MRI scanners use this property to encode spatial location into the received RF signal, through manipulation of magnetic field gradients and the RF pulse. For example, the Larmor frequency of a single proton, which is the nuclei of a hydrogen atom, while inside a 3.0 Tesla (3T) magnetic field, is 127.74MHz. During scanning, the scanner will generate a magnetic field gradient, which alters the Larmor frequency of protons along this gradient. By tuning into the correct RF frequency, we can pick up signals from one slice of tissue in the scanner. This is called slice selection. Together with frequency encoding and phase encoding, these techniques allow for gathering of RF signal that can be decoded into three-dimensional images [1, 8, 9]. Thus, in practical terms, the scan quality is most impacted by disturbances in the magnetic field gradient and RF signals. This means that MRI scanners need to be shielded from magnetic field disturbances and external RF signals.

### 3.2.2 Scanner Preparation

The MRI physicist or technician maintains the scanner and makes sure it is well calibrated. This usually includes periodically scanning phantoms and fine-tuning scanner settings. A phantom is an object made with various materials [14], which, when placed in a scanner, can mimic the response of various tissues to being scanned. Scanning the phantom assures that the data being generated stays consistent and can help identify emerging issues as the scanner ages [11]. Therefore, the person who maintains the scanner, whether it be the MRI physicist, technician, or the researcher themselves, is the person who knows best about the scanner's current conditions, which protocols will best work for acquiring the intended data, and how to avoid running into issues while operating this particular scanner. It is important, therefore, to have conversations with the magnet person throughout the scanning process to stay updated on the scanner conditions. For research-oriented scanners, this person may even serve as a liaison between different research groups, providing insight into problems already solved by others working onsite.

In clinical settings, scanner technicians have different priorities. They may change scanning parameters from scan to scan, or opt to use a different protocol altogether to finish a scan on time or to ensure visual quality is suitable for physician review. This inconsistency in scanning parameters can lead to issues during data analysis, making it both difficult to analyze while also decreasing statistical power. Frequently, clinical scanner data would be considered poor or subpar quality for neuroimaging analysis. However, for epilepsy neuroimaging research, sometimes it is necessary to use clinical data. This can still be achieved with proper dialogue with the radiology team running the scanner. For example, if there is a functional MRI scan being obtained as part of the diagnosis protocol, it would be advisable for the researcher to reach out to the lead radiologist to discuss the parameters most important for data analysis, such as repetition time (TR), field of view (FOV), and scan length. Letting the radiologist know that altering the parameters will impact data analysis and discussing alternatives for when changes are needed is helpful. For example, if time is short on an fMRI scan, it may be better to cut the scan length shorter and keep TR consistent, rather than changing TR and FOV in an attempt to maintain the same number of time points. With good communication, clinical data can become a source of useful data for research settings.

### 3.2.3 Scanner Software Settings

The most common modalities used for epilepsy research are the standard MRI, fMRI, PET, and DTI. The standard MRI is typically used to record a high-resolution structural image, which will provide the basis for subsequent co-registration operations. The aim is high visual detail, with emphasis on grey and white matter tissue distinction and minimum spatial distortion. Traditionally, magnetization-prepared rapid acquisition gradient echo (MPRAGE) is used, with spoiled gradient recalled (SPGR) becoming more prevalent later. These protocols provide good contrast between the white and grey matter and can handle air cavities and bone without much distortion.

FMRI is a blood oxygenation level-dependent (BOLD) sequence that aims to capture temporal changes at the cost of structural detail. For the typical 3T magnet, this usually is a scan with a TR of around 2 seconds and a voxel size of 3mm to 4mm. With the advent of multi-band sequences and ultra-high field magnets at 7T and 9T, it is possible to record BOLD sequences with a TR of less than one second and voxel resolution around 1 to 1.2 millimeters. Regardless of the magnet or image resolution, these echo planar imaging (EPI) sequences are prone to susceptibility artifacts, and care must be taken in the setup to avoid losing signal in important areas [6]. The two areas to watch out for are nasal cavities and ear cavities. Although the standard practice is to align the scan with the anterior commissure-posterior commissure (AC-PC) line, for temporal lobe epilepsy, it may be necessary to increase the angle to reduce signal dropout in the temporal region [4].

For diffusion-weighted imaging, it is typical to record additional field maps as DTI is particularly susceptible to field distortions. These field maps can be used to estimate distortion and provide a basis for correction. The most common of these are the phase-encode-reversed pairs or blip-up blip-down images [7].

### 3.2.4 Participant Comfort and Stabilization

After accounting for scanner settings, the next step in obtaining quality scan data is to reduce participant movement during scanning. This can be accomplished by ensuring physical and mental comfort. A comfortable participant is less likely to be adjusting position during the scan and will remove the most major movements. Physical comfort can be achieved via pillows and pads for the head, neck, back, legs, and arms, which should be used according to the participant's size and weight. For epilepsy, start with pillows around the head, then adjust the rest of the body accordingly. Around the head, pillows should be snug but not restricting; any small pressure points will grow to become uncomfortable as time goes by. We recommend getting feedback from the participant and asking specific questions for each part. For example, if the participant can feel the hardness of the scanner on the back of their head through the pillow, then more pillows might be needed. Additionally, remember to add or remove body pads so that the neck is not at an uncomfortable angle as the head coil is not movable. If any part of the neck is not touching the pad below, then neck pillows are needed. If the participant's elbows extend past the scanner bed's pads, then pads under the elbows might help. A triangular pad elevates the legs and puts the spine into a relaxed position and helps most people to be more comfortable. After pillows are set, allow some time for the participant to settle and get feedback from the participant and adjust as necessary, making sure to inform the participant that little discomforts might become unbearable as time goes. This extra time spent on comfort will translate into quality data, so it is well worth the small cost.

Beyond the pads and pillows are other physical concerns, such as remembering to ask the participant if they need to use the restroom before entering the scanner room, using earplugs to dampen scanner noise, and providing blankets for warmth.

It is important to provide mental comfort through proper briefing and safety protocols. Communicate often and between sequences to let the participant know what is coming up and how long it will take. Remind the participant that they can adjust slightly for comfort between scans. The specific instructions given are also important, such as saying "relax and try not to move your head during the scan," rather than "hold still and don't move." The latter could cause the participant to tense up and attempt to actively maintain still, which might actually cause more movement in the long term as they become exhausted after maintaining a tense pose for prolonged periods. The participant should have an emergency squeeze bulb to stop the scan at any time, but instructions should also include explicit cases where it is not needed, e.g., a bathroom break.

**TABLE 3.1**
Common sources of MRI artifact and mitigation steps [15].

| Artifact | Causes | Mitigation |
|---|---|---|
| Gibbs or ringing artifact | Fourier transform on high intensity signal changes | Increase matrix size |
| Zipper artifact | Unshielded radiofrequency signal | Close scanner door, check for electronic devices |
| Aliasing or wrap-around artifact | Field of view (FOV) too small | Increase FOV or oversample |
| Susceptibility artifact | Metal or air cavities | Proper screening and adjust slice angles |
| Ghosting artifact | Many, including motion | Check gradient field and reduce sources of motion |

After the scan, always debrief and address any concerns the participant has. Make a note if the participant failed to maintain the mental state needed for the study, such as accidentally falling asleep, or if any discomfort arises, which implies movements during the scan. Finally, all scanning centers have rigorous safety and screening protocols. These are the most important protocols to follow, as a safety incident, even a minor one, might land one in suspension of scanning privileges, during which time no data can be obtained.

### 3.2.5 Recording Additional Physiological Signals

Finally, another method of cleaning up motion artifacts involves recording physiological signals and regressing out activations that highly correlate to these non-neuronal activities. One of the most common motion artifacts is the cardioballistic artifact. This is caused by a combination of blood vessel expansion during heartbeats and lung expansion during respiration. Both of these actions contribute differently to periodic brain movements during the scan [3]. It is possible to record the heartbeat using a pulse detector and record the respiration movement with a breathing strip. These separate physiological records can be used later during the analysis to account for motion-related activations and be regressed out [2]. For epilepsy research, simultaneous EEG and fMRI may be acquired, and during such scans, the EEG can provide additional information that may be accounted for such as, but not limited to, eye movement, sleep state [10], or ictal status [12].

## 3.3 Data Preprocessing

The term "pre-processing" may refer to any number of processing steps prior to obtaining the statistical values of interest. Much of preprocessing in MRI refers to removing artifacts, cleaning up noise, and excluding subjects that exceed quality control criteria. However, in practice, teasing out unwanted signals may occur during the same step as obtaining the signal of interest, particularly during the general linear modeling (GLM) step. Thus, "pre-processing" may occur at the same time as "processing" and is not indicative of exact order.

Below, we provide an outline of typical preprocessing steps for MRI, PET, and DTI.

- Typical MRI preprocessing steps:

    1. Conversion of DICOM files to NIfTI format
    2. Quality check – exclude bad data
    3. Anatomical – Rotation and bias field correction
    4. Anatomical – Brain extraction and tissue segmentation
    5. BOLD – ICA decomposition and denoising
    6. BOLD – Motion correction, brain extraction, slice correction, and outlier detection
    7. Co-registration of anatomical and functional images and then to standard space
    8. BOLD – Extract signal from CSF and WM using co-registered and segmented masks
    9. Run GLM with motion parameters, CSF and WM signal, and outliers

- Typical PET preprocessing steps:

    1. Conversion of DICOM files to NIfTI format
    2. Quality check – exclude bad data
    3. PET – Calculate the attenuation correction factors for each slice
    4. PET – Motion correction, data normalization
    5. PET – If needed, reorient the PET data to a different orientation
    6. Co-registration of PET images to a reference anatomical
    7. Data smoothing – apply 3D spatial filters to smooth the data

- Typical DTI preprocessing steps:

    1. Conversion of DICOM files to NIfTI format
    2. Quality check – exclude bad data
    3. Anatomical – Rotation and bias field correction
    4. Anatomical – Brain extraction and tissue segmentation
    5. DWI – Check rotation and gradient directions, check tensor directions
    6. DWI – Bias field correction, eddy current correction
    7. Co-registration of Anatomical to DWI
    8. DWI – Fit the diffusion tensor [FSL or SPM]
    9. DWI – Estimate response function and fiber orientation distribution [MRtrix]
    10. Statistical analysis (e.g., fiber tractography, tensor directions, fractional anisotropy (FA), mean diffusivity (MD), and other analyses)

The following neuroimaging analysis softwares are of use in preprocessing:

– Analysis of Functional NeuroImages (AFNI) (`https://afni.nimh.nih.gov`): Suite of analysis tools for MRI, fMRI, and DWI.

– Advanced Normalization Tools (ANTs) (`https://github.com/ANTsX/ANTs`): Suite of image registration and segmentation tools capable of advanced nonlinear morphing of 2D, 3D, and 4D images.

- EEGLAB (https://sccn.ucsd.edu/eeglab/index.php): MATLAB toolbox for EEG and MEG analysis.
- FMRIB Software Library (FSL) ( https://fsl.fmrib.ox.ac.uk/fsl/fslwiki/FSL): Suite of analysis tools for MRI, fMRI, and DWI.
- FreeSurfer (https://surfer.nmr.mgh.harvard.edu/fswiki): Cortical-surface-model based suite of MRI, fMRI, and DWI analysis tools.
- MRtrix (https://www.mrtrix.org): Suite of analysis tools with emphasis on DWI processing and visualization.
- Statistical Parametric Mapping (SPM) (https://www.fil.ion.ucl.ac.uk/spm): MATLAB toolbox for analysis of MRI, fMRI, PET, SPECT, EEG, and MEG data.

### 3.3.1 Bash Scripting Introduction

In this section, it is assumed that the reader has a basic understanding of Linux/UNIX systems and command line interfaces like Bash, and although some fundamental operations will be discussed, it is not meant to be an exhaustive list. Bash is a popular shell program and is frequently included as the default command line interface for many Linux distributions such as Ubuntu. As such, it is a convenient environment to automate many processing steps. It also has robust support for text parsing and very flexible syntax for scripting, making entry into Bash scripting fairly straightforward to pick up. Some basic Bash keywords are listed in Table 3.2.

**TABLE 3.2**
Examples of basic Bash keywords.

| Command | Description |
|---|---|
| `ls` | List files in the current directory. Many parameters are available to specify how and what details are included and displayed. |
| `cd` | Change directory; changes the current working directory. |
| `rm` | Remove file. Parameters can make the action interactive or recursive. |
| `mkdir/rmdir` | Make directory; creates a new directory. Use the `-p` option to create multiple levels at once. `rmdir` removes a directory. |
| `for;done` | `for` loop. Accepts many syntaxes, including iterative loops or each object of an array. |
| `if;fi` | `if` statement. Can test for variables, files, directories, or other patterns. |
| `echo` | Echoes text to the screen, can display variables to inform the user or to debug. |
| `<variable>=` | Assigns value to the named variable, e.g., `x=1`. Bash variables are untyped and are interpreted depending on operational context. Arrays are assigned using parenthesis, e.g., `x=(1, 2, 3)`. |

These essential commands form the basic building blocks of preprocessing scripts, including loops and decision-making. Bash variables are declared with the variable name followed by the equal sign (=), and they are called by preceding the variable name with the dollar sign ($). The variable names are case-sensitive, thus `$date` and `$DATE` are different variables. Only alphanumeric and underscore characters are allowed in variable names, and the first character cannot be a number. The variable can be called implicitly, as described above, or explicitly, using curly brackets ({}), e.g., `${x}`. Common Bash commands for string or array manipulation are shown in Table 3.3, and example Bash commands for handling text files are shown in Table 3.4.

**TABLE 3.3**
Example Bash commands for string and array manipulation.

| Command | Description |
|---|---|
| `TEXT=abc-ijk_xyz` | Declaring a string |
| `ARRAY=(1 2 3 4 5)` | Declaring an array |
| `echo $TEXT` | Calling a variable |
| `echo ${ARRAY[0]}` | Calling the zeroth element in array |
| `echo ${ARRAY[@]}` or `echo ${ARRAY[*]}` | Calling all the elements in an array |
| `echo ${TEXT%_xyz}` | Truncate matching pattern from the end of the variable |
| `echo ${TEXT#abc-}` | Cut matching pattern from the beginning of the variable |
| `echo ${TEXT/ijk/opq}` | Find and replace pattern with another |

**TABLE 3.4**
Example Bash commands for handling text files.

| Command | Description |
|---|---|
| `head` | Returns the beginning line(s) of a text file. |
| `tail` | Returns the end line(s) of a text file. |
| `grep` | Returns the line(s) of text that matches a pattern. |
| `awk` | Versatile program for handling multi-column multi-row texts. |
| `sed` | Performs string substitution and manipulation on a text file. |

Bash commands follow the UNIX philosophy of modularity, being simple programs that do one job very well, and outputting results other programs can use. Thus, a great variety of tools can be used in combination to perform complex tasks. The scripting examples that follow use many such programs, including several that have been specifically developed for neuroimaging analysis. A simple online search for `bash script <what needs to be done>` will turn up multiple solutions to specific problems.

A simple Bash script is simply several of the above described terminal commands combined together. To illustrate, the first step of MRI pre-processing is to convert the DICOM files from the scanner into NIfTI format, the current standard for neuroimaging analysis. This can be accomplished using `dcm2niix`, which is a simple and straightforward program. The simplest use of `dcm2niix` is:

```
cd <DICOM folder, where .dcm files are>
dcm2niix ./
```

This can be converted to a script by creating and looping through an array of folders:

```
#!/bin/sh

DOC_PATH=~/Documents/DICOM
SUBJECTS=('S1' 'S2' 'S3' 'S4')
for i in ${SUBJECTS[@]}; do
  cd ${DOC_PATH}/$i
```

```
  dcm2niix .
done
```

The first line uses the special combination `#!` (this is called a shebang) to indicate which interpreter is to be used to run the script. The parameter `/bin/sh` means the script will be run using Bourne shell, following strict POSIX guidelines. The aim of using `/bin/sh` is to increase compatibility, and thus many advanced features of Bash will not be available through this interpreter. This simple script will loop through the array `SUBJECTS`, go into each directory, and execute the command `dcm2niix` in that directory. Next, we will expand this basic script into a real-world example.

### 3.3.2 Bash Scripting Example: Convert and Copy DICOM Files

We begin with a Bash scripting example to convert and copy DICOM files.

```
#!/bin/sh
#$ -cwd
#$ -j y
#$ -S /bin/sh
#$ -V

START_TIME=$SECONDS
### Filename: Copy_dcm2niix_2022.sh
### Make a copy of DICOM files, then convert them to nifti files
### Author: Hsiang Yeh
### email: shawn.j.yeh@gmail.com

### Files required for this step:
#   DICOM files

### Data information:
# SUBS_DCM contains the DICOM folders to be converted
# SUB is the current subject ID

### Set path to FSL on either cluster or local, comment/uncomment each line as
    needed.
# *** local: /usr/share/fsl *** cluster: /u/home9/FMRI/apps/fsl/current

FSL_PATH=/usr/share/fsl
#FSL_PATH=/u/home9/FMRI/apps/fsl/current

### Set working directory; expected directory structure is:
# DOC_PATH --- Sub1
#          |-- Sub2
#          |-- Sub3 --- nifti             <-- where data will be loaded from,
    DATA_PATH
#          |     *-- Sub3-1-nuisance.feat <-- where feat results will be created,
    RESULT_PATH
#          *-- scripts                    <-- where the script and template files
    are located
# *** Local: ~/Documents/fMRI *** Cluster: ~/data/fMRI

DOC_PATH=~/Documents/fMRI
#DOC_PATH=~/data/fMRI-EEG

# DICOM_PATH is the working path to which the DICOM files will be placed
DICOM_PATH=${DOC_PATH}/DICOM

# ORIG_DCM is the location of original DICOM files
ORIG_DCM=/media/DICOM1
```

In this example, we properly comment the script with description and expected data structure. The header starts with the same shebang: `#!/bin/sh`. The next four lines are special parameters for the Sun Grid Engine (SGE). Here, we specify to run the script from the current working directory `(-cwd)`, join the standard error and standard output streams `(-j y)`, run using the `/bin/sh` interpreter `(-S /bin/sh)`, and export all environmental variables when done `(-V)`. Running the script on a cluster computing system via SGE can be achieved simply with these parameters and minimum changes to the path variables. These four lines starting with `#$` may be omitted if there are no plans to run the script on a cluster using SGE. Additionally, a rough timer is created by marking the start and end time of the script.

```
cd "$ORIG_DCM"
SUBS_DCM=(`"ls" -d S???_*`)
for i in ${SUBS_DCM[@]}; do
  SUB=${i%%_*}
  if [ ! -d ${DICOM_PATH}/${SUB} ]; then
    echo "Copying Subject $SUB from $ORIG_DCM to $DICOM_PATH/$SUB..."
    mkdir -p ${DICOM_PATH}/${SUB}
    cp -r "$ORIG_DCM"/${SUB}_* ${DICOM_PATH}/${SUB}
  fi
  #read -p "Press any key to continue..."

  DATA_PATH=${DOC_PATH}/${SUB}/nifti
  if [ ! -d ${DATA_PATH} ]; then
    echo "Converting DICOM to Nifti for $SUB..."
    mkdir -p ${DATA_PATH}
    dcm2niix -o ${DATA_PATH} -i y -z o -x y ${DICOM_PATH}/${SUB}
  fi
  #read -p "Press any key to continue..."

done

###END of Script
END_TIME=$SECONDS
DIFF=$[${END_TIME}-${START_TIME}]
echo "Time taken: $[$DIFF / 3600] hours $[($DIFF % 3600) / 60] minutes $[$DIFF %
    60] seconds"
```

Note here that we created the subjects array `SUBS_DCM` by listing out the directories matching the pattern `???_*`, which is any three characters followed by an underscore, followed by anything. This was done by command substitution invoked by the backticks (`) substituting the output of `"ls" -d ???_*` into the array inside the parenthesis (can also accomplished via $() invocation). Since the DICOM file names are long, we truncate the string with `SUB=$i%%_*`, which removes the first underscore and everything that follows. From here, we copy the DICOM files and convert them using `dcm2niix`, this time with explicit output path. Importantly, if we find previous output results, we skip the current step, as `dcm2niix` will happily find and convert any neuroimaging files it encounters, including previous results. Thus, we have automated a simple script and saved useful notes in the comments for future reference.

Once we have converted the DICOM images to NIfTI format, we can start pre-processing the data for analysis. However, prior to starting the pre-processing, it is useful to perform a quality assessment on our data. This way, we can identify data that are below quality standards and choose to exclude them from analysis. MRIQC is a tool that can generate such a report on data quality metrics. In the next example, we write a script that organizes our data into BIDS-compliant structure, and then pass off the data to MRIQC.

### 3.3.3 Bash Scripting Example: Generate Data Quality Report Using MRIQC

Next, let us look at a Bash scripting example for generating a data quality report using MRIQC.

```
###===Header omitted for space===###

DOC_PATH=/home/syeh/Documents/fMRI
#DOC_PATH=~/data/fMRI

MRIQC_PATH=${DOC_PATH}/BIDS_files_2023

### BIDS directory structure will be created under $MRIQC_PATH as:
# MRIQC_PATH --- sub-S001
#             |-- sub-S002
#             \-- sub-S003 --- anat --- sub-S003_T1w.nii.gz
#                          |        \-- sub-S003_T1w.json
#                          \-- func --- sub-S003_task-rest_run-1_bold.nii.gz
#                                   \-- sub-S003_task-rest_run-1_bold.json

MRIQC_RPRT=${DOC_PATH}/mriqc_report_2023
if [ ! -d ${MRIQC_PATH} ]; then mkdir ${MRIQC_PATH};fi
if [ ! -d ${MRIQC_RPRT} ]; then mkdir ${MRIQC_RPRT};fi
if [ ! -e ${MRIQC_PATH}/dataset_description.json ];
then echo -e '{\n\t"Name": "2023 fMRI data",\n\t"BIDSVersion":
"1.7.0",\n\t"Authors": ["Hsiang J. Yeh",""]\n}' > ${MRIQC_PATH}/
    dataset_description.json;fi
```

BIDS is a standardized way of structuring and organizing neuroimaging data. It was developed to ensure that raw and preprocessed data from different research centers using different imaging techniques are systematically organized in a consistent manner. We create the BIDS directory structure, the output directory, and a basic dataset description file, if it does not exist yet. Then we loop through each subject and create the directory and file structure for the anatomical image and functional images.

```
cd ${DOC_PATH}
#SUBS='"ls" -d [0-9]*'

for SUB in ${SUBJECTS[@]}; do
  ## Go to working directory and run script there
  DATA_PATH=${DOC_PATH}/${SUB}/nifti

  cd ${DATA_PATH}
  echo "Working on $SUB..."
  SPGR='"ls" *_Crop_1.nii.gz'
  BOLDFILES=('"ls" *BOLD_*.nii.gz')
#  DWIFILES=('"ls" *.bval')
#  CT='"ls" *Brain*ab_*.nii.gz'
  if [ ! -d ${MRIQC_PATH}/sub-${SUB} ]; then
    echo "Copying data to MRIQC folder..."
    mkdir -p ${MRIQC_PATH}/sub-${SUB}
    mkdir ${MRIQC_PATH}/sub-${SUB}/anat
    mkdir ${MRIQC_PATH}/sub-${SUB}/func
#    mkdir ${MRIQC_PATH}/sub-${SUB}/dwi
#    mkdir ${MRIQC_PATH}/sub-${SUB}/ct
    cp ${DATA_PATH}/${SPGR} ${MRIQC_PATH}/sub-${SUB}/anat/sub-${SUB}_T1w.nii.gz
cp ${DATA_PATH}/${SPGR%_Crop_1.nii.gz}.json ${MRIQC_PATH}/sub-${SUB}/anat/sub-${
    SUB}_T1w.json
#    cp ${DATA_PATH}/${CT} ${MRIQC_PATH}/sub-${SUB}/ct/sub-${SUB}_ct.nii.gz
#    cp ${DATA_PATH}/${CT%.nii.gz}.json ${MRIQC_PATH}/sub-${SUB}/ct/sub-${SUB}_ct.
    json
  fi
```

Since this example dataset does not contain diffusion weighted (DWI) and CT images, we comment out the sections related to them. It is important to note that the script expects only one anatomical image per subject, and that the file always ends with _CROP_1.NII.GZ. This file is generated via `dcm2niix` with the `-x` (rotate and crop 3D images) option enabled. In turn, `dcm2niix` generates filenames and sidecar JSON files from the information it finds in the DICOM file. Thus, having a consistent protocol naming scheme at the scanner is important for analysis down the line.

```
  # Loop through bold files
  for ((i=1; i <= ${#BOLDFILES[@]}; i++)); do
    BOLDNUM=${i}
    if [ ! -e ${MRIQC_PATH}/sub-${SUB}/func/sub-${SUB}_task-rest_run-${i}_bold.nii
    .gz ]; then
      echo "Copying BOLD $i to MRIQC folder for SUB $SUB..."
      cp ${DATA_PATH}/${BOLDFILES[$[$i-1]]}
          ${MRIQC_PATH}/sub-${SUB}/func/sub-${SUB}_task-rest_run-${i}_bold.nii.gz
      sed -i ':a;N;$!ba;s#{\n\t"Modality": "MR",#{\n\t"TaskName": "rest",\n\t"
    Modality":
          "MR",#' ${DATA_PATH}/${BOLDFILES[$[$i-1]]%.nii.gz}.json
      cp ${DATA_PATH}/${BOLDFILES[$[$i-1]]%.nii.gz}.json ${MRIQC_PATH}/
          sub-${SUB}/func/sub-${SUB}_task-rest_run-${i}_bold.json
    fi
  done

  # Loop through dwi files
#  for ((i=1; i <= ${#DWIFILES[@]}; i++)); do
#    if [ ! -e ${MRIQC_PATH}/sub-${SUB}/dwi/sub-${SUB}_run-${i}_dwi.nii.gz ]; then
#      echo "Copying DWI $i to MRIQC folder..."
#      cp ${DATA_PATH}/${DWIFILES[$[$i-1]]}
                                    ${MRIQC_PATH}/sub-${SUB}/dwi/sub-${SUB}_run-${i}
    _dwi.bval
#      cp ${DATA_PATH}/${DWIFILES[$[$i-1]]%.bval}.bvec
                                     ${MRIQC_PATH}/sub-${SUB}/dwi/sub-${SUB}_run-${i}
    _dwi.bvec
#      cp ${DATA_PATH}/${DWIFILES[$[$i-1]]%.bval}.nii.gz
                                     ${MRIQC_PATH}/sub-${SUB}/dwi/sub-${SUB}_run-${i}
    _dwi.nii.gz
#      cp ${DATA_PATH}/${DWIFILES[$[$i-1]]%.bval}.json
                                     ${MRIQC_PATH}/sub-${SUB}/dwi/sub-${SUB}_run-${i}
    _dwi.json
#    fi
#
#  done

  #read -p "Press enter to continue.."

done
```

We then copy the BOLD images to their directory, following BIDS convention. We also insert the name of the task, in this case "rest," into the JSON file using `sed`. Now the data is ready for MRIQC. However, it is wise to first check the data with a BIDS validator.

```
cd ${DOC_PATH}
if [ ! -d ${MRIQC_RPRT}/logs ]; then
  read -p "Press enter to run MRIQC on copied files..."
  docker run -it --rm -v ${MRIQC_PATH}:/data:ro -v ${MRIQC_RPRT}:/out
                                        nipreps/mriqc:latest /data /out participant
    --no-sub
  docker run -it --rm -v ${MRIQC_PATH}:/data:ro -v ${MRIQC_RPRT}:/out
                                        nipreps/mriqc:latest /data /out group --no-
    sub
fi
```

```
###END of Script
END_TIME=$SECONDS
DIFF=$[${END_TIME}-${START_TIME}]
echo "Time taken: $[$DIFF / 3600] hours $[($DIFF % 3600) / 60] minutes $[$DIFF %
    60] seconds"
```

We run the Docker version of MRIQC, as installation of the "bare-metal" version is non-trivial. Running commands via Docker typically involves additional parameters to tell Docker where the data ought to be mounted. In this example, we mount the BIDS compliant directory structure `$MRIQC_PATH` and a directory `$MRIQC_RPRT` for the output. When completed, the results of MRIQC will be found in `$MRIQC_RPRT`.

Once the data quality has been assessed, we can start pre-processing the data. For pre-processing, first we make sure the filenames are consistent. The conversion software `dcm2niix` will generate the filename according to protocol details in the DICOM files, so inconsistent protocol details will affect the filenames. Luckily, Bash has good text parsing features, and renaming files could be as easy as one line of command:

```
for i in */nifti/*3DSPGR*.gz; do mv $i ${i%/*}/3dspgr.nii.gz; done
# Note that *3DSPGR*.gz must match only one file per subject
# or else multiple files will be moved into one
```

### 3.3.4 Bash Scripting Example: ICA Denoising

Once the files are named, next we run ICA decomposition and denoise. For this next script, we will require ANTs, FSL, and FSL's FIX automated denoising tool [13].

```
#!/bin/sh
#$ -cwd
#$ -j y
#$ -S /bin/sh
#$ -V

START_TIME=$SECONDS
### Filename: Melodic_fnirt_FIX_2022.sh
### Run Melodic with registration, mcflirt, and bet.  Then run FIX automatic noise
     removal.
### Author: Hsiang Yeh
### email: shawn.j.yeh@gmail.com

# Files required for this step:
#   Converted files in nifti format, with structural and bold sequences.

### Data information:  These fields are the names of the nifti files.
# SUBJECTS contain the subject IDs
# Structural scan is expected to be named 3dspgr.nii.gz
# BOLD images are expected to be named BOLD*.nii.gz

#SUBJECTS=('S100' 'S101' 'S102' 'S103' 'S104' 'S105' 'S106' 'S107' 'S108' 'S109')
SUBJECTS=('S100' 'S101')

### Sets path to FSL on either cluster or local, comment/uncomment each line as
    needed.
# *** Local: /usr/share/fsl *** Cluster: /u/home9/FMRI/apps/fsl/current
#FSL_PATH=/usr/local/fsl
#FSL_PATH=/u/home9/FMRI/apps/fsl/current
if [ -z "$FSLDIR" ]; then
  FSL_PATH=/home/syeh/tools/fsl
 else
  FSL_PATH=$FSLDIR
fi
```

Again, we set the header descriptions to include what the script does, and what files are needed for input. Here, we explicitly set the subject IDs that we want to run the analysis on instead of every subject we find in the directory. Alternatively, one can rename subject folders to exclude them (see below). Also, instead of always setting the `$FSL_PATH` manually, we detect if the variable `$FSLDIR` exists first, as this is the variable set by FSL when it is installed properly.

```
### Path to the design templates
MELODIC_TEMPLATE_PATH=${DOC_PATH}/scripts/Melodic_ICA_reg_mcf_for_FIX_Template.fsf
```

This template file contains pre-set parameters for MELODIC, with MCFLIRT, BET, and 5 mm smoothing. These are the default pre-processing settings for use with the standard training dataset in FIX.

```
cd ${DOC_PATH}
#SUBJECTS=('"ls" -d S[0-9]*')
```

This commented line, if uncommented, would list every directory that started with "S" followed by numbers only, and feed the result into `$SUBJECTS` to become an array of subjects to loop through. Subjects can be excluded by renaming their directory to not fit this pattern (e.g., renaming a directory from `S122` to `exclude_S122`).

```
for ((i=1; i <= ${#SUBJECTS[@]}; i++)); do
  SUB=${SUBJECTS[$[$i-1]]}
  RESULT_PATH=${DOC_PATH}/${SUB}
  DATA_PATH=${RESULT_PATH}/nifti
  cd ${DATA_PATH}

  ## Run N4BiasFieldCorrection on anat
  if [ ! -e N4_3dspgr.nii.gz ]; then
    echo "Brain extracting anatomical images..."
    bet 3dspgr.nii.gz 3dspgr_brain.nii.gz -R -m -n
    N4BiasFieldCorrection -d 3 -i 3dspgr.nii.gz -x 3dspgr_brain_mask.nii.gz -r 1 -
    o N4_3dspgr.nii.gz
    bet N4_3dspgr.nii.gz 3dspgr_brain.nii.gz -R -m
  fi

  ##Loop over each subject's BOLD files
  j=1
  for IMGNAME in ''ls' BOLD*.nii.gz'; do
# IMGNAME contains the current BOLD file
```

There are numerous ways of using `for` loops under bash. Here we highlight two alternatives for using for loops, with variables `$i` and `$j` to serve as the iteration counter. If the counter is not needed, then for `$SUB` in `${SUBJECTS[@]}`; do will just as a fine job of looping through each element of the array. Next, we run `N4BiasFieldCorrection`, which is a tool from ANTs. `N4BiasFieldCorrection` will attempt to correct lose of signal due to magnetic field distortions and inhomogeneity. These kinds of signal lose may cause white matter in one part of the brain to be less intense than grey matter in another part, which can be problematic for brain extraction tools. Because it requires a rough brain mask as input, we run `bet` (Brain Extraction Tool from FSL) before `N4BiasFieldCorrection`, followed by another `bet` on the corrected image.

```
    ##Run MELODIC with registration, mcflirt, bet
    cd ${DATA_PATH}
    if [ ! -e ${RESULT_PATH}/$SUB-${j}-mel-reg-mcf.ica ]; then
      IMGNAME=${IMGNAME%.nii.gz}
      NUMVOL='fslnvols ${DATA_PATH}/${IMGNAME}'
      VOLINFO=('fslstats ${DATA_PATH}/${IMGNAME} -v')
      TRINFO=('fslinfo ${DATA_PATH}/${IMGNAME}|grep pixdim4')
```

```
      MEL_DESIGN=${SUB}-${j}-melodic.fsf

      # regexp note: g and I flags denote (g) apply globally (all match instances)
     and (I) apply to all letter cases
      sed -e "s#=FSL_PATH#${FSL_PATH}#" -e "s#=RESULT_PATH#${RESULT_PATH}#" -e
                                  "s#=DATA_PATH#${DATA_PATH}#" -e "s#=SUB#${
    SUB}#g" -e
                                  "s#=NVOL#${NUMVOL}#" -e "s#=IMGNAME#${
    IMGNAME}#" -e
                                   "s#=SESSNUM#${j}#" -e "s#=NUMTR#${TRINFO
    [1]}#" -e
                                   "s#=TOTALVOX#${VOLINFO[0]}#"
    $MELODIC_TEMPLATE_PATH > $ {DATA_PATH}/$MEL_DESIGN
        # Here we call sed to substitute preplaced parameter key words with the
    values we generated before.
      echo "***Running MELODIC on Subject $SUB session $j***"
      feat ${DATA_PATH}/${MEL_DESIGN}
    else
      echo "Result exists!  Skipping MELODIC of $SUB session $j"
    fi
```

Here we use command substitution to store the number of volumes, volume size, and TR of the current BOLD file into their respective variables. Then we use sed to substitute preplaced parameter key words in the template file with the values from the current BOLD file. Once the design file is filled with the values we need, MELODIC ICA is run with the design file as input.

```
    if [ ! -f ${RESULT_PATH}/$SUB-${j}-mel-reg-mcf.ica/filtered_func_data_clean.
    nii.gz ]; then
      echo "Running FIX automatic ICA denoising on $SUB session $j"
      ~/tools/fix/fix ${RESULT_PATH}/${SUB}-${j}-mel-reg-mcf.ica
      ~/tools/fix/training_files/Standard.RData 15 -m
    else
      echo "Result exists!  Skipping FIX ICA denoising of $SUB session $j"
    fi

  #read -p "Press enter to continue.."
  if [ -f ${DATA_PATH}/${MEL_DESIGN} ]; then rm ${DATA_PATH}/${MEL_DESIGN}; fi
  j=$[$j+1]
  done

done
###END of Script
END_TIME=$SECONDS
DIFF=$[${END_TIME}-${START_TIME}]
echo "Time taken: $[$DIFF / 3600 ] hours $[($DIFF % 3600) / 60] minutes $[$DIFF %
    60] seconds"
```

Next, we call FIX, which is an automated ICA classifier for use with MELODIC results. We use the standard training model, which was trained using the same preprocessing steps as we specified in the design file.

These scripts are separated into different stages for which data checking is needed. After this script, the key points to check is the non-linear co-registration (FNIRT) and FIX noise component selection. If the registration is off, then all the analysis following it will be off. FSL provides a handy tool `slicesdir` to view multiple NIfTI files at once. An example usage of slicesdir while in the working `$DOC_PATH` is:

```
slicesdir */*-mel-reg-mcf.ica/reg/example_func2standard.nii.gz
```

This will generate a report including all the functional images registered to standard space, and allows one to see at a glance how each of the registration turned out.

### 3.3.5 Bash Scripting Example: Nuisance Regression

Once the results are verified, nuisance level analysis is run:

```
###===Header omitted for space===###

### Path to the FEAT design templates
NUI_FEAT_TEMPLATE_PATH=${DOC_PATH}/scripts/
    fsl600_design_RestingState_nuisance_run_segcsfwm_eigen_motion_outliers_Template
    .fsf

OUT_SUFFIX=RS-nuisance-SegCSFWM-eigen-motionscrubbed

for ((i=1; i <= ${#SUBJECTS[@]}; i++)); do
  SUB=${SUBJECTS[$[$i-1]]}
  RESULT_PATH=${DOC_PATH}/${SUB}
  cd ${RESULT_PATH}

  ##Loop over each subject's BOLD sessions
  for ICA in `"ls" -d ${SUB}-?-mel-reg-mcf.ica`;do
    ITMP=${ICA#${SUB}-}
    j=${ITMP%-mel-reg-mcf.ica} #find j
    DATA_PATH=${DOC_PATH}/${SUB}/nifti
    MEL_PATH=${DOC_PATH}/${SUB}/${ICA}
    IMGNAME=${MEL_PATH}/filtered_func_data_clean
    NUI_DESIGN=${SUB}-${j}-RS-nuisance_run.fsf
```

The nuisance analysis refers to regressing out the signals of no interest in the GLM. Although this is generally done at the same time as obtaining the statistics on the signal of interest, we choose to run the nuisance step separately. This will save time later on, when we want to look at different signals of interest on the same subject. For this step, we loop over the pre-processing folder generated by the previous script.

```
cd ${DATA_PATH}
    ## Generate motion files if not there
    if [ ! -f ${SUB}-${j}-motion6 ]; then
      echo "Generating motion parameter files..."
      extractmotion ${MEL_PATH}/mc/prefiltered_func_data_mcf.par ${SUB}-${j}
    fi

    ##Segment anatomical brain, then threshold result to make into CSF and WM
    masks
    if [ ! -f ${DATA_PATH}/3dspgr_brain_pveseg.nii.gz ]; then
      echo "Segmenting anatomical image for ${SUB}..."
      fast -t 1 -n 3 -H 0.1 -I 4 -l 20.0 -a ${MEL_PATH}/reg/standard2highres.mat
      -o ${DATA_PATH}/3dspgr_brain ${DATA_PATH}/3dspgr_brain
      fslmaths 3dspgr_brain_pve_0.nii.gz -ero -thr .9 -bin 3dspgr_CSF_mask
      fslmaths 3dspgr_brain_pve_2.nii.gz -ero -thr .9 -bin 3dspgr_WM_mask
      rm 3dspgr_brain_csf_stdspace.nii.gz
    rm 3dspgr_brain_gm_stdspace.nii.gz
    rm 3dspgr_brain_wm_stdspace.nii.gz
    rm 3dspgr_brain_mixeltype.nii.gz
    rm 3dspgr_brain_pve_1.nii.gz
    rm 3dspgr_brain_seg.nii.gz
    fi

    ##Transform CSF and WM mask into session space and extract time-series
    if [ ! -f ${DATA_PATH}/CSF_segmask-eig-seed$j.txt ]; then
      echo "Transforming and extracting CSF time series from ${SUB} session ${j
    }..."
      flirt -in 3dspgr_CSF_mask.nii.gz -ref ${MEL_PATH}/reg/example_func.nii.gz -
    applyxfm
      -init ${MEL_PATH}/reg/highres2example_func.mat -out ${SUB}-${j}-CSF_segmask
      -interp nearestneighbour
```

```
    fslmeants -i ${IMGNAME} -m ${DATA_PATH}/${SUB}-${j}-CSF_segmask --eig > $
    {DATA_PATH}/CSF_segmask-eig-seed$j.txt;
    #cat ${DOC_PATH}/scripts/norm_vec.R | R --slave --args CSF_segmask-seed$j.
  txt --no-save
    rm ${SUB}-${j}-CSF_segmask.nii.gz
    #rm CSF_segmask-seed$j.txt
  else
    echo "--Skipping CSF Time Series Extraction-- Result exists!"
  fi
  if [ ! -f ${DATA_PATH}/WM_segmask-eig-seed$j.txt ]; then
    echo "Transforming and extracting WM time series from ${SUB} session ${j
  }..."
    flirt -in 3dspgr_WM_mask.nii.gz -ref ${MEL_PATH}/reg/example_func.nii.gz -
  applyxfm
    -init ${MEL_PATH}/reg/highres2example_func.mat -out ${SUB}-${j}-WM_segmask
    -interp nearestneighbour
    fslmeants -i ${IMGNAME} -m ${DATA_PATH}/${SUB}-${j}-WM_segmask --eig >
    ${DATA_PATH}/WM_segmask-eig-seed$j.txt;
    #cat ${DOC_PATH}/scripts/norm_vec.R | R --slave --args WM_segmask-seed$j.txt
   --no-save
    rm ${SUB}-${j}-WM_segmask.nii.gz
    #rm WM_segmask-seed$j.txt
  else
    echo "--Skipping WM Time Series Extraction-- Result exists!"
  fi

##Generate outlier matrix if doesn't exist
  if [ ! -e ${DATA_PATH}/${SUB}-${j}-outliermat.txt ]; then
    echo "Running fsl_motion_outliers for Subject $SUB session $j***"
    fsl_motion_outliers --nomoco -i ${IMGNAME} -o ${SUB}-${j}-outliermat.txt
  else
    echo "Result exists!  Skipping outlier detection of $SUB session $j"
  fi
```

This section of the script generates the necessary nuisance signals for use in this step. `extractmotion` is a custom bash script which extracts the estimated six motion parameters into individual single-column text files. Next, we run FSL's segmentation program FAST, this generates the spatial masks for the CSF and WM. The masks are then used to generate eigenvectors of the CSF and WM areas of the fMRI image. Finally, we use `fsl_motion_outliers` to mark time points with excessive motion. With these files in place, we are ready to run the nuisance analysis.

```
  ##Run feat
  cd ${DATA_PATH}
  OUTPUT_DIR=${RESULT_PATH}/$SUB-${j}-${OUT_SUFFIX}.feat
  if [ ! -e ${OUTPUT_DIR} ]; then
    NUMVOL='fslnvols ${IMGNAME}'
    VOLINFO=('fslstats ${IMGNAME} -v')
    TRINFO=('fslinfo ${IMGNAME}|grep pixdim4')

    # regexp note: g and I flags denote (g) apply globally (all match instances)
   and (I)
    apply to all letter cases
    sed -e "s#=IMGNAME#${IMGNAME}#" -e "s#=OUTPUT_DIR#${OUTPUT_DIR}#" -e
     "s#=FSL_PATH#${FSL_PATH}#" -e "s#=SUB#${SUB}#" -e "s#=SESSNUM#${j}#" -e
     "s#=DATA_PATH#${DATA_PATH}#" -e "s#=NVOL#${NUMVOL}#" -e "s#=NUMTR#${TRINFO
  [1]}#" -e
     "s#=TOTALVOX#${VOLINFO[0]}#" $NUI_FEAT_TEMPLATE_PATH > ${DATA_PATH}/
  $NUI_DESIGN
    echo "***Running Nuisance step for Subject $SUB session $j***"
    feat ${DATA_PATH}/${NUI_DESIGN}
  else
    echo "Result exists!  Skipping nuisance FEAT of $SUB session $j"
```

```
    fi

  #read -p "Press enter to continue.."
  if [ -f ${DATA_PATH}/${NUI_DESIGN} ]; then rm ${DATA_PATH}/${NUI_DESIGN}; fi
  done

done
###END of Script
END_TIME=$SECONDS
DIFF=$[${END_TIME}-${START_TIME}]
echo "Time taken: $[$DIFF / 3600 ] hours $[($DIFF % 3600) / 60] minutes $[$DIFF %
    60] seconds"
```

We run the nuisance by replacing the values in the template file with the values we need. Note that for this example, the file names of nuisance signals are hardcoded into the template file. After the nuisance analysis, we can run the traditional correlational analysis, or extract time-series from ROIs from the pre-processed images for functional connectivity analysis. Example scripts of correlational analysis can be found in Runlevel2_2022.sh and Runlevel3_2022.sh files.

### 3.3.6 Bash Scripting Example: Frequency Filtering and Time-Series Extraction

For functional connectivity analysis, we extract the time-series from the fMRI after it has been scrubbed of the nuisance signals.

```
###===Header omitted for space===###

NUI_DIR=RS-nuisance-SegCSFWM-eigen-motionscrubbed.feat
OUT_PATH=${DOC_PATH}/Outgoing/Result_FIXICA_denoise_nuisance_regression

ATLAS_PATH=${DOC_PATH}/atlas
BNAME=('low')
BLSIG=('0.01')
BHSIG=('0.1')

for ((j=0; j <= $[${#BNAME[@]}-1]; j++)); do
```

Note that for this script, it is possible to include multiple bandpass filter frequency ranges by specifying additional values for `BNAME`, `BLSIG`, `BHSIG`, e.g.,s BNAME=('low' 'high'), BLSIG=('0.01' '0.1'), BHSIG=('0.1' '0.2').

```
  for SUB in ${SUBJECTS[@]}; do
   RESULT_PATH=${DOC_PATH}/${SUB}
   DATA_PATH=${RESULT_PATH}/nifti
   cd ${RESULT_PATH}

   for NUI in `"ls" -d ${SUB}-?-${NUI_DIR}`;do
    ITMP=${NUI#${SUB}-}
    i=${ITMP%-${NUI_DIR}} #find i
    FILEO=res4d
    FILEN=res4d_${BNAME[$j]}
    REG_PATH=${RESULT_PATH}/${SUB}-$i-mel-reg-mcf.ica/reg
    NUI_PATH=${RESULT_PATH}/${SUB}-$i-${NUI_DIR}

    echo "Working on $SUB session ${i} frequency band: ${BNAME[$j]}"
```

We will loop through each nuisance run from the previous script. Similar to the previous script, we find the iteration count from the directory name, and do not assume all sessions to be present and in sequential order.

```
cd ${NUI_PATH}/stats
    if [ ! -f scaled_${FILEN}.nii.gz ]; then
      TR=('fslinfo ${FILEO} |grep pixdim4')
      #echo "TR is: ${TR[1]}"

      ## Bandpass
      LOWF='echo "scale=3;1/(2*${BLSIG[$j]}*${TR[1]})"|bc -l'
      HIGHF='echo "scale=3;1/(2*${BHSIG[$j]}*${TR[1]})"|bc -l'
      echo "Applying bandpass filter (${LOWF} - ${HIGHF} sigma) on time series (TR
    =${TR[1]})
       of $SUB..."
      fslmaths ${FILEO} -bptf ${LOWF} ${HIGHF} ${FILEN} -odt float
```

Here, we use `fslmaths` to bandpass the fMRI data. First, however, we convert the low and high frequency range from Hertz to sigma, as needed by `fslmaths`. Since Bash numeric operations are limited to integer arithmetic, we call `bc` to do the necessary math.

```
  ## scale time series
      echo "Scaling time series of $SUB..."
      fslmaths ${FILEN} -Tmean -abs -bin mask
      fslmaths ${FILEN} -Tmean mn_${FILEN}_tmp
      fslmaths ${FILEN} -Tstd std_${FILEN}_tmp
      fslmaths ${FILEN} -sub mn_${FILEN}_tmp -div std_${FILEN}_tmp -add 100 -mul
    mask
       scaled_${FILEN}
      rm *${FILEN}_tmp*
    else
      echo "--Skipping bandpass and scaling--  Result exists!"
    fi

    ## Transform mask to MNI 2mm space
    if [ ! -f Shen2bold_masked.nii.gz ]; then
      echo "Transforming Shen atlas to BOLD ${i} space and masking..."
      if [ ! -f ${REG_PATH}/standard2example_func_warp.nii.gz ]; then
        echo "Generating inverse warp for $SUB session $i..."
        invwarp --ref=${REG_PATH}/example_func --out=${REG_PATH}/
    standard2example_func_warp
        --warp=${REG_PATH}/example_func2standard_warp
      fi
      applywarp --ref=scaled_${FILEN} --in=${ATLAS_PATH}/Shen_fconn_atlas_150_2mm
      --out=Shen2bold --warp=${REG_PATH}/standard2example_func_warp --interp=nn
      fslmaths Shen2bold -mas mask Shen2bold_masked -odt input
    else
      echo "--Skipping Transformation and atlas masking--  Result exists!"
fi

    ##extract time series
    if [ ! -f scaled_${FILEN}_Shen_ts.txt ]; then
      echo "Extracting residuals to Shen atlas ROIs for SUB $SUB..."
  fslmeants -i scaled_${FILEN} -o scaled_${FILEN}_Shen_ts.txt --label=
    Shen2bold_masked.nii.gz
    else
      echo "--Skipping Time Series Extraction-- Result exists!"
    fi
```

The multiple calls to `fslmaths` here is to scale the bandpass filtered data and add a constant value to the data within the brain mask. This step is essential if we want to run the correlation analysis using FSL again. Next, we transform the ROI (in this case, a 150 parcel functional connectivity defined regions based on [16]) from standard MNI space into the BOLD space, and then extract the time-series from the BOLD using the transformed ROI.

```
    ## Remove intermediate files
    if [ -f ${NUI_PATH}/stats/${FILEN}.nii.gz ];then rm ${NUI_PATH}/stats/${FILEN
    }.nii.gz; fi
    #if [ -f scaled_${FILEN}.nii.gz ];then rm scaled_${FILEN}.nii.gz; fi

    ## copy results to outgoing folder
    if [ ! -e ${OUT_PATH}/${BNAME[$j]} ]; then mkdir -p ${OUT_PATH}/${BNAME[$j]};
    fi
    if [ ! -f ${OUT_PATH}/${BNAME[$j]}/${SUB}_${i}.txt ] ; then
      echo "Copying results to outgoing folder for SUB $SUB..."
      cp scaled_${FILEN}_Shen_ts.txt ${OUT_PATH}/${BNAME[$j]}/${SUB}_${i}.txt
    else
      echo "--Skipping copy--  Result exists!"
    fi

    #read -p "Press enter to continue.."

   done #NUI loop
  done  #subject loop
done  #frequency band loop
###END of Script
END_TIME=$SECONDS
DIFF=$[${END_TIME}-${START_TIME}]
echo "Time taken: $[$DIFF / 3600] hours $[($DIFF % 3600) / 60] minutes $[$DIFF %
    60] seconds"
```

Finally, we copy the results to a folder, ready for functional connectivity analysis.

### 3.3.7 PET Preprocessing Steps

While the PET data processing steps are straightforward, conversion from either DICOM or ECAT format to BIDS compliant NIfTI format is complicated by the fact that many values needed for analysis are not stored in either DICOM or ECAT format. In the following example, we use `dcm2niix4pet` to populate the missing data fields, before running the PET analysis.

```
###===Header omitted for space===###

DOC_PATH=/home/syeh/Documents/PET
#DOC_PATH=~/data/fMRI

BIDS_PATH=${DOC_PATH}/BIDS_files_2023
PET_DICOM_PATH=${DOC_PATH}/DICOM
APPIAN_RPRT=${DOC_PATH}/appian_report_2023
if [ ! -d ${BIDS_PATH} ]; then mkdir ${BIDS_PATH};fi
if [ ! -d ${APPIAN_RPRT} ]; then mkdir ${APPIAN_RPRT};fi
if [ ! -e ${BIDS_PATH}/dataset_description.json ]; then echo -e '{\n\t"Name":
"2023 PET data",\n\t"BIDSVersion": "1.8.0",\n\t"Authors": ["Hsiang J. Yeh",""]\n}'
    >
${BIDS_PATH}/dataset_description.json;fi

cd ${DOC_PATH}

for SUB in ${SUBJECTS[@]}; do
  ## Go to working directory and run script there
  DATA_PATH=${DOC_PATH}/${SUB}/nifti

  cd ${DATA_PATH}
  echo "Working on $SUB..."
  SPGR=`"ls" *_Crop_1.nii.gz`
  if [ ! -d ${BIDS_PATH}/sub-${SUB} ]; then
```

```
    echo "Copying MRI data to BIDS folder..."
    mkdir -p ${BIDS_PATH}/sub-${SUB}
    mkdir ${BIDS_PATH}/sub-${SUB}/anat
    cp ${DATA_PATH}/${SPGR} ${BIDS_PATH}/sub-${SUB}/anat/sub-${SUB}_T1w.nii.gz
 cp ${DATA_PATH}/${SPGR%_Crop_1.nii.gz}.json ${BIDS_PATH}/sub-${SUB}/anat/sub-${
    SUB}_T1w.json
  fi
```

Because our anatomical MRI file can be converted via `dcm2niix` normally, we use that result and put it into BIDS compliant format. Next, we fill in the values missing from the DICOM files into the metadata spreadsheet.

```
  ## Run dcm2niix4pet using subject specific metadata file if found
  if [ -e ${PET_DICOM_PATH}/${SUB}/subject_metadata.xlsx ]; then
    dcm2niix4pet ${PET_DICOM_PATH}/${SUB}/ -d ${BIDS_PATH}/sub-${SUB}/pet -m
    ${PET_DICOM_PATH}/${SUB}/subject_metadata.xlsx
  else
    dcm2niix4pet ${PET_DICOM_PATH}/${SUB}/ -d ${BIDS_PATH}/sub-${SUB}/pet -m
    ${PET_DICOM_PATH}/scanner_metadata.xlsx
  fi

done

cd ${DOC_PATH}
if [ ! -e ${APPIAN_RPRT}/input_file_report.csfv ]; then
  read -p "Press enter to run APPIAN on copied files..."
  docker run --rm -it -v ${BIDS_PATH}:/data:ro -v ${APPIAN_RPRT}:/out tffunck/
    appian:latest
  bash -c "python3 /opt/APPIAN/Launcher.py -s /data -t /out"
fi
###END of Script
END_TIME=$SECONDS
DIFF=$[${END_TIME}-${START_TIME}]
echo "Time taken: $[$DIFF / 3600 ] hours $[($DIFF % 3600) / 60] minutes $[$DIFF %
    60] seconds"
```

We create a subject specific metadata file if there are specific differences, such as TimeZero or FrameTimesStart. Otherwise, we use a scanner specific metadata file. Assuming all the fields are properly converted and entered into the respective JSON files, we then run APPIAN through docker. APPIAN is a fully automated PET analysis pipeline [5]. Once called with a valid BIDS dataset, APPIAN will attempt to automatically co-register the MRI and PET images, then transform them into stereotaxic space. From there, it will apply the default ROI, perform a partial-volume effects correction, and quantification, if the proper arterial sampling data is supplied. It will then generate a report at the directory specified.

## 3.4 Summary

In this chapter, we provide practical recommendations for recording quality neuroimaging data for epilepsy research and an example preprocessing pipeline to analyze such data using custom Bash scripts. We cover best practices for scanning, with the goal of obtaining scans with the best quality signals and avoiding artifacts, as well as a brief treatment of MRI physics, scanner upkeep, communication with the radiology team, and scanner software settings for MRI. We provide an example preprocessing pipeline using Bash scripting to automate the process. A brief overview of Bash scripting is presented, followed by examples of scripts for conversion from DICOM to NifTI, organizing into BIDS data structure and evaluate data quality using MRIQC, ICA denoising using FIX and MELODIC, nuisance regression using FEAT, frequency filtering and time-series extraction, and PET image processing.

## Bibliography

[1] Sherief Abdulla and Chris Clarke. *FRCR Physics Notes.* Radiology Cafe Publishing, January 1 2020.

[2] Rasmus M. Birn. The role of physiological noise in resting-state functional connectivity. *NeuroImage*, 62(2):864–870, August 2012.

[3] Catie Chang, James P. Cunningham, and Gary H. Glover. Influence of heart rate on the BOLD signal: The cardiac response function. *NeuroImage*, 44(3):857–869, February 2009.

[4] Rolf Deichmann, Jan Gottfried, Chloe Hutton, and Robert Turner. Optimized EPI for fMRI studies of the orbitofrontal cortex. *NeuroImage*, 19(2):430–441, June 2003.

[5] Thomas Funck, Kevin Larcher, Pierrick J. Toussaint, Alan C. Evans, and Andreas Thiel. APPIAN: Automated Pipeline for PET Image Analysis. *Frontiers in Neuroinformatics*, 12, September 26 2018.

[6] Maria Luisa Gorno-Tempini, Chloe Hutton, Oliver Josephs, Rolf Deichmann, Cathy Price, and Robert Turner. Echo time dependence of BOLD contrast and susceptibility artifacts. *NeuroImage*, 15(1):136–142, January 2002.

[7] Peter Jezzard and Robert S. Balaban. Correction for geometric distortion in echo planar images from B0 field variations. *Magnetic Resonance in Medicine*, 34(1):65–73, July 1995.

[8] Michael L. Lipton. *Totally Accessible MRI.* Springer Science & Business Media, April 28 2010.

[9] Donald W. McRobbie, Elizabeth A. Moore, Martin J. Graves, and Martin R. Prince. *MRI from Picture to Proton.* Cambridge University Press, April 28 2017.

[10] Sebastian Olbrich, Christoph Mulert, Susanne Karch, Maria Trenner, Gregor Leicht, Oliver Pogarell, and Ulrich Hegerl. EEG-vigilance and BOLD effect during simultaneous EEG/fMRI measurement. *NeuroImage*, 45(2):319–332, April 2009.

[11] John D. Port and Martin G. Pomper. Quantification and Minimization of Magnetic Susceptibility Artifacts on GRE Images. *Journal of Computer Assisted Tomography*, 24(6):958–964, November 2000.

[12] Afraim Salek-Haddadi, Martin Merschhemke, Louis Lemieux, and David R. Fish. Simultaneous EEG-correlated ictal fMRI. *NeuroImage*, 16(1):32–40, May 2002.

[13] Gholamreza Salimi-Khorshidi, Gwenaëlle Douaud, Christian F. Beckmann, Matthew F. Glasser, Ludovica Griffanti, and Stephen M. Smith. Automatic denoising of functional MRI data: Combining independent component analysis and hierarchical fusion of classifiers. *NeuroImage*, 90:449–468, April 2014.

[14] John F. Schenck. The role of magnetic susceptibility in magnetic resonance imaging: MRI magnetic compatibility of the first and second kinds. *Medical Physics*, 23(6):815–850, June 1996.

[15] Yuranga Weerakkody, Ian Bickle, Mustafa Jafar, et al. MRI artifacts. Radiology Reference Article, Radiopaedia.org, November 9 2022. Accessed on January 30, 2023.

[16] Xilin Shen, Fuyuze Tokoglu, Xenophon Papademetris, R. Todd Constable. Groupwise whole-brain parcellation from resting-state fMRI data for network node identification. *Neuroimage*, 82:403–415, 2013.

# 4

# *Hypothesis Testing and Correction for Multiple Testing*

**Doug Speed**

*Center for Quantitative Genetics and Genomics, Aarhus University (Denmark)*

## CONTENTS



DOI: 10.1201/9781003254515-4

This chapter describes how to perform hypothesis testing. We begin with the statistical details of hypothesis testing, explaining how to create hypotheses, and assess their validity using a statistical test. Next, we explain correction for multiple testing, which is important to consider when performing an analysis that contains more than one test. Finally, we consider the use of hypothesis testing within a genome-wide association study (GWAS), which is a tool for investigating how genetic variants influence a heritable trait such as epilepsy. Examples for implementing hypothesis testing are demonstrated in R.

## 4.1 Hypothesis Testing

Suppose we wish to test whether a coin is fair, meaning that when it is tossed, it is equally likely to land heads or tails. We could toss the coin 100 times and record the total number of heads. If the total number is 50 (i.e., it landed heads exactly half the time), we would have no reason to suspect the coin is biased. Conversely, if the total is 100 (i.e., it always landed heads), we would certainly decide the coin is biased.

However, what do we conclude if the total number of heads is 58? This value is higher than 50, the expected number if the coin is fair, and therefore suggests that heads is more likely than tails. However, is 58 heads sufficient evidence to conclude the coin is biased? To answer this question, we must perform a hypothesis test, in order to statistically assess whether the data (in this case, the number of times the coin lands heads) are plausible under the null hypothesis (that the coin is fair).

This section begins by describing the key steps when performing hypothesis testing, then explains some special considerations.

### 4.1.1 Identify Parameters

First we must identify the parameters in whose values we are interested. If we are trying to decide whether a coin is fair, there is only one parameter, the probability that the coin lands heads. We can denote this probability using the variable $p_H$; if the coin is fair, then $p_H = 0.5$. Note that our choice to consider heads is arbitrary; it is equally valid to instead focus on the probability that the coin lands tails.

### 4.1.2 Decide Hypotheses

Having identified the parameters, we can construct the null and alternative hypotheses (denoted $H_0$ and $H_1$, respectively). The null hypothesis is the focal point of the analysis (i.e., the scenario whose validity we wish to assess), while the alternative hypothesis is the complement of the null hypothesis (i.e., contains all possible scenarios not covered by the null hypothesis).

For the coin example, the null hypothesis is $H_0 : p_H = 0.5$ (i.e., the coin is fair), while the alternative hypothesis is $H_1 : p_H \neq 0.5$ (i.e., the coin is not fair). Note that we will be performing a "two-sided" hypothesis test, because the alternative hypothesis includes both $p_H < 0.5$ and $p_H > 0.5$ (i.e., considers both scenarios where the coin is downwards and upwards biased). The alternative is to perform a "one-sided" test, for example, using the hypotheses $H_0 : p_H \leq 0.5$ and $H_1 : p_H > 0.5$.

### 4.1.3 Construct a Likelihood

We next assess how well the observed data align with the null hypothesis. Loosely speaking, if it seems reasonable that the data could have been generated under the null hypothesis, then the null hypothesis is accepted. By contrast, if it is unlikely that the data could have been generated under the null hypothesis, then the null hypothesis is rejected.

Formally, we must construct the likelihood of the observed data given values for the parameters. The likelihood is easiest to understand when the observed data come from a discrete distribution, as then it equals the probability of the observed data as a function of the model parameters. When the data come from an continuous distribution, the likelihood is instead a "density" (discussed later).

For the coin example, we observe $n_H$, the total number of heads. Note that $n_H$ is discrete, because there are a finite number of possible values ($n_H$ must be an integer between 0 and 100). As explained above, the only parameter is $p_H$, the probability that the coin lands heads. Therefore the likelihood is the probability of observing $n_H$ given $p_H$. Statistical theory tells us that when we toss a coin $n$ times, the number of heads follows a binomial distribution, whose likelihood function is

$$L(p_H|n_H) = \frac{n!}{n_H!(n-n_H)!} \times {p_H}^{n_H} \times (1-p_H)^{n-n_H} \tag{4.1}$$

where $a!$ denotes the "factorial of $a$," and equals $a \times (a-1) \times \ldots \times 2 \times 1$ (for example, $3! = 3 \times 2 \times 1 = 6$). Note that we write $L(p_H|n_H)$ instead of $L(n_H|p_H)$, because it is conventional to consider the likelihood a function of the parameters, given the data (even though we compute it by considering the probability of the data, given the parameters).

Fully understanding the derivation of Eq. 4.1 is complicated (it requires us to consider how many different sequences of $n$ coin tosses result in $n_H$ heads). However, we can easily check that the formula seems sensible. For example, suppose we had tossed the coin only twice (instead of 100 times). In this case, there would be four possible sequences, head-then-head, head-then-tail, tail-then-head and tail-then-tail, which correspond to observing a total of two, one, one and zero heads, respectively. If the coin is fair, then the four possible sequences are equally likely, and thus each has a 25% chance of occurring. Therefore, the probabilities of observing $n_H = 0$, $n_H = 1$, and $n_H = 2$ are 0.25, 0.5, and 0.25, respectively. We see that these three probabilities match those given by Eq. 4.1 if we set $n = 2$ and $p_H = 0.5$, then evaluate $L(p_H|n_H)$ for $n_H$ equal to 0, 1 and 2.

Figure 4.1 plots the likelihood function for a binomial distribution with $n = 100$ and $p_H = 0.5$. We see that the most likely value for $n_H$ is 50, yet the probability of this is relatively low (0.080). This means that if the coin is fair, there is only an 8% chance that exactly 50 of the tosses will land heads. And in fact, this probability is only slightly higher than the chances of observing 49 or 51 heads (both 0.079).

### 4.1.4 Compute a $p$-value

Suppose that 58 of the 100 tosses were heads ($n_H = 58$). If the null hypothesis is true, the probability of observing 58 heads is 0.022 (this value comes from setting $n = 100$, $p_H = 0.5$ and $n_H = 58$ in Eq. 4.1). This sounds very small, so we might be tempted to automatically reject the null hypothesis and conclude that the coin is biased. However, this would be ignoring the fact that all outcomes are individually unlikely (as mentioned above, the most likely outcome, $n_H = 50$, has probability only 0.080). Instead, we must compute a $p$-value, which corresponds to the probability of observing an outcome at least as extreme as the outcome we observed if the null hypothesis is true.

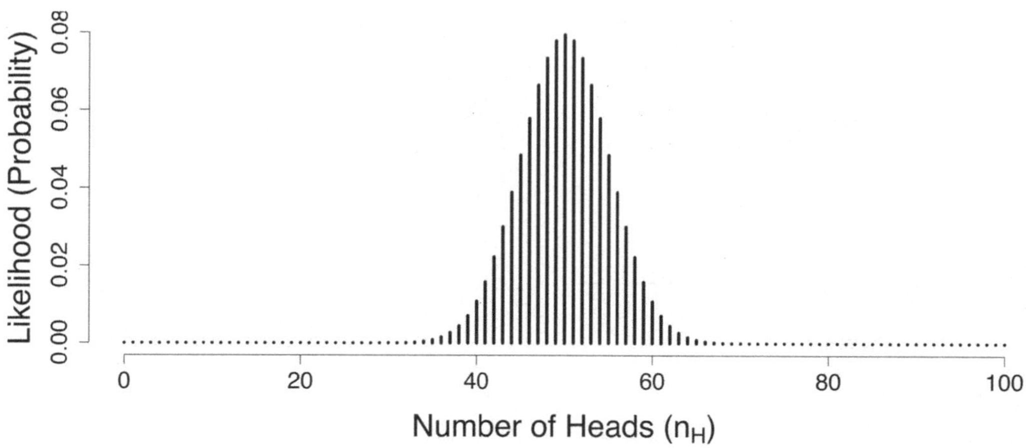


**FIGURE 4.1**
When tossing a coin $n$ times, the total number of heads $n_H$ follows a binomial distribution with parameters $n$ and $p_H$, where $p_H$ is the chance each toss is heads. This figure shows the likelihood function for a binomial distribution with $n = 100$ and $p_H = 0.5$. There are 101 vertical bars, reflecting that $n_H$ must be an integer between 0 and 100, whose heights mark the probabilities of the possible observations.

The $p$-value corresponding to observing $n_H = 58$ is $2\mathbb{P}(n_H \geq 58|p_H = 0.5)$, twice the probability of observing 58 or more heads if the null hypothesis is true. We can calculate $\mathbb{P}(n_H \geq 58|p_H = 0.5)$ using Eq. 4.1 (specifically, we first use the equation to calculate the probabilities $\mathbb{P}(n_H = 58)$, $\mathbb{P}(n_H = 59)$, ..., $\mathbb{P}(n_H = 99)$, $\mathbb{P}(n_H = 100)$, then we compute their sum). We obtain that $\mathbb{P}(n_H \geq 58|p_H = 0.5) = 0.067$, and thus the $p$-value corresponding to observing $n_H = 58$ is $2 \times 0.067 = 0.133$.

The reason we calculate $2 \times \mathbb{P}(n_H \geq 58)$ is to appreciate that when performing a two-sided hypothesis test, both high and low values of $n_H$ are extreme and give us reason to reject the null hypothesis. It is evident from Figure 4.1 that, under the null hypothesis, the distribution of $n_H$ is symmetrical about the expected value ($n_H = 50$). It therefore follows that $\mathbb{P}(n_H \geq 58) = \mathbb{P}(n_H \leq 42)$, and thus the $p$-value can be interpreted as the probability that the total number of heads is eight or more away from the expected value (if the null hypothesis is true). Note that the symmetry also ensures that $p$-value corresponding to observing $n_H = 58$ is the same as that corresponding to observing $n_H = 42$.

If we instead perform a one-sided hypothesis test, there are two things to consider. Firstly, we no longer multiply by two when computing the $p$-value. Secondly, the extreme observations are only those within the "tail opposite the null hypothesis." To illustrate these two points, suppose that we are performing a one-sided test using the hypotheses $H_0 : p_H \leq 0.5$ and $H_1 : p_H > 0.5$. Now only high values of $n_H$ are considered extreme (whereas for the two-sided test, both low and high values of $n_H$ were considered extreme). The $p$-value corresponding to observing $n_H = 58$ is now $\mathbb{P}(n_H \geq 58|p_H = 0.5) = 0.067$ (whereas for the two-sided test, it was twice this value). Meanwhile, the $p$-value corresponding to $n_H = 42$ is now $\mathbb{P}(n_H \geq 42|p_H = 0.5) = 0.956$. Note that we continue to calculate the probabilities assuming $p_H = 0.5$, because this is the value that results in the highest $p$-values (of those consistent with the null hypothesis).

Figure 4.2 plots the $p$-values corresponding to all possible values of $n_H$, when performing either a two-sided test (using the hypotheses $H_0 : p_H = 0.5$ and $H_1 : p_H \neq 0.5$) or a one-sided test (using the hypotheses $H_0 : p_H \leq 0.5$ and $H_1 : p_H > 0.5$).

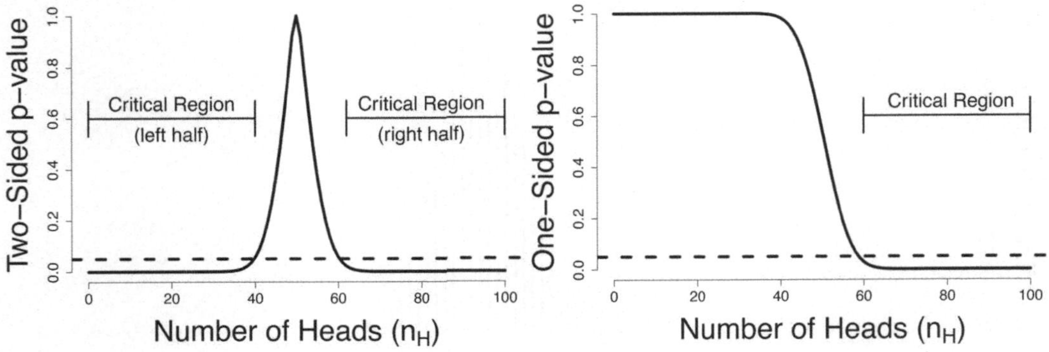


**FIGURE 4.2**
This figure shows $p$-values for the coin example. (Left panel) $p$-values for a two-sided test (using the hypotheses $H_0 : p_H = 0.5$ and $H_1 : p_H \neq 0.5$). (Right panel) $p$-values for a one-sided test (using the hypotheses $H_0 : p_H \leq 0.5$ and $H_1 : p_H > 0.5$). The segments mark the critical regions when using the significance threshold $\alpha = 0.05$ (note that for the two-sided test, the critical region has two parts).

### 4.1.5 Decide Whether to Reject the Null Hypothesis

We will reject the null hypothesis if the $p$-value is sufficiently small that we consider the outcome unlikely to have occurred were the null hypothesis true. To make this decision, we must set $\alpha$, the significance threshold; we will then reject the null distribution if the $p$-value is below $\alpha$. In medical science, the most common significance threshold is $\alpha = 0.05$; i.e., we consider an event unlikely if the chance of observing the event or something more extreme is less than 5%. Note that if performing multiple tests, we should use a lower threshold, as explained in the next section.

For the coin example, we observed $n_H = 58$, for which the corresponding $p$-value was 0.133. This $p$-value is above $\alpha = 0.05$, so we conclude that there is insufficient evidence to reject the null hypothesis. Note that it would be tempting to instead conclude that the null hypothesis is true, but this terminology is not correct. This is because being unable to prove a hypothesis is false is different to proving the hypothesis is true. To demonstrate this point, suppose we used the same data but instead tested the hypotheses $H_0 : p_H = 0.52$ and $H_1 : p_H \neq 0.52$. With these new hypotheses, the $p$-value corresponding to $n_H = 58$ equals 0.271, which is again above $\alpha = 0.05$. We would clearly end up with a contradiction if each analysis declared that the corresponding null hypothesis was true (i.e., the first analysis would declare that $p_H = 0.5$, while the second analysis would declare that $p_H = 0.52$).

### 4.1.6 Positives and Negatives

If we decide to reject the null hypothesis, our finding is "positive," while if we instead decide not to reject the null hypothesis, our finding is "negative." A positive finding can be either a "true positive," if it is the correct conclusion, or a "false positive," if it is incorrect. Similarly, a negative finding can be either a "true negative" or a "false negative." Table 4.1 illustrates these options for the coin example.

### 4.1.7 Critical Regions

Given a significance threshold, the critical region is the set of observations that lead to rejection of the null hypothesis. Figure 4.2 shows critical regions for the coin example, when the significance threshold is $\alpha = 0.05$. We see that when performing a two-sided

**TABLE 4.1**
Possible outcomes when performing a hypothesis test to determine if a coin is fair.

| | Negative Finding (Do Not Reject $H_0$) | Positive Finding (Reject $H_0$) |
|---|---|---|
| Coin is Fair | True Negative | False Positive |
| Coin is Biased | False Negative | True Positive |

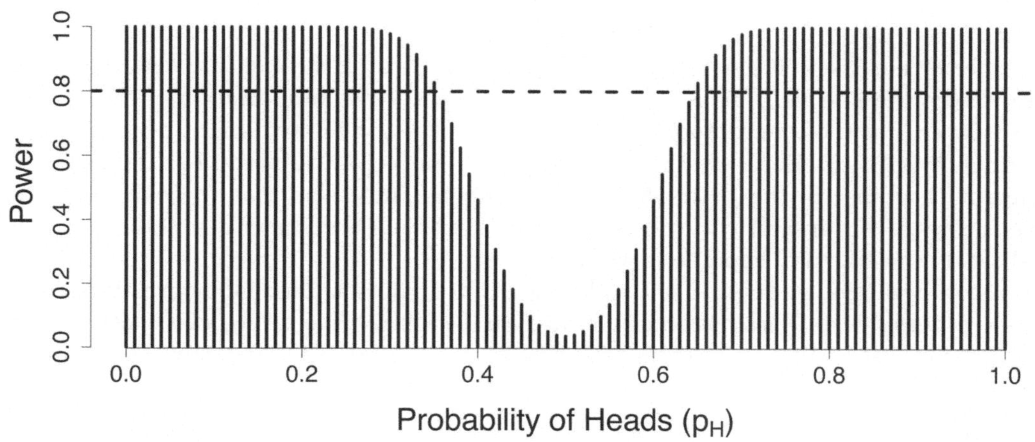


**FIGURE 4.3**
The power of a hypothesis test is the probability of rejecting the null hypothesis if the alternative hypothesis is true. This figure shows how, for the coin example, the power depends on $p_H$, the probability that the coin lands heads (values correspond to using the hypotheses $H_0 : p_H = 0.5$ and $H_1 : p_H \neq 0.5$, and the significance threshold $\alpha = 0.05$). The horizontal line marks 80% power.

test (using the hypotheses $H_0 : p_H = 0.5$ and $H_1 : p_H \neq 0.5$), the critical region is the set $\{0, 1, \ldots, 38, 39, 61, 62, \ldots, 99, 100\}$ (i.e., $n_H \leq 39$ or $n_H \geq 61$). Meanwhile, when performing a one-sided test (using the hypotheses $H_0 : p_H \leq 0.5$ and $H_1 : p_H > 0.5$), the critical region is the set $\{59, 60, \ldots, 99, 100\}$ (i.e., $n_H \geq 59$).

### 4.1.8 Power

The power of a hypothesis test (for a given significance threshold $\alpha$) is the probability of rejecting the null hypothesis when the alternative hypothesis is true. Prior to performing an experiment, it is good practice to estimate the power. Typically, this involves picking a selection of values for the parameters, and for each value computing the probability that we reject the null hypothesis (i.e., that the observed data will lie within the critical region).

For the coin example, we might first consider what would happen if the true value of $p_H$ is 0.6. When performing a two-sided test using the significance threshold $\alpha = 0.05$, we reject the null hypothesis if $n_H \leq 39$ or $n_H \geq 61$. Therefore, the power of the test will be $\mathbb{P}(n_H \leq 39 | p_H = 0.6) + \mathbb{P}(n_H \geq 61 | p_H = 0.6) = 0.462$. We thus know that if $p_H = 0.6$, there is a 46% chance that our hypothesis test will correctly reject the null hypothesis. We could then repeat the calculations for $p_H$ equal to 0.7, 0.8, and 0.9.

Figure 4.3 reports estimates of power for various values of $p_H$. A hypothesis test is generally considered to be well-powered if its power is 80% or higher. We see that for the current experiment (where we toss a coin 100 times), we have at least 80% power provided the true value of $p_H$ is below 0.35 or above 0.65. The advantage of performing the power analysis prior to the experiment is that if the power estimates are unsatisfactory (i.e., lower than we desire), we can adjust the experimental design. For example, if we consider a 46% chance of rejecting the null hypothesis when $p_H = 0.6$ too low, then we can decide to increase the number of tosses.

### 4.1.9 Reporting Results

When reporting results from a hypothesis test, the main focus is the overall conclusion (i.e., whether or not the null hypothesis is rejected). However, the test should, as a minimum, also report the *p*-value. This is because the *p*-value provides an indication of the strength of evidence. For the coin example, both $n_H = 51$ and $n_H = 58$ would lead us to not reject the null hypothesis. However, the corresponding *p*-values (0.920 and 0.133, respectively), make it clear that in the latter case, there was some indication that the null hypothesis was incorrect (but insufficient evidence to reject), while in the former case, there was little indication that the null hypothesis was false.

As well as the *p*-value, it is good practice to report additional information about the hypothesis test. These can include an explanation for the choice of hypotheses, the assumptions used when constructing the likelihood, or details of any power calculations.

### 4.1.10 Continuous Data

Consider a new experiment, where instead of tossing a coin, we measure how long we must wait for a bus to arrive. Suppose we measure the waiting time for the bus 100 days in a row, and let $W$ denote the total waiting time (in minutes). The bus company has advertised that the average time to wait for a bus is ten minutes. We wish to use our observed data ($W$) to test whether the company's claim is accurate.

To perform the hypothesis test, we follow the same steps outlined above. Therefore, we begin by identifying the parameters and deciding the null and alternative hypotheses. Here, the parameter of interest is the mean time to wait for a bus, which we denote $w$, while we choose the hypotheses $H_0 : w = 10$ and $H_1 : w \neq 10$.

The next step is to construct the likelihood. This requires us to assume a distribution for the waiting time for each bus. Let's suppose this is exponential distributed with mean $w$. Statistical theory then tells us that the total waiting time is gamma distributed with shape parameter 100 and scale parameter $w$. Figure 4.4 illustrates the exponential and gamma distributions.

The gamma distribution can produce an infinite number of different values and is therefore an example of a continuous distribution. The chance of any specific value is infinitesimally small, and so it is no longer meaningful to compute the probability of the observed data. For this reason, the likelihood function reports the "density" of different values (whereas for discrete distributions, the likelihood reports probabilities). Loosely speaking, the density of a value is like a probability, in that it is non-negative and higher densities indicate (regions of) more probable values. More formally, the density is a function such that the probability of the observed data being between two values equals the area under the density function between those two values. For example, Figure 4.4 shows that for a gamma distribution with shape parameter 100 and scale parameter 10, there is a 38% chance that the observed value is between 950 and 1050.

The likelihood function of a gamma distribution with shape parameter 100 and scale parameter $w$ is

$$L(w|W) = \frac{W^{99} \exp\left(-W/w\right)}{\Gamma(100)\, w^{100}}$$

where $\Gamma(x)$ is the gamma function (too complicated to explain here).

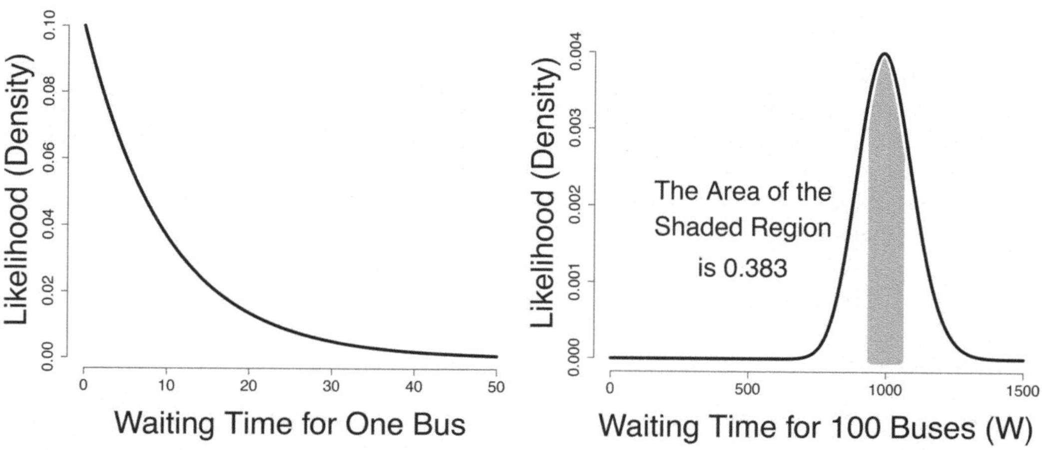


**FIGURE 4.4**
(Left panel) Likelihood function for an exponential distribution with mean 10. (Right panel) Likelihood function for a gamma distribution with shape parameter 100 and scale parameter 10 (which is the distribution obtained by summing 100 draws from an exponential distribution with mean 10). The area of the shaded region is the probability that a draw from a gamma distribution (with shape parameter 100 and scale parameter 10) is between 950 and 1050.

Suppose that the total waiting time is 803 minutes, and we wish to compute the corresponding $p$-value. We are performing a two-sided test (because the alternative hypothesis includes both $w < 10$ and $w > 10$), and so we must identify in which side of the distribution the observed data lie. Under the null hypothesis, the expected value of $W$ is 1000 (this is because, under the null hypothesis, the expected waiting time for each bus is 10, so the expected sum of 100 waiting times is 1000). Therefore, the observed data lie on the "left side," and so the $p$-value is $2\mathbb{P}(W \leq 803|w = 10)$, twice the probability of observing a value less than or equal to 803 when $w = 10$. By integrating the likelihood function between 0 and 803, we find that $\mathbb{P}(W \leq 803|w = 10) = 0.019$, and thus the $p$-value corresponding to observing $W = 803$ is 0.037.

The $p$-value from the two-sided test is below the significance threshold $\alpha = 0.05$, and therefore, we decide to reject the null hypothesis (i.e., we conclude that the waiting time advertised by the bus company is incorrect). Note that if we are only concerned whether the waiting is longer than advertised, it would be more appropriate to perform a one-sided test, using the hypotheses $H_0 : w \leq 10$ and $H_1 : w > 10$. In this case, the $p$-value corresponding to $W = 803$ would be $\mathbb{P}(W \geq 803|w = 10) = 0.981$, because extreme values are those in the right tail (the tail opposite the null hypothesis), and we would not reject the null hypothesis.

As explained above, when reporting the results, we should not only state the conclusion (i.e., sufficient or insufficient evidence to reject the null hypothesis), but additional details such as the $p$-value and the number of observations. It would also be good to mention the assumption that the waiting time for each individual bus was exponentially distributed (if we doubted the validity of this assumption, we could repeat the analysis using different distributions, or perform a follow-up analysis to assess whether the exponential assumption is justified).

### 4.1.11 Likelihood Ratio Testing

A likelihood ratio hypothesis test compares $L_0$ and $L_1$, the maximum likelihoods under the null and alternative hypotheses, respectively. The test will reject the null hypothesis if the likelihood ratio $L_1/L_0$ is significantly above one (i.e., if the alternative hypothesis results in significantly better model fit than the null hypothesis). A likelihood ratio test requires that the null hypothesis is "nested" within the alternative hypothesis. This means that the null hypothesis must be a special case of the alternative hypothesis, obtained by constraining parameters of the alternative hypothesis, and ensures that $L_1/L_0 \geq 1$.

The steps for performing a likelihood ratio test match those described above, except when computing the $p$-value. For this step, it is necessary to compute $L_1/L_0$, then a $p$-value corresponding to $\lambda = 2\log(L_1/L_0)$ (because $\lambda$ is a monotonic function of $L_1/L_0$, the $p$-value for $\lambda$ matches the $p$-value for $L_1/L_0$). The reason we compute $\lambda$ is because this has a known distribution under the null hypothesis. Specifically, when performing a two-sided null test, $\lambda$ has a chi-square distribution with $d$ degrees of freedom, where $d$ is the number of fixed parameters. Meanwhile, when performing a one-sided test, $\lambda$ has a mixture distribution; with probability half, $\lambda$ is chi-square distributed with $d$ degrees of freedom, otherwise it equals zero.

To perform a likelihood ratio test for the coin example, we might choose the hypotheses $H_0 : p_H = 0.5$ and $H_1 : p_H \in [0, 1]$. Note that the alternative hypothesis is slightly different to that used previously, because it allows $p_H$ takes any value (whereas before the alternative hypothesis allowed for any value except 0.5). This change ensures the null hypothesis is nested within the alternative hypothesis. As a reminder, the likelihood of the observed data is given by setting $n_H = 58$ and $n = 100$ in Eq. 4.1.

It is straightforward to calculate the maximum likelihood under the null hypothesis, because under the null hypothesis, $p_H$ must equal 0.5. Therefore, we obtain

$$L_0 = \frac{100!}{58! \times 42!} \times 0.5^{58} \times 0.5^{42}$$

Figure 4.5 shows that, under the alternative hypothesis, the likelihood is maximized when $p_H = 0.58$ (this can be shown formally using calculus). Therefore, we obtain

$$L_1 = \frac{100!}{58! \times 42!} \times 0.58^{58} \times 0.42^{42}$$

Next we compute the likelihood ratio

$$\frac{L_1}{L_0} = \left(\frac{0.58}{0.5}\right)^{58} \left(\frac{0.42}{0.5}\right)^{42} = 3.62$$

Loosely speaking, this ratio indicates that we are 3.62 times more likely to observe the data under the alternative hypothesis than under the null hypothesis.

We are performing a two-sided test, and so the distribution of $\lambda = 2\log(L_1/L_0)$ under the null hypothesis is chi-squared with one degree of freedom. The observed value of $\lambda$ is $2\log(3.62) = 2.57$, and so the corresponding $p$-value is 0.109 (this is the probability that a draw from a chi-squared distribution with one degree of freedom is greater or equal to 2.57). Therefore, if we continue to use the significance threshold $\alpha = 0.05$, we conclude that there is insufficient evidence to reject the null hypothesis. Note that if we had instead observed $n_H = 42$, we would obtain the same observed value of $\lambda$, and therefore the same $p$-value.

Suppose we instead perform a one-sided test using the hypotheses $H_0 : p_H \leq 0.5$ and $H_1 : p_H \in [0, 1]$. Now the distribution of $\lambda$ under the null hypothesis is either chi-squared with one degree of freedom or fixed to zero (with each possibility equally likely). When

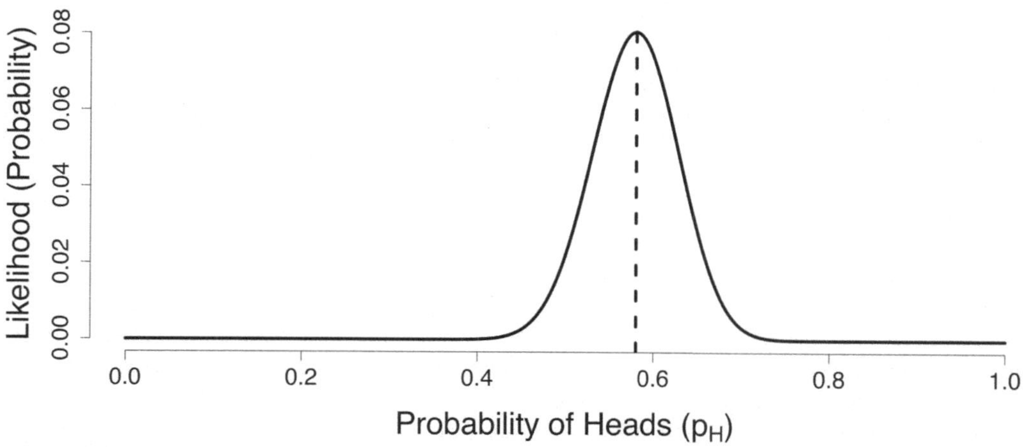


**FIGURE 4.5**
Suppose that we toss a coin 100 times and observe 58 heads. This figure shows how the likelihood depends on $p_H$, the probability that each toss is heads. We see that the likelihood is maximized when $p_H = 0.58$.

$n_H = 58$, the observed value of $\lambda$ remains 2.57, but now the corresponding $p$-value is 0.054 (i.e., half the $p$-value obtained when performing a two-sided test). By contrast, when $n_H = 42$, the observed value of $\lambda$ becomes zero, and the corresponding $p$-value is one. This reflects that when $n_H = 42$, the likelihood is maximized when $p_H = 0.42$, a value consistent with both the null and alternative hypotheses, and therefore $L_0$ and $L_1$ are equal.

### 4.1.12 Permutation Testing

Permutation testing provides a way to compute a $p$-value without specifying a likelihood. The idea is that if we can generate additional observations under the null hypothesis, we can then obtain an empirical $p$-value by comparing how often the additional observations are at least as extreme as the original observation.

For the coin example, we could perform a permutation test by obtaining a fair coin, then repeatedly tossing this 100 times. Suppose we performed $K$ repetitions, and let $n_H^k$ denote the number of heads obtained on the $k$th repetition. The permutation $p$-value is

$$2 \times \frac{1 + \sum_{k=1}^{K} I(n_H^k \geq n_H)}{1 + K},$$

where the indicator function $I(\ldots)$ takes value one if its argument is true, and zero if its argument is false. The fraction is the proportion of times all observations (i.e., both those from permutations and the original observation) are at least as extreme as the original observation. Note that this is the permuted $p$-value corresponding to a two-sided test (using the hypotheses $H_0 : p_H = 0.5$ and $H_1 : p_H \neq 0.5$); if instead we are performing a one-sided test (using the hypotheses $H_0 : p_H \leq 0.5$ and $H_1 : p_H > 0.5$), we do not multiply the fraction by two.

The main advantage of computing a permutation $p$-value is the simplicity. In the example above, it was not necessary to know the distribution of the number of heads obtained when tossing the coin. However, the main disadvantage is the computational burden. In particular, to obtain a precise $p$-value (e.g., accurate to three decimal places), we must perform thousands of permutations.

### 4.1.13 Other Statistical Tests

The likelihood ratio test is a flexible framework for hypothesis testing as its generality accommodates many statistical scenarios for which hypothesis testing may be required. However, it is important to note that there are tens, possibly hundreds of different statistical tests, of which the likelihood ratio test is only one. Most of these tests are designed for specific situations (i.e., types of experiments). However, the basic principle of the tests are the same: they each compute a test statistic, whose distribution under the null hypothesis is known (either exactly or approximately), and can therefore be converted into a $p$-value. Furthermore, if two tests can be applied to the same data, they are usually "asymptotically equivalent," meaning that given sufficient sample size, they will reach the same conclusion (i.e., both reject the null hypothesis, or both find insufficient evidence to reject the null hypothesis). This subsection summarizes some of the most common hypothesis tests.

The *one-sample t-test* is used to test whether the mean of a random variable is significantly different to a specified value. Its test statistic takes the form $t = (\bar{X} - \mu)/s$, where $\bar{X}$ is the mean of the observed data, $\mu$ is the specified value and $s$ is the sample standard deviation. Under the null hypothesis, $t$ is assumed to have a $t$ distribution (the $t$ distribution is symmetric and bell-shaped, similar to the normal distribution). If the null hypothesis is correct (i.e., the mean of the random variable equals $\mu$), then we expect $\bar{X}$ to be close to $\mu$, in which case $t$ will to be close to zero and the corresponding $p$-value will be close to one. By contrast, a large value for $t$ (either large positive or large negative) and therefore a small corresponding $p$-value, arises when $\bar{X}$ is substantially different from $\mu$, and thus provides evidence to reject the null hypothesis. We could have used a one-sample $t$-test above to analyze data from the bus example, in which case $\bar{X} = 8.03$ (the average waiting time of the 100 buses), $\mu = 10$ (the average waiting time advertised by the bus company), and $s$ is an estimate of the variation in bus waiting times (which can be calculated from the individual waiting times of the 100 buses). Note that the $t$-test does not require an assumed distribution for the random variable (e.g., that the bus waiting times are exponentially distribution) and is therefore appropriate to use when we are uncertain of its distribution (conversely, if we were confident of the distribution, we would expect a test that accommodated this information to be more powerful).

The *two-sample t-test* is used to test for differences between the means of two random variables. Now the test statistic takes the form $t' = (\bar{X} - \bar{X}')/s'$, where $\bar{X}$ and $\bar{X}'$ are the observed means of the two random variables, and $s'$ is an estimate of the pooled standard deviation. As with the one-sample $t$-test, values of $t'$ close to zero are consistent with the null hypothesis (that the two random variables have the same mean), while large values for $t'$ provide evidence to reject the null hypothesis. To provide an example, suppose we wished to compare the waiting times of two buses. We could record 100 waiting times for the first bus, and 100 waiting times for the second bus, and use a two-sample $t$-test to test for a difference between the average waiting times of the two buses. Note that there is no requirement to collect the same number of observations for each bus (e.g., we could still use a two-sample $t$-test if we only recorded 50 waiting times for the second bus).

The *paired t-test* matches the one-sample $t$-test except that each observation is the difference between a pair of random variables. For example, suppose each of the 100 waiting times corresponded to a different driver. The bus company subsequently introduces operational changes (e.g., a new training system) and repeats the experiment using the same 100 drivers. They can then test the impact of the operational changes by analyzing the differences in waiting time (with times matched based on drivers). This approach is expected to be more powerful than using a two-sample $t$-test that ignores the pairing of observations, because it controls for driver-specific effects (e.g., if some drivers tend to be late more often than others).

*Analysis of variance (ANOVA)* can be considered a generalized version of the two-sample $t$-test to allow for more than two groups. It is used to test for differences between the average effects of different groups (usually three or more). Its test statistic compares the variance within groups to the variance between groups. If the groupings are informative, then we would expect the between-group variance to be high relative to the within-group variance.

Statistical tests are referred to as "parametric tests" if they make assumptions regarding the distribution of the data. For example, the one-sample $t$-test is a parametric test because it assumes that the mean of the random variable is normally distributed. Ideally, a parametric test should only be used if its distribution assumptions are reasonable. The one-sample $t$-test, for instance, is most appropriate when the random variable is approximately normally distributed (because the mean of a sample of normally distributed random variables will also be normally distributed).

It is often difficult to verify the assumptions of a parametric test. In this case, it may be better to use a "non-parametric test." Perhaps the most simple non-parametric test is the *sign test*, which can be viewed as a non-parametric alternative to the paired $t$-test. Specifically, the sign test records the proportion of times the difference between the pair of random variables is positive (i.e., the value for the first random variable is larger than the second); if the proportion is significantly greater or less than 0.5, this implies consistent differences between the two random variables. The sign test is non-parametric because it does not make assumptions regarding the distributions of the random variables (instead, it relies only on the fact that if the pairs of random variables are similar, their differences are equally likely to be positive and negative).

More advanced non-parametric tests often involve rankings. For example, the *Mann-Whitney-Wilcoxon test* is a non-parametric alternative to the two-sample $t$-test. It starts by replacing observed values by their ranks (i.e., the smallest observed value is replaced by 1, the second smallest is replaced by 2, and so on), then computes a test statistic based on the difference between the average ranks for each random variable. If the two random variables are similar, then we would expect their average ranks to be equal, and thus a large test statistic is evidence to reject the null hypothesis that the two random variables are alike. The *Kruskal Wallis test* generalizes the Mann-Whitney-Wilcoxon test when there are more than two groups (analogous to how ANOVA generalizes the two-sample $t$-test).

These other statistical tests are often difficult to code, and it is therefore more convenient to use ready-made functions. Section 4.5.2 explains how each of the above tests can be performed within R [11].

### 4.1.14 Bayesian Hypothesis Testing

So far, this section has focused on "classical" hypothesis testing, in which inferences are based entirely on the observed data. The alternative is to perform a "Bayesian" hypothesis test, which combines information from the observed data with external knowledge about the parameters. Specifically, a Bayesian hypothesis test incorporates a "prior distribution," which describes our beliefs about the values of parameters before performing the experiment.

The first three steps when performing a Bayesian hypothesis test are the same as for a classical hypothesis test (i.e., we identify parameters, decide the null and alternative hypotheses and construct a likelihood). The next step is to specify prior distributions corresponding to the null and alternative hypothesis. The final step is to compute a "Bayes Factor," which measures the relative support for each hypothesis (and is the Bayesian equivalent of a $p$-value).

Let $D$ and $\theta$ denote the observed data and the parameters of interest, respectively, and let $L(\theta|D)$ denote the likelihood of the observed data given the parameters. Let $\pi(\theta|H_0)$ denotes the prior distribution for $\theta$ under the null hypothesis, while $\pi(\theta|H_1)$ denotes the

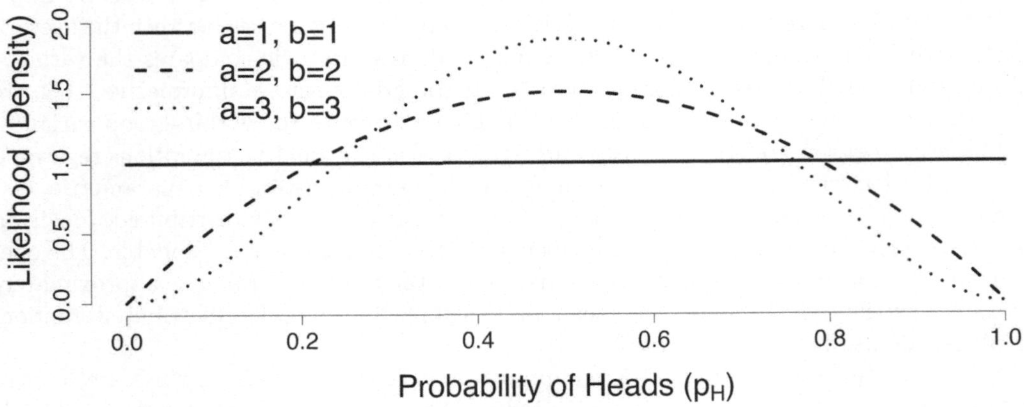


**FIGURE 4.6**
The beta distribution is a continuous distribution whose values are between 0 and 1. It is parameterized by the shape parameters $a$ and $b$. This figure shows the likelihood function for three pairs of values.

prior distribution for $\theta$ under the alternative hypothesis. The Bayes Factor is

$$BF = \frac{\int L(\theta|D)\pi(\theta|H_1)d\theta}{\int L(\theta|D)\pi(\theta|H_0)d\theta} \tag{4.2}$$

A Bayes Factor above one indicates that the alternative hypothesis should be preferred over the null hypothesis (and vice versa).

Consider the example of testing whether a coin is fair using the hypotheses $H_0 : p_H = 0.5$ and $H_1 : p_H \neq 0.5$. The only prior distribution compatible with the null hypothesis is a discrete distribution where $p_H$ must equal 0.5. The density of this distribution is written as $\pi(p_H|H_0) = \delta_{\{0.5\}}$, where $\delta_{\{a\}}$ is a function whose value is zero everywhere except 0.5, and whose integral is one. By contrast, many prior distributions are compatible with the alternative hypothesis. One possibility is to use a beta distribution, which is described in Figure 4.6.

Suppose we choose to represent $\pi(p_H|H_1)$ using a beta distribution with shape parameters $a = 3$ and $b = 3$. As is clear from Figure 4.6, this choice would reflect a prior belief that $p_H$ is more likely to be close to 0.5, than close to 0 or 1. The density for this distribution is

$$\pi(p_H|H_1) = \frac{{p_H}^2(1-p_H)^2}{\beta(3,3)} \quad \text{where} \quad \beta(a,b) = \frac{\Gamma(a)\Gamma(b)}{\Gamma(a+b)}$$

To compute the Bayes Factor corresponding to observing $n_H = 58$, we enter the densities for these two prior distributions into Eq. 4.2, as well as the likelihood function from Eq. 4.1. After some rearrangement and canceling of terms, we obtain

$$BF = \frac{\int {p_H}^{58+2}(1-p_H)^{42+2}/\beta(3,3)dp_H}{\int {p_H}^{58}(1-p_H)^{42}\delta_{\{0.5\}}dp_H} = \frac{\beta(61,45)/\beta(3,3)}{0.5^{100}} = 0.778$$

A Bayes Factor less than one indicates that the data support the null hypothesis more than the alternative hypothesis. Therefore, we would conclude that the null hypothesis is more likely to be true than the alternative hypothesis.

Bayesian hypothesis testing has a number of advantages over classical hypothesis testing. Firstly, we almost always have some prior information about the parameter values, and so it is preferable to include this in the analysis (instead of drawing inferences only from the observed data). Secondly, Bayesian hypothesis testing measures support for each hypothesis, whereas classical hypothesis testing only measures support against the null hypothesis. It is for this reason that Bayesian hypothesis tests sometimes refers to the two hypotheses as $H_1$ and $H_2$, or as Models 1 and 2, to reflect that they are treated as equals (whereas classical hypothesis testing focuses on the null hypothesis). Thirdly, Bayesian hypothesis testing is very flexible. In general, we can test any pair of hypothesis, provided we can identify corresponding prior distributions. For example, this means that the two hypotheses do not need to be complements, but can instead overlap.

Despite these advantages, classical hypothesis testing is generally more popular than Bayesian hypothesis testing for several reasons. Firstly, a $p$-value is easier to interpret than a Bayes Factor. Secondly, it is often hard to know which prior distribution best describes our beliefs about the parameter values. Thirdly, until Bayesian hypothesis testing becomes mainstream, it may continue to be regarded with skepticism.

## 4.2 Multiple Testing

In the previous section, we used the significance threshold $\alpha = 0.05$. However, it is only appropriate to use this threshold when performing a single hypothesis test. To understand why, suppose that instead of testing whether a single coin is fair, we now wish to test whether each of 20 coins is fair. We therefore perform the experiment described above for 20 coins in a row (i.e., we toss each coin 100 times, record the total number of heads, and compute the corresponding $p$-value). Suppose all 20 coins are fair, and we continue to use the significance threshold $\alpha = 0.05$. The probability of obtaining a true negative (i.e., finding no evidence that the coin is biased) for a single coin is $1 - 0.05 = 0.95$. Therefore, the probability of obtaining true negatives for all 20 coins is $0.95^{20} = 0.358$. It follows that the chance of obtaining one or more false positive (i.e., concluding that at least one coin is biased) is $1 - 0.358 = 0.642$. In general, such a high chance of a false positive is not acceptable. It is for this reason that, when performing multiple tests, it is necessary to reduce the significance threshold (e.g., if we repeat the above calculations using $\alpha = 0.01$ and $\alpha = 0.005$, respectively, the probability of one or more false positives reduces to 0.182 and 0.095).

### 4.2.1 Family-Wise Error Rate and False Discovery Rate

Suppose we are performing $T$ hypothesis tests. The *family-wise error rate (FWER)* is the probability of observing one or more false positives (i.e., of incorrectly rejecting the null hypothesis at least once). Meanwhile, the *false discovery rate (FDR)* is the expected proportion of times we incorrectly reject the null hypothesis (i.e., the probability that a positive is a false positive).

When accounting for multiple testing, some studies try to control the FWER. This approach aims to keep the number of false positives to a minimum (ideally zero). By contrast, other studies seek to control the FDR. This approach considers that it is more important to control the relative number of false positives than the absolute number. For example, suppose that a study reports 100 positives, of which 98 are true positives and two are false positive; with respect to the FWER, this could be viewed as a poor outcome

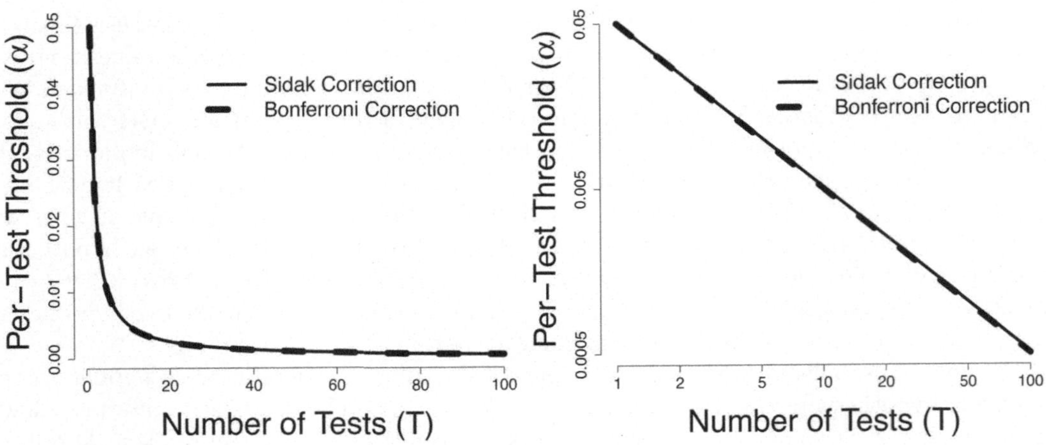


**FIGURE 4.7**
Sidák and Bonferroni corrections corresponding to a family-wise error rate threshold $\alpha_{\text{FWER}} = 0.05$. In both plots, the curves show how the per-test significance threshold $\alpha$ depends on the number of tests $T$. In the right panel, the logarithmic scale is shown for each axis.

(because the study failed to avoid any false positives, but with respect to the FDR, this could be considered a good outcome (because only 2% of the positives were false positives).

### 4.2.2 Controlling the Family-Wise Error Rate

Let $\alpha_{\text{FWER}}$ denote the desired FWER (commonly, we set $\alpha_{\text{FWER}} = 0.05$, so that there is at most a 5% chance of observing one or more false positives). Sidák, Bonferroni and Holm correction are three methods for ensuring the FWER is no higher than $\alpha_{\text{FWER}}$.

*Sidák correction* [12] uses the (per-test) significance threshold $\alpha = 1 - (1 - \alpha_{\text{FWER}})^{\frac{1}{T}}$, which ensures that the FWER equals $\alpha_{\text{FWER}}$ when the $T$ tests are independent. To understand why, note that when performing $T$ independent tests, the FWER is $1-(1-\alpha)^T$ (at the start of this section, we derived this formula for $\alpha = 0.05$ and $T = 20$).

*Bonferroni correction* [3] uses $\alpha = \alpha_{\text{FWER}}/T$ [3], which ensures that the FWER is at most $\alpha_{\text{FWER}}$ (regardless of whether the $T$ tests are independent). The proof of this is not straightforward, but follows from a theorem called Boole's Inequality.

As shown in Figure 4.7, Bonferroni and Sidák correction are typically very similar, reflecting that $1 - T\alpha_{\text{FWER}}$ is a good approximation of $(1 - \alpha_{\text{FWER}})^T$ when $\alpha_{\text{FWER}}$ is small. However, the major difference between the two approaches is that whereas Bonferroni correction guarantees control of the FWER, this is not the case for Sidák correction (specifically, Sidák correction can lead to inflated FWER in the unusual scenario that the tests are negatively dependent).

A common criticism of both Sidák and Bonferroni correction is that they are conservative (tend to over-correct) when the multiple tests are correlated. This issue is discussed further in the next section.

*Holm correction* [6] is more complicated than Sidák and Bonferroni correction, because it does not use a single significance threshold. Instead, let $P_1, P_2, \ldots, P_T$ denote the $p$-values from the $T$ tests, ordered from smallest to largest; Holm correction rejects the null hypothesis for the $T'$ tests with lowest $p$-values, where $T'$ is the highest integer such that $P_t < \alpha_{\text{FWER}}/(T + 1 - t)$ for $t = 1, 2, \ldots, T'$. For example, if $P_1 < \alpha_{\text{FWER}}/T$ and $P_2 <$

$\alpha_{\text{FWER}}/(T-1)$, but $P_3 \geq \alpha_{\text{FWER}}/(T-2)$, then $T' = 2$, and so Holm correction determines that there is sufficient evidence to reject the null hypothesis for the two tests with lowest $p$-values, but insufficient evidence to reject the null hypothesis for the remaining $T-2$ tests. Holm correction ensures that the FWER is at most $\alpha_{\text{FWER}}$ (like Bonferroni correction, this is regardless of whether the $T$ tests are independent).

Holm correction is at least as powerful than Bonferroni correction, because any test rejected based on Bonferroni correction will also be rejected based on Holm correction (e.g., if Bonferroni correction rejects the null hypothesis twice, this means that both $P_1$ and $P_2$ are less than $\alpha_{\text{FWER}}/T$, in which case $P_t < \alpha_{\text{FWER}}/(T+1-t)$ for both $t=1$ and $t=2$, and so $T'$ will be at least 2). For this reason, Holm correction should be more popular than Bonferroni correction. However, in practice, this is not the case, which likely reflects the complexity of Holm correction (both to perform and to explain).

### 4.2.3 Controlling the False Discovery Rate

Let $\alpha_{\text{FDR}}$ denote the desired FDR (e.g., setting $\alpha_{\text{FDR}}$ corresponds to requiring that at least 95% of the positives are expected to be true positives). The most common method for controlling the FDR is the *Benjamini–Hochberg* procedure [1], which has similarities to Holm correction. If $P_1, P_2, \ldots, P_T$ denote the ordered $p$-values from the $T$ tests, the Benjamini–Hochberg procedure rejects the null hypothesis for the $T^*$ tests with lowest $p$-values, where $T^*$ is the highest integer such that $P_t < t \times \alpha_{\text{FDR}}/T$ for $t = 1, 2, \ldots, T^*$. For example, if $P_1 < 1 \times \alpha_{\text{FDR}}/T$ and $P_2 < 2 \times \alpha_{\text{FDR}}/T$, but $P_3 \geq 3 \times \alpha_{\text{FDR}}/T$, then $T^* = 2$ and the Benjamini–Hochberg procedure determines that there is sufficient evidence to reject the null hypothesis for the two tests with lowest $p$-values, but insufficient evidence to reject the null hypothesis for the remaining $T-2$ tests. The Benjamini–Hochberg procedure ensures that the FDR is at most $\alpha_{\text{FDR}}$, provided the $T$ tests are independent. The *Benjamini–Yekutieli* procedure [2] modifies the Benjamini–Hochberg procedure to allow for the case when the tests are not independent (specifically, $T^*$ becomes the highest integer such that $P_t < t/c(T) \times \alpha_{\text{FDR}}/T$ for $t = 1, 2, \ldots, T^*$, where $c(T) = \sum_{i=1}^{m} 1/i$).

### 4.2.4 Examples of Multiple Testing

Multiple testing generally occurs for studies that involve multiple analyses (e.g., this was the case above when testing whether each of 20 coins is fair). However, multiple testing also occurs when a study performs a single analysis that involves more than one comparison. For example, suppose having tossed a coin 100 times, we tested both whether it was fair ($p_H = 0.5$) and whether heads were three times more likely than tails ($p_H = 0.75$); in this case, we would have performed two tests (not one). Occurrences of multiple testing can also be less obvious. For example, suppose that having tested whether a coin is fair based on 100 tosses ($n = 100$), we decided the power was insufficient, and therefore we repeat the analysis with 200 tosses ($n = 200$); even if we only report results from the second analysis, it remains that two tests were performed.

## 4.3 Genome-Wide Association Studies

A genome-wide association study (GWAS) is a common way to investigate the genetic factors affecting a phenotype. In medical sciences, GWAS are typically used to investigate diseases. The aim is to find genetic variants that influence disease risk, information that will help us, for example, identify drug targets, predict high-risk individuals, and develop personalized treatments.

In essence, a GWAS is a regression problem, where we seek to understand how predictors (the genetic variants) influence an outcome (the phenotype of interest). Commonly, the genetic variants are single-nucleotide polymorphisms (SNPs), which are perhaps the most basic type of genetic variant. DNA comprises a long sequence of nucleotides, each of which is either adenine, cytosine, guanine or thymine (abbreviated as A, C, G, and T, respectively). Most DNA loci exhibit no variation (e.g., at a particular locus, all people have nucleotide A). By contrast, a SNP is a locus where at least two different nucleotides are observed (e.g., some people have nucleotide A, while others have nucleotide G). Note that we usually restrict to SNPs that are biallelic (exactly two nucleotides are observed), common (each nucleotide is observed in at least 1% of people), and autosomal (do not lie on the sex chromosomes). There are approximately 10 M biallelic, common, autosomal SNPs in the human genome, each of which has a reference and an alternative allele [13]. Each of these SNPs can be coded as 0, 1, or 2, based on the number of copies of the alternative allele. For example, if a SNP has reference allele A and alternative allele G, then the codings 0, 1, & 2 correspond to individuals with allele pairs AA, AG, and GG, respectively.

A GWAS involves recruiting individuals, each of whom are measured for the phenotype and recorded for a large number of SNPs (e.g., 1 M). In the mathematics below, we assume there are $n$ individuals and $m$ SNPs, and that the length-$n$ vector $Y$ contains the phenotypes, while the $n$ times $m$ matrix $X$ contains the SNP values (i.e., $Y_i$ is the phenotype of the $i$th individual, while $X_{i,j}$ is their value for the $j$th SNP).

### 4.3.1 Testing Single-Nucleotide Polymorphisms for Association with the Phenotype

A simple method for testing whether SNP $j$ is associated with the phenotype is via the linear model

$$\mathbb{E}[Y_i] = \mu + \beta_j X_{i,j}, \tag{4.3}$$

where $\mu$ is the intercept and $\beta_j$ is the SNP's effect size. The null and alternative hypotheses are $H_0 : \beta_j = 0$ and $H_1 : \beta_j \neq 0$, respectively. The least squares estimate of $\beta_j$ is

$$\hat{\beta}_j = \frac{Cov(X_j, Y)}{Var(X_j)}, \tag{4.4}$$

the covariance between the SNP and the phenotype divided by the variance of the SNP. The likelihood ratio test statistic is

$$\lambda_j = n\text{log}(1 - r_j^2) \approx nr_j^2, \tag{4.5}$$

where $r_j$ is the correlation between the SNP and the phenotype. The corresponding $p$-value, $P_j$, can be obtained by comparing $\lambda_j$ to a chi-squared distribution with one degree of freedom.

### 4.3.2 Genome-Wide Significance Threshold

When performing a human GWAS, the genome-wide significance threshold is usually set to $5 \times 10^{-8}$ [10]. This means that when testing SNP $j$, we will reject the null hypothesis (i.e., declare the SNP associated) if $P_j < 5 \times 10^{-8}$. This threshold can be motivated by assuming there are approximately 1 M SNPs, then using Bonferroni correction with $\alpha_{\text{FWER}} = 0.05$ (i.e., $5 \times 10^{-8} = 0.05/1\,000\,000$).

The threshold $5 \times 10^{-8}$ has often been described as conservative, because it fails to appreciate that the tests are not independent [8]. Specifically, neighboring SNPs tend to be highly correlated (due to something called linkage disequilibrium), and therefore neighboring $p$-values will also be correlated. For example, if $P_j$ is small (large), then $P_{j-1}$ and $P_{j+1}$ are likely to also be small (large). Conversely, $5 \times 10^{-8}$ can also be viewed as anti-conservative, reflecting that it is now common for GWAS to test more than 1 M SNPs (e.g., if they sequence individuals, use imputation, or include both common and rare SNPs) [4].

One way to obtain a more accurate genome-wide significance threshold is via permutation testing. We can repeat the GWAS using permuted outcomes (i.e., having shuffled the elements of $Y$). The $p$-values from the permuted GWAS will be sampled under the null hypothesis for each SNP (because the permutation will ensure that $\beta_j = 0$ for all SNPs). However, importantly, the $p$-values from the permuted GWAS will retain their correlation structure (i.e., correlated SNPs will continue to have similar $p$-values). For example, to find a genome-wide significance threshold that ensures $\alpha_{\text{FWER}} = 0.05$, we could perform 1 000 permuted GWAS, record for each the minimum $p$-value across all SNPs, then select the 50th smallest of these minima.

### 4.3.3 Power of a Genome-Wide Association Study

When using the genome-wide significant threshold $5 \times 10^{-8}$, a SNP will be declared associated if the corresponding chi-squared test statistic exceeds 29.7 (because there is a $5 \times 10^{-8}$ chance that a draw from a chi-squared distribution with one degree of freedom exceeds 29.7). It therefore follows from Eq. 4.5, that SNP $j$ will be declared associated if $r_j^2$, its squared correlation with the phenotype, exceeds approximately $29.7/n$. Note that $r_j^2$ also denotes the proportion of phenotypic variation explained by SNP $j$ (e.g., $r_j^2 = 0.01$ indicates the SNP explains 1% of phenotypic variation).

The above inequality allows us to quickly estimate the power of a GWAS given its sample size. For example, Figure 4.8 shows that if the GWAS has $n = 1000$, it will declare associated SNPs whose squared correlation with the phenotype exceeds approximately 0.03 (i.e., explains at least 3% of phenotypic variation), whereas if the GWAS has $n = 50\,000$, it will declare associated SNPs whose squared correlation exceeds approximately 0.0006 (i.e., explains at least 0.06% of phenotypic variation). Conversely, we can use the inequality as a guide for deciding GWAS sample size. For example, if our primary aim is to detect SNPs with a very large impact on the phenotype (e.g., those that explain at least 1% of phenotypic variation), we require at least 3000 individuals, whereas if we are interested in also detecting SNPs with a more modest impact (e.g., those explaining between 0.01% and 1% of phenotypic variation), we require at least 300 000 individuals.

The squared correlation between SNP $j$ and the phenotype is

$$r_j^2 = \frac{Cov(X_j, Y)^2}{Var(X_j)Var(Y)}. \tag{4.6}$$

It follows from Eq. 4.4, that

$$r_j^2 = \frac{\hat{\beta}_j^2 \times Var(X_j)}{Var(Y)}. \tag{4.7}$$

When analyzing human data, we tend to observe $Var(X_j) \approx 2f_j(1 - f_j)$, where $f_j$ is the minor allele frequency of SNP $j$ (this approximation is known as Hardy-Weinberg Equilibrium [5, 14]). It therefore follows that

$$\lambda_j \propto n \times \hat{\beta}_j^2 \times f_j(1 - f_j), \tag{4.8}$$

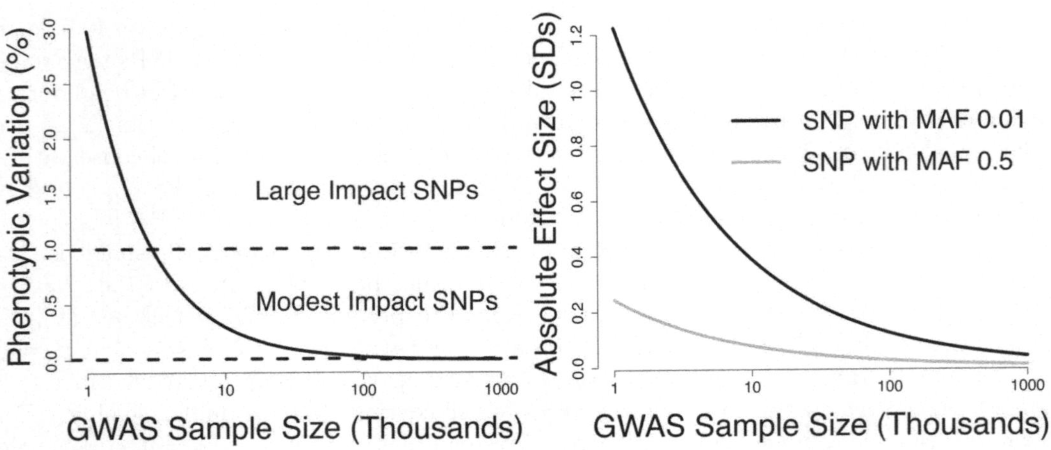


**FIGURE 4.8**
(Left panel) Illustration of how the required proportion of phenotypic variation explained by a SNP depends on the GWAS sample size. The lines mark the thresholds for genome-wide significance when testing SNPs for association with a phenotype (i.e., a $p$-value $< 5 \times 10^{-8}$). (Right panel) Illustration of how the required absolute effect size of a SNP (whose units are standard deviations of the phenotype) depends on the GWAS sample size; lines indicate whether the SNP has minor allele frequency (MAF) of 0.01 or 0.5. For example, for a GWAS of 10 000 individuals, a genome-wide significant SNP will explain at least 0.3% of phenotypic variation; if the SNP has MAF 0.01 (0.5), then this corresponds to an absolute effect size of at least 0.07 (0.39) standard deviations.

and so the test statistic for SNP $j$ depends on both its effect size and minor allele frequency (as well as the sample size). This means that if two SNPs have the same effect size, we will have higher power to detect the more common SNP. For example, Figure 4.8 shows that for a SNP with $f_j = 0.01$ to be declared associated, the effect size threshold is approximately five times larger than for a SNP with $f_j = 0.5$.

### 4.3.4 Genome-Wide Association Studies of the Epilepsies

In 2014, the International League Against Epilepsy (ILAE) Consortium published results from three epilepsy GWAS [7]. In total, the consortium analyzed data from 8,696 epilepsy patients (of whom 2,606 had genetic generalized epilepsy, 5,310 had focal epilepsy, and 780 were unclassified) and 26,157 population controls. Their first GWAS compared all epilepsy patients against controls ($n = 34,853$), their second compared genetic generalized epilepsy patients against controls ($n = 28,763$), while their third compared focal epilepsy patients against controls ($n = 31,467$). After imputation, each individual was recorded for approximately 6 million biallelic, common, autosomal SNPs.

For each GWAS, the consortium tested SNPs for association with the phenotype using an advanced version of Eq. 4.3 (specifically, they added a random effect to the linear model, designed to capture the contribution of population structure and familial relatedness [9]). They set the genome-wide significance threshold to $1.66 \times 10^{-8}$, obtained by applying Bonferroni correction to the regular genome-wide significance threshold (i.e., $1.66 \times 10^{-8}$ equals $5 \times 10^{-8}$ divided by three, the total number of GWAS performed). This means that the consortium, in effect, used Bonferroni correction twice (once to allow for testing of multiple SNPs, and once to allow for testing of multiple phenotypes).

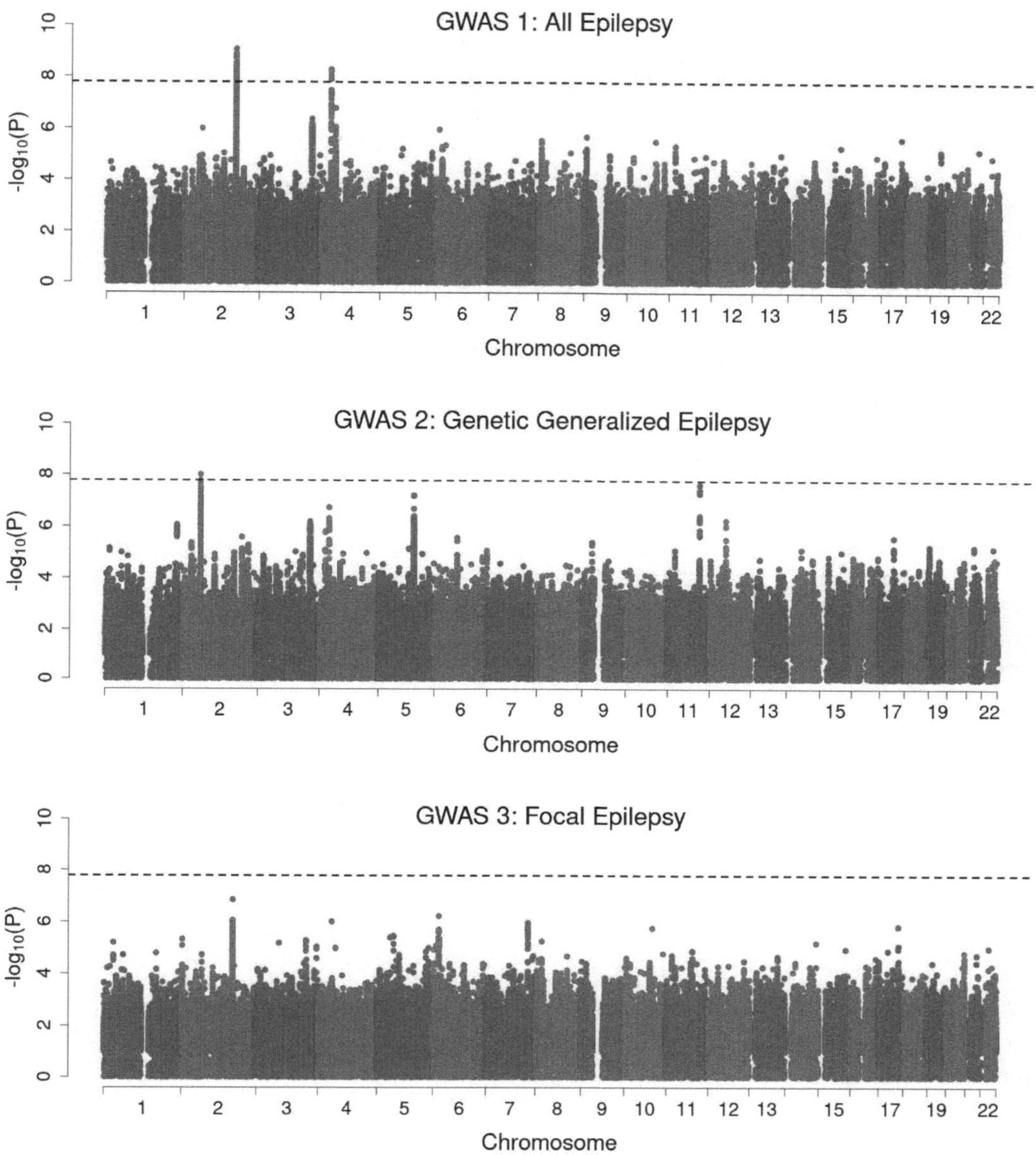


**FIGURE 4.9**
Results from the ILAE GWAS of (top panel) all epilepsies, (middle panel) genetic generalized epilepsies, and (bottom panel) focal epilepsies. Each point reports the $-\log_{10}$ $p$-value from testing a SNP for association with the phenotype. The horizontal lines mark the genome-wide significance threshold. (Color version available in electronic supplement.)

The results from the three GWAS are shown in Figure 4.9. In total, three loci achieve genome-wide significance; two of these are for the GWAS of all epilepsy (on Chromosomes 2 and 4), while the third is for the GWAS of genetic generalized epilepsy (on Chromosome 2). We note that had the consortium not corrected for multiple GWAS (i.e., continued to use the standard genome-wide threshold $5 \times 10^{-8}$), there would be an additional significant loci for genetic generalized epilepsy (on Chromosome 11).

## 4.4 R Example: Coin and Bus Examples

This section provides R codes for performing some of the analyses used in the coin and bus examples in Section 4.1 [11].

### 4.4.1 Plot the Likelihood Curve for the Coin Example

First we make the binomial likelihood function defined by Eq. 4.1.

```
# Make the likelihood function
binom_like = function(pH, nH, n) {
  return(factorial(n) / factorial(nH) / factorial(n - nH) * pH ^ nH * (1 - pH) ^ (
    n - nH))
}
```

We can check our likelihood function is sensible by using it to confirm that when tossing a fair coin twice (i.e., $p_H = 0.5$ and $n = 2$), the probabilities of obtaining 0, 1 and 2 heads are 0.25, 0.5 and 0.25, respectively.

```
# Check our function is sensible
> binom_like(pH = 0.5, nH = c(0, 1, 2), n = 2)
[1] 0.25 0.50 0.25
```

We can now plot the likelihood function for the coin example (i.e., replicate Figure 4.1).

```
# Use our function to plot the likelihood curve
nHs <- 0:100
xl <- "Number of Heads"
yl <- "Likelihood (Probability)"
plot(nHs, binom_like(pH = 0.5, nH = nHs, n = 100), type = "h", xlab = xl, ylab =
    yl)
```

Note that instead of creating our own likelihood function, we could have used the built-in function `dbinom()`.

```
# Plot the likelihood curve using the built-in function dbinom()
nHs <- 0:100
xl <- "Number of Heads"
yl <- "Likelihood (Probability)"
plot(nHs, dbinom(nHs, 100, 0.5), type = "h", xlab = xl, ylab = yl)
```

### 4.4.2 Compute an Exact $p$-value for the Coin Example

Suppose we are performing a two-sided hypothesis test using the hypotheses $H_0 : p_H = 0.5$ and $H_1 : p_H \neq 0.5$. We can now use our likelihood function to compute the $p$-value corresponding to observing $n_H = 58$. As a reminder, the $p$-value equals $2\mathbb{P}(n_H \geq 58 | p_H = 0.5)$, twice the probability of observing 58 or more heads if the null hypothesis is true.

```
# Compute the p-value corresponding to observing 58 heads
sum <- 0
for (x in 58:100) {
  sum <- sum + binom_like(pH = 0.5, nH = x, n = 100)
```

```
}

> 2 * sum
[1] 0.1332106
```

Note that instead of using our own likelihood function, we could have used the built-in function `pbinom()`.

```
# Compute the p-value using the built-in function pbinom()
> 2 * pbinom(57.5, 100, .5, lower = F)
[1] 0.1332106
```

Be aware that if we instead used the code `2 * pbinom(58, 100, .5, lower = F)`, R would return $2\mathbb{P}(n_H > 58|p_H = 0.5)$, which would be incorrect (because the $p$-value should consider values "at least as extreme" as that observed, and not just values "more extreme").

### 4.4.3 Compute a Permutation $p$-value for the Coin Example

We continue to perform a two-sided hypothesis test (using the hypotheses $H_0 : p_H = 0.5$ and $H_1 : p_H \neq 0.5$), but now compute the $p$-value corresponding to observing $n_H = 58$ via permutation testing. Specifically, we use the built-in function `rbinom()` to simulate experiments where we toss a fair coin 100 times, then we count how often the simulations result in at least 58 heads. As a reminder, the permutation $p$-value is $2 \times \frac{1+\sum_{k=1}^{K} I(n_H^k \geq n_H)}{1+K}$, where $K$ is the total number of repetitions and $n_H^k$ is the number of heads on the $k$th repetition.

```
# Compute the p-value using 10000 permutations
K <- 10000
record <- rep(NA, K)
for (i in 1 : K){
  record[i] <- rbinom(1, 100, .5)
}

> 2 * (1 + sum(record >= 58)) / (1 + K)
[1] 0.1367863
```

Note that the code above is stochastic (due to the use of the function `rbinom()`), and therefore your permutation $p$-value will likely be slightly different from the one shown here (and slightly different from 0.133, the exact $p$-value).

### 4.4.4 Key Functions Used in the Bus Example

We can use the built-in functions `dexp()` and `dgamma()` to compute the likelihood functions of the exponential and gamma distributions. For example, we can replicate Figure 4.4 using the following code:

```
par(mfrow=c(1,2))

# Plot the likelihood curve for an exponential distribution with mean 10
x <- 0:50000 / 1000
xl <- "Waiting Time for One Bus"
yl <- "Likelihood (Density)"
plot(x, dexp(x, 1 / 10), type = "l", xlab = xl, ylab = yl)

# Plot the likelihood curve for a gamma distribution with shape 100 and scale 10
x <- 0000:150000/100
xl <- "Waiting Time for 100 Buses (W)"
yl <- "Likelihood (Density)"
```

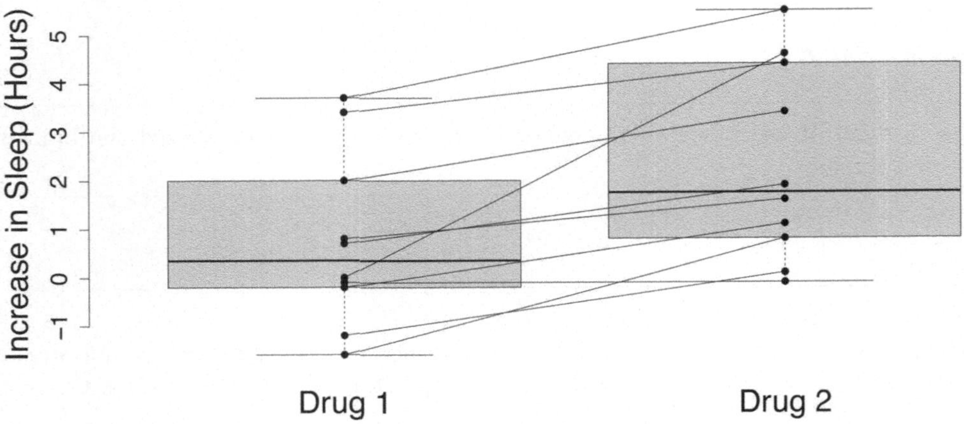


**FIGURE 4.10**
The ten lines indicate the increase in hours sleep when each patient is prescribed either Drug 1 or 2. The boxes report the median, inter-quartile range and extreme values for each drug.

```
plot(x, dgamma(x, 100, 1/10), type = "l", xlab = xl, ylab = yl)
```

We can compute a $p$-value corresponding to observing $W = 803$ using the built-in function `pgamma`.

```
# Compute the p-value corresponding to observing W=803
> 2 * pgamma(803, 100, 1/10, lower = T)
[1] 0.0372783
```

Note that we used 1/10 in the above scripts (instead of 10), because the functions `dexp()`, `dgamma()` and `pgamma()` expect to be provided with the rate parameter, which for the exponential distribution, is the inverse of the mean, and for the gamma distribution is the inverse of the scale parameter.

## 4.5 R Code: Parametric and Non-parametric Hypothesis Testing

This section provides `R` code for performing the other parametric and non-parametric hypothesis tests described in Section 4.1.13 [11]. The codes make use of the pre-installed `R` dataset named `sleep`, which reports the hours increase in sleep for ten patients given Drugs 1 and 2 (the datapoints are plotted in Figure 4.10).

### 4.5.1 Parametric Tests

We note that across the 20 datapoints, the mean increase in sleep is 1.54 hours. We can use the one-sample $t$-test to assess whether this mean is different from zero.

```
# Test whether the mean increase in sleep is different to zero
> t.test(sleep$extra)

One Sample t-test
```

```
data: sleep$extra
t = 3.413, df = 19, p-value = 0.002918
alternative hypothesis: true mean is not equal to 0
95 percent confidence interval: 0.5955845 2.4844155
```

The $p$-value is 0.002, so based on the usual significance threshold ($\alpha = 0.05$) we reject the null hypothesis that the mean increase in sleep is zero. Note that this is a two-sided test (because we are testing whether the mean is greater or less than zero). To instead perform a one-sided test, we would use one of the following two codes:

```
# Use one-sample t-test to assess whether mean sleep increase is greater than zero
t.test(sleep$extra, alternative = "greater")

# Test whether the mean increase in sleep is less than zero
t.test(sleep$extra, alternative = "less")
```

We note that when given Drug 1, the mean increase in sleep is 0.75 hours, whereas when given Drug 2, the mean increase is 2.33 hours. We can use the two-sample $t$-test to assess whether these means are different:

```
# Use two-sample t-test to assess whether mean sleep increase depends on drug
    choice
> t.test(sleep$extra ~ sleep$group)

Welch Two Sample t-test
data:  sleep$extra by sleep$group
t = -1.8608, df = 17.776, p-value = 0.07939
alternative hypothesis: true difference in means between group 1 and group 2 is
    not equal to 0
95 percent confidence interval: -3.3654832  0.2054832
```

The $p$-value is 0.08, so based on the usual significance threshold ($\alpha = 0.05$) we do not reject the null hypothesis that the mean increase in sleep is the same for Drugs 1 and 2.

Because each individual is recorded for each drug, it is valid to use the paired $t$-test to assess whether the mean increases in sleep are different for Drugs 1 and 2.

```
# Use paired t-test to assess whether mean sleep increase depends on drug choice
sleep2 <- reshape(sleep, direction = "wide", idvar = "ID", timevar = "group")
> t.test(Pair(extra.1, extra.2) ~ 1, data = sleep2)

Paired t-test
data:  Pair(extra.1, extra.2)
t = -4.0621, df = 9, p-value = 0.002833
alternative hypothesis: true mean difference is not equal to 0
95 percent confidence interval: -2.4598858 -0.7001142
```

Now the $p$-value is 0.003, so based on the usual significance threshold ($\alpha = 0.05$) we reject the null hypothesis that the mean increase in sleep is the same for Drugs 1 and 2. The fact that we reject the null hypothesis when using the paired $t$-test, but not when using the two-sample $t$-test, demonstrates the potential advantage of using a paired $t$-test. Specifically, the increase in power reflects that analyzing the difference between paired datapoints reduces the impact of confounders (in this case, sources of variation in sleep increase unrelated to drug choice).

Alternatively, we can use ANOVA to assess whether the mean increase in sleep depends on drug choice.

```
# Use ANOVA to assess whether mean sleep increase depends on drug choice
> summary(aov(sleep$extra ~ sleep$group))
```

```
              Df Sum Sq Mean Sq F value Pr(>F)
sleep$group  1  12.48  12.482   3.463 0.0792 .
Residuals   18  64.89   3.605
```

The $p$-value is 0.08, so based on the usual significance threshold ($\alpha = 0.05$) we do not reject the null hypothesis that the mean increase in sleep is the same for Drugs 1 and 2. Note that the $p$-value from ANOVA is very similar to that from the two-sample $t$-test, reflecting that the two tests are asymptotically equivalent (when applied to data with only two groups).

### 4.5.2 Non-Parametric Tests

First we use the Mann-Whitney-Wilcoxon test to assess whether the increase in sleep is different for Drugs 1 and 2.

```
# Use Mann-Whitney-Wilcoxon test to assess whether sleep increase depends on drug
    choice
> wilcox.test(sleep$extra ~ sleep$group)

Wilcoxon rank sum test with continuity correction
data:  sleep$extra by sleep$group
W = 25.5, p-value = 0.06933
alternative hypothesis: true location shift is not equal to 0
```

The $p$-value is 0.07, so based on the usual significance threshold ($\alpha = 0.05$) we do not reject the null hypothesis that the increase in sleep is similar for Drugs 1 and 2. This $p$-value from the Mann-Whitney-Wilcoxon test (0.07) is similar to that from the two-sample $t$-test (0.08), which is to be expected considering the former is a non-parametric version of the latter. The difference between the two $p$-values reflects that the Mann-Whitney-Wilcoxon test considers only the rankings of values, whereas the two-sample $t$-test considers their actual values. This can be demonstrated by showing that the results of the Mann-Whitney-Wilcoxon test are identical if the values are replaced by their rankings.

```
# Repeat the Mann-Whitney-Wilcoxon test replacing actual values with rankings
ranks = rank(sleep$extra)
> wilcox.test(ranks ~ sleep$group)

Wilcoxon rank sum test with continuity correction
data:  ranks by sleep$group
W = 25.5, p-value = 0.06933
alternative hypothesis: true location shift is not equal to 0
```

Alternatively, we can use the Kruskal Wallis test to assess whether the increase in sleep depends on drug choice.

```
# Use Kruskal Wallis test to assess whether mean sleep increase depends on drug
    choice
> kruskal.test(sleep$extra ~ sleep$group)

Kruskal-Wallis rank sum test
data:  sleep$extra by sleep$group
Kruskal-Wallis chi-squared = 3.4378, df = 1, p-value = 0.06372
```

The $p$-value is 0.07, so based on the usual significance threshold ($\alpha = 0.05$) we do not reject the null hypothesis that the increase in sleep is similar for Drugs 1 and 2. Note that the $p$-value from the Kruskal Wallis test is very similar to that from the Mann-Whitney-Wilcoxon test, reflecting that the two tests are asymptotically equivalent (when applied to data with only two groups).

## 4.6 Summary

In this chapter, we introduce readers to the problem of hypothesis testing by providing an accessible and in-depth discussion of various aspects of the statistical procedures behind single and multiple testing. We review several of the most common procedures used to correct for the problem of multiple comparisons, and end with an application of hypothesis testing to a genome-wide association study in epilepsy.

## Bibliography

[1] Yoav Benjamini and Yosef Hochberg. Controlling the false discovery rate: a practical and powerful approach to multiple testing. *Journal of the Royal Statistical Society: Series B (Methodological)*, 57(1):289–300, 1995.

[2] Yoav Benjamini and Daniel Yekutieli. The control of the false discovery rate in multiple testing under dependency. *Annals of Statistics*, pages 1165–1188, 2001.

[3] C. Bonferroni. *Studi in onore del Professore Salvatore Ortu Carboni.* Bardi, 1935.

[4] João Fadista, Alisa K. Manning, Jose C. Florez, Leif Groop. The (in)famous GWAS P-value threshold revisited and updated for low-frequency variants. *European Journal of Human Genetics*, 24:1202–1205, 2016.

[5] Godrey H. Hardy. Mendelian proportions in a mixed population. *Science*, 28:49–50, 1908.

[6] Sture Holm. A simple sequentially rejective multiple test procedure. *Scandinavian Journal of Statistics*, pages 65–70, 1979.

[7] International League Against Epilepsy Consortium on Complex Epilepsies. Genetic determinants of common epilepsies: a meta-analysis of genome-wide association studies. *Lancet Neurology*, 13:893–903, 2014.

[8] Randall C. Johnson, George W. Nelson, Jennifer L. Troyer, James A. Lautenberger, Bailey D. Kessing, Cheryl A. Winkler, Stephen J. O'Brien. Accounting for multiple comparisons in a genome-wide association study (GWAS). *BMC Genomics*, 11, 2010.

[9] Christoph Lipper, Jennifer Listgarten, Ying Liu, Carl M. Kadie, Robert I. Davidson, David Heckerman. FaST linear mixed models for genome-wide association studies. *Nature Methods*, 8:833–835, 2011.

[10] Itsik Pe'er, Roman Yelensky, David Altshuler, Mark J. Daly. Estimation of the multiple testing burden for genomewide association studies of nearly all common variants. *Genetic Epidemiology*, 32:381–385, 2008.

[11] R Core Team. *R: A Language and Environment for Statistical Computing.* R Foundation for Statistical Computing, Vienna, Austria, 2022.

[12] Zbynek Sidak. Rectangular confidence regions for the means of multivariate normal distributions. *Journal of the American Statistical Association*, 62:626–633, 1967.

[13] The International HapMap 3 Consortium. Integrating common and rare genetic variation in diverse human populations. *Nature*, 467:52–58, 2010.

[14] W. Weinberg. Über den Nachweis der Vererbung beim Menschen. *Jahreshefte des Vereins fur Vaterländische Naturkunde in Württemberg*, 64:368–382, 1908.

# Part II

# Statistical Inference

# 5

# *Introduction to Linear, Generalized Linear, and Mixed-Effects Models*

**Omar Vazquez**

*Department of Statistics, University of California, Irvine (USA)*

**Xiangmin Xu**

*Department of Anatomy and Neurobiology, University of California, Irvine (USA)*

**Zhaoxia Yu**

*Department of Statistics, University of California, Irvine (USA)*

## CONTENTS



Outcomes in neuroscience research, including studies of epilepsy, are often not normally distributed; nor are they independent with each other. For example, in a study of patients with epilepsy, counts of seizures might be repeatedly collected from the same subject. In this chapter, we first review linear models and then introduce generalized linear models for non-normal data and mixed-effects models for handling dependency due to repeated measurements or clustered data. Robust procedures, such as generalized estimating equations (GEE), are also covered. Examples are provided in an application to single neuron data using the `R` programming language.

DOI: 10.1201/9781003254515-5

## 5.1 Linear Models

Linear models are perhaps the most commonly used regression models for studying the relationship between clinical covariates and a continuous patient outcome such as seizure duration, cognitive scores, or standardized well-being scores. They serve as the foundation for advanced methods. As an example, a linear model can be considered as a neural network with linear activation. From a theoretical point of view, linear models cover models corresponding to tools familiar to scientists in many areas. As elaborated below, one-sample t-tests, two-sample t-tests, and F-tests from ANOVA, discussed also in Chapter 4, can all be regarded as test statistics from their corresponding linear models. We further discuss several extensions of linear models to model non-continuous responses via generalized linear models (Section 5.2) and to account for data dependency in repeated or clustered measurements via mixed-effects models (Section 5.3) and generalized estimating equations (Section 5.4). We also briefly discuss Bayesian methods (Section 5.5) and model diagnostics (Section 5.6). Each extension is illustrated by an application to the single neuron data described in Section 5.2.1, including relevant code from R.

### 5.1.1 Linear Models for One-Sample t-test, Two-Sample t-test, and One-Way ANOVA

To see how linear models provide a unified framework for many familiar tools, including several of those discussed in Chapter 4, consider the one-sample problem, which is often described as the problem of inferring the population mean, denoted by $\mu$, based on a random sample. Let $Y_1, \ldots, Y_n$ denote a random sample (e.g. of patient seizure durations) from a distribution with mean $\mu$ and variance $\sigma^2$. A reasonable estimator for the population mean is the sample mean

$$\bar{Y} = \frac{1}{n}\sum_{i=1}^{n} Y_i.$$

Although the population variance $\sigma^2$ is not of primary interest, it is critical to quantify the uncertainty in using $\bar{Y}$ as an estimate of the population mean. An unbiased estimator of $\sigma^2$ is the sample variance $\hat{\sigma}^2 = \frac{1}{n-1}\sum_{i=1}^{n}(Y_i - \bar{Y})^2$. The t-test statistic for $H_0 : \mu = \mu_0$ is defined as

$$T = \frac{\bar{Y} - \mu_0}{se(\bar{Y})}$$

where the standard error of $\bar{Y}$ is $se(\bar{Y}) = \sqrt{\frac{1}{n}\hat{\sigma}^2}$. If, in addition to the assumption of independence, $\epsilon_i \sim N(0, \sigma^2)$, $i = 1, \ldots, n$ is assumed, then the t-test statistic follows a t distribution with $n - 1$ degrees of freedom when $H_0$ is true. This test, also known as "Student's t-test," was first derived by the British statistician William Sealy Gosset under the pseudonym "Student" in (Student, 1908). It plays a critical role in making inference of the population mean. The assumption of normality is not essential if the sample size is large enough, say $n > 30$.

To recognize that the one-sample problem is a special case of linear models, we rewrite the assumption that $Y_1, \ldots, Y_n$ is a random sample from a population with mean $\mu$ and variance $\sigma^2$ as follows:

$$Y_i = \beta_0 \times 1 + \epsilon_i$$

where $\epsilon_i$'s are independent and identically distributed from the same distribution with mean 0 and variance $\sigma^2$, and $\mu$ is replaced by $\beta_0$ for the sake of consistent notations with more general linear models.

Next consider the two-sample problem of comparing patient outcomes in a clinical trial with randomly assigned anti-seizure medication or placebo, with $n_0$ observations from the control group and $n_1$ observations from the treatment group. Let $x_i$ be the binary indicator of treatment, i.e., $x_i = 1$ if the observed outcome $Y_i$ is from the anti-seizure treatment group and $x_i = 0$ otherwise. The linear model corresponding to the two-sample problem is

$$Y_i = \beta_0 + x_i \times \beta_1 + \epsilon_i, \; i = 1, \ldots, n_0, n_0 + 1, \ldots, n_0 + n_1, \tag{5.1}$$

where $\beta_0$ is the population mean of the reference group, which is the placebo group in this setting, and $\beta_0 + \beta_1$ is the population mean of the anti-seizure medication group. The random errors $\epsilon_i$'s are assumed to be independent. The two-sample t-test, which tests the null hypothesis $H_0 : \beta_1 = 0$ of no effect of the anti-seizure treatment, can also be derived by standardizing the least square estimate of the coefficient $\beta_1$. In particular, the t-test under the assumption of a homogeneous variance of the random errors is the equal-variance two-sample t-test, whereas dropping this restriction leads to the two-sample t-test with unequal variances. Similar to the one-problem problem, the t-test statistic follows a t-distribution approximately when the assumption of normality is dropped.

The model in 5.1 can be extended for multiple, say $K$, treatments, each of which could represent a distinct medication or dosage received. Specifically, we create one indicator variable, also known as a dummy variable, for each treatment:

$$Y_i = \beta_0 + x_{i1} \times \beta_1 + \ldots + x_{iK} \times \beta_K + \epsilon_i, \; i = 1, \ldots, \sum_{k=0}^{K} n_k,$$

where $n_0$ denotes the number of observations in the control / placebo group, $n_k$, $k = 1, \ldots, K$, denotes the number of observations from treatment $k$, and $x_{ik} = 1$ if the $i$th observation is from the $k$th treatment, and zero otherwise. The coefficients are parameters of the means, with $\beta_0$ being the population mean of the control/reference group, and $\beta_k$, $k = 1, \ldots, K$, being the difference in population mean between the $k$th treatment and the control group. When the random errors are independently and identically distributed (i.i.d.) from a normal distribution, one can construct an F distributed test statistic to test whether any of the $K$ has a treatment effect, i.e., $H_0 : \beta_1 = \cdots = \beta_K = 0$. The exact same statistic can be derived by the one-way analysis of variance (ANOVA), which compares the means of the $(K + 1)$ levels, including $K$ treatments and the control, of a factor by assessing the variance attributable to two sources: randomness and the factor.

### 5.1.2 Multiple Linear Regression and Beyond Linear Models

As shown above, linear models can be considered as a unified tool for several familiar inference tools. This is achieved by creating dummy variables (taking values of 0 and 1) to represent categorical information such as treatment group. For example, in the one-way ANOVA with a control group and $K$ treatment groups, we create a set of $K$ dummy variables, each of which is often known as an explanatory / independent/ predictive variable in the linear model. Multiple factors and their interactions can be investigated through a similar strategy. The inclusion of continuous variables such as age allows inference for the continuous variables or adjustment for their effects. In a generic form of a linear model with $p$ explanatory variables, we have

$$Y_i = \beta_0 + x_{i1} \times \beta_1 + \ldots + x_{ip} \times \beta_p + \epsilon_i, \; i = 1, \ldots, n, \tag{5.2}$$

where $n$ is the total number of observations and the coefficients $\beta_1, \ldots, \beta_p$ are either of direct scientific interest or correspond to variables whose effects should be accounted for.

A limitation of traditional linear models is that they allow predicted values to take any real number, which may not always be suitable for outcomes like binary, proportional, or count data. Additionally, these types of data often violate the assumption of constant variance (homoscedasticity). For example, count data like neural spikes in a time window tend to have increasing variance with the mean. In fact, the Poisson distribution, commonly used for count data, assumes that mean and variance are equal. Next, we introduce a more general framework that can model a broader range of outcome types.

## 5.2 Generalized Linear Models

Epilepsy research often seeks to examine the association between clinical covariates and a non-continuous outcome, which cannot be analyzed using linear regression. For instance, patient survival, epilepsy diagnosis, or remission status can only have two values (yes/no). Another outcome of interest is the number of seizures recorded in a given time period, which is a count variable. Generalized linear models (GLM) offer a unified approach for analyzing various outcome types [7, 8]. It includes the conventional linear regression (for continuous response variables) and several other commonly used models, such as logistic regression (for binary outcomes) and Poisson regression (for count data), as special cases. We will demonstrate the concept using logistic regression.

Consider the $i$th of $n$ observations. Let $Y_i$ denote the binary outcome (e.g. epilepsy diagnosis with "yes" coded as the value one) and $X_i = (X_{i1}, \cdots, X_{ip})$ be a vector of $p$ covariates such as age, gender, family history of epilepsy, etc. Because $Y_i$ is binary, a natural choice of distribution is the Bernoulli distribution with the "success probability" $\pi_i$, where $\pi_i = E(Y_i|X_i)$ is the probability that $Y_i$ takes the value 1, i.e. the $i$th patient is diagnosed with epilepsy, conditional on the covariates $X_i$. The logistic regression model links the logit-transformed success probability to a linear function of the covariates, i.e.,

$$logit(\pi_i) = log\left(\frac{\pi_i}{1-\pi_i}\right) = \beta_0 + X_{i1} \times \beta_1 + \ldots + X_{ip} \times \beta_p. \tag{5.3}$$

The logit transformation ensures that the estimated success probability is always between 0 and 1, thus preventing undesired fitted values. Note that the distribution of $Y_i$ is completely determined by the coefficients $\beta_0, \ldots, \beta_p$. The maximum likelihood method is often used to estimate and make inference on the parameters.

In general, a GLM is characterized by two components. The first is the distribution imposed on $Y_i$, which is a member of the exponential family, or extended versions to model variance in a flexible way. This family is not only mathematically tractable but also encompasses useful distributions for frequently observed quantities, such as the Poisson distribution for count data. The second component is the link function $g()$ that connects the expected value of the outcome to a linear function of the explanatory variables as follows:

$$g(E(Y_i|X_i)) = \beta_0 + X_{i1} \times \beta_1 + \ldots + X_{ip} \times \beta_p.$$

### 5.2.1 Example: Overview of Single Neuron Data

The examples in this chapter are drawn from a dataset of human single neuron activity published* by [2] and made available online. Previous versions of this dataset have been

*available at https://dandiarchive.org/dandiset/000004/draft

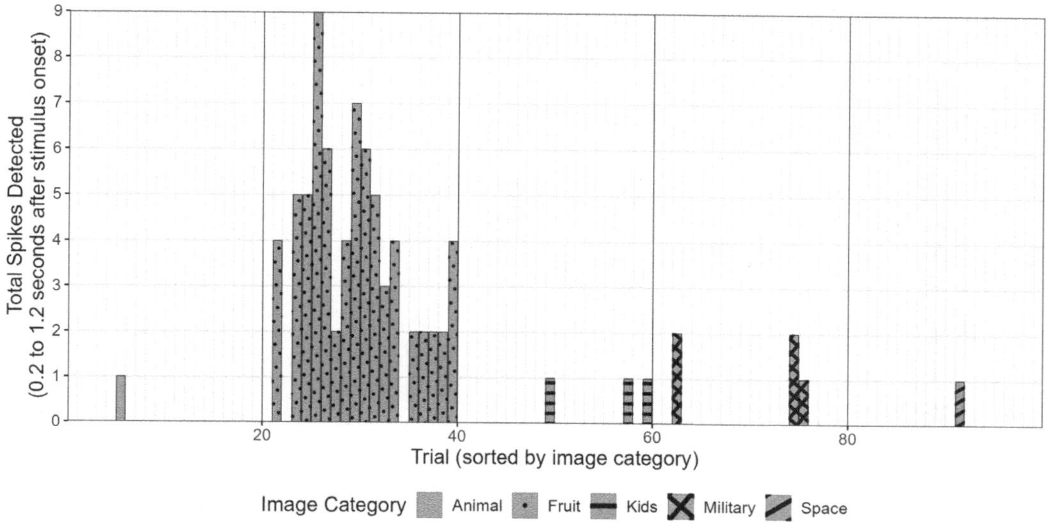


**FIGURE 5.1**
Plot of neuron spike counts, with trials sorted by the category of image shown to the patient, for a visual-selective neuron during the 100 trials in the learning phase of the session.

analyzed in various studies such as [11], which contains more technical details on the experimental setup and data pre-processing. We present a brief summary below.

Single neuron recordings were obtained from the medial temporal lobe of 59 epilepsy patients who had volunteered for the study as part of their planned invasive intracranial monitoring for epilepsy. The participants underwent a memory task, which consisted of a learning phase where they were presented with 100 images from five distinct visual categories, followed by a recognition phase where they were shown 50 new and 50 previously seen images and asked to identify whether each image was new or old from the learning phase. Some participants had multiple sessions with different images from different sets of five visual categories.

In total, the data contains the behavioral responses and neuron spikes of 59 patients over 87 sessions, for a total of 1863 neurons recorded across all sessions. Two patients with two sessions each are excluded from the analysis shown in this chapter due to constraints on data pre-processing.

There are repeated measurements on each subject at the trial level, with each trial corresponding to a different image in the memory task, as well as at the session level, where there are 35 subjects with one session each, 18 subjects with two sessions each, and the remaining four with three sessions each. Therefore, random effects may be included at the subject level as well as at the session level, as demonstrated in Section 5.3. Each session corresponds to a single patient.

### 5.2.2 Example of GLM: Modeling Neuron Spike Counts

We will start by considering a scenario where GLM is appropriate. Neurons may exhibit selective firing for certain types of stimuli, such as so-called visual-selective neurons that fire for specific visual categories of images. To assess this for a single neuron, we count the number of spikes detected during a one-second window starting 200 milliseconds after the image stimulus was presented to the patient, for each trial in the learning phase.

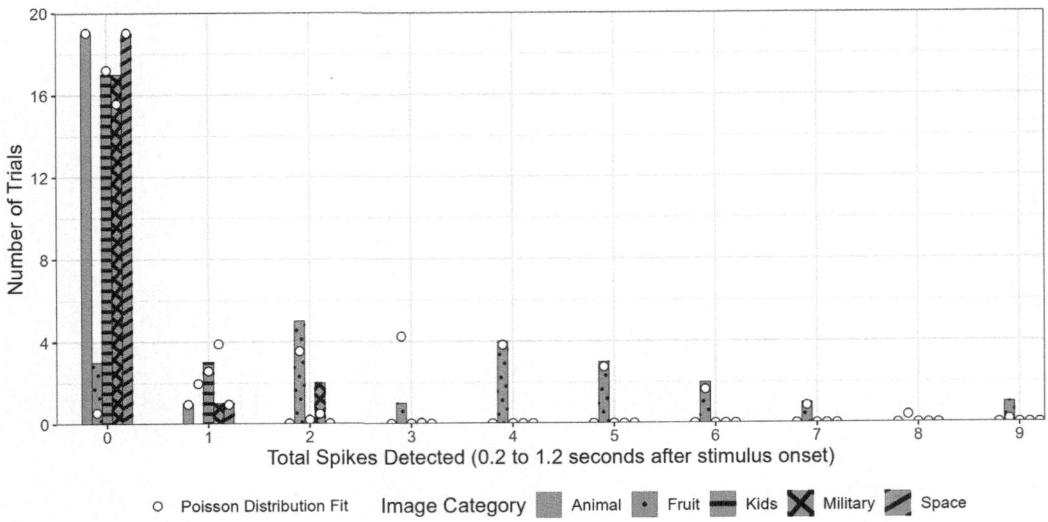


**FIGURE 5.2**
Histogram of the number of spikes detected from a visual-selective neuron in the learning phase trials, between 0.2 and 1.2 seconds after the chosen patient was shown an image, grouped by image category. The black points indicate the expected frequencies from a Poisson distribution, calculated using the mean spike count for each image category. There are 20 total trials for each of the five image categories, making a total of 100 trials.

To quantify the association between these neuron spike counts and the visual category of the image, we use a Poisson GLM as the response variable represents count data. For illustration purposes, the analysis is limited to only the learning phase trials, where all images are new to the patient; otherwise the interaction between image type and category (new vs old images) would need to be modeled as well. For the selected neuron, there are 100 learning trials, with each of the five visual categories appearing in 20 of these trials. The first six rows of the data are presented below:

```
trial_number n_spikes image_categ
           1        0      Animal
           2        0        Kids
           3        0       Fruit
           4        0       Space
           5        0       Space
           6        4       Fruit
```

Figure 5.1 shows that the chosen neuron fires more frequently in trials where the patient is shown images of fruit compared to any other visual category. This is evident in the histogram of spike counts (Figure 5.2), which shows that most of the trials in other categories had no spikes detected within the time window. By comparing the observed and predicted frequencies for the spike counts grouped by image category, it can be seen that the Poisson distribution provides an adequate fit to the data.

We fit a Poisson GLM with log-link function in order to quantify the association between the neuron's spike counts (`n_spikes`) and the image category (`image_categ`):

```
poisson_fit <- glm(n_spikes ~ image_categ, data = chosen_neuron_data,
                   family = poisson())
```

**TABLE 5.1**
Poisson GLM estimates for regression of neuron spike counts on image category, with log link function. The baseline group is trials with animal images.

| Coefficient | Estimate | Std. error | t-stat | p-value | Lower 95% CI | Upper 95% CI |
|---|---|---|---|---|---|---|
| Intercept | −3.00 | 1.00 | −3.00 | 0.00 | −5.86 | −1.51 |
| Fruit | 4.28 | 1.01 | 4.25 | 0.00 | 2.77 | 7.15 |
| Kids | 1.10 | 1.15 | 0.95 | 0.34 | −0.96 | 4.11 |
| Military | 1.61 | 1.10 | 1.47 | 0.14 | −0.22 | 4.56 |
| Space | 0.00 | 1.41 | 0.00 | 1.00 | −3.23 | 3.23 |

We can test whether the image category is a significant predictor of the neuron spikes to determine whether this is a visual-selective neuron. We choose a $\chi^2$ test, evaluated by `anova(poisson_fit, update(poisson_fit, n_spikes ~ 1), test = "Chisq")`. The first two arguments to the `anova()` function are the two models to be compared, i.e. the full model with image category as a predictor and the reduced model with only the intercept, while `test` specifies the type of test statistic to calculate. In this case, the association is highly significant ($p < 2.2 \times 10^{-16}$), as was suggested by Figure 5.1.

From the Poisson model estimates in Table 5.1, we see that, when compared to the baseline group of animal images, the average neuron spike counts are only significantly different for the fruit category. Specifically, after transforming the coefficient estimates from the log-link scale to the response scale, fruit image trials are associated with an increase of $(e^{4.28} - 1) \approx 71$ times the average neuron spikes recorded when compared to animal image trials, for this neuron. The corresponding 95% confidence interval is roughly (15, 1270).

The GLM generalizes the conventional LM in several ways. However, both of them share a foundational assumption – independence between all the observations. This assumption is often violated in practice. For instance, repeated measurements on the same subject lead to dependent observations. To handle such dependence, mixed-effects models are introduced, which incorporate random effects into the model framework.

## 5.3 Linear Mixed-Effects Models and Generalized Linear Mixed-Effects Models

Data acquired in epilepsy research often includes multiple outcome measurements for each patient, and this clustering of the data violates the independence assumption of GLMs. For example, a clinical trial may assess seizure counts at multiple follow-up times for each patient after administering a randomly assigned treatment or placebo. Linear mixed-effects models (LME) and generalized linear mixed-effects models (GLMM) are generalizations of linear models and GLMs, respectively, that allow for repeated measurements.

### 5.3.1 Example of LME: Modeling Patient Response Time

We first use the single neuron data from the 59 patients described in Section 5.2.1 to motivate the use of linear mixed-effects models. In this analysis, the goal is to investigate the association between the time it takes for patients to respond whether they believe an image is new or old and the type of image. We first log-transform the patient response times since their distribution is highly skewed, and this changes the interpretation of our

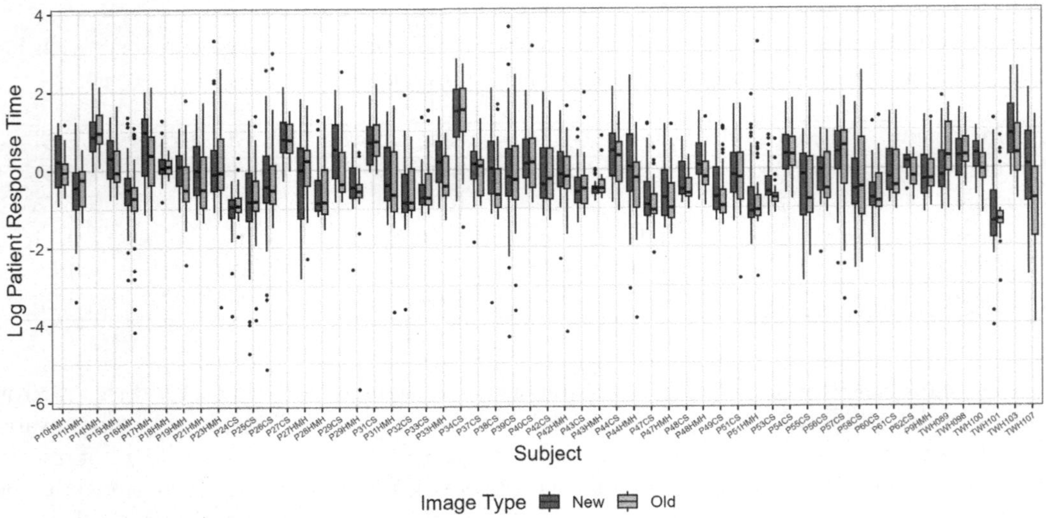


**FIGURE 5.3**
Side-by-side boxplots of log patient response times (measured in seconds) grouped by image type, over the last 50 trials in each session.

regression coefficients to be in terms of percent change in response time. We also restrict the analysis to the last 50 trials of the recognition phase, since the first few trials tend to last longer as patients become more familiar with the task. In total, there were 4150 trials (observations) from 57 patients over 83 sessions, with 22 patients having data for more than one session (see Section 5.2.1). The first six rows of the data are presented below:

| subject_id | session_id | trial_number | sex | age | image_type | resp_conf | log_resp_time |
|---|---|---|---|---|---|---|---|
| P24CS | CS24_59 | 51 | F | 57 | Old | confident | -0.9546340 |
| P24CS | CS24_59 | 52 | F | 57 | New | confident | -2.6529798 |
| P24CS | CS24_59 | 53 | F | 57 | Old | confident | -0.3153863 |
| P24CS | CS24_59 | 54 | F | 57 | New | confident | -0.6894082 |
| P24CS | CS24_59 | 55 | F | 57 | Old | confident | -0.9450246 |
| P24CS | CS24_59 | 56 | F | 57 | Old | confident | -0.9679709 |

Boxplots of the log-transformed patient response times grouped by subject and image type (Figure 5.3) show substantial variation in the average response time between subjects. This clustering is evidence of correlated observations within the same subject. We therefore account for the dependency due to repeated measurements by including a random subject-specific effect $u_i$ for observations from subject $i$ in a linear mixed-effect model:

$$Y_{ij} = \beta_0 + X_{ij,1} \times \beta_1 + \ldots + X_{ij,p} \times \beta_p + u_i + \epsilon_{ij}, \ i = 1, \ldots, 57; \ j = 1, \ldots, n_i \qquad (5.4)$$

where $Y_{ij}$ is the log response time for subject $i$ and trial $j$ (`log_resp_time`), $n_i$ is the number of measurements from subject $i$, and the covariates $X_{ij,1}, \ldots, X_{ij,p}$ include dummy variables for image type (`image_type`). Mathematically, this is equivalent to creating dummy/indicator variables $Z_{ij,k}$, $k = 1, \ldots, 57$ where $Z_{ij,k} = 1$ if $k = i$ and $Z_{ij,k} = 0$ otherwise:

$$Y_{ij} = \beta_0 + X_{ij,1} \times \beta_1 + \ldots + X_{ij,p} \times \beta_p + Z_{ij,1} \times u_1 + \ldots + Z_{ij,57} \times u_{57} + \epsilon_{ij} \qquad (5.5)$$

Thus, $Z_{ij,k}$ is the indicator for whether an observation is from patient $k$. When fitting the LME through a software package, what is needed is the cluster ID variable (in this case `subject\_id`), and the corresponding dummy variables will be created internally by the software. For example, using the `lmer()` function in the `lme4` package for `R`, we run†

```
lme_fit <- lmer(log_resp_time ~ sex + age + image_type * resp_conf + (1 | subject_
    id), data = resp_time_data)
```

where random effects for a given predictor and clustering are included in the model formula by using the format `(predictor | cluster_ids)`.

In the framework of linear mixed-effects models, the coefficients $\beta = (\beta_0, \ldots, \beta_p)$ are parameters with fixed but unknown values. In this example, fixed-effects variables include image type, which is the variable of interest, and covariates we would like to adjust for: patient age, sex, and self-reported response confidence. Exploratory plots of the distribution of the log response time grouped by image type (Figure 5.4) indeed suggest that on average patient responses are slower for new images. Grouping by response confidence as well (Figure 5.5) reveals that the same trend is present within "confident" and "probably" confidence levels, although the average difference seems to be larger for high-confidence trials. We also see that patient responses in high-confidence trials were typically faster than in low-confidence trials, which makes intuitive sense. This leads us to include an interaction between image type and response confidence as fixed-effects in our model.

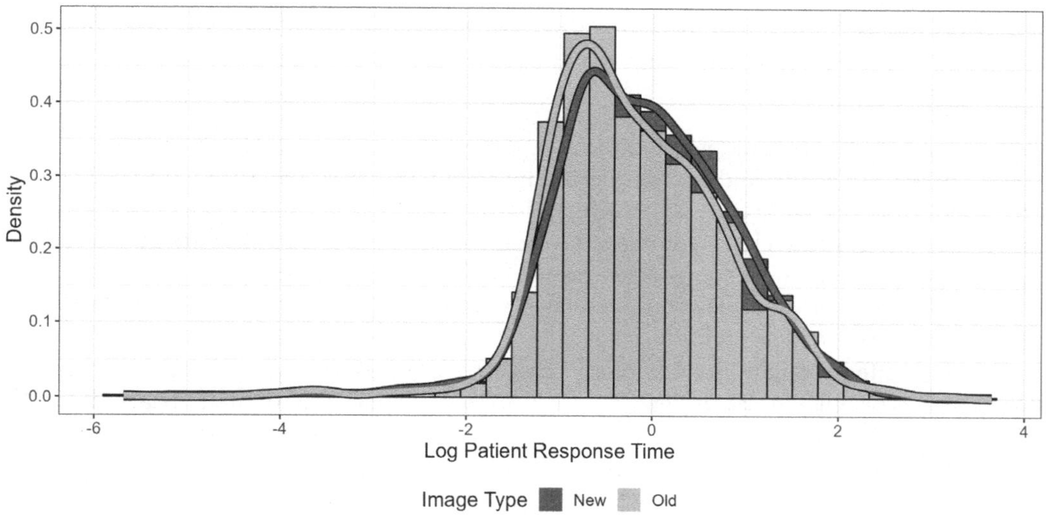


**FIGURE 5.4**
Histograms of log patient response times grouped by image type, for the last 50 trials in each session. Response times were originally measured in seconds.

The random effects $u_1, \ldots, u_{57}$, on the other hand, are treated as independent random variables from a common distribution. Typically, this is a normal distribution centered at zero, with a variance to be estimated from the data: $N(0, \sigma_u^2)$. It is worth noting that, just like the residuals $\epsilon_{ij}$'s, the values of the subject-specific means $u_i$'s are not of direct interest. Further, they are quantities specific to randomly selected units, such as patients, rather than quantities representing population characteristics. The random-effect $u_i$ represents the deviation between the overall intercept $\beta_0$ and the intercept specific to the $i$th subject. For this reason, $u_1, \ldots, u_{57}$ are also known as random intercepts.

†For numerical ID variables, it is important to convert to factors before using the `lmer()` function.

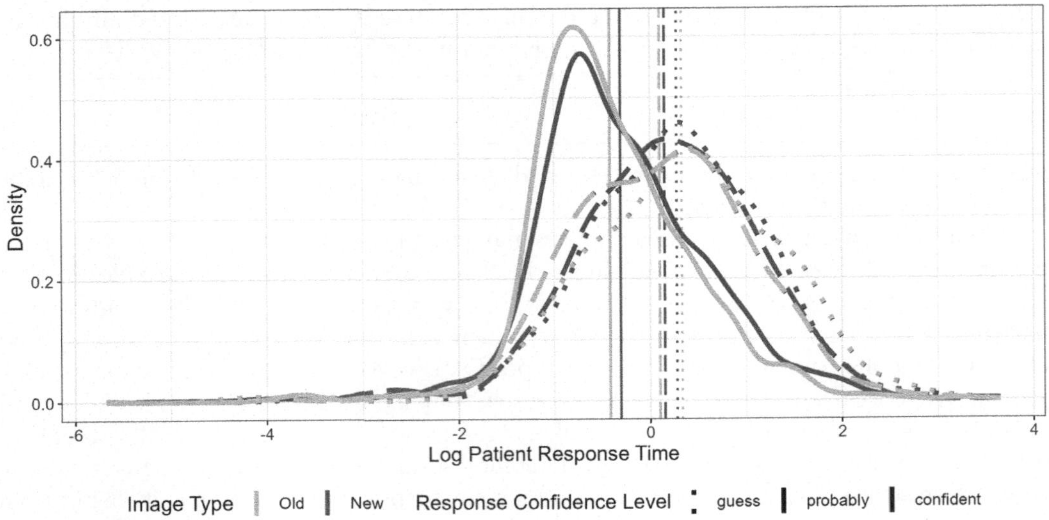


**FIGURE 5.5**
Smoothed histograms of log patient response times grouped by image type and response confidence level, for the last 50 trials in each session. Vertical lines indicate the group averages. Response times were originally measured in seconds.

In some situations, random slopes for a given covariate might also be necessary. This can be assessed visually and by conducting likelihood-based comparisons. The boxplots in Figure 5.3 shows that there is far less variation in the effect of image type across subjects, suggesting that random slopes for image type may not be necessary. In addition, after adding random slopes there was a convergence issue. Therefore, random slopes are not used in this example. For further examples on mixed-effects models with random slopes, we recommend reading our recent article [12].

Random effects might involve more than one level. Recall that there were multiple sessions of recordings for 22 patients, with each session consisting of many trials. Thus, the data has a nested structure of clusters: trials are nested within sessions, and sessions are nested within patients. We therefore fit a nested random-effects model

```
lme_fit <- lmer(log_resp_time ~ sex + age + image_type * resp_conf +
                (1|subject_id/session_id), data = resp_time_data)
```

where the slash between the two cluster id variables indicates that clusters of `session_id` are nested within clusters of `subject_id`.

The `summary(lme_fit)` command provides an overview of the estimated fixed effect coefficients and random effect variances. The fixed effects alone can be extracted through `fixef(lme_fit)`, and we compute 95% Wald confidence intervals for all the fixed effects through the `confint()` function, specifying `method="Wald"`. A summary of the linear mixed-effects model results is presented in Table 5.2. The reference groups for the dummy variables are females, old images, and "guess" confidence levels. Interaction terms are denoted by a colon separating the two dummy variable names.

First, we note that image type is significantly associated with log response time ($\chi^2$ test, $p = 0.002$) after controlling for response confidence, sex, and age, although the direction and significance varies between confidence levels. Within "guess"-level trials, new images are associated with a 0.06 decrease in log response time on average, all else constant, which translates to a roughly $100\% \times \left(e^{-0.06} - 1\right) \approx -6\%$ change in patient response times,

**TABLE 5.2**
Linear mixed-effects model estimates for regression of log patient response times in the last 50 trials of each session, including subject-specific and session-specific random intercepts. The baseline groups are females, old images, and "guess" response confidence.

| Coefficient | Estimate | Std. error | t-stat | Lower 95% CI | Upper 95% CI |
|---|---|---|---|---|---|
| Intercept | −0.05 | 0.20 | −0.25 | −0.43 | 0.34 |
| Sex (Male) | 0.27 | 0.12 | 2.26 | 0.04 | 0.51 |
| Age | 0.01 | 0.00 | 1.94 | 0.00 | 0.02 |
| Image Type (New) | −0.06 | 0.05 | −1.20 | −0.16 | 0.04 |
| Probably | −0.31 | 0.06 | −5.38 | −0.42 | −0.19 |
| Confident | −0.83 | 0.05 | −17.41 | −0.93 | −0.74 |
| New:Probably | 0.12 | 0.07 | 1.69 | −0.02 | 0.27 |
| New:Confident | 0.17 | 0.06 | 2.79 | 0.05 | 0.29 |

although this effect is not statistically significant. On the other hand, within "probably" and "confident"-level trials, new images are associated with $100\% \times \left(e^{-0.06+0.12} - 1\right) \approx +6\%$ and $100\% \times \left(e^{-0.06+0.17} - 1\right) \approx +11\%$ changes in average patient response times, respectively, but only the latter is statistically significant. This is consistent with the trends shown in Figure 5.5.

### 5.3.2 Example of GLMM: Modeling Proportions of Selective Neurons

We showed how to extend LM to LME to account for data dependency in Section 5.3.1. In a very similar fashion, to account for data dependency, the GLM has been extended to generalized linear mixed-effects models (GLMM) (Breslow and Clayton, 1993; Liang and Zeger, 1986; Stiratelli et al., 1984; Wolfinger and O'connell, 1993; Zeger and Karim, 1991; Zeger and Liang, 1986):

$$E(Y_i|X_i) = g(\beta_0 + X_{i1} \times \beta_1 + \ldots + X_{ip} \times \beta_p + Z_{ij,1} \times u_1 + \ldots + Z_{ij,57} \times u_{57}) \quad (5.6)$$

The random-effects terms in LME (Eq. 5.4) and GLMM (Eq. 5.6) play the same role; they explicitly model the dependence structure by specifying subject-specific or other relevant random effects and their joint distribution. With appropriate assumptions on the distribution of the outcome variables $Y_i$ and the mean assumption specified in equation (5.6), likelihood-based approaches are often used for parameter estimation.

As mentioned in the Poisson GLM example of Section 5.2.2, visual-selective neurons preferentially fire for specific visual categories of images. We first identify these neurons by labeling each with whether image category is a significant predictor of the number of neuron spikes detected between 0.2 and 1.2 seconds after stimulus onset in the learning phase, using a Poisson GLM as in the example and a $\chi^2$ test at a 0.05 significance level. One natural question that arises is whether the proportion of neurons that are visual-selective is stable across sessions. In order to investigate whether this proportion varies with patient age, sex, or the combination of image categories available in the session, we use a binomial GLMM with logit link function. The first few rows of the data are shown below (output of `image_categs` truncated):

```
subject_id session_id sex age image_categs
P24CS      CS24_59    F   57 Houses, Landscapes, Mobility, Phones, Small animal
P24CS      CS24_60    F   57 Animal, Fruit, Kids, Military, Space
P25CS      CS25_61    F   36 Houses, Landscapes, Mobility, Phones, Small animal
P25CS      CS25_63    F   36 Animal, Fruit, Kids, Military, Space
P26CS      CS26_64    F   56 Houses, Landscapes, Mobility, Phones, Small animal
P26CS      CS26_66    F   56 Animal, Fruit, Kids, Military, Space
```

```
prop_selective_visual n_neurons
0.2857143          21
0.2727273          22
0.0000000           8
0.0000000          14
0.1818182          33
0.2727273          11
```

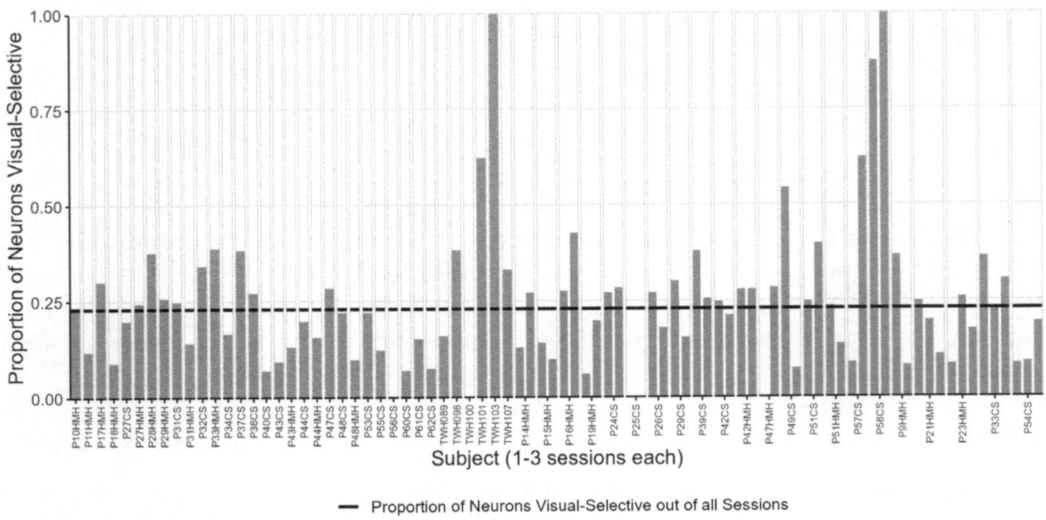


**FIGURE 5.6**
Barchart of the proportion of neurons selective for the visual category of the images, out of all neurons detected in the session. Selectivity for each neuron is determined by a $\chi^2$ test for whether image category is significantly associated with neuron spike counts between 0.2 and 1.2 seconds after stimulus onset, as in the Poisson GLM example (Section 5.2.2). The dashed line indicates the total proportion selective out of all the detected neurons. On the $x$-axis, sessions are grouped by subject and sorted by the number of sessions per subject.

We include subject-specific random intercepts since many patients had two or three sessions of the experiment. Figure 5.6 also shows some evidence of subject-level clustering in the proportions, although this can be difficult to evaluate because the total number of detected neurons varies substantially between sessions. In the same figure we see a few apparent outlier sessions, specifically three sessions with more than 75% of detected neurons classified as visual-selective. This may be explained by the fact that these sessions have a small number of detected neurons: three, eight, and two, in the order that they appear in Figure 5.6. Since, however, the binomial GLMM weights sessions according to their total number of detected neurons, it is not a major concern here. Lastly, plots of the proportion of visual-selective neurons against patient age and sex (Figure 5.7) suggest that those two covariates are not associated with the proportion.

Note that in order to fit the binomial GLMM with the proportions as the response variable we need to specify the corresponding group sizes as weights:

```
glme_fit <- glmer(prop_selective_visual ~ age + sex + image_categs +
                    (1 | subject_id),
                  weights = aggregate_selectivity$n_neurons,
                  data = aggregate_selectivity, family = "binomial")
```

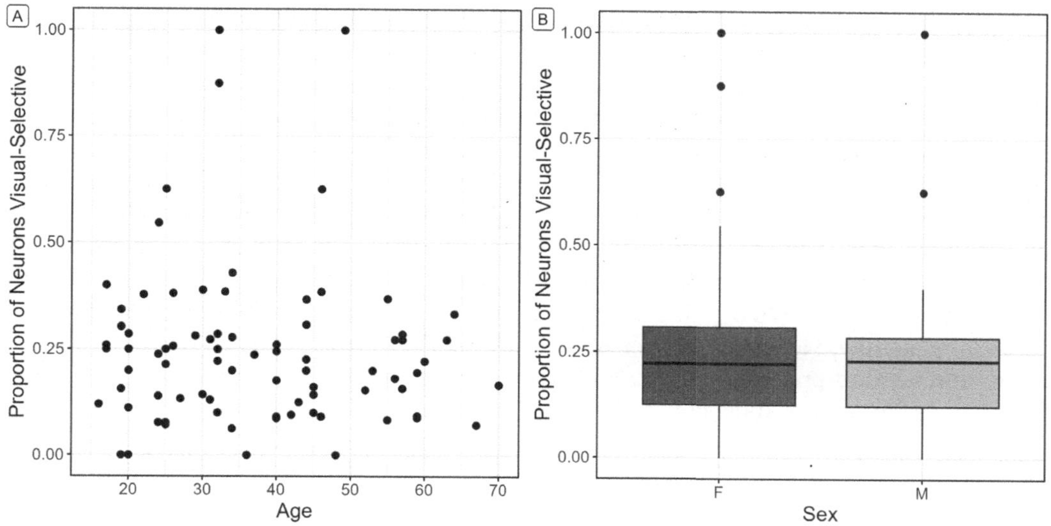


**FIGURE 5.7**
(Left panel) Scatterplot of patient age and the proportion of visual-selective neurons in the session, with no clear trend and a few notable outliers. (Right panel) Boxplots of the proportion of visual-selective neurons in a session, grouped by patient sex. The binomial GLMM results indicate that neither covariate is a significant predictor of the proportion.

Otherwise, the response variable in the model formula should be two columns of counts:

```
cbind(prop_selective_visual * n_neurons, n_neurons * (1 - prop_selective_visual))
```

In either case the model estimates are identical, and a $\chi^2$ test, evaluated by `anova(glme_fit, update(glme_fit, prop_selective_visual ~ (1 | subject_id)))`, shows that none of the covariates are significantly associated with the proportion of visual-selective neurons ($p = 0.17$), which suggests that the proportion is stable across sessions.

**TABLE 5.3**
Binomial GLMM estimates for regression of visual-selective neuron proportions, including subject-specific random intercepts, with logit link function. The baseline group of image categories is (Animals, Fruit, Kids, Military, Space), while the second group is (Animals, Cars, Food, People, Spatial) and the third group is (Houses, Landscapes, Mobility, Phones, Small animal).

| Coefficient | Estimate | Std. error | z-stat | p-value | Lower 95% CI | Upper 95% CI |
|---|---|---|---|---|---|---|
| Intercept | −0.93 | 0.31 | −2.99 | 0.00 | −1.54 | −0.32 |
| Age | −0.01 | 0.01 | −1.50 | 0.13 | −0.02 | 0.00 |
| Sex (Male) | −0.07 | 0.17 | −0.41 | 0.68 | −0.40 | 0.26 |
| Image Group 2 | 0.26 | 0.18 | 1.43 | 0.15 | −0.09 | 0.61 |
| Image Group 3 | −0.06 | 0.16 | −0.34 | 0.74 | −0.38 | 0.27 |

The model results in Table 5.3 further illustrate that none of the covariates are significantly associated with the proportion of visual-selective neurons. For example, among typical subjects, neurons from males are associated with a 0.07 decrease in the log-odds of being visual-selective, or equivalently a $100\% \times \left(e^{-0.07} - 1\right) \approx -7\%$ change in the odds, when compared to females. The corresponding 95% confidence interval is (-33%, 30%), which contains 0% as expected.

The interpretation of the fixed effects for GLMM is complicated by both the random effects and non-linear link functions. A variable like image category, which varies across repeated measurements for the same subject, has a subject-specific interpretation, i.e. the expected change due to the covariate while holding all other effects (fixed and random) constant. However, for variables that do not change (like gender) strictly speaking, there is no valid subject-specific or population-average interpretation [5]. In either case, a reasonable interpretation of the fixed effects for GLMMs might be in terms of comparing "typical individuals," i.e. individuals with a value of zero for their random intercept in this case, or, more generally, values of zero for all of their random effects. This is distinct from the more familiar interpretation in terms of population averages, due to the role of the link function. In linear mixed-effects models, which use the identity link, both interpretations are equivalent.

## 5.4 Generalized Estimating Equations (GEE)

Compared to LME, the computation involved in GLMM with non-normal data is substantially more challenging, both in computational speed and stability. As a result, several strategies have been developed to approximate the likelihood [1]. A robust alternative is the generalized estimating equation (GEE) approach [13]. GEE makes assumptions based on the first two moments rather than imposing explicit distributional assumptions. The idea of GEE is to estimate coefficients using a "working" correlation structure, which does not have to be identical to the unknown underlying true correlation. An incorrect correlation structure, while it would not bias the parameter estimates, would affect the estimate of their variance. Thus, a correction is applied to obtain consistent estimates of variance and covariance. However, cautions need to be taken, as the two approaches might lead to different estimates and interpretations. The correction procedure in GEE relies on aggregated information across subject-level data; as a result, the accuracy of GEE results may be questionable when the number of subjects is small.

### 5.4.1 Example of GEE: Modeling Patient Response Time

We fit generalized estimating equations using the `geeglm()` function in the `geepack` package. The syntax is similar to that of `glm()`, now with the working correlation structure specified via `corstr`. Some common choices are "independence," which assumes that all observations are independent, and "exchangeable," which assumes that observations within the same cluster have a common correlation. The latter is equivalent to the marginal correlation structure of a linear mixed-effects model with random intercepts at the cluster level. Observations in different clusters are always assumed to be independent, with the cluster IDs specified via `id`. It is important to be sure to supply cluster IDs as factor variables, otherwise `geeglm` may not run. Lastly, in order for `geeglm()` to accurately detect the clusters, the data should be sorted by cluster ID so that the clusters form contiguous blocks of rows.

The fitted model from `geeglm()` works with the usual `coef()`, `summary()`, and `anova()` functions, but notably not with `confint()`. The asymptotic $(1-\alpha)\%$ confidence interval for an individual regression coefficient can be calculated from the output of `summary()`, however, as Estimate $\pm z_{1-\alpha/2} \times$ Std. Error, where $z_{1-\alpha/2}$ is the $(1-\alpha/2)$-

quantile of the standard normal distribution. Also, note that `summary()` provides Wald statistics for each regression coefficient. These are simply squared t-statistics, and under the model assumptions each has an asymptotic $\chi_1^2$ distribution.

We revisit the regression of log patient response times on image type and response confidence from Example 5.3.1, now fitting a GEE instead of a linear mixed-effects model. The clustering of log patient response times in Figure 5.3 suggests that an independence correlation structure is not likely to fit the data well, so an exchangeable working correlation structure would be preferable. We choose to cluster at the subject level since it seems reasonable to assume that subjects are independent, while it would be less justifiable to assume that trials across different sessions, even for the same subject, are independent. The GEE results for both correlation structure choices are presented in Table 5.4 for comparison.

```
gee_fit_exch <- geeglm(log_resp_time ~ sex + age + image_type * resp_conf,
                       id = as.factor(resp_time_data$subject_id),
                       corstr = "exchangeable", data = resp_time_data)
```

**TABLE 5.4**
GEE estimates for regression of log patient response times in the last 50 trials of each session, using independence and exchangeable working correlation structures for patient-level clusters. The baseline groups are females, old images, and "guess" response confidence.

| | Independence | | | Exchangeable | | |
|---|---|---|---|---|---|---|
| Coefficient | Estimate | Std. error | p-value | Estimate | Std. error | p-value |
| Intercept | −0.15 | 0.21 | 0.47 | −0.11 | 0.23 | 0.62 |
| Sex (Male) | 0.30 | 0.11 | 0.01 | 0.26 | 0.12 | 0.03 |
| Age | 0.01 | 0.00 | 0.06 | 0.01 | 0.00 | 0.08 |
| Image Type (New) | −0.07 | 0.07 | 0.28 | −0.07 | 0.07 | 0.27 |
| Probably | −0.24 | 0.09 | 0.01 | −0.22 | 0.08 | 0.01 |
| Confident | −0.73 | 0.10 | 0.00 | −0.74 | 0.10 | 0.00 |
| New:Probably | 0.13 | 0.08 | 0.10 | 0.16 | 0.08 | 0.04 |
| New:Confident | 0.19 | 0.08 | 0.02 | 0.18 | 0.07 | 0.01 |

For linear models, the regression coefficients from GEEs have the same population-averaged interpretation as the fixed effect coefficients from linear mixed-effects models. For example, using the estimates from the exchangeable working correlation structure, within "confident"-level trials, new images are associated with a roughly $-0.07 + 0.18 = 0.11$ increase in log patient response time, or a $100\% \times \left(e^{-0.07+0.18} - 1\right) \approx +11\%$ increase in patient response time, all else constant, on average. This difference is statistically significant at the $\alpha = 0.05$ level.

Under our model assumptions, the GEE estimates and standard errors in Table 5.4 will approach their true values as the number of subjects increases, regardless of the chosen working correlation structure, and we do see that the standard errors are fairly similar when comparing independence and exchangeable structures. The working correlation structure has a larger effect on some of the coefficient estimates, however, most notably sex and the interaction between new images and "probably"-level confidence trials. Given our moderate sample size of 57 patients, we should exercise caution about relying on large-sample approximations, especially for working correlation structures that are poor fits to the data.

Lastly, we can compare the GEE estimates in Table 5.4 with the corresponding linear mixed-effects model estimates in Table 5.2. Although several variables have similar coefficient estimates between the GEE and LME, others such as the dummy variable for "confident"-level confidence trials differ substantially. The standard errors are also fairly close for all covariates except that same dummy variable. The same set of variables are significant for the LME and GEE except for the interaction between new images and "probably"-level confidence trials, which is marginally significant for only the GEE.

### 5.4.2 Example of GEE: Modeling Proportions of Selective Neurons

We now revisit the regression of proportions of visual-selective neurons from Example 5.3.1, where we previously fit a binomial generalized linear mixed-effects model with logit link function, and now fit a GEE instead. We choose an exchangeable working correlation structure and subject-level clustering. Table 5.5 contains the resulting estimates.

```
gee_fit <- geeglm(prop_selective_visual ~ age + sex + image_categs,
                  id = as.factor(aggregate_selectivity$subject_id),
                  weights = aggregate_selectivity$n_neurons,
                  family = "binomial", corstr = "exchangeable",
                  data = aggregate_selectivity)
```

**TABLE 5.5**
Binomial GEE estimates for regression of visual-selective neuron proportions with logit link function and exchangeable working correlation structure. Clustering is at the patient level. The baseline group of image categories is (Animal, Fruit, Kids, Military, Space), while the second group is (Animals, Cars, Food, People, Spatial) and the third group is (Houses, Landscapes, Mobility, Phones, Small animal).

| Coefficient | Estimate | Std. error | Wald-stat | p-value | Lower 95% CI | Upper 95% CI |
|---|---|---|---|---|---|---|
| Intercept | −0.90 | 0.30 | 9.13 | 0.00 | −1.48 | −0.31 |
| Age | −0.01 | 0.00 | 3.61 | 0.06 | −0.02 | 0.00 |
| Sex (Male) | −0.04 | 0.17 | 0.06 | 0.81 | −0.37 | 0.29 |
| Image Group 2 | 0.25 | 0.20 | 1.67 | 0.20 | −0.13 | 0.64 |
| Image Group 3 | −0.08 | 0.18 | 0.19 | 0.67 | −0.42 | 0.27 |

None of the covariates in Table 5.5 are significantly associated with the proportion of visual-selective neurons. This is the same result as in Example 5.4.2, but the coefficient estimates for GEE have a different interpretation from the fixed effects of GLMM. For example, on average across subjects, neurons from males are associated with a 0.04 decrease in the log-odds of being visual-selective, or equivalently a $100\% \times \left(e^{-0.04} - 1\right) \approx -4\%$ change in the odds, when compared to females. This effect is not significant, as illustrated by the large p-value of 0.81, or, equivalently, the fact that the asymptotic 95% confidence interval of roughly $(-31\%, 33\%)$ does contain 0%. The interpretation of GEE estimates is in terms of population averages, since we are estimating the coefficients of a marginal model, as opposed to the GLMM, which is specified as a subject-specific model, conditional on the subject's random effects. Again, the difference in interpretation is specific to GLMMs due to the role of the link function.

## 5.5 Bayesian Estimates

The analysis we have presented thus far is the frequentist version, which assumes the coefficients corresponding to random effects are random variables from a distribution, rather than fixed. In the Bayesian counterpart, all the coefficients are treated as random variables from distributions, the parameters of which are either given or treated as hyperparameters that follow some hyperpriors. Compared to the frequentist approach, the Bayesian approach has several advantages. For example, the Bayesian approach can naturally address the intractable computation involved in GLMM by using sampling rather than relying on closed-forms or asymptotic approximations that may be invalid with limited sample sizes. An additional attractive feature is that the Bayesian approach not only computes point estimates and large-sample confidence intervals but also fully characterizes the uncertainty in estimation by means of computing the posterior distribution.

Below we provide the Bayesian version of our analysis. We fit Bayesian LMEs and GLMMs using the `brm()` function in the `brms` R package. The syntax for this function is similar to that of `lme4`, except for how binomial response variables are specified. Using flat uninformative priors, the results for the fixed effects in each example are similar to those estimated by maximum likelihood (ML) and restricted maximum likelihood (REML).

### 5.5.1 Example: Modeling Patient Response Time

For the LME of log patient response time, the posterior means and 95% credible intervals closely match the REML estimates from `lmer`, due in part to the large amount of trials available across all the sessions.

```
blme_fit <- brm(log_resp_time ~ sex + age + image_type * resp_conf +
               (1 | subject_id) + (1 | session_id), data = resp_time_data,
              iter = 2500, warmup = 500, chains = 4)
```

**TABLE 5.6**
Bayesian linear mixed-effects model results for regression of log patient response times in the last 50 trials of each session, including subject-specific and session-specific random intercepts. Posterior estimates are based on flat priors and four Markov chains, each with 2000 post-burnin MCMC iterations. The baseline groups are females, old images, and "guess" response confidence.

| Coefficient | Mean | SD | Lower 95% CI | Upper 95% CI | $n_{\text{eff}}$ | $\hat{R}$ |
|---|---|---|---|---|---|---|
| Intercept | −0.05 | 0.20 | −0.45 | 0.34 | 9125.96 | 1 |
| Sex (Male) | 0.28 | 0.12 | 0.04 | 0.52 | 7880.41 | 1 |
| Age | 0.01 | 0.00 | 0.00 | 0.02 | 9939.64 | 1 |
| Image Type (New) | −0.06 | 0.05 | −0.16 | 0.04 | 8501.14 | 1 |
| Probably | −0.31 | 0.06 | −0.42 | −0.20 | 8743.23 | 1 |
| Confident | −0.83 | 0.05 | −0.93 | −0.74 | 9292.58 | 1 |
| New:Probably | 0.13 | 0.07 | −0.02 | 0.27 | 7810.54 | 1 |
| New:Confident | 0.17 | 0.06 | 0.05 | 0.28 | 8549.51 | 1 |

### 5.5.2 Example: Modeling Neuron Spike Counts

For the Poisson GLM of neuron spikes, the posterior means and 95% credible intervals have similar values to the ML estimates from `glm()`.

```
bglm_fit <- brm(n_spikes ~ image_categ, data = chosen_neuron_data,
               family = poisson, iter = 2500, warmup = 500, chains = 4)
```

**TABLE 5.7**
Bayesian Poisson GLM results for regression of neuron spike counts on image category, with log link function. Posterior estimates are based on flat priors and four Markov chains, each with 2000 post-burnin MCMC iterations. The baseline group is trials with animal images.

| Coefficient | Mean | SD | Lower 95% CI | Upper 95% CI | $n_{\text{eff}}$ | $\hat{R}$ |
|---|---|---|---|---|---|---|
| Intercept | −3.63 | 1.32 | −6.64 | −1.68 | 1289.05 | 1 |
| Fruit | 4.90 | 1.32 | 2.94 | 7.96 | 1298.98 | 1 |
| Kids | 1.57 | 1.47 | −0.91 | 4.82 | 1411.32 | 1 |
| Military | 2.13 | 1.40 | −0.12 | 5.38 | 1342.84 | 1 |
| Space | 0.06 | 1.82 | −3.60 | 3.76 | 1443.30 | 1 |

### 5.5.3 Example: Modeling Proportions of Selective Neurons

For the GLMM of proportions of visual-selective neurons, the posterior means and 95% credible intervals have quite similar values to the ML estimates from `glmer()`.

```
bglme_fit <- brm(n_selective_visual | trials(n_neurons) ~ age + sex +
                   image_categs + (1 | subject_id),
                 data = aggregate_selectivity, family = binomial,
                 iter = 2500, warmup = 500, chains = 4)
```

**TABLE 5.8**
Bayesian binomial GLMM results for regression of visual-selective neuron proportions, including subject-specific random intercepts, with logit link function. Posterior estimates are based on flat priors and four Markov chains, each with 2000 post-burnin MCMC iterations. The baseline group of image categories is (Animal, Fruit, Kids, Military, Space), while the second group is (Animals, Cars, Food, People, Spatial) and the third group is (Houses, Landscapes, Mobility, Phones, Small animal).

| Coefficient | Mean | SD | Lower 95% CI | Upper 95% CI | $n_{\text{eff}}$ | $\hat{R}$ |
|---|---|---|---|---|---|---|
| Intercept | −0.94 | 0.34 | −1.61 | −0.27 | 7968.97 | 1 |
| Age | −0.01 | 0.01 | −0.02 | 0.00 | 7820.90 | 1 |
| Sex (Male) | −0.07 | 0.19 | −0.45 | 0.29 | 7084.13 | 1 |
| Image Group 2 | 0.26 | 0.19 | −0.11 | 0.63 | 9479.96 | 1 |
| Image Group 3 | −0.05 | 0.17 | −0.38 | 0.28 | 10086.57 | 1 |

One advantage of using Bayesian GLMMs is the ease with which we can form prediction intervals, by sampling from the posterior predictive distribution for each session and estimating the corresponding 95% credible intervals. This is done using `predict(bglme_fit)`, and the results are plotted in Figure 5.8 below, which further illustrates how the model takes into account the high level of uncertainty in the outlier sessions with small numbers of recorded neurons. For those sessions, the prediction intervals are quite large and almost cover the entire range between zero and one.

## 5.6 Model Diagnostics

Model diagnostics is a critical but also challenging step in statistical modeling. The purpose of model diagnostics is to assess models, more specifically, the assumptions that each

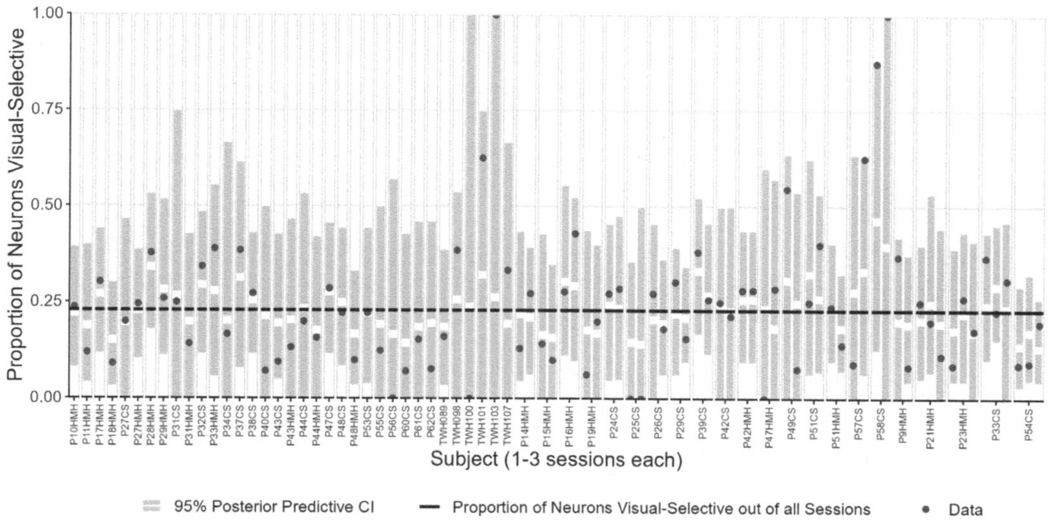


**FIGURE 5.8**
Plot of the 95% Bayesian prediction intervals for the proportion of neurons selective for the visual category of the images in each session, from a binomial GLMM fit. The dots are the observed proportion in the session, while the dashed line indicates the total proportion selective out of all the detected neurons. Sessions are grouped by subject and sorted by the number of sessions per subject.

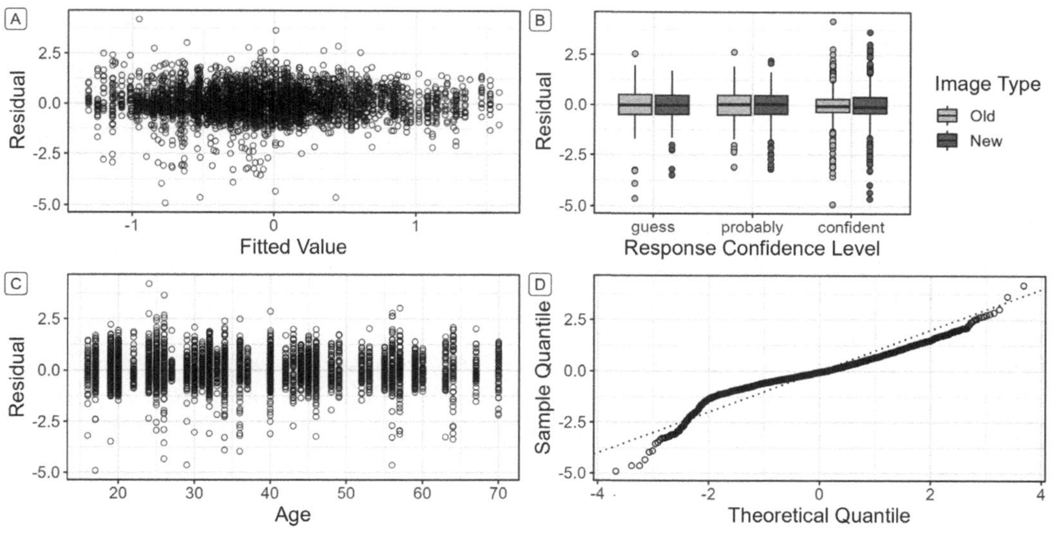


**FIGURE 5.9**
Plots of the LME residuals against (top left panel) fitted values, (top right panel) image type and response confidence level, and (bottom left panel) patient age, as well as (bottom right panel) a normal quantile-quantile plot. None of these diagnostic plots show strong evidence against the model assumptions.

statistical model makes. Below we show how to use residuals, the difference between the observed and predicted values, to check for constant variance and normality.

Residual diagnostic plots can be used to asses how well a model fits the data and, for linear models, whether the normal distribution assumption for the errors is reasonable. Linear model or LME residuals are often plotted against fitted values or covariates to check for any trends that would indicate a misspecified model. Residual plots for GLMs and GLMMs tend to be less informative when there is a non-continuous response variable, particularly for binomial models. They may exhibit patterns even when the model is correctly specified.

With mixed-effects models fit using `lme4` or generalized estimating equation fits from `geepack`, the residuals and fitted values can be easily extracted using the usual `residuals()` and `fitted()` functions. Alternatively, we can use `plot()` on the fitted model object, with various options to customize the resulting diagnostic plot.

For example, Figure 5.9 contains plots of the LME residuals for the regression of log patient response times from Example 5.3.1. The residuals remain centered around zero, with roughly constant spread, for different fitted values and covariate values. The suggests that the model provides an adequate fit to the data, and it is not necessary to consider, for example, including a quadratic term for patient age as an additional predictor in the model. The quantile-quantile plot shows a slight skew in the distribution of the residuals, but otherwise they are fairly close to normal.

Robust methods have been proposed to overcome many limitations of the conventionally used parametric methods. For these robust alternatives, such as resampling or rank based methods, and semiparametric methods, we direct the reader's attention to related articles [3, 4, 6, 9, 10, 13].

## 5.7 Summary

Linear models, also known as linear regression, were introduced to the scientific community more than two centuries ago. In the past fifty years, extensions have been developed for non-normal responses and correlated outcomes, as linear models are often not adequate to analyze data from real studies. In this chapter, we illustrated how linear models, generalized linear models, and generalized linear mixed-effects models can be used in single neuron spike datasets. Specialized regression models for various scenarios are covered in other chapters. For instance, Cox proportional hazard regression model for survival data is covered in Chapter 6, spatio-temporal models and scalar on image regression for spatial data in Chapter 7, autoregressive moving average models for time-series data in Chapter 9, and penalized regression for high-dimensional data to prevent overfitting in Chapter 12.

## Bibliography

[1] Benjamin M Bolker, Mollie E Brooks, Connie J Clark, Shane W Geange, John R Poulsen, M Henry H Stevens, and Jada-Simone S White. Generalized linear mixed models: A practical guide for ecology and evolution. *Trends in Ecology & Evolution*, 24(3):127–135, 2009.

[2] N Chandravadia, D Liang, AGP Schjetnan, A Carlson, M Faraut, JM Chung, CM Reed, B Dichter, Uri Maoz, SK Kalia, et al. A NWB-based dataset and processing pipeline

of human single-neuron activity during a declarative memory task. *Scientific Data*, 7(1):1–12, 2020.

[3] Somnath Datta and Glen A Satten. Rank-sum tests for clustered data. *Journal of the American Statistical Association*, 100(471):908–915, 2005.

[4] Sandipan Dutta and Somnath Datta. A rank-sum test for clustered data when the number of subjects in a group within a cluster is informative. *Biometrics*, 72(2):432–440, 2016.

[5] Garrett M Fitzmaurice, Nan M Laird, and James H Ware. *Applied Longitudinal Analysis*. John Wiley & Sons, 2012.

[6] Ulrich Halekoh and Søren Højsgaard. A Kenward-Roger approximation and parametric bootstrap methods for tests in linear mixed models–the R package pbkrtest. *Journal of Statistical Software*, 59:1–32, 2014.

[7] Peter McCullagh and John A Nelder. *Generalized Linear Models*. Routledge, 2019.

[8] John Ashworth Nelder and Robert WM Wedderburn. Generalized linear models. *Journal of the Royal Statistical Society: Series A (General)*, 135(3):370–384, 1972.

[9] B Rosner and D Grove. Use of the Mann-Whitney U-test for clustered data. *Statistics in Medicine*, 18(11):1387–1400, 1999.

[10] Bernard Rosner, Robert J Glynn, and Mei-Ling Ting Lee. Incorporation of clustering effects for the Wilcoxon rank sum test: a large-sample approach. *Biometrics*, 59(4):1089–1098, 2003.

[11] Ueli Rutishauser, Shengxuan Ye, Matthieu Koroma, Oana Tudusciuc, Ian B Ross, Jeffrey M Chung, and Adam N Mamelak. Representation of retrieval confidence by single neurons in the human medial temporal lobe. *Nature Neuroscience*, 18(7):1041–1050, 2015.

[12] Zhaoxia Yu, Michele Guindani, Steven F Grieco, Lujia Chen, Todd C Holmes, and Xiangmin Xu. Beyond t test and ANOVA: applications of mixed-effects models for more rigorous statistical analysis in neuroscience research. *Neuron*, 110(1):21–35, 2022.

[13] Scott L Zeger, Kung-Yee Liang, and Paul S Albert. Models for longitudinal data: a generalized estimating equation approach. *Biometrics*, pages 1049–1060, 1988.

# 6

# *Survival Analysis*

**Fei Jiang**

*Department of Epidemiology & Biostatistics, University of California, San Francisco (USA)*

**Elan Guterman**

*Department of Neurology, University of California, San Francisco (USA)*

## CONTENTS



This chapter reviews motivations, statistical concepts, and practical implementation of survival analysis. These methods are used across a broad range of disciplines when researchers are interested not only in whether an event occurs but also in the duration of time it takes for the event to occur. In epilepsy research, common events of interest may include seizure recurrence after epilepsy surgery, readmission after a hospitalization for status epilepticus or a seizure cluster, or death. This chapter introduces basic quantities of interest in survival analysis, their estimation procedures, and important hypothesis tests. We specifically explore nonparametric and semiparametric survival models and their application

DOI: 10.1201/9781003254515-6 

to the field of epilepsy using real-world data from a randomized controlled trial. Examples of concepts discussed in this chapter are demonstrated in the R programming language.

## 6.1 Introduction

Survival analysis, also known as time-to-event analysis, is an important statistical method used when we are not only interested in studying whether an event occurs but also how quickly. The fundamental goal of a survival analysis is to determine the amount of time that will pass before an event occurs, use this to calculate the probability that the event will occur within a given time period, and assess whether the rate of occurrence differs between populations.

The term "survival analysis" follows from its original use in studies predicting life expectancy. Researchers were interested in predicting the duration of an individual's life and determining the probability an individual would survive (or conversely, die) during a certain period of time. While there are many statistical methods that can model the distribution of this duration of time, many of these models collapse when the rate is skewed – for example, if there are many events early in the follow-up period and relatively few events later in the follow-up period – or when an individual does not have the event of interest and the duration of time until the event is therefore missing. Survival analyses are specifically designed to address these unique scenarios.

In this chapter, we provide an overview of the statistical methods used for survival analyses. The chapter begins with a review of the unique measurements and structure of time-to-event data necessary for setting up a rigorous survival analysis. This is followed by a discussion of the different methods for modeling survival. These sections focus heavily on Kaplan-Meier estimation, Cox proportional hazard regression, and accelerated failure time models using a real-world randomized controlled trial as an example for understanding these varied and important approaches to epilepsy research. Examples of code are provided from a survival data analysis package available in R.

## 6.2 Measurements in Survival Analysis

In this section, we first review the structure of time-to-event data employed in survival analysis.

### 6.2.1 Defining the Outcome

We will use a randomized controlled trial of surgical resection for children with drug-resistant epilepsy to illustrate the potential use of survival analyses in epilepsy research. In this trial, Dwivedi et al. [3] randomized 116 children with drug-resistant epilepsy to one of two treatments: surgical resection of a seizure focus or continued medical therapy. The primary outcome was freedom from seizures at 12 months, which can be reframed in the context of a survival analysis as the time until a participant experienced their first breakthrough seizure after randomization. The trial selected time-to-seizure as the primary outcome, however, survival analyses can be used to model the occurrence or the recurrence of any event that is binary and occurs once [1]. In research related to epilepsy, other common examples of events of interest may include readmission after hospitalization for status epilepticus or a seizure cluster, prescription of a second antiseizure medication, or death.

### 6.2.2 Defining the Baseline

Researchers aim to measure the period of time between the start of the follow-up period and the outcome occurring. The start of the follow-up period is the baseline. By definition, the baseline is a time when all individuals are event-free and theoretically at risk of experiencing the event. Typically, it is defined by the onset of an exposure of interest, and thus it is dictated by the research question and defined uniquely for each study. In this example, Dwivedi et al. were conducting a randomized trial to study the effect of surgical resection, thus they selected the time of randomization as their baseline. Researchers interested in examining survival among individuals with epilepsy could instead select a different baseline, such as time since a diagnosis of epilepsy or time since an individual was born (i.e. chronological age).

It is important to ensure the baseline timepoint is clearly and consistently identified across all subjects so statistical comparisons are valid. For example, the month that an individual underwent surgery for temporal lobe epilepsy is reliably recorded in the electronic medical record and consistently collected as part of a clinical trial. Thus, researchers who are studying whether surgery leads to better seizure control can confidently identify this date for all individuals. In contrast, the time when an individual developed epilepsy is difficult to identify using data from the electronic medical record. In circumstances where the date of the exposure is more challenging to pinpoint, it is important to have specific definitions that can be used for the entire study population. Researchers who use administrative claims data might define incident epilepsy as the first time that seizure is included as a billing code in an insurance claim, or they may use natural language processing to identify the first date that epilepsy was entered into an encounter note in the electronic medical record. These definitions use available information to define a plausible, discrete time when an individual developed epilepsy that can be used consistently for the entire study population to minimize bias in the results.

### 6.2.3 Defining Time

The time that passes between the baseline and the outcome can be measured in days, months, or years. The measure of time should be relevant to the research question and feasible with the dataset. It is possible to use measures other than time as the "time scale," although that is beyond the scope of this chapter. Common terms to describe the time between the baseline and the outcome are *progression-free survival*, a term that originates from the field of oncology to describe the time between baseline and cancer progression, and *overall survival time*, which is used to describe the time between baseline and death. Progression-free survival is a popular endpoint because it occurs at faster rate than death and researchers can have adequate statistical power to detect an effect with a smaller sample size and shorter follow up period.

### 6.2.4 Censoring Mechanism

One challenge of survival data is the presence of individuals who do not experience the event of interest during the study period. This phenomenon is called censoring. Censoring may arise in the following ways:

**TABLE 6.1**
Summary of different types of censoring in survival analysis.

| Left censoring | Interval censoring | Right censoring |
|---|---|---|
| Event occurred before time A | Event occurred between time A and B | Event occurred after time B |
| Subject with epilepsy had first lifetime seizure before the study began but unclear when first lifetime seizure occurred | Subject died between annual assessment at year 2 and year 3 but unclear when death occurred | Subject alive at the end of the study or lost to follow up but unclear when death occurred |

- Administrative censoring: Individuals who did not experience the outcome by the end of the study (but are still at risk in the future);
- Lost to follow-up: Individuals who leave the study during the follow-up period (either because they are lost tofollow-up or they intentionally withdraw from the study); or
- Competing event: Individuals who experience a different (competing) event that makes the outcome impossible.

We can use the randomized controlled trial of epilepsy surgery [3] as an example. An individual who was administratively censored would have been followed for 12 months and seizure-free at the end of the study. An individual who was lost to follow up may have withdrawn from the study six months after enrollment. An individual who experienced a competing event may have died from a procedural complication one month after surgery and researchers would not know whether the individual would have had a recurrent seizure if they had instead survived.

In each of these scenarios, researchers do not have a precise measure of the duration between randomization and seizure occurrence. However, they do know that the individual was seizure-free at the time of censoring. Rather than excluding these individuals because their data is incomplete, survival analyses include these individuals and incorporate these data into the model via censoring.

There are three types of censoring that describe when censoring occurred relative to the study period (Table 6.1). This is important because the methods for handling censoring depend upon the type of censoring present. Left censoring occurs when the event takes place before the beginning of the study. Interval censoring occurs when the event takes place between study visits. Right censoring occurs when the event takes place after the end of the study. Right censoring is the most common type of censoring in medical studies.

Standard survival analysis methods are valid only if the censoring is "non-informative," which means that individuals who are censored have the same rate of the event as those who are not censored thus their missing data carries no additional information about survival in the study population. Conversely, informative censoring implies that individuals who are censored have a different rate of the event thus incomplete information about these individuals biases the results of the study. For example, informative censoring occurs when patients who withdraw from a study have more severe disease than those who remain enrolled.

In some circumstances, the period of time between an exposure and the event occurring is so short or long that individuals are "missed" and excluded from the study population. This is called truncation. For example, an individual who has sudden unexpected death in epilepsy (SUDEP) in association with their first seizure cannot inform a survival analysis estimating death among individuals with epilepsy because the individual never has an opportunity to receive a diagnosis of epilepsy and enter the study before they die. It is important to recognize when truncation can lead to selection bias and influence the validity of the results.

## 6.3 Structuring Data for a Survival Analysis

To perform a survival analysis, researchers must have two pieces of information for each individual: survival time and a censoring indicator. Survival time refers to the amount of time an individual is followed during a study and reflects the amount of time between the baseline of the study and the end of the follow-up period when either the outcome or censoring occurs. The censoring indicator is a dichotomous variable indicating whether the outcome was observed or the individual was censored. Conventionally, the censoring indicator is set to 1 when the event was observed and 0 when the individual was censored.

Figure 6.1 visualizes these data for eight hypothetical participants in the randomized controlled trial. The baseline is the time of randomization and indicated by the circle on the left side of each line. Survival time is indicated by the line extending right from the circle. In Figure 6.1 (left panel), the $x$-axis is calendar time, because individuals are randomized at different times, the lines start at different x-coordinates for each individual. In a survival analysis, however, calendar time is often not the relevant time scale. Instead, the data can be reset so that the baseline is aligned for each individual, as demonstrated in Figure 6.1 (right panel). In addition to survival time, Figure 6.1 (right panel) also includes a marker for whether the individual had the outcome (marked with an "x") or was censored (marked with a diamond). In this example, there were three individuals who had seizure and five individuals who were censored. Among the five individuals who were censored, we could imagine that two individuals died during the study while they were seizure-free, one individual was lost to follow up, and two individuals were seizure-free at the end of the study.

We can transform Figure 6.1 (right panel) into a table to visualize how the variables are incorporated in the survival analysis (Table 6.2). The key variables are defined as follows:

- **ID**: number used to uniquely identify individuals in the study;
- **Survival time**: the number of months between randomization and an individual having a first seizure or being censored;
- **Censored**: indicator of whether an individual was censored (Censored = 0) or experienced a seizure (Censored = 1) during the study period; and
- **Group**: indicator of treatment assignment as surgical resection (Group = 1) or medical therapy (Group = 0).

To address any underlying differences in the baseline characteristics of the two treatment groups, the investigators also collected data about the following variables:

- **Age at onset**: age when individual developed epilepsy (in years);
- **Seizure type**: indicator of whether the individual has focal to bilateral tonic clonic (Seizure Type = 1) or focal seizures (Seizure Type = 0);
- **Family history**: indicator of whether an individual has a family member with epilepsy (Family History = 1) or not (Family History = 0);

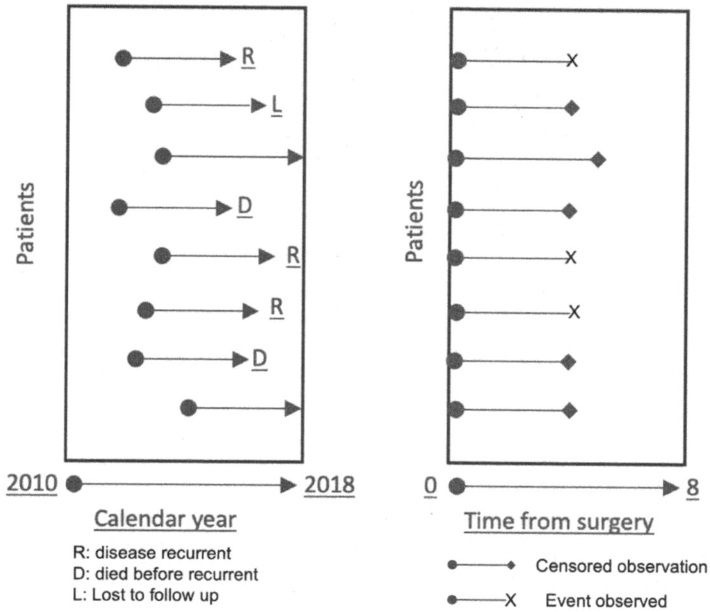


**FIGURE 6.1**
Definition of survival times for eight hypothetical patients in randomized controlled trial can be defined relative to (left panel) calendar time, versus (right panel) time from surgery. (Color version available in electronic supplement.)

- **Age**: age of the patient at the time of enrollment in the study (in years); and
- **Female sex:** indicator of whether the sex of the patient is female (Female Sex = 1) or male (Female Sex = 0).

## 6.4 Basic Quantities of Survival Models

Next, we describe two fundamental quantities in survival analysis, the survival function and hazard function.

### 6.4.1 The Survival Function

Survival data are generally described and modeled in terms of two related quantities, namely the survival function and the hazard function. The survival function is denoted $S(t)$ and describes the probability that an event will occur after a specific point in time. More specifically, let $T$ be a random variable that records the time to the event of interest. The survival function evaluating the probability that the event will have occurred after time $t$ can be written as

$$S(t) = \Pr(T > t),$$

**TABLE 6.2**
Variables used in the survival analysis illustrative example, shown for the first ten patients.

| | Survival outcome | | Baseline covariates | | | | | |
|---|---|---|---|---|---|---|---|---|
| ID | Survival Time | Censored | Group | Age at onset | Seizure type | Family history | Age | Gender |
| 1 | 1 | 1 | 1 | 5 | 0 | 0 | 11 | M |
| 2 | 2 | 1 | 1 | 7 | 0 | 1 | 15 | F |
| 3 | 2 | 1 | 1 | 0.005 | 0 | 0 | 16 | M |
| 4 | 12 | 0 | 0 | 1.5 | 0 | 0 | 4 | F |
| 5 | 12 | 0 | 0 | 0.25 | 0 | 1 | 6 | M |
| 6 | 12 | 0 | 0 | 0.008 | 0 | 0 | 3 | M |
| 7 | 2 | 1 | 1 | 0.5 | 0 | 0 | 15 | M |
| 8 | 12 | 0 | 0 | 0.67 | 1 | 0 | 14 | M |
| 9 | 12 | 0 | 0 | 4.5 | 0 | 0 | 5 | F |
| 10 | 12 | 0 | 0 | 0.5 | 1 | 0 | 6 | M |

The goal of a survival analysis is to describe the survival experience of a cohort by estimating the survival function across all individuals in the population at any given time $t$. For the randomized trial of surgical resection, the survival function describes whether participants remained seizure-free after surgery or randomization at a specified time $t$, and the primary analysis compares the survival probability of those who underwent surgical resection with those who received medical therapy.

### 6.4.2 The Hazard Function

Another important quantity in a survival analysis is the hazard function. The hazard function is denoted as $h(t)$ or $\lambda(t)$. It is an alternative way to describe the distribution of survival time. Intuitively, the hazard function describes whether an individual who is event-free at a given time t experiences the event within an infinitely short period of time after t. It is defined as follows:

$$h(t) = \lim_{\delta \to 0} \frac{\Pr(t < T \leq t + \delta | T \geq t)}{\delta}.$$

Put another way, it represents the rate at which an event is occurring at any given instant in time. Here, we need to emphasize that $h(t)$ is rate and not a probability though it is fundamentally tied to the probability of survival. We can see the relationship between the hazard function and the survival function through a different way of calculating the hazard function:

$$h(t) = -\frac{d\log\{S(t)\}}{dt}.$$

We can also describe the distribution of survival time by the cumulative hazard function $H(t)$, which is an integral of the hazard function over time interval $[0, t]$. The relationship between the cumulative hazard function and the survival function is described as follows:

$$H(t) = -\log\{S(t)\}.$$

This equation demonstrates that the survival function is inversely correlated with the cumulative hazard function, that is the greater probability of survival is associated with lower hazard of the event.

## 6.5 Nonparametric, Semiparametric, and Parametric Survival Models

The survival function can be estimated using different methods depending on what is known, or assumed, about the survival functions. These methods can be classified into nonparametric, semiparametric, and parametric models.

A nonparametric model is directly derived from observed survival time in the data and there are no prespecified parameters about survival or any model covariates. Kaplan-Meier estimation is an example of a nonparametric method. Nonparametric models are robust to model misspecification because they are not making any assumptions about the variables estimating survival. However, the estimates can be more difficult to interpret and parameter estimation is less statistically efficient, which means larger sample sizes are needed to estimate the parameters.

A semiparametric model does not fully specify the distribution of survival but does specify aspects of survival time as well as parameters of any model covariates. A Cox proportional hazards model is an example of a semiparametric model. Semiparametric models are less robust to model misspecification than the nonparametric models, but the estimates are easier to interpret and parameter estimation is more statistically efficient than non-parametric models.

A parametric model fully specifies the distribution of survival. An accelerated failure time model is an example of a parametric model that models survival according to different probability distributions. Parametric models are sensitive to model selection – in other words, the model can lead to biased estimates of survival if the probability distribution is incorrectly specified. However, the model parameters are easy to interpret and efficient to estimate when the model is correctly specified.

## 6.6 Nonparametric Survival Models and the Kaplan-Meier Estimator

The Kaplan-Meier (KM, or product-limit) method [7] is a nonparametric method of determining the probability of survival. It does not impose any assumptions about the distribution of survival and describes the probability of survival by aggregating data from each individual in the study population. Suppose that $N$ patients have events during the follow-up at distinct times $t_1 < t_2 \ldots, < t_N$. The probability of being event free at time $t_j$ is calculated recursively by the following equation

$$\widehat{S}(t_j) = \widehat{S}(t_{j-1}) \left(1 - \frac{d_j}{n_j}\right). \tag{6.1}$$

In this model, the survival at baseline $\widehat{S}(t_0)$ equals 1, $d_j$ is the number of events that occur at time $t_j$, and $n_j$ is the number of individuals at risk right at time $t_j$, that is the number of patients who have not yet experience the event before $t_j$. If no event occurs at time at $t_j$ (regardless of whether censoring occurrs), $d_j$ equals 0 and hence $S(t_j) = S(t_{j-1})$. Therefore, the estimated survival function becomes a step function with one step change every time that an event occurs. When no observations have been censored, this estimator reduces to the ratio of the number of individuals who are event-free at time t divided by the number of individuals who entered the study.

The variation of the KM estimator can often estimated by the Greenwood's formula [4] as follows

$$\widehat{\text{var}}\{\widehat{S}(t)\} = \{\widehat{S}(t)\}^2 \sum_{t_j \le t} \frac{d_j}{n_j(n_j - d_j)}. \tag{6.2}$$

Based on the variation estimator, we construct the $(1-\alpha)\%$ confidence interval for the survival function as

$$\left[\widehat{S}(t) - z_{1-\alpha/2}\sqrt{\widehat{\text{var}}\{\widehat{S}(t)\}}, \widehat{S}(t) + z_{1-\alpha/2}\sqrt{\widehat{\text{var}}\{\widehat{S}(t)\}}\right],$$

where $z_{1-\alpha/2}$ is the $(1-\alpha/2)100\%$ quantile of the standard normal distribution. When $\alpha = 0.05$, $z_{1-\alpha/2}$ is approximately 1.96.

### 6.6.1 Construct Kaplan-Meier Estimator Using R

We can use the R package `survival` [13] to provide an example of KM estimation using data from all participants in the randomized trial of surgical resection [3]. We also use R packages `survminer` [8] and `ggplot2` [14] to create graphs of the estimated survival curves. To construct the KM estimator, take the following steps:

Step 1. Load `survival`, `survminer`, and `ggplot2` packages into R session.

Step 2. Construct the KM estimator for the two treatment groups separately.

Step 3. Summarize the estimated results.

```
# Load packages
library(survival)
library(ggplot2)
library(survminer)

# Estimate the survival function
fits <- survfit(Surv(survtime, censor) ~ Group, data = Dsurv)

# Summarize result
> summary(fits)

                Group=0
 time n.risk n.event survival std.err lower 95% CI upper 95% CI
    1     59      48   0.1864  0.0507      0.10941        0.318
    2     11       6   0.0847  0.0363      0.03664        0.196
    3      5       2   0.0508  0.0286      0.01688        0.153
    6      3       2   0.0169  0.0168      0.00243        0.118

                Group=1
 time n.risk n.event survival std.err lower 95% CI upper 95% CI
    1     57       6    0.895  0.0406        0.819        0.978
    2     51       1    0.877  0.0435        0.796        0.967
    3     50       1    0.860  0.0460        0.774        0.955
    4     49       2    0.825  0.0504        0.732        0.929
    5     47       2    0.789  0.0540        0.690        0.903
    8     45       1    0.772  0.0556        0.670        0.889
```

In the above R script, we use `survfit()` to construct the estimator of the survival function among those who received medical therapy (Group = 0) and those who underwent

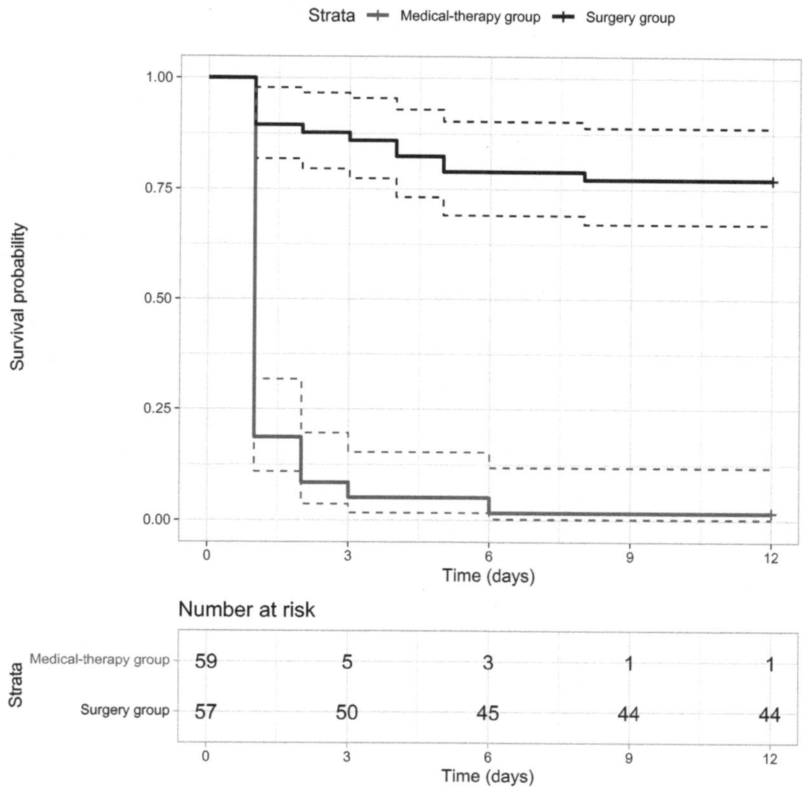


**FIGURE 6.2**
Kaplan-Meier curves describing the probability of seizure freedom with surgical resection (black line) and medical therapy (gray line). The solid lines are the calculated estimates and the dashed lines are the associated 95% confidence intervals.

surgical resection (Group = 1). We use the `summary()` function to print out the estimated results as two tables. Each row indicates the month (`time`), the number of individuals who are seizure free and thus are at risk of the primary outcome (`n.risk`), the number of individuals who had a breakthrough seizure during that month (`n.event`), the survival function (`survival`), the standard error of the survival function (`std.err`) and the 95% confidence interval of the survival function (`lower 95% CI`, `upper 95% CI`). Of note, these tables only include a row for each month a seizure occurred (because the survival probability does not change during the months where all individuals remain event-free).

The function `ggsurvplot()` plots a KM curve to visualize the survival function and summarize the estimated result. The argument `risk.table = T` is included so that the output includes a risk table at the bottom of the graph to communicate the number of individuals at risk at each time point. This allows readers to determine whether the number at risk is decreasing due to seizure occurrence or censoring.

```
ggsurv <- ggsurvplot(fits , data= Dsurv, conf.int =TRUE, risk.table =T,  ggtheme =
     theme_light(), pval = F, conf.int.style = "step", legend.lab = c('Medical-
    therapy group', 'Surgery group'), palette= gray(seq(0.5, 0, len = 2)), xlab =
    'Time (days)')
print(ggsurv)
```

The KM curves (Figure 6.2) illustrate that the probability of seizure freedom differs between those who underwent surgical resection and those who received medical therapy. Because the survival estimates and associated 95% confidence intervals are always higher among those who underwent surgical resection, we conclude that surgical resection leads to a higher probability of seizure freedom than medical therapy.

### 6.6.2 Comparing Survival Using the Log-Rank Test

KM curves do not provide a test to determine whether differences visualized in the graph are statistically significant. The log-rank test [12] is the most widely used statistic to determine whether those graphical differences in survival reach statistical significance. The log-rank test is typically used to accompany KM curves because it similarly does not make assumptions about the underlying distribution of the outcome.

The log-rank test is testing the null hypothesis that there is no difference in the probability of survival between two or more groups. Suppose there are different groups of individuals who are event-free at time $t_i$. We calculate the observed number of events that occur during time $t_i$ in each group and the expected number of events that occur during time $t_i$ assuming there is no difference in the probability of survival between groups (the null hypothesis). We then sum the observed and expected number of events that occur over the entire study period for each group separately and use a chi-square distribution to compare the difference. Let $O_i$ be the total observed events, $E_i$ be the total expected events, and $g$ be the number of groups. The test statistics used in the log-rank test is described by the following equation:

$$\chi^2 = \sum_{i=1}^{g} \frac{(O_i - E_i)^2}{E_i}.$$

Let $\chi^2_{1-\alpha}(g-1)$ be the $(1-\alpha)100\%$ quantile of a chi-square distribution with $g-1$ degrees of freedom and $\alpha$ be the nominal Type I error. If $\chi^2 > \chi^2_{1-\alpha}(g-1)$, we reject the null hypothesis and conclude there is a statistically significant difference in the probability of survival across groups.

### 6.6.3 Performing the Log-Rank Test Using R

We can implement the log-rank test in R using the function `survdiff()` from the `survival` library. We can use data from the randomized trial and examine differences in the probability of seizure freedom between the two intervention groups. The output includes the observed and expected number of events as well as the resulting $\chi^2$ statistic. In this example, $\chi^2 = 93.3$, which follows a chi-square distribution with one degree of freedom, and the associated p-value is $< 2e-16$, which is smaller than 0.05 allowing us to conclude that the difference in probability of seizure freedom between those who underwent surgical resection and received medical therapy is statistically significant.

```
surv_diff <- survdiff(Surv(survtime, censor) ~ Group, data = Dsurv)

> print(surv_diff)

         N Observed Expected (O-E)^2/E (O-E)^2/V
Group=0 59       58     29.4      27.9      93.3
Group=1 57       13     41.6      19.7      93.3

 Chisq= 93.3  on 1 degrees of freedom, p= <2e-16
```

## 6.7 Semiparametric and Parametric Survival Models

We discussed KM estimators and the log-rank test considering only one independent variable, the intervention group. However, it is common to have multiple variables influencing survival. For example, the randomized trial of [3] considered age at epilepsy onset, seizure type, family history of epilepsy, age at randomization, and sex as variables that influence seizure freedom and excluding these variables from the model may introduce bias if they are not equally balanced across the two intervention groups. Semiparametric and parametric methods for estimating survival are useful in these scenarios because they provide an opportunity to incorporate covariates into the model. Furthermore, the log-rank test only determines whether the probability of survival is different between groups. These additional methods help to quantify that difference and indicate which group has a higher versus lower probability of survival function. In this section, we will describe the most widely used semiparametric and parametric methods to examine survival. For all models described in this section, we assume observations are independent of each other, censoring occurs solely as right-censoring, censoring is uninformative, covariates are present at baseline, and covariates are time-independent. Comprehensive discussions on the models that do not satisfy the above assumptions can be found in [9].

### 6.7.1 Cox Proportional Hazard Regression Model

The Cox proportional hazard (PH) model [2] is a common regression model used to estimate survival in the context of more than one independent variable. It is a semiparametric model because the independent variables have known parameters but survival, the outcome, does not follow a known distribution. The model incorporates the baseline hazard function when all covariates are zeros $h_0(t)$ which is the nonparametric component of the model and a p-dimensional covariate vector $x = (x_1, ..., x_p)$ in which each covariate is associated with a parameter $(\beta_1 \ldots, \beta_p)$ that explains the effect of $x$ on the hazard of the event. The model is described by the following equation:

$$h(t, \mathbf{x}) = h_0(t)\exp(\beta_1 x_1 + \beta_2 x_2, \ldots, +\beta_p x_p).$$

One key assumption of the Cox model is that survival curves of different strata have hazard functions that are proportional over the time. Suppose we have a Cox model with one independent variable specifying treatment assignment and no additional covariates which can be described as follows:

$$h(t, \mathbf{x}) = h_0(t)\exp(\beta_0 + \beta x)$$

Using the randomized trial as an example, the variable $x$ could indicate randomization to medical therapy ($x = 0$) or surgical resection ($x = 1$). Under the proportional hazards assumption, the hazard functions describing survival in the two groups are proportional. Unlike a typical regression model, the regression function does not contain a consistent intercept term. The intercept term in a Cox model is $log\{h_0(t)\}$, which varies over time. The model is primarily used to compare the hazard rate of an event between two groups. The output of a Cox model is $\exp(\beta)$, which is the hazard ratio and defined as the hazard of one group divided by the hazard of the other group.

### 6.7.2 Fitting a Cox Proportional Hazards Model Using R

We can implement the Cox model using data from the randomized trial and the `coxph()` function in R. First, we use the `coxph()` function to estimate the hazard function for those randomized to medical therapy ($x = 0$) and those randomized to surgical resection ($x = 1$) without considering covariates.

```
coxfits <- coxph(Surv(survtime, censor) ~ Group, data = Dsurv)

> summary(coxfits)

  n= 116, number of events= 71

          coef exp(coef) se(coef)      z Pr(>|z|)
Group -2.70845   0.06664  0.33549 -8.073 6.86e-16 ***
---

      exp(coef) exp(-coef) lower .95 upper .95
Group   0.06664      15.01   0.03453    0.1286

Concordance= 0.837  (se = 0.025 )
Likelihood ratio test= 90.15  on 1 df,   p=<2e-16
Wald test            = 65.17  on 1 df,   p=7e-16
Score (logrank) test = 94.04  on 1 df,   p=<2e-16
```

The first portion of the output includes the estimator for the effect of surgical resection on the hazard of seizure (`coef`), the hazard ratio for surgical resection (`exp(coef)`), the standard error of the effect estimator (`se(coef)`), the normalized effect estimator (`z`), and the p-value testing whether the effect of treatment is nonzero (`Pr(>z)`).

The second portion of the output indicates the hazard ratio for surgical resection (hazard of group 1 divided by the hazard of group 0 (`exp(coef)`), the hazard ratio for medical therapy (the inverse of hazard ratio for surgical resection (`exp(-coef)`), and the 95% confidence interval of the hazard ratio for surgical resection (`lower .95`, `upper .95`). If the 95% confidence interval includes one then the hazards are considered equivalent and we cannot reject the null hypothesis. If the 95% confidence interval does not include one then the difference in hazards reach statistical significance and we can reject the null hypothesis at the 0.05 significance level. If the exposure is a continuous as opposed to dichotomous variable, then the hazard ratio describes the relative hazard of a one-unit change in the exposure. In this example, the estimated hazard ratio of 0.067 is less than one and the 95% confidence interval does not include one; thus, we can conclude that those who underwent surgical resection had lower hazard of seizure recurrence than those who received medical therapy.

The third portion of the output indicates the concordance, the likelihood ratio test, the Wald test, and the score test. Concordance quantifies the accuracy of the Cox model in predicting survival. A higher value indicates better performance of the model. The likelihood ratio test, Wald test, and score test determine whether the proposed model fits the data better than the null model in which all coefficients are set to zero.

Next, we will fit a multivariable Cox model in which there are multiple covariates in addition to treatment status, and add baseline covariates to the above model to evaluate the effect of surgical resection on seizure freedom after adjustment for other variables.

```
coxcovfits <- coxph(Surv(survtime, censor) ~ Group + Age + Gender + Diag+
    Family_hist, data = Dsurv)

> summary(coxcovfits)

  n= 116, number of events= 71
```

```
                 coef exp(coef) se(coef)      z Pr(>|z|)
Group        -2.64315   0.07114  0.33642 -7.857 3.94e-15 ***
Age           0.03541   1.03605  0.02994  1.183   0.2369
Gender       -0.09338   0.91085  0.26343 -0.354   0.7230
Diag          0.64308   1.90233  0.26032  2.470   0.0135 *
Family_hist -0.02383   0.97645  0.43808 -0.054   0.9566
---
```

The estimated hazard ratio of 0.071 continues to be less than one after adjustment, which reinforces the conclusion that surgical resection leads to lower hazard of seizure recurrence and higher probability of seizure freedom over time. The output also includes the effect of each covariate on seizure freedom and indicates that seizure type is also associated with the hazard of seizure. Those with focal to bilateral tonic clonic seizures have higher hazard of seizure than those with focal seizures.

### 6.7.3 Testing the Proportional Hazards Assumption Using R

The Cox model relies on the proportional hazards assumption and it is important to test whether this assumption holds. This can be done by using `cox.zph()`, which checks the proportionality assumption using Schoenfeld residuals against transformed time:

```
testcov.ph <- cox.zph(coxcovfits)

> testcov.ph
                chisq df    p
Group        0.000127  1 0.99
Age          2.536964  1 0.11
Gender       0.091886  1 0.76
Diag         0.349206  1 0.55
Family_hist 0.090737  1 0.76
GLOBAL       4.561780  5 0.47
```

The p-values for all covariates and the model (`GLOBAL`) are large, which suggest that the proportional hazard assumption holds and the effect estimators are valid in our analysis. In contrast, a function that had resulted in small p-values would have suggested time-dependent coefficients and potential violation of the proportional hazards assumption, which could threaten the validity of results from the Cox model.

### 6.7.4 Accelerated Failure Time Model

Survival curves derived from KM estimation and Cox models are useful for comparing survival that is observed during a defined study period. However, these methods do not draw conclusions about survival that falls beyond the follow up period. This is where parametric survival models are useful. The term parametric implies the model specifies a distribution, or parameter, for the survival function and any covariates.

An accelerated failure time (AFT) model is a parametric survival model frequently used for survival analysis. One key assumption of an AFT model is that the effect of a covariate is to accelerate or decelerate the life course of a disease by some constant. The standard AFT model estimates the logarithm of survival time $T$ as follows:

$$\log(T) = \beta_0 + \beta_1 x_1 + \beta_2 x_2, \ldots, +\beta_p x_p + \epsilon. \tag{6.3}$$

In Eq. (6.3), there is a random error $\epsilon$ that quantifies the variability in $\log(T)$ that is not explained by $\beta_0+\beta_1 x_1+\beta_2 x_2, \ldots, +\beta_p x_p$. The distribution of the survival curve is specifying the relationship between $\epsilon$ and $T$. In other words, for any given $\epsilon$, there is a corresponding distribution for $T$. The coefficient for each covariate estimates the effect of the variable on survival time and the exponentiated coefficients are defined as time ratios. We can transform the above equation to demonstrate how an AFT model is estimating survival as a function of the baseline survival function multiplied by an acceleration factor. Let $T_0 = \exp(\epsilon)$, we can easily see that

$$T = \exp(\beta_0 + \beta_1 x_1 + \beta_2 x_2, \ldots, +\beta_p x_p)T_0,$$

and therefore,

$$\begin{aligned} S(t) &= \Pr(T > t) \\ &= \Pr\left[T_0 > \exp\{-(\beta_0 + \beta_1 x_1 + \beta_2 x_2, \ldots, +\beta_p x_p)\}t\right] \\ &= S_0(\psi t), \end{aligned}$$

where $S_0$ is the survival function for $T_0$, namely the baseline survival function, and $\psi \equiv \exp\left\{-(\beta_0 + \beta_1 x_1 + \beta_2 x_2, \ldots, +\beta_p x_p)\right\}$ is an "acceleration factor". Here the exponentiated coefficients, $\exp(\beta_j)$'s, are referred to as time ratios. A coefficient $\beta_j > 0$ or the time ratio $\exp(\beta_j) > 1$ for the $j$th covariate implies that increasing the value of $x_j$ will increase the probability of survival, and accordingly "decelerate" the rate of the event and prolong the time to event. Conversely, a time ratio $\exp(\beta_j) < 1$ implies that increasing the value of $x_j$ will decrease the probability of survival, "accelerate" the rate of the event, and shorten the time to event.

Three common probability distributions used to model survival are exponential, Weibull, and log-normal distributions. Exponential distributions are used to describe a scenario where the hazard of survival is constant over time. Weibull and log-normal distributions can be adjusted to describe multiple different probability distributions and are useful for providing this flexibility. $T$ is often specified with a Weibull distribution when $\epsilon$ has an extreme value distribution while $T$ is often specified with a log-normal distribution when $\epsilon$ follows a normal distribution. Figure 6.3 displays the hazard functions and the survival functions from different parametric models. We can see that the exponential distribution often gives a constant hazard function and the log-normal distribution yields a decreasing hazard, while the Weibull distribution can have both increasing and decreasing hazards by choosing different model parameters.

AFT models are useful for multiple reasons. They provide information about survival beyond the observed follow up period. They are more statistically efficient than a Cox model because they are fully parametric and there is less variation in the estimates. They do not assume proportional hazards so can be used when data are in violation of this assumption. Furthermore, when survival follows a Weibull distribution, AFT models also satisfy the proportional hazards assumption. Therefore, parameters of an AFT model that follow a Weibull distribution can be interpreted as hazard ratios or time ratios, a property that does not hold true for other distributions.

In practice, however, it can be difficult to identify an appropriate distribution for the data. It is important to recognize that failing to do so can threaten the validity of the model and result in biased survival estimates.

### 6.7.5 Fitting an Accelerated Failure Time Model Using R

We can implement an AFT model in `R` using data from the randomized trial and the `survreg()` function. We first fit an AFT model that follows a log-normal distribution and has treatment assignment as the only independent variable.

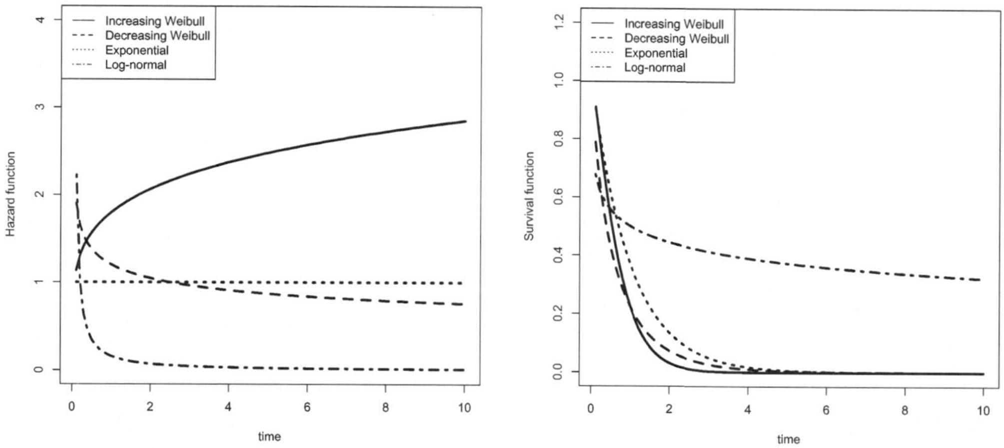


**FIGURE 6.3**
(Left panel) Hazard function and (right panel) survival function under different parametric models.

```
regfits <- survreg(Surv(survtime, censor) ~ Group, data = Dsurv,
  dist = 'lognormal')

> summary(regfits)

               Value Std. Error      z       p
(Intercept)   0.2163     0.1287   1.68   0.093
Group         2.5792     0.2216  11.64  <2e-16
Log(scale)   -0.0121     0.0913  -0.13   0.895

Scale= 0.988

Log Normal distribution
Loglik(model)= -146.2   Loglik(intercept only)= -201.7
  Chisq= 110.92 on 1 degrees of freedom, p= 6.2e-26
Number of Newton-Raphson Iterations: 6
n= 116
```

The output includes a value quantifying the effect of surgical resection on seizure freedom, the coefficient 2.58, which is positive and has an associated p-value $< 2e - 16$ allowing us to reject the null hypothesis and conclude that surgical resection leads to a higher probability of seizure freedom. The output also includes the logarithm of the scale parameter in the log-normal distribution (`Log(scale)`), which describes the variability in $\log(T_0)$, and the estimated scale parameter (0.988). `Loglik(model)` is the log-likelihood of the fully parameterized AFT model, while `Loglik(intercept only)` is the log-likelihood of the null model when $\beta_1 =, \ldots, = \beta_p = 0$. The last p-value of $6.2 \times 10^{-26}$ is comparing the fit of these two models and the low value indicates the full model fits the data significantly better than the null model.

Next, we will fit a multivariable AFT model and add baseline covariates to the above model to evaluate the effect of surgical resection on seizure freedom after adjusting for baseline covariates:

```
regcovfits <- survreg(Surv(survtime, censor) ~ Group + Age + Gender + Diag +
    Family_hist, data = Dsurv, dist = 'lognormal')

> summary(regcovfits)

               Value Std. Error      z        p
(Intercept)  0.7393     0.2826  2.62  0.0089
Group        2.5513     0.2119 12.04 < 2e-16
Age         -0.0331     0.0227 -1.46  0.1453
Gender       0.0106      0.2002  0.05  0.9579
Diag        -0.8475     0.2079 -4.08 4.6e-05
Family_hist  0.1594     0.3554  0.45  0.6538
Log(scale)  -0.1000     0.0904 -1.11  0.2684

Scale= 0.905

Log Normal distribution
Loglik(model)= -136.6   Loglik(intercept only)= -201.7
  Chisq= 130.1 on 5 degrees of freedom, p= 2.3e-26
Number of Newton-Raphson Iterations: 6
n= 116
```

The output recapitulates findings from the KM curve, Cox models, and AFT models above. Surgical resection leads to improved seizure freedom with a value of 2.55 and corresponding p-value $< 0.05$, and focal to bilateral tonic clonic (as opposed to focal) seizures are associated with decreased seizure freedom.

### 6.7.6 Comparing Survival Distributions for an Accelerated Failure Time Model

Selecting the appropriate distribution to describe survival is crucial for fitting a valid AFT model. A misspecified model can lead to biased results, and incorrect conclusions. Deviance residual plots are a useful graphical tool to compare models specifying different distributions. When a selected model matches the true distribution of the data, the deviance residuals will vary evenly around zero. When a selected model does not match the distribution of the data, the deviance residuals will move away from zero.

We can compare the fit of a log-normal and Weilbull distribution for the randomized trial data using the `residuals()` function from `survival` library:

```
# Log-normal AFT model
regcovfits <- survreg(Surv(survtime, censor) ~ Group + Age + Gender + Diag +
    Family_hist, data = Dsurv, dist = 'lognormal')
plot(residuals(regcovfits, method = 'deviance'), ylab = 'Deviance')

# Weibull AFT model
wregcovfits <- survreg(Surv(survtime, censor) ~ Group + Age + Gender + Diag +
    Family_hist, data = Dsurv, dist = 'weibull')
plot(residuals(wregcovfits, method = 'deviance'), ylab = 'Deviance')
```

The output includes two graphs which plot the deviance residuals from the fitted results. The plots demonstrate that the deviance residuals from the log-normal model are more evenly distributed and closer to zero than the deviance residuals from the Weibull model. This confirms that the log-normal distribution is a better fit than the Weibull distribution for modeling seizure freedom in this study population (Figure 6.4).

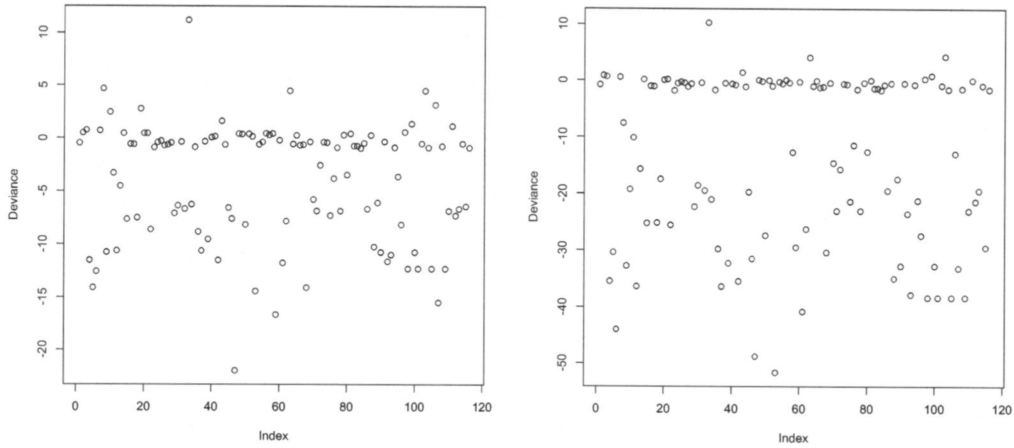


**FIGURE 6.4**
(Left panel) Deviance residuals from the log-normal model. (Right panel) Deviance residuals for the Weibull model. The x-axes in the figures are the subject indices.

## 6.8 Summary

Survival analysis is an important tool for any research question that intends to estimate the rate of an event in different populations. The methods discussed in this chapter can be used to estimate the probability of seizure freedom, hospital readmission, or death taking nonparametric, semiparametric, and fully parametric approaches. Each of these approaches have important strengths and limitations. For additional statistical methods in survival analysis, such as censored quantile regressions and trasnformation models, we point the reader to further reading resources [5, 6, 10, 11, 15, 16].

## Bibliography


[1] Leila DAF Amorim and Jianwen Cai. Modelling recurrent events: a tutorial for analysis in epidemiology. *International Journal of Epidemiology*, 44(1):324–333, 2015.

[2] David R Cox. Regression models and life-tables. *Journal of the Royal Statistical Society: Series B (Methodological)*, 34(2):187–202, 1972.

[3] Rekha Dwivedi, Bhargavi Ramanujam, P Sarat Chandra, Savita Sapra, Sheffali Gulati, Mani Kalaivani, Ajay Garg, Chandra S Bal, Madhavi Tripathi, Sada N Dwivedi, et al. Surgery for drug-resistant epilepsy in children. *New England Journal of Medicine*, 377(17):1639–1647, 2017.

[4] Major Greenwood et al. A report on the natural duration of cancer *A Report on the Natural Duration of Cancer*, 88(7), 1926.

[5] Fei Jiang, Qing Cheng, Guosheng Yin, and Haipeng Shen. Functional censored quantile regression. *Journal of the American Statistical Association*, 115(530):931–944, 2020.

[6] Fei Jiang and Sebastien Haneuse. A semi-parametric transformation frailty model for semi-competing risks survival data. *Scandinavian Journal of Statistics*, 44(1):112–129, 2017.

[7] Edward L Kaplan and Paul Meier. Nonparametric estimation from incomplete observations. *Journal of the American Statistical Association*, 53(282):457–481, 1958.

[8] Alboukadel Kassambara, Marcin Kosinski, Przemyslaw Biecek, and S Fabian. Package 'survminer'. *Drawing Survival Curves using 'ggplot2'(R package version 03 1)*, 2017.

[9] John P Klein and Melvin L Moeschberger. *Survival Analysis: Techniques for Censored and Truncated Data*, volume 1230. Springer, 2003.

[10] Roger Koenker and Olga Geling. Reappraising medfly longevity: a quantile regression survival analysis. *Journal of the American Statistical Association*, 96(454):458–468, 2001.

[11] Limin Peng and Yijian Huang. Survival analysis with quantile regression models. *Journal of the American Statistical Association*, 103(482):637–649, 2008.

[12] Richard Peto, MCetal Pike, Philip Armitage, Norman E Breslow, DR Cox, SV Howard, N Mantel, K McPherson, J Peto, and PG Smith. Design and analysis of randomized clinical trials requiring prolonged observation of each patient. ii. analysis and examples. *British Journal of Cancer*, 35(1):1–39, 1977.

[13] Terry M Therneau and Thomas Lumley. Package 'survival'. *R Top Doc*, 128(10):28–33, 2015.

[14] Hadley Wickham, Winston Chang, and Maintainer Hadley Wickham. Package 'ggplot2'. *Create elegant data visualisations using the grammar of graphics. Version*, 2(1):1–189, 2016.

[15] Donglin Zeng and DY Lin. Maximum likelihood estimation in semiparametric regression models with censored data. *Journal of the Royal Statistical Society: Series B (Statistical Methodology)*, 69(4):507–564, 2007.

[16] Donglin Zeng and DY Lin. Semiparametric transformation models with random effects for joint analysis of recurrent and terminal events. *Biometrics*, 65(3):746–752, 2009.

# 7

# *Graph and Network Control Theoretic Frameworks*

**Ankit N. Khambhati**

*Department of Neurological Surgery, University of California, San Francisco (USA)*

**Sharon Chiang**

*Department of Neurology, University of California, San Francisco (USA)*

## CONTENTS



This chapter provides an overview of network and graph estimation in epilepsy. We start by conceptualizing the notion of a graph and its role in the analysis of neural signals. We present a framework for intuiting and defining nodes and edges for various data sources commonly encountered in the field. We discuss the distinction between undirected and directed graphs and provide a brief overview of common methods used for their estimation, including correlation and coherence measures, Gaussian graphical models, Poisson graphical models, Bayesian networks, and sparse methods for graph estimation. We then turn to an overview of graph theory and measures for quantifying graph topological properties, followed by a discussion of graph dynamics and perturbation of network topology. Examples are provided along with sample data in a Python-based Jupyter notebook available in the repository that accompanies this book. This chapter demonstrates how a practitioner can employ network estimation and graph theoretic tools to study the architecture of the epileptic network.

DOI: 10.1201/9781003254515-7

## 7.1 What Is a Graph and Why Use It?

Conventional diagnosis of epilepsy aims to delineate abnormal brain *tissue* that impacts normal brain function and drive seizures, yet the notion of labeling epilepsy as a disorder of brain *networks* is clouded and generic [48]. What constellation of brain structures precipitate a seizure? How might a seizure in one area of the brain disrupt normal function in another part of the brain? Which brain areas project, or feed, into the seizure focus? How are these processes expressed across biological scales of single neurons, neuronal populations, and gross functional brain systems? Though definitive answers to these questions remain elusive, they are unified by the common goal to describe how different areas of the epileptic brain are structurally or functionally related over one or more instances in time [66].

Measurements drawn from different points of interconnected and dynamic systems, such as those derived from neuroimaging or electrophysiology studies of the brain, are inherently relational. For instance, measurements at points made in close spatial proximity may sample overlapping populations of neurons and measurements at points separated by longer spatial distances could be linked by white-matter connections that run between them. Beyond relationships in space, measurements from neural systems also exhibit interdependence in time. Measurements from a single brain area at nearby points in time are more likely to reflect one state of the system, such as wakefulness, and measurements at a later point in time may reflect an entirely different state, such as sleep. Whether the individual measurements for a neuroscience experiment span a spatial axis, a time axis, or both, these data points are drawn from complex interconnected systems that typically defy assumptions of statistical independence.

*Graph theory* provides a mathematical language for describing relationships between data points through a mathematical object called a graph, $G$. A point, or *node*, on the graph refers to a fundamental unit in the neural system, such as a single neuron or a single brain region and is represented by $v$. Any two nodes, $v_i$ and $v_j$, in $G$ may be linked by an *edge*, which encodes a context-dependent association between them – such as a direct anatomical connection, an indirect functional interaction, or possibly the similarity in their respective gene expression pattern – and is represented by $e_{ij}$. Collectively, the $N$ number of nodes of a graph make up a set $V$, where $V = \{v_1, v_2, \ldots, v_N\}$, and the pattern of $N^2$ possible edges spanning the $N$ nodes make up a set $E$. Accordingly, a graph that reflects a single context of the relationships present in the system is defined as $G = (V, E)$. An alternate mathematical representation of the graph that does not rely on set notation is the *adjacency matrix* $A$, which has a square shape with dimensions $N$x$N$ and in which the entry $a_{ij}$ corresponds to the edge $e_{ij}$ that connects node $i$ ($v_i$) with node $j$ ($v_j$). The adjacency matrix may also be unraveled into its *edge vector* representation which has a single column and $N^2$ rows. For the remainder of this chapter, we will refer to the graph in terms of its adjacency matrix and edge vector representations.

A graph representation of the neural system is a mathematical abstraction or model of brain anatomy and its inter-regional communication (Figure 7.1). As a mathematical object, a bevy of tools may be used to analyze the organization of a brain graph [14] and those tools remain largely agnostic to the biological processes reflected by the graph's nodes and edges. This marriage between graph theory and neuroscience opens a new frontier of network neuroscience for neural circuit analysis that allows the researchers to understand how organized patterns of interconnections shape neural dynamics, brain function, and behavior [5].

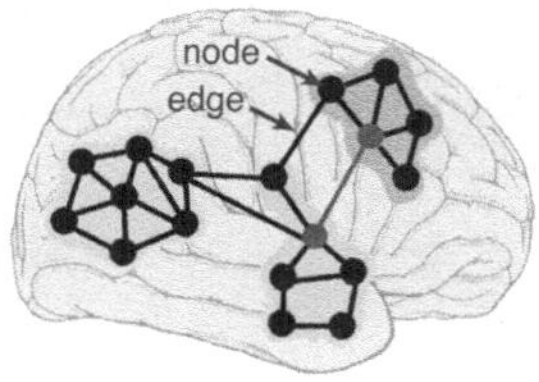


**FIGURE 7.1**
Graph representation of brain network connectivity. Nodes (dark circles) sample various brain regions and edges (dark lines) reflect structural or functional connections between nodes. (Color version available in electronic supplement.)

### 7.1.1 Graphical Abstraction of the Brain Network

You have in hand a neural data set with rich spatial or temporal structure; how do you next model that data using a graph (Figure 7.2)? A primary objective is to frame the graphical model in terms of the scientific question at hand [7]. First, consider what the graph nodes represent, such as individual microelectrode sensors recording action potentials, macroelectrode sensors recording local field potentials, or fMRI voxels recording BOLD signal. In some cases sensor or voxel data might be inverted to recover discrete, underlying neural sources or aggregated into more coarse regions-of-interest (ROIs) defined by an anatomical or functional brain atlas; in either case, the resulting neural sources or ROIs could also serve as nodes in the graph model.

With the graph nodes defined, our attention turns to defining the graph edges. Imaging modality of the source data will constrain how the edges are defined [15]. Anatomical neuroimaging modalities, such as magnetic resonance imaging (MRI) or diffusion tensor imaging (DTI), enable the construction of a *structural graph*. These graphs may indicate the presence or absence of physical connections in the brain, such as white-matter fibers, axonal projections, or synaptic junctions. In contrast, functional neuroimaging and electrophysiology modalities, such as functional MRI (fMRI), electroencephalography (EEG), electrocorticography (ECoG), or magnetoencephalography (MEG), are used to measure *functional graphs*. While a structural network maps the possible paths that signals *could* travel, a functional network provides a momentary glimpse into which paths were actually traversed by the signal [64]. A functional graph projects the physical links between nodes in the brain network as a shadow-on-the-wall through correlated or synchronized signal fluctuations across network nodes. Thus, functional graphs tend to encode time-dependent communication patterns across the network.

## 7.2 Undirected Graphs

Graph representations of structural and functional edges are built using specialized mathematical tools. Structural and functional edges imply that interconnected brain regions are co-mingled in their interactions within the brain circuit. Structural and functional edges are *undirected*, such that the presence of edge $e_{ij}$ linking node $v_i$ to node $v_j$ necessarily implies the presence of a symmetrically positioned edge $e_{ji}$ linking node $v_j$ to node $v_i$. An undirected graph results in a symmetric adjacency matrix where $A = A^T$. Without loss of generality, how do we measure the presence of edge $e_{ij}$?

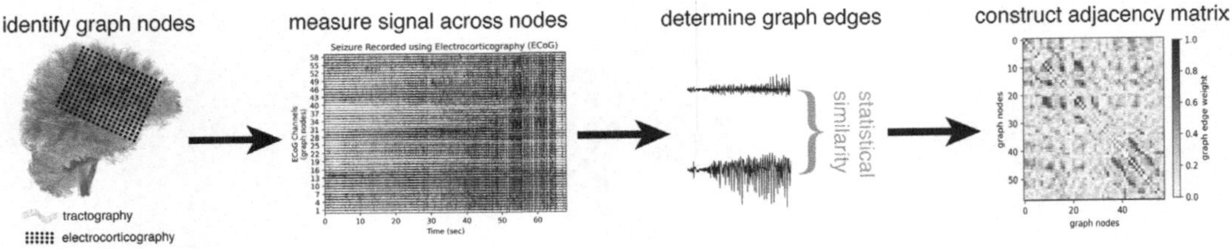


**FIGURE 7.2**
Methodological pipeline for constructing a graph model of the brain network. Schematic depicts functional graph modeling of the seizure network for a patient with drug-resistant epilepsy undergoing electrocorticographic monitoring. A graph node is a single ECoG sensor and a graph edge is the amount of statistical similarity of signal fluctuations recorded between each pair of graph nodes. (Color version available in electronic supplement.)

There exists no single correct way to estimate links between brain regions [5]. Suppose for example if one wished to construct a graph relating various fruits and one node was an apple and another node were a pear; one might draw an edge linking the two fruits on the basis of their shared oval shape, their tendency to harbor seeds, or their color. Yet, one might not be able to draw an edge between the fruits on the basis of flavor. A broad variety of features may be used to describe the relationship between the two fruits; similarly, a vast library of statistical metrics may be used to identify physiologically relevant features from structural or functional data and compare those features between brain regions.

### 7.2.1 Correlational Models

How does one translate the measurement samples or features derived from two graph nodes into an edge? The answer lies in the notion that the edge represents the relationship or likelihood that the measurement samples between the two nodes are meaningfully linked. A similarity statistic may be calculated to discern the extent to which measurement samples obtained from node $v_i$ are linked to samples obtained from node $v_j$. A naive index for $e_{ij}$ might be the number of times a specific item appears in a list of repeated measurement samples at $v_i$ and at $v_j$. A more rational method uses the *Jaccard Index* [33], defined as

$$J_{v_i v_j} = \frac{|v_i \cap v_j|}{|v_i \cup v_j|}, \tag{7.1}$$

and quantifies the similarity between sample sets observed at $v_i$ and $v_j$ as the ratio between the number of unique sample items found in both sets and the unique number of sample items aggregated across both sets. This and other more complex bag-of-words methods are effective for quantifying similarity in categorical data where nodal measurements are discrete items and are sampled in arbitrary order.

**Similarity in the Time Domain:** Sample order is a defining feature of sequential data, such as a time-series, and must be considered when measuring a graph edge. For sequential measurements, such as a raster of action potential firing, *correlational* methods quantify the intersection between ordered lists by assessing their item-wise overlap. One interpretation of a correlation is that it summarizes the statistical interaction effect between two random variables. Pearson correlation coefficient is among the most well-known correlation metrics and is an aggregate measure of the normalized pairwise product between two ordered lists, defined as

$$r_{v_i v_j} = \frac{\sum_{t=1}^{T}(v_i(t) - \overline{v_i})(v_j(t) - \overline{v_j})}{\sqrt{\sum_{t=1}^{T}(v_i(t) - \overline{v_i})}^2 \sqrt{\sum_{t=1}^{T}(v_j(t) - \overline{v_j})}^2}, \tag{7.2}$$

where $t$ indexes each observed sample in the ordered list, $T$ refers to a window size over which the metric is computed, and $\overline{v}$ corresponds to the mean sample value at node $v$. Graph edges based on the Pearson correlation reflects the co-variation (or co-variance) between measurements at nodes $v_i$ and $v_j$ normalized by the product of their respective standard deviations $\sigma_{v_i}$ and $\sigma_{v_j}$ or more compactly

$$r_{v_i v_j} = \frac{\text{cov}(v_i, v_j)}{\sigma_{v_i}\sigma_{v_j}}. \tag{7.3}$$

Correlation values closer to 1, −1, or 0 indicate strong positive, negative, or lack of linear relationship between measurements at nodes $v_i$ and $v_j$, respectively. Yet, this approach assumes that interactions between nodes occur instantaneously – with zero lag or zero time-delay. The cross-correlation function overcomes this limitation by measuring delayed interactions between nodes and is defined as

$$r_{v_i v_j}(\tau) = \frac{\sum_{t=1}^{T}(v_i(t) - \overline{v_i})(v_j(t+\tau) - \overline{v_j})}{\sqrt{\sum_{t=1}^{T}(v_i(t) - \overline{v_i})}^2 \sqrt{\sum_{t=1}^{T}(v_j(t) - \overline{v_j})}^2}, \tag{7.4}$$

which shifts the measurement samples at one node with respect to the other by a lag $\tau$ and computes the correlation, $r_{v_i v_j}(\tau)$, between the shifted data and the unshifted data. Note that the cross-correlation function generalizes to the Pearson correlation metric when $\tau = 0$. The magnitude, sign, and lag of the correlation values can impact the functional interpretation of an inferred edge, but we leave this as a thought exercise to the reader and provide guidance as follows. Practitioners may wish to use the magnitude of the correlation value if they simply wish to quantify the presence of an association between two nodes. Alternatively, the sign of the correlation may be retained if a distinction between synergistic (positive correlations) and antagonistic (negative correlations) interactions is desired. For delayed interactions, it may be desirable to quantify an edge as the peak correlation value across lags or as the lag at which the peak correlation occurs (Figure 7.3). While there is flexibility in the choice of a correlation-based statistic, there are limitations to consider [31, 43].

Correlational methods carry three key assumptions: (i) measurement samples at each node are normally distributed, (ii) measurement samples between nodes have a linear relationship (i.e. may be written in the form $v_j = av_i + b$ where $a$ and $b$ are arbitrary scalar values), and (iii) sequential measurement samples drawn from a node are independent (i.e. the data sample observed during one draw from the node is a poor predictor of the data sample observed during the next draw from the same node). Non-parametric alternatives to the Pearson correlation coefficient, such as the *Spearman correlation coefficient*, relax assumptions of normality and linearity by replacing the value of the measurement samples by their rank ordering in the measurement set. Unlike the Pearson correlation, the Spearman correlation quantifies the extent to which measurement samples between two nodes exhibit a similar ranking by evaluating the presence of monotonic relationships between nodes and it is invariant to the magnitude and scale of the measurement samples. Spearman correlation is one of many non-linear methods – including mutual information, transfer entropy, and non-linear correlation – that extract higher-order statistical relationships commonly present in neural systems [53]. In spite of their strengths, non-linear methods must also comply with the assumption of statistical independence, which is described next.

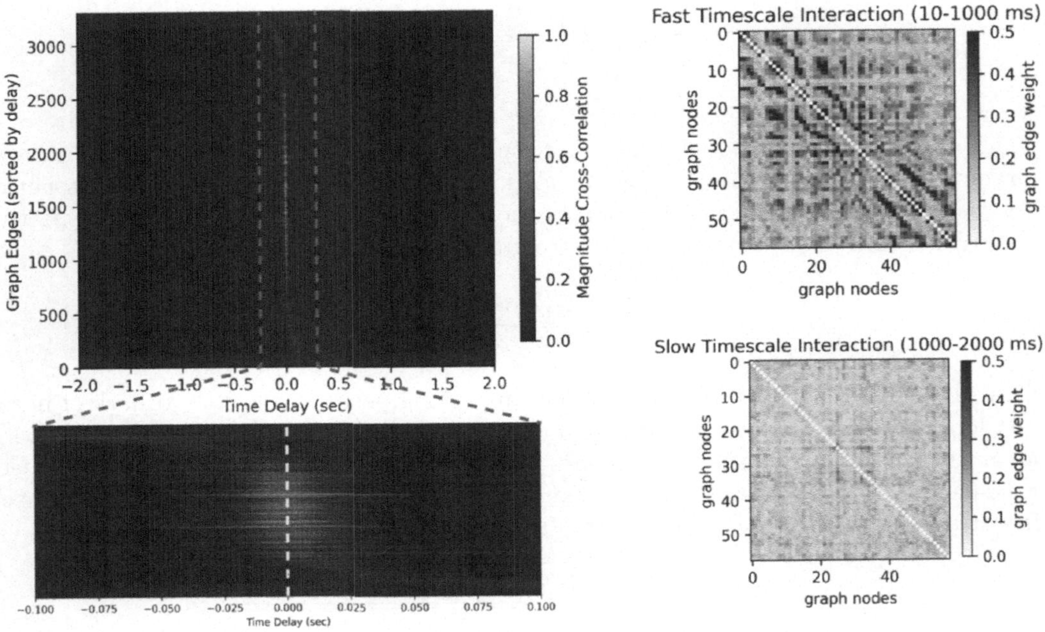


**FIGURE 7.3**
(Left panel) Distribution of lagged cross-correlation for all possible graph edges during the first 10 seconds of a seizure; (inset) majority of graph edges capture fast nodal interactions that occur within 25 ms and few interactions unfold more slowly over 100 ms. (Right panel) Adjacency matrix representations of functional connectivity during a seizure, created by imposing different constraints on the range of allowable lag values. (Top right panel) Faster functional connectivity involves a different portion of the graph nodes than (bottom right panel) slower functional connectivity. (Color version available in electronic supplement.)

Spurious correlations may be found if the data exhibit *autocorrelation* [4] – a statistical phenomenon that occurs when data samples measured from a single node are statistically related based on the order in which those samples were measured. Autocorrelation is a property of the underlying system that indicates periodicity, which is the presence of cycles or occurrence of drift. Autocorrelation can confound correlational measurements. For example, assume that you have separately recorded the single neuron activity in two subjects continuously over several days and wish to confirm the likely hypothesis that the firing pattern of a neuron in one subject is functionally independent, or shows zero correlation, with the firing pattern of a neuron in the other subject. As it happens, the subjects sleep and wake at the same times of the day and exhibit similar circadian behaviors, which modulates neurons in both subjects independently. You might measure a strong correlation in the activity between neurons collected across the two subjects and falsely conclude that the neurons are functionally connected and mutually interact despite the fact that one subject has no relation to the other subject – outside of common sleep patterns. In more complex data sets, sources of autocorrelation may not be as obvious and tools that help identify autocorrelation should be employed before measuring correlation between nodes. Surrogate data testing methods can help mitigate the influence of autocorrelation on correlation between nodes, and we discuss these methods later in the chapter.

**Similarity in the frequency-domain:** Functional neural data is often transformed into the frequency-domain to extract cyclical patterns, such as brain oscillations [17]. Statistical similarity metrics that operate in the frequency-domain can be used to quantify how signal oscillations are *synchronized* between two nodes [25]. Similar to correlation-based methods used in the time-domain, a variety of frequency-based methods exist to quantify different forms of synchrony in the data. To help define these forms of synchrony, we first introduce the analytic signal representation of filtered, or band-limited, time-series data from a single node $v_i$ as follows

$$v_i(t, f) = A(t, f) \cdot e^{i\theta(t,f)}, \tag{7.5}$$

where $A(t, f)$, and $\theta(t, f)$, is the instantaneous amplitude, and the instantaneous phase, of oscillatory activity within the frequency band $f$ at time $t$. Components of the analytic signal can be used to measure statistical similarity in the frequency-domain.

Amplitude correlation is one measure of a graph edge that quantifies correlation in the time-domain [65], as discussed earlier in this chapter, between the amplitude data $A_i(t, f)$ of node $v_i$ and the amplitude data $A_j(t, f)$ of node $v_j$. Intuitively, the amplitude correlation is used to describe whether the presence or strength of band-limited oscillations is similar between nodes. Note that amplitude correlation does not take signal phase $\theta$ into consideration.

Phase locking value (PLV) is a separate measure of a graph edge that is invariant to amplitude information and quantifies similarity in the phase structure of band-limited oscillations between nodes [13, 39]. Specifically, PLV quantifies the stability or consistency of the phase offset between the oscillations of two nodes $v_i$ and $v_j$ and is defined as

$$\text{PLV}_{v_i v_j}(f) = e^{i(\theta_i(t,f) - \theta_j(t,f))}, \tag{7.6}$$

and is strictly bounded between 0 (no phase locking) and 1 (perfectly phase locked).

Unlike the PLV, which is invariant to differences in oscillation amplitude between nodes, coherence is a similarity measure that weighs PLV by the combined strength of oscillation amplitudes between nodes [16, 39]. Coherence is defined as

$$\text{PLV}_{v_i v_j}(f) = |\sum_{t=1}^{T} e^{i(\theta_i(t,f) - \theta_j(t,f))}|, \tag{7.7}$$

and is strictly bounded between 0 (no coherence) and 1 (maximal coherence). Intuitively, nodes that exhibit greater coherence must have a consistent phase relationship and strong oscillatory activity within a spectral frequency band.

### 7.2.2 Gaussian Graphical Models

The bivariate association measures described above have several strengths that motivate their popularity in the estimation of undirected graphs, including ease of interpretation and lack of assumptions about the distribution of variables. However, they come with a few disadvantages. Bivariate measures, while simple to interpret, capture pairwise associations between nodes, and generally do not account for higher-order interactions or indirect relationships; moreover, they do not allow for formal statistical inference about graph structure. Graphical models, on the other hand, provide a statistical framework for the estimation of graphs that captures conditional dependencies between nodes, allowing for higher-order interactions and indirect relationships to be considered. The use of graphical models also provides a statistical framework that is amenable to formal statistical inference about the network structure, including hypothesis testing and model selection across candidate graphs.

Gaussian graphical models (GGMs), also known as Gaussian networks or Gaussian Markov random fields, are a type of probabilistic graphical model that represents the dependencies between variables using a graph structure. A GGM models the joint distribution of the variables (nodes) in the graph using a multivariate Gaussian distribution; inference on the inverse covariance matrix of the multivariate Gaussian distribution, also called the *precision matrix*, then yields the estimated edges of the graph. The elements of the precision matrix represent the partial correlations between the nodes. Specifically, non-zero entries indicate that an edge is present between two nodes, while zero entries indicate that an edge is absent between two nodes. In a GGM, if an edge is estimated to be present between two nodes, this means that the two nodes are conditionally dependent given all other nodes in the graph. conversely, if an edge is absent, this means that the two nodes are conditionally independent given all other nodes.

GGMs can be estimated in various ways. Maximum likelihood estimation (MLE) methods find the value of the precision matrix $\mathbf{\Omega}$ that maximizes the log-likelihood of the GGM,

$$L(\mathbf{\Omega}|\mathbf{X}) = -0.5 * n * \log(\det(\mathbf{\Omega})) - 0.5 * \mathrm{tr}(\mathbf{\Sigma} * \mathbf{\Omega}),$$

where $X$ is the matrix of variables modeled in the graph, $n$ is the number of observations for each node, $\Omega$ is the precision matrix, det is the determinant, $\Sigma$ is the covariance matrix, and tr is the trace. One method used to enforce sparsity in graphical models is statistical regularization. Regularization is especially important when estimating graphical models with a large number of nodes, as fitting a high-dimensional graphical model without enforcement of sparsity may lead to overfitting. Regularization enforces sparse estimation of network edges by adding a penalty term to the loss function, which shrinks or sets some edges to zero, thus decreasing overfitting. One of the most popular methods used for regularization of graphical models is L1 regularization, also known as LASSO (Least Absolute Shrinkage and Selection Operator). Similar to its use in regularized regression (Chapter 12), LASSO adds the absolute value of the magnitude of the coefficients as a penalty term to the loss function. In the context of GGMs, graphical LASSO allows for estimation of a sparse precision matrix. The degree of sparsity is controlled by a regularization parameter, which can be adjusted to minimize prediction error or to maximize a measure of model fit. Such models can be fit using the `GraphicalLasso()` class in `scikit-learn` in Python.

Alternatively, GGMs can be estimated via Bayesian methods. In general, Bayesian estimation methods specify a prior distribution, such as a Wishart prior, on the precision matrix $\Omega$. The posterior distribution of $\Omega$ is then updated via Bayes' rule. If a conjugate prior such as a Wishart prior is imposed on the precision matrix, then the posterior can be analytically derived as a multivariate Gaussian distribution and Markov chain Monte Carlo (MCMC) methods can be used to sample from the posterior distribution of the precision matrix [21]. Furthermore, continuous shrinkage priors for precision matrices, first proposed by [68], can be used and allow scalability of the methods to larger graphs. These priors have also been extended to methods that allow the estimation of multiple graphs [54, 60]. In recent years, Bayesian methods for graphical models have been successfully employed in neuroimaging applications, particularly for the estimation of functional brain connectivity networks based on fMRI data; see, for example, [42, 61, 70], and references therein.

### 7.2.3 Poisson Graphical Models

A key assumption in Gaussian graphical models is that the joint distribution of the nodes is multivariate Gaussian. However, many data sources acquired in epilepsy are ill-suited to be modeled by Gaussian distributions. For example, data sources that involve count data, such as spike counts acquired from electroencephalography or single neuron recordings are not reasonably assumed to be Gaussian.

Given that a reasonable distribution for modeling count data in the univariate case is the Poisson distribution, one area of methodological graphical models research in modeling count data is the area of Poisson graphical models and related models. The original Poisson graphical model (PGM), in contrast to the GGM, assumes that the conditional distribution of each node, given the rest of the nodes, is univariate Poisson. There is then a unique joint distribution which factors according to the node-conditional distributions [9]. This seems like a good candidate for modeling multivariate count data; however, a major drawback of the PGM is that it only models non-positive conditional dependencies between variables, i.e., competitive relationships between nodes. This limits the practical applicability of the PGM, especially for many data sources in epilepsy such as neural count data, in which we expect both positive and negative dependencies between the variables. To address this drawback, various alternative models have been proposed, including the use of a Winsorized Poisson distribution [35] and truncated PGMs [3]. Other approaches to address the restriction of non-negative dependencies in the original PGM have been proposed and we refer the reader to those sources [20, 29, 32]. Alternatively, non-Poisson approaches are also available for modeling graphs based on count data, such as Gaussian copula [47] and nonparametric approaches [57].

## 7.3 Directed Graphs

Unlike the undirected graph, a *directed* graph is used to convey sequential association, information flow, or causal influence between nodes [8, 26]. Specifically, for two nodes $v_i$ and $v_j$, without loss of generality, a directed edge may be defined as $e_{ij}$, where $v_i$ is a leader node that precedes or influences $v_j$ the follower node, and $e_{ij} \neq e_{ji}$. Note that the existence of edge $e_{ij}$ is *not* mutually exclusive from the existence of edge $e_{ji}$ – one possibility is that one node exclusively influences the other or that both nodes influence each other and their association is bi-directional. Directed edges form the basis for *effective* graph models, which may be measured by applying causal inference tools to functional neuroimaging or electrophysiology data [27] – modalities also used to model functional edges – or by applying external perturbation, such as neurostimulation, to individual nodes and quantifying the effects of the perturbation at the other non-perturbed nodes [36, 45]. Thus, effective graphs can provide a rich quantitative description of directed interactions between nodes, but this capability may come at the cost of additional computational complexity needed to infer this information.

There are various methods that can be used to estimate directed graphs, including structural equation models, dynamic causal models, vector autoregressive models, Granger causality, and Granger graphical models. Bayesian networks are another approach for estimating directed graphs, which is discussed below. Vector autoregressive models and Granger causality are discussed in Chapter 8.

### 7.3.1 Bayesian Networks

A directed graphical model (DGM), also known as a *Bayesian network*, *causal model*, or *belief network*, is a type of probabilistic graphical model (PGA) that allows for the estimation of directed graphs. In a DGM, the edges between nodes are represented by a directed acyclic graph (DAG). This means that the relationships between nodes have directionality, where each edge indicates a causal relationship betwen the variables, with the additional assumption that there are no directed cycles in the graph. More specifically, the main property of DAGs is the *ordered Markov property*; i.e., the assumption that each node depends only on its immediate parents (the nodes that directly influence it in the graph), and that contingent on its parents, it is statistically independent of the predecessors to the parents. This is a generalization of the Markov property discussed in Chapter 8 from sequences to graphs. Each node in the graph, then, can be written to have a conditional probability distribution that quantifies the relationship between that parent and its node, so that the joint distribution of the DAG can be decomposed into the conditional probability distributions.

There are several algorithms that can be used to learn the structure of directed graphical models. These include *constraint-based methods*, which evaluate statistical dependencies and conditional independence relationships to determine the presence or absence of edges in the network, and *score-based methods*, which compare the model fit of different candidate network structures to find the network that best fits the data. Examples of constraint-based methods include the Peter and Clark (PC) algorithm and Fast Causal Inference (FCI) algorithm [62, 63]. The PC algorithm starts with a complete undirected graph, and recursively deletes edges based on conditional independence, while the FCI algorithm is an extension of the PC algorithm that allows for latent and selection variables into the learned network structure. Score-based methods, on the other hand, search through different configurations of edges and select the best fit network structure based on optimization of metrics such as the Akaike Information Criterion (AIC), Bayesian Information Criterion (BIC), or likelihood-based scores.

## 7.4 Preservation of Edge Strength

An edge may be *unweighted* and indicate the presence or absence of a connection as a binary number $a_{ij} \in \{0, 1\}$. Unweighted edges are frequently used to model structural connections that have a direct anatomical correlate, such as the presence of a white-matter fiber and are physically present in the system. Alternatively, a *weighted* edge may be used to encode the strength or probability of a network connection using a continuous value, which is often bounded such that $0 <= a_{ij} <= 1$. Weighted edges are commonly used in scenarios where the amount of connectivity or interactivity may be meaningfully graded between different node pairs [14]. Functional and effective connectivity graph models tend to define weighted edges that are probabilistic in nature since these models are based on statistical inference of relatedness across multiple channels of brain recordings. Choosing to define a graph with or without weighted edges may also impact the types of post-hoc analysis tools that may be used. As the prevalence of weighted graph models has grown, many graph theoretic tools originally built to analyze unweighted graphs have been extended so that they may be applied to weighted graphs.

At this stage of the graph modeling process, the inferred graph may contain spurious edges measured by chance and driven by undesirable noise in the underlying signal. Spurious edges in a weighted graph can be removed by thresholding the graph edges via a critical threshold $\alpha$ such that $a_{ij} = 0$ if $a_{ij} < \alpha$ – a procedure that yields a sparse, weighted graph. The sparse, weighted graph may be further converted to a binary, unweighted graph by imposing the criteria that $a_{ij} = 1$ if $a_{ij} >= \alpha$. Indeed, determination of the optimal critical threshold $\alpha$ is non-trivial. One approach is to assume a constant noise-level across all graph edges and evaluate the network structure parametrically across a range of critical thresholds (Figure 7.4). Another statistically grounded approach is to set the Type 1 error rate (commonly 5%) of false positive graph edges under the null hypothesis that no edge exists between two nodes. This approach involves thresholding the graph such that edges with a weight greater than $\alpha$ occur with probability below the Type 1 error rate. To control for multiple hypothesis tests that occur due to large number of graph edges in a network, more conservative statistical hypothesis testing that restricts the family-wise rate of Type 1 errors should be used.

Thus far, our treatment of spurious edges has relied on a fixed critical threshold that is uniformly applied across the network. A more rigorous treatment is to assume that graph edge weights depend on the statistical signal properties unique to each node and derive a separate threshold for each graph edge, such that $a_{ij} = 0$ if $a_{ij} < \alpha_{ij}$. We next describe methods that the practitioner can use to define edge-specific critical thresholds $\alpha_{ij}$.

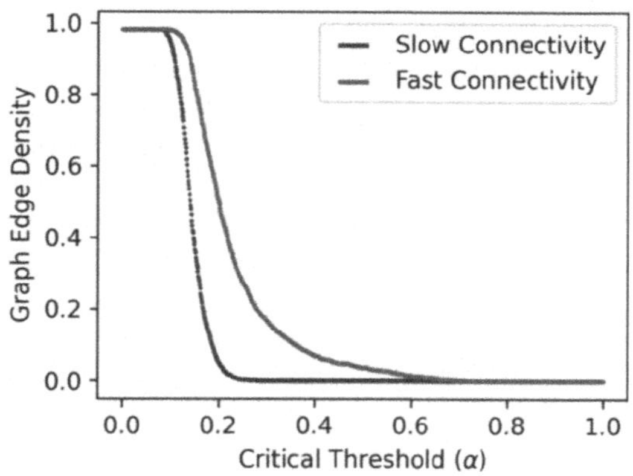


**FIGURE 7.4**
Survival analysis of graph edge density (fraction of possible graph edges observed) by varying the critical threshold $\alpha$ for a graph constructed using either slow (blue) or fast (red) cross-correlation lag values. Denser graph structure is observed for fast connectivity compared to slow connectivity, which contains weaker edges that are more rapidly explained away during $\alpha$ titration. (Color version available in electronic supplement.)

### 7.4.1 Null Models for Surrogate Time-Series

Graph models should be compared against null graph models measured from surrogate time-series in which meaningful statistical structure is disrupted. Graph connectivity measures presented in this chapter are based on similar patterns of brain activity fluctuation, and surrogate data generation procedures should aim to disrupt relationships *between* time-series of two nodes while preserving the structure of the time-series at each node as much as possible [4, 6, 56]. We next build upon this idea by presenting three different methods for generating surrogate datasets underlying the null graph model (Figure 7.5).

*Random shuffle* is a null model applied to each node's time-series that preserves the distribution (mean, variance, and higher-order moments) of its constituent values but disrupts its sequential structure and smoothness. A simple implementation of the random shuffle null model involves permuting the order of the values in each nodal time-series uniformly. By removing the ordinal property of each node's time-series, this approach penalizes graph edge measures that rely on similar patterns of time-series fluctuation between nodes. While the random shuffle null model diminishes correlations between nodal time-series, a pitfall is that it also destroys the autocorrelation, which contributes to the smoothness or oscillatory nature, of each node's time-series. Autocorrelation can artificially inflate the correlational structure of the time-series between two nodes by generating oscillations independently at each node that intermittently coincide and give the appearance of synchronized activity pattern. Thus, more conservative null models that preserve autocorrelation in surrogate time-series data are warranted.

The *phase shuffle* null model preserves the distribution statistics and autocorrelation structure of each node's time-series. This model first projects the time-series $v_i(t)$ of a single node into the frequency-domain through the Fourier transform. Next, the magnitude and phase corresponding to each frequency are extracted from the Fourier coefficients – the magnitudes reflect how strongly an oscillation is represented in the time-series and the phases indicate how those oscillations are ordered relative to one another. Therefore, permutation of the relative phase information uniformly across frequencies disrupts the order in which those oscillations appear in the time-series. Lastly, an inverse Fourier transform is applied to the set of magnitudes and scrambled phases to reconstruct a phase shuffled surrogate representation of the original time-series. Extensions of this method that better preserve the power spectral density and other non-linear properties of each node's time-series data exist, and we refer the reader to [40] to explore these topics further.

Surrogate time-series are next used to construct a null distribution of edge weights for each pair of network nodes. A critical threshold based on each edge's null distribution may be used in conjunction with multiple hypothesis testing to determine whether a specific edge is weighted more strongly than expected by the null distribution. This pruning approach compares the true graph model to the null graph model at the level of individual edges. Alternatively, surrogate edges may be combined to reconstitute a surrogate graph, which can be used to evaluate relational structure, or topology, across the broader network.

## 7.5 Graph Topology

In conventional neural data analysis, nodes of a brain network are studied based upon their anatomical position in physical space. A graph model explains away this physical representation and projects brain network nodes into an abstract functional position in topological space. While a physical representation of the brain is based upon three-dimensional geometric relationships between nodes, a topological representation of the brain is based upon edge connectivity between nodes. In other words, nodes that are located far from each other in physical space may be positioned more closely in topological space based on the overall arrangement of the graph's edges. A network's topology is thought to play an important role in the routing, distribution, and processing of information. Generative network models typically weigh the benefits of efficiency and redundancy against costs of heightened metabolism and energy consumption when considering the addition or arrangement of nodes and connections in a complex system [1, 10]. Functioning of the system can be characterized through metrics that resolve the spatial arrangement of connectivity at multiple topological scales of the graph [15, 19].

### 7.5.1 Local Scale

Local graph topology describes patterns of connectivity across edges that link an individual node to other nodes in the graph. A commonly described feature of a node is whether it is centralized, or behaves as a *'hub'*, in the network. Hub nodes receive and project a higher density of connections in the network than non-hub nodes. *Degree centrality* is a simple topological measure of a node's hubness and is defined as the total number or, for a

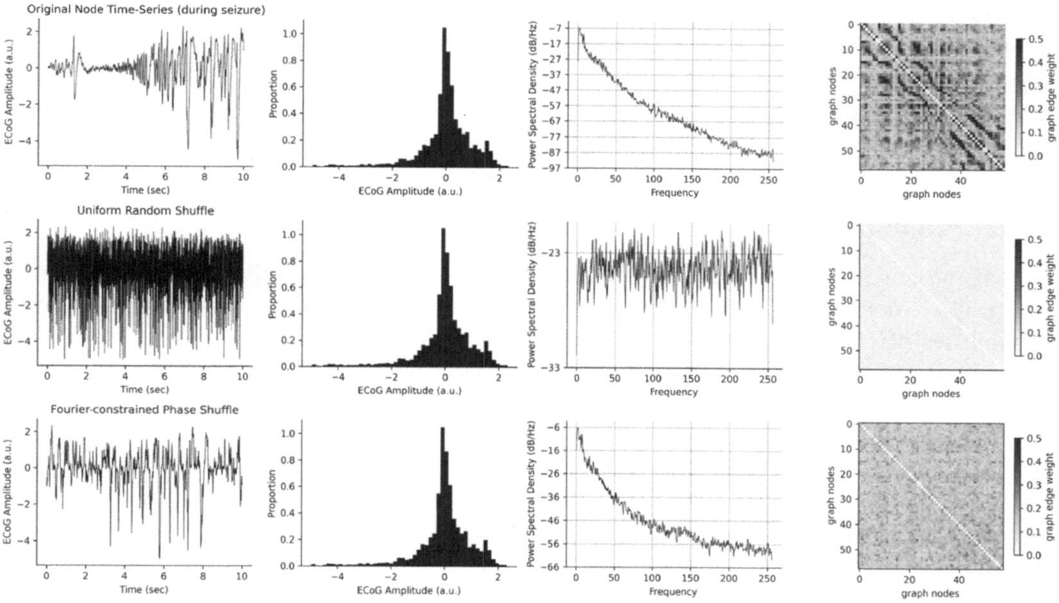


**FIGURE 7.5**
Effects of surrogate time-series methods on signal statistics and graph structure. (First column; top) Example ECoG signal during a seizure from a node in the seizure-onset zone, and temporally corrupted versions of the signal using (middle) random shuffle and (bottom) phase shuffle surrogate models. (Second column) Original and surrogate models show identical distribution of signal amplitudes. (Third column) Phase shuffling preserves the shape of the power spectrum from the original signal whereas the spectral statistics are destroyed using the random shuffle. (Fourth column) Shuffled models destroy the pairwise relationships between nodes observed using in the original signal. Phase shuffling retains stronger graph edges than random uniform shuffling. (Color version available in electronic supplement.)

weighted graph the average weight, of network connections stemming from that node [51]. Degree centrality $D$ for a node $v_i$ is defined as

$$D_i = \frac{1}{N} \sum_{j=1}^{N} A_{ij}. \tag{7.8}$$

In a directed graph, the node degree measure may be further dichotomized into the node's *in-degree* and *out-degree*, which measure the connections either projecting into the node or emanating from the node respectively. Degree considers the relationship of a node with its immediate, or first-order, topological neighbors. Yet, more complex notions of node centrality consider a node's extended relationships with its neighbors, its neighbors' neighbors, and beyond. *Clustering coefficient* is one such example that measures the fraction of a node's neighbors that are themselves connected neighbors of one another and indicates the level of engagement of a node with other nodes in its local neighborhood. A broader measure of nodal importance is *betweenness centrality*, which assesses the role of a node as a waypoint or facilitator of information travel between other nodes in the network and is defined for a fully connected graph – one in which a path exists from every node to every other node through the pattern of graph edges [51]. Betweenness centrality of a node is calculated as the fraction of shortest paths that exist between every pair of nodes that traverse that node; excluding paths in which that node is the starting node or terminal node in the path. A node with high betweenness centrality may not necessarily also have high degree centrality, however it may be an equally critical junction point within the network. Indeed, this example illustrates the notion that individual nodes can have varied roles in the context of local and global functioning of a networked system.

### 7.5.2 Global Scale

Global measures of graph topology describe patterns of connectivity across all edges in the graph collectively. This scale of measurement characterizes the broader functional capabilities of the interconnected system. The simplest such measurement is the overall connectivity of the graph, which is defined as the density or average weight of connections present between all node pairs in the graph. Graph connection density quantifies the amount of interaction or resources available for information transmission within the network, but it is unable to characterize whether those resources are allocated effectively [1]. *Average path length* is a measure related to the shortest path metric that quantifies the mean distance between nodes in topological space and is calculated as the minimum number of nodes that need to be traversed to reach each node from every other node in the network [71]. For the brain network, path length is a particularly important measure for weighing the cost of a connection existing between two geometrically distant nodes against the length of the path between the two nodes in topological space. It follows that the overall efficiency of the network can be calculated as the inverse of the path length statistic. Intuitively, the connection density of a network necessarily imposes a constraint on path length since every additional connection will always shorten the path between at least two nodes in the network. Thus, great care should be taken to account for the effects of connection density when interpreting the prevalence of more complex global graph features.

### 7.5.3 Meso Scale

Situated between the local scale and global scale is the mesoscale organization involving groups of nodes. *Assortativity* is a basic network property that emerges when nodes tend to preferentially connect to other nodes with similar characteristics [2, 11, 15]. For example, nodes that are relevant for a specific cognitive function may exhibit a strong preference to maintain close ties to each other. In epilepsy, graph nodes involved in the seizure onset typically display preferential connectivity to each other in a manner that forms a tightly interconnected *rich club* (Figure 7.6).

Assortativity is the basis for *modularity*, a form of mesoscale organization that is commonly observed in the brain network and refers to the clustering of nodes into modules, where nodes within a module are highly connected to each other and are sparsely connected to nodes that occupy other modules [49, 50]. Nodes can be assigned into modules by optimizing the following modularity cost function **Q**:

$$Q = \sum_{ij} [A_{ij} - \gamma P_{ij}] \delta(g_i, g_j) \,, \tag{7.9}$$

where node $i$ is assigned to community $g_i$, node $j$ is assigned to community $g_j$, the Kronecker delta $\delta(g_i, g_j) = 1$ if $g_i = g_j$ and it equals 0 otherwise, $\gamma$ is the *structural resolution parameter*, and $P_{ij}$ is the expected weight of the edge connecting node $i$ to node $j$ under a specified null model. A default structural resolution parameter of $\gamma = 1$ is commonly used, but it is important to consider the formation and dissolution of modular structure across multiple topological scales by parametrically varying the value of $\gamma$. Lastly, the

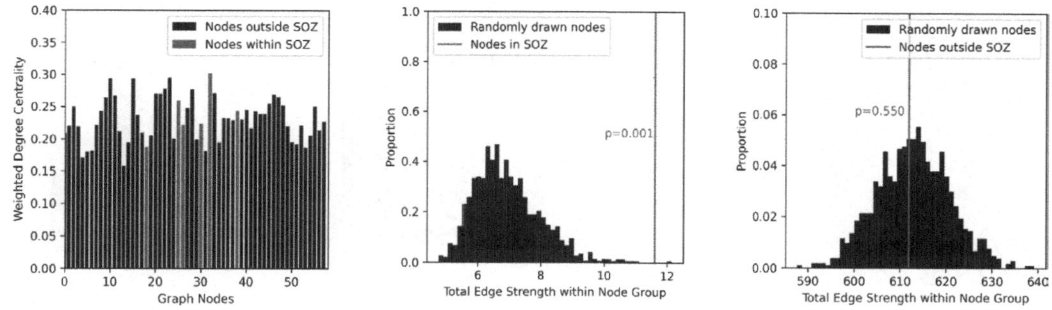


**FIGURE 7.6**
Graph topology involving nodes within and outside of the seizure-onset zone (SOZ). (Left panel) Weighted degree centrality across nodes of a functional graph constructed during initial phase of a seizure. Nodes within the SOZ (red) exhibit no difference in their degree of connectivity to the rest of the network compared to nodes outside the SOZ (black). (Middle panel) Total edge weight linking nodes identified as belonging to the SOZ (red) compared to a null distribution in which nodes were randomly reassigned to the SOZ (black). Edges among SOZ nodes are substantially stronger than chance sampling. (Right panel) Similarly, total edge weight linking nodes identified as belonging outside the SOZ (red) is no different than chance sampling. (Color version available in electronic supplement.)

Newman-Girvan model is commonly chosen as a null graph model [49, 55] and it is defined as follows:

$$P_{ij} = \frac{k_i k_j}{2m} \tag{7.10}$$

where $k_i = \sum_j A_{ij}$ is the strength of node $i$ and $m = \frac{1}{2}\sum_{ij} A_{ij}$ is the average strength over all connections. The Louvain algorithm is a popular method used to optimize the modularity cost function and assign nodes to modules [34].

It is also possible for the mesoscale organization of the network to be *disassortative*, where like nodes tend to repel one another and stronger connections manifest between nodes that are functionally dissimilar [11]. This topological feature may be observed in the brain when nodes of a single functional brain system exhibit strong cross-modal interaction or integration with nodes of another functional brain system. In between assortative and disassortative topology lies *core-periphery organization*, in which nodes of a single module are highly connected to each other – forming a network core – and also highly connected to nodes of other modules that are far less densely connected to each other – forming a network periphery [12, 23]. Core-periphery structure reflects a top-down integrative topology in which the network core consolidates information that is either projected to or received from the network periphery. Methods to resolve disassortative and core-periphery structure include the weighted stochastic block model [11]. On the whole, these mesoscale structures demonstrate that a single network may be comprised of various sub-networks that have their own diverse topologies that coexist and contribute distinct functions that are combined at the global scale of the network (Figure 7.7).

## 7.6 Dynamics on Graphs

How is the topology of a graph related to the physical flow or dynamics of processes that move from one node to the next within a graph? Graph connectivity is a useful tool to

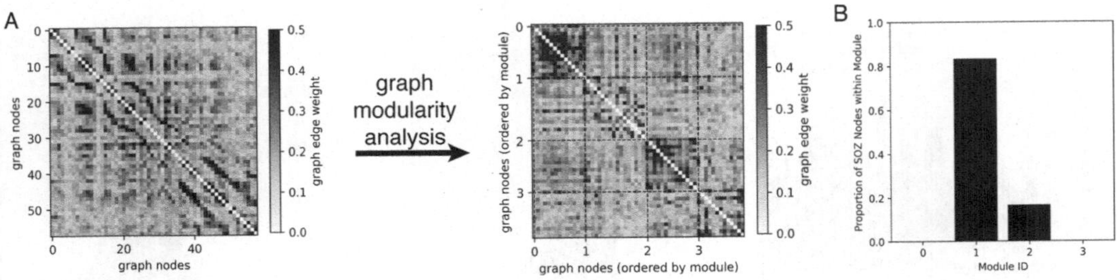


**FIGURE 7.7**
Modular topological structure of the epileptic brain network. (Left and middle panels) Identification of network modules in a functional graph constructed during initial phase of a seizure. Rows and columns of the (left panel) original adjacency matrix are (middle panel) re-ordered according to the module assignment of the corresponding nodes. Edges between nodes within the same module (block diagonal) have greater weight than edges between nodes of different modules (off block diagonal). (Right panel) Nodes contained within the seizure onset zone tend to occupy a single module, which suggests that other nodes within the module may be complicit or directly impacted during the onset of the seizure. (Color version available in electronic supplement.)

characterize diffusive dynamics in the brain, such as those involving the spread of an epileptic seizure through different brain regions. Generative models that can simulate diffusion dynamics can be valuable for pinpointing seizure starting points and critical waypoints and bottlenecks that support the rich and diverse repertoire of seizure dynamics observed in an individual. *Master stability function* [28, 52] is an important generative model for epilepsy that aims to quantify the diffusion of dynamical processes that manifest as a result of oscillations and synchronization, which are phenomena that are often studied in neuroscience and epilepsy. In the framework of the master stability function, each node in the network is characterized as a dynamical system and the state of a node at a single point in time is governed by the prior history of the node's state dynamics and the influence of state dynamics at other nodes which are mediated by the network's connectivity. Formally, these concepts are defined in the master stability function as follows:

$$\dot{x_i}(t) = f(x_i(t)) + \sigma(t)\sum_{j=1}^{N} A_{ij}(t)(x_j(t) - x_i(t)), \tag{7.11}$$

where $x_{v_i}(t)$ represents the dynamical state of node $v_i$, $f$ is a function describing the node's independent state dynamics, $\sigma$ is a diffusion constant, $A(t)$ is an $N \times N$ adjacency matrix of connection weights between $N$ network nodes. A variety of questions pertaining to epilepsy may be asked using this model, including: Given the current state at each node, how those states change over time, and how the nodes are interconnected, what is the state of each node at a future point in time? How does the network's topological pattern of connectivity affect the nodes' state dynamics? How likely is it that node dynamics will synchronize or coalesce into a seizure-like pattern? Which nodes or connections are most important for promoting synchronization or desynchronization? Which parts of the network could be removed or ablated to better control nodal dynamics? To understand the relationship between nodal dynamics and network topology, there exists a simple solution to the master stability function under assumptions of linear dynamical coupling [28] and is given by

$$\dot{x}(t) = -\mathcal{L}x(t), \tag{7.12}$$

where $\mathcal{L}$ is the graph Laplacian whose entries $l_{ij}$ quantify how easily a node's dynamics can diffuse between nodes $i$ and $j$. The Laplacian matrix $\mathbf{L}$ is computed as the difference between the rank-1 matrix of node degree centrality values $\mathbf{D}$ and the network adjacency matrix $\mathbf{A}$, such that $\mathbf{L} = \mathbf{D} - \mathbf{A}$. The solution to the master stability function suggests that a node's state changes based on the connections it forms with other nodes where nodes engage in a game of tug-of-war as the dynamics of each node synchronizes and desynchronizes with other nodes in the network [30, 69]. For some network topologies, nodes are able to stabilize and reach a dynamical equilibrium more or less quickly than other network topologies. For a given network configuration, the potential for dynamics at each node to achieve equivalence around an arbitrary state $q(t)$ such that $q(t) = x_1(t) = x_2(t) = ... = x_N(t)$ is the network's *synchronizability* $S$, which is a global topological measure [18, 69]. Synchronizability is quantified by the eigenvalues of $\mathcal{L}$ such that

$$S = \frac{\lambda_2}{\lambda_{\text{max}}}, \tag{7.13}$$

where $\lambda_2$ and $\lambda_{\text{max}}$ are the second-smallest and largest eigenvalues of $\mathcal{L}$, respectively. Larger values of $S$ correspond to greater potential for the dynamics occurring within a network to stably synchronize or reach a fixed attractor point. For epilepsy, this dynamical system lens can be used to quantify the brain network's stability in the period leading up to a seizure [59], the propensity for seizures to spread to and synchronize healthy regions of the brain network [37], or potentially the responsiveness of the brain network to treatment [38, 58].

## 7.7 Perturbation of Network Topology

Earlier, we touched upon the concept of network centrality to illustrate the concept that, even in large networks, individual nodes can be key players in the organization and functioning of the underlying system. In some cases, those key nodes can be the source of dysfunctional dynamics and sought to be removed. It may also be possible that additional nodes or edges are needed to enhance the functioning of the network or to make the network more redundant and resilient to attack [18, 41, 67]. Conceptually, by disrupting a node's relationship with the network, either by severing or remapping its connectivity, the practitioner can evaluate the functional significance or role of that node in the context of the surrounding network [22]. Here, we highlight methods to perturb network structure to make predictions about the result of interventions on network organization and function.

An emerging trend is to perturb the network by pursuing a virtual resection of graph nodes within an individual's brain network model and the consequential impact on the dynamical stability of the system [37, 41]. Specifically, we might ask the question, "Which nodes of the network naturally regulate how feasible it is for the system to reach a stably synchronized state?" An answer to this question can be reached by independently perturbing the connectivity of graph nodes in the network model and measuring the fractional change, termed control centrality, in the network's synchronizability property [37]. How should the node's connectivity be perturbed? One approach is to simply zero all the connections that emanate from the node. A caveat is that this perturbation doesn't necessarily isolate the impact of the node in question because the network's connection density, the network's degree distribution, and the node's degree centrality would have also changed. To protect the original network's connection density and the node's degree centrality, one can uniformly permute the distribution of a node's connections to the other nodes in the network. A more conservative modification would entail a complete degree-preserving permutation and edge re-weighting to retain the degree distribution of all the nodes of the original network [44, 46]. A rewiring of node $v_i$ of the adjacency matrix is represented as $\hat{A}^{v_i}$. Fractional change of a network property, such as synchronizability, due to the perturbation is formally defined as

$$CC_{v_i} = \frac{f(\hat{A}^{v_i}) - f(A)}{f(A)}, \tag{7.14}$$

where $CC_{v_i}$ refers to the control centrality obtained after perturbing the connectivity of node $v_i$ and calculating an arbitrary network property measurement $f$ for a network with adjacency matrix $A$. The magnitude and directionality of a node's control centrality indicates its specific role in contributing to the network property of interest. Specifically, a node may contribute synergistically ($CC_i < -\epsilon$), antagonistically ($CC_i > \epsilon$), or not at all ($-\epsilon < CC_i < \epsilon$) to the network property. To determine the boundaries posed by $\epsilon$, the upper and lower extremities of the null distribution associated with the node's control centrality must be computed using a surrogate graph model [24]. For the synchronizability network feature, the control centrality could identify a node as a synchronizer (contributing synergistically), a desynchronizer (contributing antagonistcally), or belonging to the bulk (not contributing).

In this regard, the graph model can be seen as an *in silico* platform for simulation and insight into the theoretical and functional effects of targeted intervention. While the perspective provided here is heavily centered on the individual contributions of nodes, more biologically and clinically plausible extensions – such as those that perturb edges rather than nodes or groups of nodes within a single brain region rather than individual nodes – may be derived. Perturbation methods showcase the potential next frontier for the role of graph models as an investigative tool in clinical and research workflows of epilepsy.

## 7.8 Summary

The use of graph and network estimation methods may provide valuable insights into the connectivity and complex dynamics of the brain network among individuals with epilepsy. In this chapter, we have explored various aspects related to the representation of the brain as a network, including graph estimation methods, graph theory, methods for sparsifying graphs, graph dynamics, and perturbation of graph topology. Combination of graph and network control theoretic frameworks with other statistical and machine learning methods offers an approach for advancing knowledge about spatiotemporal dynamics in epilepsy.

## Bibliography

[1] Sophie Achard and Ed Bullmore. Efficiency and cost of economical brain functional networks. *PLoS Computational Biology*, 3(2):e17–e17, 2007.

[2] Réka Albert and Albert-László Barabási. Statistical mechanics of complex networks. *Reviews of Modern Physics*, 74(1):47–97, 2002.

[3] Genevera I Allen and Zhandong Liu. A local Poisson graphical model for inferring networks from sequencing data. *IEEE Transactions on Nanobioscience*, 12(3):189–198, 2013.

[4] Mohammad R Arbabshirani, Eswar Damaraju, Ronald Phlypo, Sergey Plis, Elena Allen, Sai Ma, Daniel Mathalon, Adrian Preda, Jatin G Vaidya, Tülay Adali, and Vince D Calhoun. Impact of autocorrelation on functional connectivity. *NeuroImage*, 102:294–308, November 2014.

[5] Danielle S Bassett, Ankit N Khambhati, and Scott T Grafton. Emerging frontiers of neuroengineering: A network science of brain connectivity. *Annual Reviews of Biomedical Engineering*, 19:327–352, 2017.

[6] Danielle S Bassett, Mason A Porter, Nicholas F Wymbs, Scott T Grafton, Jean M Carlson, and Peter J Mucha. Robust detection of dynamic community structure in networks. *Chaos (Woodbury, N.Y.)*, 23(1):013142–013142, 2013.

[7] Danielle S Bassett and Olaf Sporns. Network neuroscience. *Nature Neuroscience*, 20(3):353–364, 2017.

[8] Demian Battaglia, Annette Witt, Fred Wolf, and Theo Geisel. Dynamic effective connectivity of inter-areal brain circuits. *PLoS Computational Biology*, 8(3):1–20, 2012.

[9] Julian Besag. Spatial interaction and the statistical analysis of lattice systems. *Journal of the Royal Statistical Society: Series B (Methodological)*, 36(2):192–225, 1974.

[10] Richard F Betzel, Andrea Avena-Koenigsberger, Joaquín Goñi, Ye He, Marcel A de Reus, Alessandra Griffa, Petra E Vértes, Bratislav Mivsic, Jean Philippe Thiran, Patric Hagmann, Martijn van den Heuvel, Xi Nian Zuo, Edward T Bullmore, and Olaf Sporns. Generative models of the human connectome. *NeuroImage*, 124:1054–1064, 2016.

[11] Richard F Betzel, John D Medaglia, and Danielle S Bassett. Diversity of meso-scale architecture in human and non-human connectomes. *Nature Communications*, 9(1):346, December 2018.

[12] Stephen P Borgatti and Martin G Everett. Models of core/periphery structures. *Social Networks*, 21:375–395, 1999.

[13] Ricardo Bruña, Fernando Maestú, and Ernesto Pereda. Phase locking value revisited: Teaching new tricks to an old dog. *Journal of Neural Engineering*, 15(5):056011, October 2018.

[14] Edward T Bullmore and Danielle S Bassett. Brain graphs: Graphical models of the human brain connectome. *Annual Review of Clinical Psychology*, 7(1):113–140, April 2011.

[15] Edward T Bullmore and Olaf Sporns. Complex brain networks: Graph theoretical analysis of structural and functional systems. *Nature Reviews. Neuroscience*, 10(3):186–98, 2009.

[16] TH Bullock, MC Mcclune, JZ Achimowicz, VJ Iragui-Madoz, RB Duckrow, and SS Spencer. EEG coherence has structure in the millimeter domain: Subdural and hippocampal recordings from epileptic patients. *Electroencephalography and Clinical Neurophysiology*, 95(3):161–177, 1995.

[17] György Buzsáki. *Rhythms of the Brain*. Oxford University Press, Oxford; New York, 2006.

[18] Guanrong Chen and Zhisheng Duan. Network synchronizability analysis: A graph-theoretic approach. *Chaos*, 18(3):1–10, 2008.

[19] Sharon Chiang and Zulfi Haneef. Graph theory findings in the pathophysiology of temporal lobe epilepsy. *Clinical Neurophysiology*, 125(7):1295–1305, 2014.

[20] Julien Chiquet, Stephane Robin, and Mahendra Mariadassou. Variational inference for sparse network reconstruction from count data. In *International Conference on Machine Learning*, pages 1162–1171. PMLR, 2019.

[21] Adrian Dobra, Alex Lenkoski, and Abel Rodriguez. Bayesian inference for general Gaussian graphical models with application to multivariate lattice data. *Journal of the American Statistical Association*, 106(496), 2011.

[22] Alan Edelman and N Raj Rao. Random matrix theory. *Acta Numerica*, 14:233–297, May 2005.

[23] Martin G Everett and Stephen P Borgatti. Peripheries of cohesive subsets. *Social Networks*, 21(4):397–407, 1999.

[24] Joshua Faskowitz, Richard F Betzel, and Olaf Sporns. Edges in brain networks: Contributions to models of structure and function. *Network Neuroscience*, 6(1):1–28, 2022.

[25] Pascal Fries. Rhythms for cognition: Communication through coherence. *Neuron*, 88(1):220–235, 2015.

[26] Karl J Kj Friston. Functional and effective connectivity: A review. *Brain Connectivity*, 1(1):13–36, January 2011.

[27] KJ Friston, L Harrison, and W Penny. Dynamic causal modelling. *NeuroImage*, 19(4):1273–1302, August 2003.

[28] S. Gómez, A. Díaz-Guilera, J. Gómez-Gardeñes, C. J. Pérez-Vicente, Yamir Moreno, Alex Arenas, Sergio Gomez, Albert Diaz-Guilera, Jesus Gomez-Gardeñes, Conrad J. Perez-Vicente, Yamir Moreno, Alex Arenas, S. Gómez, A. Díaz-Guilera, J. Gómez-Gardeñes, C. J. Pérez-Vicente, Yamir Moreno, and Alex Arenas. Diffusion dynamics on multiplex networks. *Physical Review Letters*, 110(2):028701–028701, July 2013.

[29] Fabian Hadiji, Alejandro Molina, Sriraam Natarajan, and Kristian Kersting. Poisson dependency networks: Gradient boosted models for multivariate count data. *Machine Learning*, 100:477–507, 2015.

[30] Zhiwei He, Xingang Wang, Guo-Yong Zhang, and Meng Zhan. Control for a synchronization-desynchronization switch. *Physical Review E*, 90(1):012909–012909, July 2014.

[31] R Matthew Hutchison, Thilo Womelsdorf, Elena A Allen, Peter A Bandettini, Vince D Calhoun, Maurizio Corbetta, Stefania Della Penna, Jeff H Duyn, Gary H Glover, Javier Gonzalez-Castillo, Daniel A Handwerker, Shella Keilholz, Vesa Kiviniemi, David A Leopold, Francesco de Pasquale, Olaf Sporns, Martin Walter, and Catie Chang. Dynamic functional connectivity: Promise, issues, and interpretations. *NeuroImage*, 80:360–378, October 2013.

[32] David I Inouye, Eunho Yang, Genevera I Allen, and Pradeep Ravikumar. A review of multivariate distributions for count data derived from the Poisson distribution. *Wiley Interdisciplinary Reviews: Computational Statistics*, 9(3):e1398, 2017.

[33] Paul Jaccard. The distribution of the flora in the alpine zone. *New Phytologist*, 11(2):37–50, February 1912.

[34] Lucas G S. Jeub, Marya Bazzi, Inderjit S Jutla, and Peter J Mucha. A generalized Louvain method for community detection implemented in MATLAB, 2016.

[35] Mark S Kaiser and Noel Cressie. Modeling Poisson variables with positive spatial dependence. *Statistics & Probability Letters*, 35(4):423–432, 1997.

[36] Corey J Keller, Christopher J Honey, Pierre Me, Laszlo Entz, Istvan Ulbert, and Ashesh D Mehta. Mapping human brain networks with cortico-cortical evoked potentials. *Philosophical Transactions of the Royal Society B*, 369:1–14, 2014.

[37] Ankit N Khambhati, Kathryn A Davis, Timothy H Lucas, Brian Litt, and Danielle S Bassett. Virtual cortical resection reveals push-pull network control preceding seizure evolution. *Neuron*, 91(5):1170–1182, 2016.

[38] Lohith G Kini, John M Bernabei, Fadi Mikhail, Peter Hadar, Preya Shah, Ankit N Khambhati, Kelly Oechsel, Ryan Archer, Jacqueline Boccanfuso, Erin Conrad, Russell T Shinohara, Joel Stein, Sandhitsu Das, Ammar Kheder, Timothy H Lucas, Kathryn A Davis, Danielle S Bassett, and Brian Litt. Virtual resection predicts surgical outcome for drug resistant epilepsy. *Brain: A Journal of Neurology*, pages 1–14, 2019.

[39] Jean-Philippe Lachaux, Eugenio Rodriguez, Jacques Martinerie, and Francisco J Varela. Measuring phase synchrony in brain signals. *Human Brain Mapping*, 8:194–208, 1999.

[40] Gemma Lancaster, Dmytro Iatsenko, Aleksandra Pidde, Valentina Ticcinelli, and Aneta Stefanovska. Surrogate data for hypothesis testing of physical systems. *Physics Reports*, 748:1–60, July 2018.

[41] Adam Li, Chester Huynh, Zachary Fitzgerald, Iahn Cajigas, Damian Brusko, Jonathan Jagid, Angel O Claudio, Andres M Kanner, Jennifer Hopp, Stephanie Chen, Jennifer Haagensen, Emily Johnson, William Anderson, Nathan Crone, Sara Inati, Kareem A Zaghloul, Juan Bulacio, Jorge Gonzalez-Martinez, and Sridevi V Sarma. Neural fragility as an EEG marker of the seizure onset zone. *Nature Neuroscience*, 24(10):1465–1474, October 2021.

[42] J Lukemire, S Kundu, G Pagnoni, and Y Guo. Bayesian joint modeling of multiple brain functional networks. *Journal of the American Statistical Association*, 116(534):518–530, 2021.

[43] Daniel J Lurie, Daniel Kessler, Danielle S Bassett, Richard F Betzel, Michael Breakspear, Shella Kheilholz, Aaron Kucyi, Raphaël Liégeois, Martin A Lindquist, Anthony Randal McIntosh, Russell A Poldrack, James M Shine, William Hedley Thompson, Natalia Z Bielczyk, Linda Douw, Dominik Kraft, Robyn L Miller, Muthuraman Muthuraman, Lorenzo Pasquini, Adeel Razi, Diego Vidaurre, Hua Xie, and Vince D Calhoun. Questions and controversies in the study of time-varying functional connectivity in resting fMRI. *Network Neuroscience*, 4(1):30–69, January 2020.

[44] Sergei Maslov and Kim Sneppen. Specificity and Stability in Topology of Protein Networks. *Science*, 296(5569):910–913, May 2002.

[45] Riki Matsumoto, Dileep R Nair, Eric LaPresto, Imad Najm, William Bingaman, Hiroshi Shibasaki, and Hans O Lüders. Functional connectivity in the human language system: a cortico-cortical evoked potential study. *Brain*, 127(10):2316–2330, 2004.

[46] R Milo, S Shen-Orr, S Itzkovitz, N Kashtan, D Chklovskii, and U Alon. Network Motifs: Simple Building Blocks of Complex Networks. *Science*, 298(5594):824–827, October 2002.

[47] Abdolreza Mohammadi, Fentaw Abegaz, Edwin van den Heuvel, and Ernst C Wit. Bayesian modelling of Dupuytren disease by using Gaussian copula graphical models. *Journal of the Royal Statistical Society. Series C (Applied Statistics)*, pages 629–645, 2017.

[48] Dileep R Nair, Armin Mohamed, Richard Burgess, and Hans Lüders. A critical review of the different conceptual hypotheses framing human focal epilepsy. *Epileptic Disorders: International Epilepsy Journal with Videotape*, 6(2):77–83, 2004.

[49] MEJ Newman and M Girvan. Finding and evaluating community structure in networks. *Physical Review E - Statistical, Nonlinear, and Soft Matter Physics*, 69(2 2):1–15, February 2004.

[50] Mark EJ Newman. Modularity and community structure in networks. *Proceedings of the National Academy of Sciences*, 103(23):8577–8582, 2006.

[51] Mark EJ Newman. *Networks: An Introduction*. Oxford University Press, 2010.

[52] Louis M Pecora and Thomas L Carroll. Master Stability Functions for Synchronized Coupled Systems Louis. *Physical Review Letters*, 80(10), 1998.

[53] Ernesto Pereda, Rodrigo Quian Quiroga, and Joydeep Bhattacharya. Nonlinear multivariate analysis of neurophysiological signals. *Progress in Neurobiology*, 77(1-2):1–37, September 2005.

[54] CB Peterson, F Stingo, and M Vannucci. Bayesian inference of multiple Gaussian graphical models. *Journal of the American Statistical Association*, 110(509):159–174, 2015.

[55] Mason a. Porter, Jukka-Pekka Onnela, and Peter J Mucha. Communities in networks. *American Mathematical Society*, 56(9):0–26, 2009.

[56] James A Roberts, Alistair Perry, Anton R Lord, Gloria Roberts, Philip B Mitchell, Robert E Smith, Fernando Calamante, and Michael Breakspear. The contribution of geometry to the human connectome. *NeuroImage*, 124:379–393, 2016.

[57] Arkaprava Roy and David B Dunson. Nonparametric graphical model for counts. *The Journal of Machine Learning Research*, 21(1):9353–9373, 2020.

[58] Brittany H Scheid, John M Bernabei, Ankit N Khambhati, Sofia Mouchtaris, Jay Jeschke, Dani S Bassett, Danielle Becker, Kathryn A Davis, Timothy Lucas, Werner Doyle, Edward F Chang, Daniel Friedman, Vikram R Rao, and Brian Litt. Intracranial electroencephalographic biomarker predicts effective responsive neurostimulation for epilepsy prior to treatment. *Epilepsia*, 63(3):652–662, March 2022.

[59] Kaspar A Schindler, Stephan Bialonski, Marie-Therese Horstmann, Christian E Elger, and Klaus Lehnertz. Evolving functional network properties and synchronizability during human epileptic seizures. *Chaos (Woodbury, N.Y.)*, 18(3):033119–033119, 2008.

[60] E Shaddox, FC Stingo, CB Peterson, S Jacobson, C Cruickshank-Quinn, K Kechris, et al. A Bayesian approach for learning gene networks underlying disease severity in COPD. *Statistics in Biosciences*, pages 1–27, 2018.

[61] Daniel Spencer, Rajarshi Guhaniyogi, and Raquel Prado. Joint Bayesian estimation of voxel activation and inter-regional connectivity in fMRI experiments. *psychometrika*, 85(4):845–869, 2020.

[62] Peter Spirtes and Clark Glymour. An algorithm for fast recovery of sparse causal graphs. *Social Science Computer Review*, 9(1):62–72, 1991.

[63] Peter Spirtes, Clark N Glymour, and Richard Scheines. *Causation, Prediction, and Search.* MIT Press, 2000.

[64] Olaf Sporns. Structure and function of complex brain networks. *Dialogues in Clinical Neuroscience*, 15(3):247–262, September 2013.

[65] Ramanujan Srinath and Supratim Ray. Effect of amplitude correlations on coherence in the local field potential. *Journal of Neurophysiology*, 112(4):741–751, August 2014.

[66] William Stacey, Mark Kramer, Kristin Gunnarsdottir, Jorge Gonzalez-martinez, Kareem Zaghloul, Sara Inati, Sridevi Sarma, Jennifer Stiso, Ankit N. Khambhati, Danielle S Bassett, Rachel J Smith, Virginia B Liu, Beth A Lopour, and Richard Staba. Emerging roles of network analysis for epilepsy. *Epilepsy Research*, 159(October 2019):106255–106255, 2019.

[67] G Tononi, O Sporns, and GM Edelman. Measures of degeneracy and redundancy in biological networks. *Proceedings of the National Academy of Sciences*, USA, 96(6):3257–3262, 1999.

[68] H Wang. Scaling it up: Stochastic search structure learning in graphical models. *Bayesian Analysis*, 10(2):351–377, 2015.

[69] Xiao Fan Wang and Guanrong Chen. Synchronization in scale-free dynamical networks: Robustness and fragility. *IEEE Transactions on Circuits and Systems I: Fundamental Theory and Applications*, 49(1):54–62, 2002.

[70] R Warnick, M Guindani, EB Erhardt, EA Allen, VD Calhoun, and M Vannucci. A Bayesian approach for estimating dynamic functional network connectivity in fMRI data. *Journal of the American Statistical Association*, 113(521):134–151, 2018.

[71] DJ Watts and SH Strogatz. Collective dynamics of 'small-world' networks. *Nature*, 393(6684):440–442, 1998.

# 8

# Time-Series Analysis

**Sharon Chiang**

*Department of Neurology, University of California, San Francisco (USA)*

**John Zito**

*Department of Statistics, Rice University (USA)*

**Vikram R. Rao**

*Department of Neurology, University of California, San Francisco (USA)*

**Marina Vannucci**

*Department of Statistics, Rice University (USA)*

## CONTENTS



Time-series analysis is useful for many applications in epilepsy. From data sources including seizure recording devices, patient seizure diaries, functional MRI and EEG, time-series analysis forms the foundation of inference and prediction in many data streams. This chapter reviews several classical statistical models in time-series analysis that have

DOI: 10.1201/9781003254515-8

been used in epilepsy research to date. We first review foundations of linear time-series models for univariate time-series data, including autoregressive moving average and conditional heteroskedasticity models. Next, we cover several multivariate time-series models, including vector autoregressive and vector autoregressive moving average models. We discuss incorporation of brain states into time-series models and cover state-space models, including dynamic linear models and hidden Markov models, as well as nonlinear extensions via regime-switching models. We end by highlighting concepts in circular data analysis, which can be used to investigate cycles in time-series data. Examples are provided in the R programming language using a simulated dataset motivated by chronic ambulatory electrocorticography collected from the Responsive Neurostimulation System (RNS® System) (NeuroPace, Inc., Mountain View, CA).

## 8.1 Introduction

Time-series methods are useful for the analysis of time-series data, or data collected over successive timepoints. Multiple sources of data inherent in epilepsy practice involve time-series data, including electroencephalography (EEG) and intracranial electrocorticography (ECoG) data, neural spike trains, blood oxygen level dependent (BOLD) signal from functional magnetic resonance imaging (fMRI), and clinical seizures from patient-reported seizure diaries. Analysis of data collected over time is typically either in the frequency domain (Chapter 9) or in the time domain.

This chapter focuses on non neural network-based statistical methods for analyzing time-series data in the time domain. Frequency domain analysis methods are covered in Chapter 9 and neural networks are covered separately in the context of language models in Chapter 13. In Section 8.2, we present four classical linear models for time-series analysis (autoregressive, moving average, autoregressive moving average, and autoregressive integrated moving average models). In Section 8.3, we describe conditional heteroskedasticity models, for use when the time-series has time-varying variance. In Section 8.4, we present vector autoregressive methods used to model multivariate time-series, which are used for data with multiple time-series such as that encountered with multiple channels in EEG or multiple voxels in fMRI. Extensions to vector autoregressive moving average models are briefly discussed. In Section 8.5, we discuss state-space models, including dynamic linear models and hidden Markov models, as well as extensions to nonlinear cases via regime-switching models. Last, in Section 8.6, we review circular statistics, which can be used to summarize data that contains direction, such as time-series data. Implementation of these methods is demonstrated in R using a simulated dataset of interictal epileptiform discharges (IEDs) motivated by the RNS System.

## 8.2 Univariate Linear Time-Series Models

A time-series $y_t$ is defined as a *linear process* if, given a white noise process $\epsilon_t$, we can write the current value of the time-series as a linear combination of the white noise terms plus a common mean. Special cases of linear time-series processes include the autoregressive integrated moving average (ARIMA) class of models, which model the autocorrelations present in time-series data, and exponential smoothing models, which use weighted averages of past observations to predict future observations. In this section, we discuss building blocks of ARIMA models, including autoregressive (AR), moving average (MA), autoregressive moving average (ARMA), and ARIMA models. Extensions to seasonal ARIMA (SARIMA), which are a variation of ARIMA models that take into account seasonality, and exponential smoothing methods, can be found in [23].

**Example 8.2.1. (Example: Overview of simulated dataset)** The examples in this chapter are based on time-series of simulated $z$-transformed hourly IED counts, motivated by continuous electrocorticography data collected by the RNS System [45]. The RNS System is a closed-loop responsive neurostimulator which automatically detects and records, among other data, the number of IED counts per hour from each of two leads that are implanted in the brain. In the examples that follow, for Patients 1–3, we will let $y_t$ denote the $z$-transformed hourly IED counts from the first lead, and let $x_t$ denote the $z$-transformed hourly IED counts from the second lead of each example patient. For context, we refer in this chapter to the left hippocampus as being the location for lead 1 and the right hippocampus as being the location for lead 2. Later examples in the chapter involve a four-variate time-series of IED counts (Patient 4) and univariate time-series of rescaled seizure times (Patient 5). `R` code and simulated data to replicate examples are available from the repository accompanying the book.

```
# Load simulated patients for data examples
load('~/Example1.RData') # Example Patient 1
load('~/Example2.RData') # Example Patient 2
load('~/Example3.RData') # Example Patient 3
load('~/Example4.RData') # Example Patient 4
load('~/Example5.RData') # Example Patient 5
```

### 8.2.1 Stationarity

When applying the ARIMA class of models to time-series data, our first task is to evaluate whether the time-series is stationary, or whether the properties of the time-series do not depend on time. If it is not, transformations should be applied to make the time-series stationary.

A linear time-series process $y_t$ is said to be *strictly stationary* if a shift in time does not cause a change in the shape of a distribution. However, the definition of strict stationarity rarely applies in practice. Therefore, a weaker form of stationarity, or *weak, or wide-sense stationarity*, is often assumed, which means that the time-series fluctuates with constant covariance around a fixed level (Figure 8.1). Most epilepsy datasets are also not weakly stationary. For example, in many individuals with epilepsy, clinical and electrographic seizures may occur at specific phases of fluctuation in interictal epileptiform discharge rate [3] and the distribution of seizure occurrences may vary depending on the phase of interictal spiking. In BOLD fMRI time-series data, various non-neural contributors may render the signal non-stationary, including tscanner drift, hardware instabilities, head motion, and other physiological fluctuations such as blood pressure or respiratory variation [28].

To evaluate if data are stationary, several approaches are often employed:

1. **Graph the data**. Plot the time-series to evaluate for obvious trends or seasonal effects. If there is an obvious trend or seasonal effect, then the data are likely non-stationary.
2. **Calculate summary statistics.** Calculate the mean and variance for subsets of the data and check for differences across time. If statistically significant differences

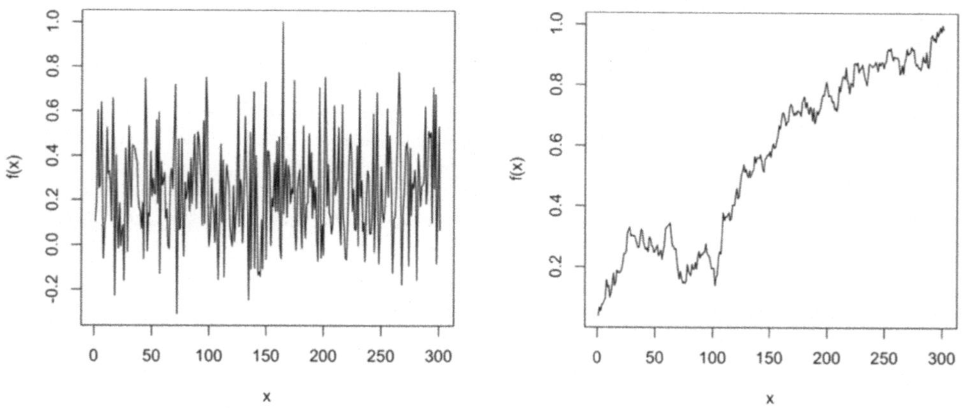


**FIGURE 8.1**
Example of (left panel) stationary and (right panel) non-stationary time-series.

in the mean or variance are present across subsets of the time-series, then the data are likely non-stationary.

3. **Look at the autocorrelation function (ACF) plot.** If the ACF plot decays slowly, this suggests the data is non-stationary.
4. **Conduct a unit-root statistical test to evaluate for stationarity.** A *unit root test* tests the null hypothesis that the time-series is non-stationary and contains a unit root, which is a characteristic of a time-series that makes it non-stationary. The number of unit roots corresponds with the number of differencing operations that are required to make the time-series stationary. One of the most commonly employed unit root tests is the Augmented Dickey-Fuller test, which can be implemented in `R` with the `ur.df()` function from the `urca` library [42].

### 8.2.2 Autoregressive Models

An autoregressive (AR) process models the current value of the time-series as a linear combination of $p$ past values of the time-series. This allows us to capture "long-term" trends in time-series data. In the example of modeling hourly IED counts, this allows us to model hourly IED counts at any given time point as a linear function of $p$ past IED counts. The number of prior time points $p$ is called the *order* of the AR model. Mathematically, this is written as:

$$y_t = a + c_1 y_{t-1} + c_2 y_{t-2} + \ldots + c_p y_{t-p} + \epsilon_t, \tag{8.1}$$

where $y_t$ is the value of the time-series at the $t$-th time point, $a$ is an intercept, the $c_l$ are regression coefficients, and $\epsilon$ is noise.

How do we determine what the order of the AR process should be, as well as if an AR process is appropriate? Two main plots that should be examined are the autocorrelation function (ACF) and partial autocorrelation function (PACF) plots. The autocorrelation at lag $k$ tells us how correlated an observation in the time-series is with observations at $k$ prior values, and the ACF plot is a bar graph that shows the correlation between the present value of the time-series with each lagged past value (the first past value, the second past value, up to the $p$th past value). The partial autocorrelation at lag $k$ tells us how correlated an observation in the time-series is with observation at $k$ prior values after removing the effect of correlations at shorter lags, and the PACF plot shows the partial correlation between each value of the time-series and its lagged values. The ACF and PACF plots are evaluated together to determine whether an AR process is appropriate, as well as the order of the process. In an AR process, we should see a gradual decrease in the ACF plot and a sharp drop after $p$ lags in the PACF plot.

**Example 8.2.2. (Fitting an AR process)** To demonstrate usage of the ACF and PACF for evaluating the suitability and order of AR process for modeling a time-series, let us return to the left hippocampal time-series $y_t$ of Example Patient 1. We can plot the ACF and PACF functions using the `acf()` and `pacf()` functions from the `stats` package in `R`:

```
# Plot ACF and PACF
y <- Example1$y
acf(y)
pacf(y)
```

Figure 8.2 shows the ACF and PACF plot for $y$. The ACF plot shows a gradually decreasing trend, whereas we see a sharp drop in the PACF plot, which drops below the 95% confidence bounds after three lags. This suggests that an AR(3) process would be appropriate for the time-series. In particular, for an AR process, the PACF should be equal to zero past the order of the models, so the number of non-zero partial autocorrelations gives the order of the AR model.

To fit an AR(3) process in `R`, we can use the `arima()` function from the `stats` package. The `arima()` function contains a parameter `order` which allows for specification of the order of a general ARIMA process as $(p, d, q)$, where $p$ is the AR order. The other parameters are $q$, which is the MA order (discussed in Section 8.2.3), and $d$ is the degree of differencing (discussed in Section 8.2.5). For an AR(3) process, we fit:

```
# Fit AR(3) process
ar_process <- arima(y, order = c(3,0,0))
ar_process
```

This yields the following AR(3) model:

$$y_t = -0.035 + 0.49y_{t-1} - 0.23y_{t-2} + 0.36y_{t-3} + \epsilon_t. \tag{8.2}$$

### 8.2.3 Moving Average Models

In contrast to an autoregressive process, a moving average (MA) process models the current value of the time-series as a linear combination of $p$ past *error values*. The MA component allows us to capture sudden "shocks" in the time-series in which the error of the observed compared to the predicted value may be large. Specifically, the IED count at time $t$ is modeled as a weighted moving average of the past forecast *errors*, rather than of the forecasted variable (IED counts) itself. The number of past error values that it depends on, $q$, defines the *order* of the MA process. The MA($q$) model is expressed as:

$$y_t = b + \epsilon_t + d_1\epsilon_{t-1} + d_2\epsilon_{t-2} + \ldots + d_q\epsilon_{t-q}, \tag{8.3}$$

where $y_t$ is the value of the time-series at the $t$-th time point, $b$ is an intercept, the $d_l$ are coefficients, and $\epsilon$ is white noise with expected value $\mathbb{E}[\epsilon_t] = 0$ and variance $\sigma^2$.

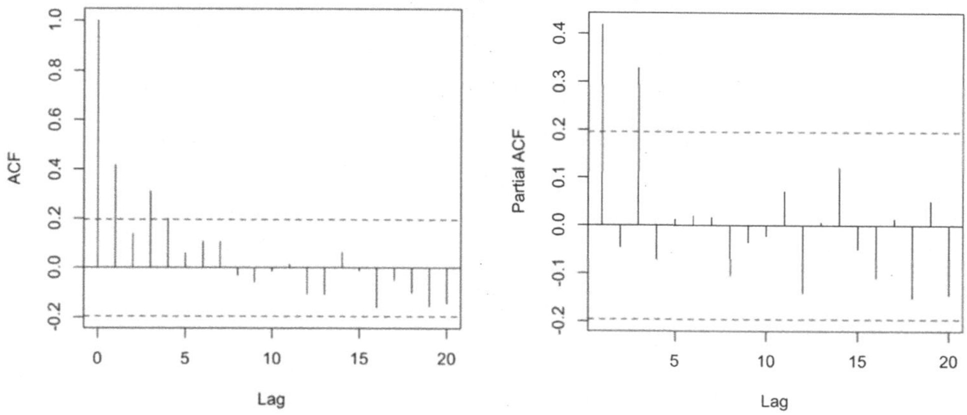


**FIGURE 8.2**
(Left panel) ACF and (right panel) PACF plots for left hippocampal IED counts of simulated patient.

To determine whether an AR or MA process is appropriate for a time-series, we look again at the ACF and PACF plots. For an MA model, we should see the opposite of the AR model: the PACF should not sharply drop past the order of the model, but instead gradually decrease to zero, while there should be a sharp drop after $q$ lags in the ACF plot. Specifically, in a MA process, the ACF should have non-zero autocorrelations only at lags involved in the model, so the number of non-zero autocorrelations gives the order of the MA model.

**Example 8.2.3. (Fitting an MA process)** To illustrate the determination of the order of an MA process, let us examine the ACF and PACF plots of the right hippocampal time-series $x_t$ of Example Patient 1. Figure 8.3 shows that the ACF plot drops sharply below the 95% confidence bounds after the first lag, while the PACF plot gradually decreases toward zero. This suggests that a MA(1) process would be appropriate for the time-series.

To fit an MA(1) process, we can use again the `arima()` function, specifying the third element of the `order` parameter as $q = 1$:

```
# Fit MA(1) process
x <- Example1$x
ma_process <- arima(x, order = c(0,0,1))
ma_process
```

This yields the following MA(1) model:

$$y_t = -0.0038 + 0.29\epsilon_{t-1} + \epsilon_t. \tag{8.4}$$

### 8.2.4 Autoregressive Moving Average Models

An autoregressive moving average (ARMA) model is simply the combination of autoregressive and moving average models. In other words, according to an ARMA($p, q$) model, the current value of the time-series depends on prior values of the time-series as well as external factors captured in random noise. This allows us to incorporate both long-term trends (AR) and sudden shocks (MA) in our model of the time-series data.

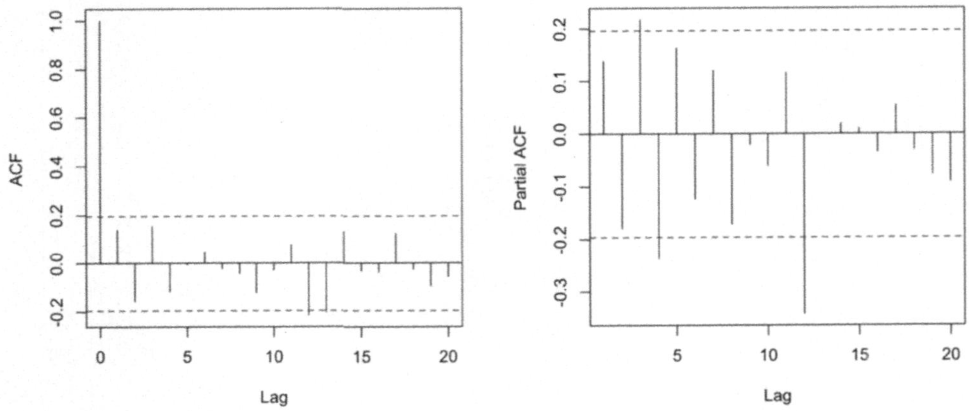


**FIGURE 8.3**
(Left panel) ACF and (right panel) PACF plots for right hippocampal IED counts of simulated patient.

To model a time-series $y_t$ as an ARMA$(p, q)$ process, we express this as:

$$y_t = \delta + c_1 y_{t-1} + c_2 y_{t-2} + \ldots + c_p y_{t-p} + d_1 \epsilon_{t-1} + d_2 \epsilon_{t-2} + \ldots + d_q \epsilon_{t-q} + \epsilon_t. \quad (8.5)$$

The order of the autoregressive process, $p$, and of the moving average process, $q$, can be determined by looking at the ACF and PACF plots to see where the cutoff is for each. Alternatively, a grid search can be performed in which the ARMA model is fit for various values of $p$ and $q$, and the model chosen based on the combination of $p$ and $q$ that minimizes an information criterion, such as the Akaike information criterion (AIC) or Bayesian information criterion (BIC).

**Example 8.2.4. (Selecting the order of an ARMA model using a grid search)** Suppose we want to fit an ARMA($p$, $q$) model to the left hippocampal time-series $y_t$ from Example Patient 2. One approach is to fit the ARMA model over a grid of values of $p$ and $q$ using maximum likelihood and calculate the AIC, then to select the model that minimizes the AIC. Here, suppose we fit values of $p$ and $q$ over a grid (for example, up to an order of 4):

```
# Select order of ARMA model over a grid
y <- Example2$y
p_max <- 4
q_max <- 4
aic_grid <- matrix(NA, p_max, q_max)
for (p in 1:p_max){
  for (q in 1:q_max){
    arima_out <- arima(y, order = c(p,0,q), method = "ML")
    aic_grid[p,q] <- arima_out$aic
  }
}
which(aic_grid == min(aic_grid), arr.ind = TRUE)
```

This yields values of $p = 2$ and $q = 3$ minimizing the AIC, i.e., an ARMA(2, 3) model. This is fit by specifying $p$ and $q$ in the `order` argument in `arima()`:

```
# Fit ARMA(2,3) model
arima_model <- arima(y, order = c(2,0,3))
arima_model
```

which gives the following ARMA(2,3) model:

$$y_t = -0.004 + 0.73y_{t-1} + -0.73y_{t-2} + 0.07\epsilon_{t-1} + 0.07\epsilon_{t-2} + 1\epsilon_{t-3} + \epsilon_t. \quad (8.6)$$

### 8.2.5 Autoregressive Integrated Moving Average Models

The models in Sections 8.2.2–8.2.4 assume that the time-series is stationary, with a constant mean and variance over time. If, however, evaluation suggests that this assumption is not true, then data should be transformed prior to applying these models, which leads to the discussion of Autoregressive Integrated Moving Average (ARIMA) models. *Differencing* is a common approach to transform non-stationary time-series into stationary ones. It removes temporal dependence, such as from trends or seasonality, by subtracting the previous observation from the current observation:

$$\triangle y_{t-1} = y_t - y_{t-1} \quad (8.7)$$

Differencing can either be used to remove trends, where the mean of the time-series varies over time, or seasonality, where there are cycles that repeat over time. It is important to note that although differencing can help make data stationary, it can also introduce autocorrelations. Therefore, it is important to examine the data after each differencing step to evaluate if further transformations are needed.

ARIMA models are essentially ARMA models fitted on differenced time-series. In an ARIMA$(p, d, q)$ model, $p$ is the order of the autoregressive process, $d$ is the number of times that the data have to be differenced to produce a stationary time-series, and $q$ is the order of the moving average process.

**Example 8.2.5. (Fitting an ARIMA model)** Suppose we have determined that first-order differencing yields a stationary time-series to the right hippocampal time-series $x_t$ from Example Patient 2. First, we difference the data using the `diff()` function in R:

```
# Difference data
x <- Example2$x
differenced_data <- diff(x)
```

We then fit an ARIMA model to the first-order differenced data using the `arima()` function, specifying the values of $p$ and $q$ from Example 8.2.4:

```
# Fit ARIMA model to differenced data
p <- 2 # AR order
q <- 3 # MA order
arima_model <- arima(differenced_data, order = c(p, 0, q))
arima_model$coef
```

Determining the order of differencing, $d$, prior to fitting an ARIMA model is an essential step in analysis. Order of differencing is determined by sequentially differencing the data. If, after taking the first differencing value, the resulting differenced values are still not stationary using the approaches discussed in Section 8.2.1, then we difference again to find the second differencing values, and so forth until the differenced data is stationary. The following are common measures employed after each differencing step to determine how many differencing steps are needed:

1. Visual inspection: Plot the time-series data and its differenced values, to determine how many times the data needs to be differenced to remove any trends and seasonality.

2. Unit root tests: Perform a unit root test, such as the Augmented Dickey-Fuller test, at each order of differencing to identify the order of differencing that yields the most stationary time-series.
3. PACF plot: The PACF plot shows us how correlated observations in the time-series are, while controlling for the effect of correlations at intermediate lags. Thus, if the PACF plot exhibits a sharp decline after a certain lag, this suggests that differencing at that order may be appropriate.
4. Measures of model fit: Information criteria such as the AIC or BIC can be used to compare ARIMA models with different orders of differencing. Lower AIC or BIC values indicate better model fit.

Although beyond the scope of this chapter, Bayesian versions of ARIMA are also available and are discussed in detail elsewhere [57].

### 8.2.6 Model Diagnostics

Model diagnostics are an important component to evaluating how well the choice of an ARIMA captures the patterns in the time-series data. Several model diagnostic measures are commonly assessed in time-series data, which are complementary and often considered in combination to provide a comprehensive evaluation of how appropriate the ARIMA model is for the data. These diagnostic measures include:

1. Residual analysis: Similar to linear models, generalized linear models, and mixed-effects models (Chapter 5), a central tool in model diagnostics is *residual analysis.* For ARIMA models, the residuals are calculated as $y_t - \hat{y}_t$, where $\hat{y}_t$ is the predicted value of $y$ based on the ARIMA model. If the model is correctly specified, the residuals should have properties of white noise; i.e., independent normal random variables with zero mean and a common variance. To check these properties, approaches that are usually taken include plotting the residuals over time to look for patterns; checking for autocorrelation and heteroskedasticity of the residuals; and checking for normality.
2. Ljung-Box test: The Ljung-Box test is an omnibus test of independence that can be used in residual analysis to test the null hypothesis that the residuals are independently distributed, against the alternative hypothesis that there is autocorrelation in the residuals. If the null hypothesis is rejected in favor of the alternative, then the test suggests that there is evidence that the residuals are not independent.
3. Information criteria: Information criteria such as the AIC or BIC can be used to compare ARIMA models and provide a trade-off between model fit and complexity. Lower values of AIC or BIC indicate better model fit.
4. Mean square error (MSE): The mean square error is calculated as the mean squared difference between the observed and predicted values of the time-series. Lower MSE values indicate better model fit. Of note, MSE can be influenced by the scale of the data and should not be used as the sole measure of model fit.

How do we know which goodness of fit measures are most pertinent to our application? One way to think about this is to consider whether inference or prediction is the main direction of interest. The first three measures above can be considered measures of in-sample predictive error, whereas the last measure can be considered a measure of out-of-sample predictive error. If understanding the direct of past values and error terms on the current observation of the time-series is the task of interest, then the first three measures may be more useful; if the ARIMA model is to be used for prediction, such as in the case of seizure forecasting, then measures of out-of-sample predictive error such as MSE may be more useful.

**Example 8.2.6. (Testing for independence of residuals with the Ljung-Box test)** The test statistic for the Ljung-Box test is

$$Q = n(n+2)\sum_{k=1}^{m} \frac{p_k^2}{n-k}, \tag{8.8}$$

where $n$ denotes the number of samples, $p_k$ is the sample autocorrelation at lag $k$, and $m$ is the total number of lags being tested. The test compares the null hypothesis that the residuals are independently distributed against the alternative hypothesis that there is autocorrelation in the residuals. We reject the null hypothesis if $Q > \chi^2_{1-\alpha,h}$, where $\chi^2_{1-\alpha,h}$ denotes the value of the chi-square distribution table for significance level $\alpha$ and $h$ degrees of freedom. When applying the Ljung-Box test to the residuals from an ARIMA model, we set the degrees of freedom $h$ to $m - p - q$, where $p$ is the AR order and $q$ is the MA order in the ARIMA model.

To apply the Ljung-Box test to residuals from the ARIMA model fit from Example 8.2.5, we can calculate residuals using `residuals()` and use the `Box.test()` function from the `stats` package on the calculated residuals:

```
# Ljung-Box test
k <- log(length(x)) # Set k to the desired lag order; for example, log(T)
residuals <- residuals(arima_model)
ljung_box_test <- Box.test(residuals, lag = k, type = "Ljung-Box")
ljung_box_test
```

In the above example, $k$ is set to the desired maximum lag order that should be considered when evaluating autocorrelation in the residuals. There are various empirical suggestions on selecting the appropriate value for $k$, including $k = \ln(T)$ [51], $k = 5$ [35], $k = 20$ [49], and $k = \min\{10, T/5\}$ [23], where $T$ is the length of the time-series, while another suggestion is to consider the length of the time-series, using a small value of $k$ for time-series that are relatively short (less than 500 values) and larger values for longer time-series [21].

## 8.3 Conditional Heteroskedasticity Models

ARIMA models model current observations of the time-series as a function of the long-term trend (AR) and sudden disruptions (MA). These are good models for time-series with long-term trends and occasional sudden disruptions, but for which the *variance* of the time-series is relatively constant, or homoskedastic. What if, however, the variance of the time-series itself has patterns that we want to account for?

There are two broad classes of models that can be used to model time-series data in which the variance changes over time (also referred to as *heteroskedastic* time-series data): conditional heteroskedasticity models, which includes autoregressive conditionally heteroskedastic (ARCH) and generalized autoregressive conditionally heteroskedastic (GARCH) models, and stochastic volatility models. Although these classes of models, which originated in the field of finance and have traditionally been used to characterize volatility in financial markets, have been used less frequently in epilepsy literature to date, these methods can be used to model non-stationary time-series that exhibit time-varying variance, with periods of relatively high variance and periods of relatively low variance. For example, if we look at the time-series of seizure counts over time, we might hypothesize that times in which anti-seizure medicines are being uptitrated might be characterized by greater variance in seizure counts prior to uptitration and lower variance after uptitration. Such conditional heteroskedasticity models have also been used to estimate dynamic functional connectivity between regions involved in the resting-state network in individuals with epilepsy using functional MRI [10], or to model the volatility of EEG signal to quantify seizure dynamics [15]. The primary difference between conditional heteroskedasticity and stochastic volatility models is that the former models variance as a deterministic function of model parameters and past data, whereas the latter models variance as a random variable. In this section, we briefly cover conditional heteroskedasticity models. The field of stochastic volatility models itself is vast and an excellent review can be found in [4], with examples of their applications to epilepsy including the extraction of volatility features to decode memory states [44].

### 8.3.1 Autoregressive Conditional Heteroskedasticity Models

The ARCH($p$) process, proposed by [14], can be thought of as an AR model applied to the variance of the time-series. Let us consider the simplest ARCH process to model the variance of a time-series, or an ARCH(1) process. We say that $y_t$ follows an ARCH(1) process if:

$$\text{Var}(y_t \mid y_{t-1}) := \sigma_t^2 = \alpha_0 + \alpha_1 y_{t-1}^2.$$

Looking at this equation, this says that, in an ARCH(1) process, the time-varying variance of the time-series is a function of a constant term $\alpha_0$ plus one lagged squared value of the time-series at time $t-1$. We also see that relatively larger values of $y_{t-1}^2$ will yield a larger value of the variance at time $t$ under the ARCH framework; in other words, the variance of $y_t$ tends to be predictable at time $t$ following large values at time $t-1$ than following small values at time $t-1$.

More generally, $y_t$ follows an ARCH($p$) process if its variance at time $t$ depends on its values at the prior $p$ times:

$$\text{Var}(y_t \mid y_{t-1}, \ldots, y_{t-p}) = \sigma_t^2 = \alpha_0 + \sum_{i=1}^{p} \alpha_i y_{t-i}^2.$$

The order $p$ of the ARCH model can be selected using the PACF of $y_t^2$ [51]. For example, if the PACF of $y_t^2$ suggests an AR($m$) process, then an ARCH($m$) process may be appropriate.

There are several assumptions inherent to ARCH models which should be considered when applying these models to epilepsy data. For example, the ARCH model assumes that positive and negative values of $y_t$ have the same effect on the variance, because the variance depends on the square of the value. In some applications, this may not be the case. It may also not be the case that variance of a given time-series tends to be more predictable following large values than small values at the previous time point.

### 8.3.2 Generalized Autoregressive Conditional Heteroskedasticitiy Models

A GARCH process is a generalization of an ARCH process which incorporates both autoregressive and moving average components [5]. Specifically, in contrast to an ARCH process, which models the variance at time $t$ as a function of the prior squared observations of the time-series, a GARCH($p$, $q$) process models the variance at time $t$ as a function of $p$ prior squared observations as well as $q$ prior variances. For example, to model a time-series

$y_t$ as a GARCH(1, 1) process, we write:

$$\text{Var}(y_t \mid y_{t-1}, \ldots, y_{t-m}) = \sigma_t^2 = \alpha_0 + \alpha_1 y_{t-1}^2 + \beta_1 \sigma_{t-1}^2.$$

Similar to ARCH models, GARCH models assume that large values of $y_{t-1}^2$ or $\sigma_{t-1}$ lead to large values of $\sigma_t$, leading to a phenomenon known as volatility clustering, where large values of the variance or of the time-series itself tend to be followed by large values of the variance. More generally, $y_t$ follows a GARCH($m$, $n$) process if

$$\text{Var}(y_t \mid y_{t-1}, \ldots, y_{t-m}) = \sigma_t^2 = \alpha_0 + \sum_{i=1}^{m} \alpha_i y_{t-i}^2 + \sum_{j=1}^{n} \beta_j \sigma_{t-j}^2.$$

where the order ($m$,, $n$) of the GARCH process can be determined similarly to the approach to determining the order of an ARMA process (Section 8.2.4).

## 8.4 Multivariate Linear Time-Series Models

In multivariate time-series analysis, we observe a vector of $n$ time-series $\mathbf{y}_t = [y_{1,t}, y_{2,t}, \ldots, y_{n,t}]^T$. Instead of modeling each component time-series $y_{i,t}$ separately using the methods described above, multivariate analysis aims to model the joint dynamics of all $n$ time-series together. This task, for instance, arises in functional connectivity studies when each $y_{i,t}$ represents the time-series of fMRI measurements taken at each voxel [18]. In this case, the task of interest is estimation of the interactions between different brain regions, which requires a model that can capture the dependence structure among the individual time-series.

Vector autoregressive (VAR) and vector autoregressive moving average (VARMA) models are two examples of multivariate time-series models which can be used for this purpose and are straightforward multivariate generalizations of the ARMA models we have already seen. [36] gives a book-length treatment of these topics from a frequentist point of view, and [25] gives an excellent introduction to the Bayesian analysis of VAR models. There are several software implementations of these and other multivariate time-series methods; we provide a few examples based on the `R` packages `vars` [43], `BVAR` [32], and `MTS` [52].

### 8.4.1 Vector Autoregressive Models

Similar to the AR model, the vector autoregressive (VAR) model expresses an $n$-dimensional vector time-series $\mathbf{y}_t$ as a linear combination of its $p$ most recent lagged values. As in the AR model, the integer $p$ is called the *order* of the VAR, and we denote a $p$th-order VAR for an $n$-dimensional time-series with VAR$_n(p)$. Mathematically, the VAR$_n(p)$ model is given by

$$\mathbf{y}_t = \mathbf{a} + \mathbf{\Phi}_1 \mathbf{y}_{t-1} + \mathbf{\Phi}_2 \mathbf{y}_{t-2} + \ldots + \mathbf{\Phi}_p \mathbf{y}_{t-p} + \boldsymbol{\varepsilon}_t, \quad \boldsymbol{\varepsilon}_t \overset{\text{iid}}{\sim} \text{N}_n(\mathbf{0}, \mathbf{\Sigma}), \tag{8.9}$$

where $\mathbf{a}$ is an $n \times 1$ intercept vector, each $\mathbf{\Phi}_l$ is an $n \times n$ coefficient matrix, $\boldsymbol{\varepsilon}_t$ is an $n \times 1$ vector of regression errors, and $\text{N}_n(\mathbf{0}, \mathbf{\Sigma})$ denotes the mean-zero multivariate normal distribution with $n \times n$ covariance matrix $\mathbf{\Sigma}$. To see how this model encodes dependencies among the individual time-series in $\mathbf{y}_t$, we can write the implied regression equation for each series as:

$$y_{i,t} = a_i + \sum_{l=1}^{p} \sum_{j=1}^{n} \phi_l^{(i,j)} y_{j,t-l} + \varepsilon_{i,t}, \tag{8.10}$$

where $a_i$ is the $i$th element of the vector $\mathbf{a}$, $\phi_l^{(i,j)}$ is the entry in the $i$th row and $j$th column of the matrix $\mathbf{\Phi}_l$, and $\varepsilon_{i,t}$ is the $i$th element of the vector $\boldsymbol{\varepsilon}_t$. In this way, we see that the $\text{VAR}_n(p)$ models each time-series $y_{i,t}$ as an ordinary multiple linear regression that depends both on its own lagged values (as in the univariate AR model) as well as the lagged values of the other series in $\mathbf{y}_t$. Further dependencies are introduced by allowing the error terms $\varepsilon_{i,t}$ in these regressions to be correlated according to the covariance matrix $\mathbf{\Sigma}$.

**Parameter Estimation:** Once the lag order $p$ has been specified, we can estimate the coefficients $\mathbf{a}$, $\mathbf{\Phi}_1$, ..., $\mathbf{\Phi}_p$ and the error covariance matrix $\mathbf{\Sigma}$ in several ways. From a classical or frequentist point of view, we can estimate them using ordinary least squares (OLS) or the method of maximum likelihood (MLE) in a manner very similar to how ordinary (multivariate) linear regression models are estimated. The `vars` package in `R` fits VAR models using OLS and reports the coefficient estimates on an equation-by-equation basis as in Eq. (8.10). Below is the `R` output when we fit a $\text{VAR}_2(2)$ to the bivariate IED time-series from Example Patient 2:

```
# Fit VAR
library(vars)
my_var_model <- VAR(Example2, p = 2, type = "const")

> summary(my_var_model)

Estimation results for equation y:
===================================
y = y.l1 + x.l1 + y.l2 + x.l2 + const

       Estimate Std. Error t value Pr(>|t|)
y.l1   0.396508   0.099982   3.966 0.000144 ***
x.l1   0.728145   0.913977   0.797 0.427668
y.l2  -0.241902   0.101350  -2.387 0.019020 *
x.l2  -0.592927   0.890045  -0.666 0.506948
const -0.008084   0.096918  -0.083 0.933703
---

Estimation results for equation x:
===================================
x = y.l1 + x.l1 + y.l2 + x.l2 + const

       Estimate Std. Error t value Pr(>|t|)
y.l1   0.005510   0.009807   0.562    0.576
x.l1   1.451038   0.089654  16.185  < 2e-16 ***
y.l2   0.009626   0.009942   0.968    0.335
x.l2  -0.475366   0.087307  -5.445  4.2e-07 ***
const  0.014193   0.009507   1.493    0.139
---
Signif. codes:  0 '***' 0.001 '**' 0.01 '*' 0.05 '.' 0.1 ' ' 1

Covariance matrix of residuals:
         y        x
y 0.859238 0.002577
x 0.002577 0.008268
```

From a Bayesian point of view, inference in the VAR is conducted by placing priors on the VAR coefficients $\mathbf{\Phi} = \{\mathbf{a}, \mathbf{\Phi}_1, ..., \mathbf{\Phi}_p\}$ and the covariance matrix $\mathbf{\Sigma}$ and sampling from the posterior distribution given a sample of observed data. We can do this with the `BVAR` package, which implements the methods of [17] for prior specification:

```
# Fit Bayesian VAR
library(BVAR)
my_bvar_model <- bvar(Example2, lags = 2)
```

```
> summary(my_bvar_model)

Numeric array (dimensions 5, 2) of coefficient values from a BVAR.
Median values:
                y      x
constant    0.002  0.022
y-lag1      0.411  0.007
x-lag1      0.309  1.161
y-lag2     -0.207  0.010
x-lag2     -0.189 -0.192

Numeric array (dimensions 2, 2) of variance-covariance values from a BVAR.
Median values:
      y     x
y 0.830 0.004
x 0.004 0.010
```

We see that the point estimates (posterior medians) are close but not identical to the OLS estimates. This reflects the influence of the prior distribution, which introduces a degree of shrinkage to the estimation.

In Bayesian inference, we write down a prior probability distribution for the model's parameters which summarizes our beliefs about how the model behaves before we see any data. Once the data arrive, we update our beliefs by using Bayes' theorem to calculate a posterior distribution. The `BVAR` package implements a class of *hierarchical Minnesota priors* [34] for the VAR coefficients, and it returns a posterior approximation based on Markov chain Monte Carlo (MCMC) sampling. The prior on the VAR coefficients is a multivariate normal distribution with the following mean and covariance:

$$E\left(\phi_l^{(i,j)}\right) = \begin{cases} 1 & i=j,\, l=1 \\ 0 & \text{else} \end{cases} \tag{8.11}$$

$$\text{cov}\left(\phi_s^{(i,j)},\, \phi_r^{(k,l)}\right) = \begin{cases} \frac{\lambda^2}{s^2}\frac{1}{\psi_j}\Sigma^{(i,k)} & l=j, r=s \\ 0 & \text{else.} \end{cases} \tag{8.12}$$

The prior mean is one for the coefficient on each variable's first *own* lag and zero otherwise. So our prior belief is centered on the VAR being a random walk for each variable: $y_{i,t} = a_i + y_{i,t-1} + \varepsilon_{i,t}$. The prior covariance controls how tight or loose our beliefs are about the prior mean, and it also controls cross-variable shrinkage. We see for instance that as $s$ gets large and we consider coefficients on far away lags, the prior automatically gets tighter ($1/s^2$) around the mean belief that these coefficients are zero. The main tuning parameter is $\lambda$, which controls the overall level of tightness. Instead of fixing this, we will endow it with a prior as well and estimate it. The $\psi_j$ are variable-specific hyperparameters that could also be estimated, but the default procedure is to fit an AR($p$) to each series $y_{j,t}$ and then fix $\psi_j$ at the resulting estimate of the residual variance.

To complete the model, we place an inverse Wishart prior on $\boldsymbol{\Sigma}$ and a gamma prior on $\lambda$. With the priors and tuning parameters specified, the default call to `bvar()` uses an MCMC algorithm to approximate the posterior of the VAR parameters:

$$p(\boldsymbol{\Phi},\, \boldsymbol{\Sigma},\, \lambda \,|\, \mathbf{y}_{1:T}) = \frac{\overbrace{p(\mathbf{y}_{1:T} \,|\, \boldsymbol{\Phi},\, \boldsymbol{\Sigma})}^{\text{from (8.9)}}\ \overbrace{p(\boldsymbol{\Phi} \,|\, \boldsymbol{\Sigma},\, \lambda)}^{\text{Minnesota prior}}\ p(\boldsymbol{\Sigma})p(\lambda)}{p(\mathbf{y}_{1:T})}. \tag{8.13}$$

Armed with this approximation, we can use summaries like posterior means and medians to produce point estimates of the VAR parameters, and we can calculate Bayesian credible intervals to quantify our posterior uncertainty about the parameters. As we saw, the

**TABLE 8.1**
Criteria for VAR lag order selection.

| Name | Formula |
|---|---|
| Final prediction error | $\text{FPE}(p) = \left(\frac{T+np+1}{T-np-1}\right)^n \lvert\hat{\mathbf{\Sigma}}_T^{(p)}\rvert$ |
| Akaike's information criterion | $\text{AIC}(p) = \ln\lvert\hat{\mathbf{\Sigma}}_T^{(p)}\rvert + \frac{2}{T}pn^2$ |
| Hannan-Quinn | $\text{HQ}(p) = \ln\lvert\hat{\mathbf{\Sigma}}_T^{(p)}\rvert + \frac{2\ln\ln T}{T}pn^2$ |
| Schwarz | $\text{SC}(p) = \ln\lvert\hat{\mathbf{\Sigma}}_T^{(p)}\rvert + \frac{\ln T}{T}pn^2$ |

Bayesian and frequentist estimates can be similar, especially as the sample size gets large and the data overwhelm the influence of the prior, but important differences between the two approaches may emerge when comparing interval estimates for uncertainty quantification. We will see this more clearly in the discussion of forecasting below.

**Lag Order Selection:** Unlike the univariate AR model, analysis of the VAR model does not usually proceed from inspecting the (partial) autocorrelation function. For a multivariate time-series, we have a (P)ACF for each constituent series $y_{i,t}$, as well as cross-correlation functions (CCFs) between each pair of series. Inspecting all of these (P)ACFs and CCFs becomes unwieldy, especially as the number of time-series $n$ grows. Instead, we will choose the order of the VAR by refitting the model for many values of $p$ and then selecting the lag order $\hat{p}_T$ that minimizes some criterion, just as we did in Example 8.2.4.

The four criteria commonly considered in VAR order selection are listed in Table 8.1. All four are implemented in the `vars` package, and Chapter 4 in [36] offers detailed discussion. Each criterion involves the maximum likelihood estimate (MLE) of the VAR error covariance matrix $\mathbf{\Sigma}$, and we denote this estimate by $\hat{\mathbf{\Sigma}}_T^{(p)}$, with the superscript $(p)$ to remind us which lag order was applied to compute the estimate.

Ultimately, which criterion we choose to minimize will depend on how we intend to use the estimated VAR model. One advantage of the Hannan-Quinn and Schwarz criteria is that they deliver lag order estimators that are consistent for the "true" lag order. That is, if our time-series $\mathbf{y}_t$ does in fact follow a stationary VAR with lag order $p_0$, then as the sample size grows ($T \to \infty$), $\hat{p}_T$ will converge in probability to $p_0$. A lag order estimator based on FPE or AIC does not have this property.

However, it may be the case that our data do not follow a stationary VAR, in which case there is no such thing as a "true lag order" for which $\hat{p}_T$ could be consistent. Nevertheless, we may still wish to fit a VAR to our data because it will be a convenient approximation that can generate useful forecasts. In this case, the Hannan-Quinn and Schwarz criteria may not deliver lag orders that are optimized for forecasting. It is for this reason that it may still be useful to consider the FPE and Akaike criteria despite the fact that they will not identify the correct lag order in general. They may still deliver superior forecasts.

The `vars` package gives us the option of specifying a maximum lag order and selection criterion. It will then return a model fit with a lag order that minimizes the chosen criterion over the grid we have chosen. Here are results applied to the bivariate IED time-series from Example Patient 3:

```
var_model_HQ  <- VAR(Example3, type = "const", lag.max = 50, ic = "HQ")
var_model_SC  <- VAR(Example3, type = "const", lag.max = 50, ic = "SC")
var_model_AIC <- VAR(Example3, type = "const", lag.max = 50, ic ="AIC")
var_model_FPE <- VAR(Example3, type = "const", lag.max = 50, ic ="FPE")

> c(var_model_HQ$p, var_model_SC$p, var_model_AIC$p, var_model_FPE$p)
 HQ(n)   SC(n) AIC(n) FPE(n)
     4       2      9      9
```

We see several things. Firstly, HQ/SC and AIC/FPE give quite different results. AIC and FPE give the same lag order, which is consistent with the fact that they are asymptotically equivalent, and in this case the sample size is fairly large. If our goal is to learn the true underlying model, then HQ/SC are consistent for the true lag order in large samples. If our goal is to use the VAR as a black box for forecasting, regardless whether or not the VAR model is actually the correct one, then AIC/FPE may be better suited to this task.

The methods described above are most readily applicable when we are estimating a VAR model from a classical point of view. From a Bayesian point of view, one way to select the lag order is to treat it as yet another hyperparameter. In other words, we could augment our prior with another hyperprior on the lag order and estimate it along with all of the other hyperparameters.

**Forecasting:** Once we have selected the lag order and estimated the parameters of a $\text{VAR}_n(p)$ model, we can put it to one of its most basic uses: forecasting future values of the time-series $\mathbf{y}_t$ – in our application, forecasting future IED counts. The `vars` and `BVAR` packages both provide functions for predicting future values $\hat{\mathbf{y}}_{T+h|T}$, as well as functions for generating fan charts. Fan charts are time-series plots that display both the point forecasts of future values, as well as the bounds of prediction intervals to visualize the uncertainty around the forecast. As we forecast values farther into the future, these plots tend to "fan out" to reflect our increasing uncertainty.

We can use the `predict()` function to generate forecasts from the VAR model:

```
# Generate predictions from VAR model
horizon <- 30
var_fcast <- predict(my_var_model, n.ahead = horizon)
bvar_fcast <- predict(my_bvar_model, horizon = horizon,
                      conf_bands = (1 - seq(0.1, 0.9, 0.1)) / 2)
```

Once we have the forecasts, we can visualize them by plotting fan charts as:

```
# Plot fancharts
fanchart(var_fcast, nc = 2, xlim = c(T-50, T+horizon), cis = seq(0.1, 0.9, 0.1))
plot(bvar_fcast, t_back = 50, orientation = 'h', area = TRUE)
```

The results are displayed in Figure 8.4. We see that the point forecasts are very similar between the classical and the Bayesian approach, but the uncertainty around the point forecasts is different. This highlights a key difference between the two approaches which can have important implications for practice. In general, the interval estimates are calculated differently, they incorporate different information, and they have different interpretations. The classical intervals are of the form $\hat{y}_{i,T+h} \pm z\,(1-\alpha/2)\,\hat{\sigma}_i(T+h)$; they typically only acknowledge uncertainty coming from the model itself ($\varepsilon_t$) and not the sampling distributions of the coefficient estimates or the tuning parameters; and they have the usual frequentist interpretation that they cover the true value of $y_{T+h}$ in $100 \times (1-\alpha)\%$ of hypothetical samples. The Bayesian intervals are even-tailed intervals based on posterior quantiles; they acknowledge uncertainty coming from both the sampling model and the parameters (and hyperparameters); but they do not necessarily have frequentist coverage guarantees. They are *credible intervals* that reflect our ex-post degree-of-belief about future data. Neither kind of interval is strictly preferred in general, but for small-to-medium sample sizes they can paint different pictures of the uncertainty around the point forecast.

**Granger Causality:** We say that one time-series $y_t$ Granger causes another time-series $x_t$ if $y_t$ is useful for predicting $x_t$. In other words, if a forecast of $x_t$ that includes lagged values of $y_t$ is better than a forecast that ignores $y_t$, then $y_t$ is Granger causal or *predictive* for $x_t$. To formalize this, let $f(x_t \,|\, \mathcal{D}_{1:t-1}, y_{1:t-1})$ denote the optimal forecast of $x_t$ based on

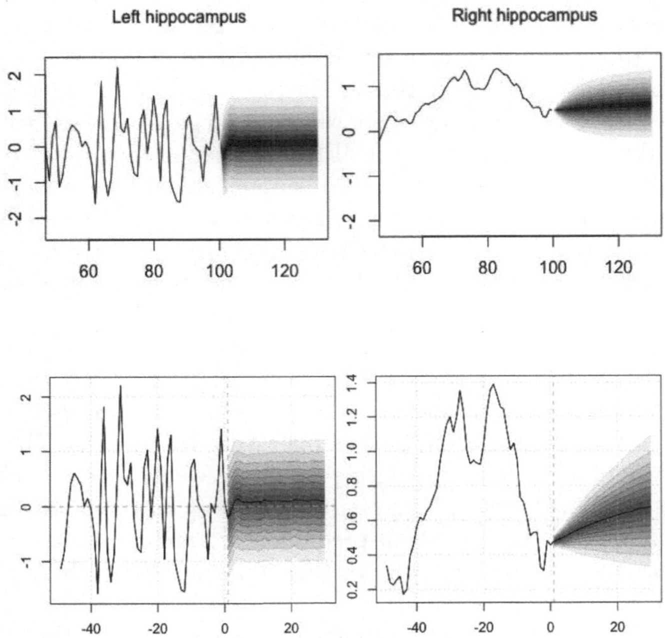


**FIGURE 8.4**
Fan charts showing predicted IED counts from vector autoregressive model fit with (top panel) ordinary least squares and (bottom panel) Bayesian vector autoregressive model.

the history of $y_t$ and all other past information, and let $f(x_t \,|\, \mathcal{D}_{1:t-1})$ denote the optimal forecast of $x_t$ based on all past information except past information about $y_t$. We say $y_t$ is Granger causal for $x_t$ if including $y_t$ in the forecast decreases the variance of the forecast error:

$$\text{var}\left[x_t - f(x_t \,|\, \mathcal{D}_{1:t-1}, y_{1:t-1})\right] < \text{var}\left[x_t - f(x_t \,|\, \mathcal{D}_{1:t-1})\right].$$

Since Granger first proposed this idea in [20], there has been much discussion about whether or not it truly captures a notion of $y_t$ "causing" $x_t$. But nevertheless, it is a useful notion for assessing the predictive relevance of $y_t$ for $x_t$, and this is an important issue to confront in multivariate time-series analysis. The goal of multivariate time-series analysis is to model the joint dynamics of several time-series in the hope that this will deliver better results than if each series were modeled independently, ignoring their potential dependencies. However, if a set of time-series do not in fact have any meaningful relationships with one another, a multivariate model may generate misleading results. So how can we test for whether a multivariate model is needed?

This is a difficult question to answer in general, and [48] offer an excellent review of history and recent advances in Granger causality. The original work in this area was restricted to pairs of time-series that follow a VAR, and in this case the notion of Granger causality is straightforward. If $x_t$ and $y_t$ follow a VAR$_2(p)$ given by

$$\begin{aligned} y_t &= a_y + \sum_{l=1}^{p} \phi_l^{(yy)} y_{t-l} + \sum_{l=1}^{p} \phi_l^{(yx)} x_{t-l} + \varepsilon_{y,t} \\ x_t &= a_x + \sum_{l=1}^{p} \phi_l^{(xx)} x_{t-l} + \sum_{l=1}^{p} \phi_l^{(xy)} y_{t-l} + \varepsilon_{x,t}, \end{aligned}$$

then $y_t$ Granger causes $x_t$ if at least one of the $\phi_l^{(xy)}$ is nonzero. A test of Granger causality compares the null hypothesis that $\phi_1^{(xy)} = \phi_2^{(xy)} = ... = \phi_p^{(xy)} = 0$ against the alternative that at least one is nonzero, and this can be performed with an $F$-test that is implemented in the `vars` package:

```
my_test <- causality(my_var_model, cause = "y")

> my_test$Granger

  Granger causality H0: y do not Granger-cause x

data:  VAR object my_var_model
F-Test = 0.8884, df1 = 2, df2 = 186, p-value = 0.4131
```

In order to be valid, this test assumes that we know the correct lag order. Since the lag order is an unknown that we usually have to estimate, this setting provides another use case for the *consistent* lag order selection criteria that we studied earlier. AIC/FPE may be optimized for prediction, but there are no theoretical guarantees that they will identify the correct lag order, even in large samples.

Furthermore, the test assumes that there are no other unmeasured time-series that might confound the relationship between $x_t$ and $y_t$. This assumption is very unrealistic, and so in general what we wish to do is fit a full VAR with all relevant variables included, and then having controlled for these extra time-series, assess Granger causality between a pair of variables $i$ and $j$. In the context of the full VAR model in (8.9), variable $y_{i,t}$ Granger causes $y_{j,t}$ if $\phi_l^{(j,i)} \neq 0$ for at least one $1 \leq l \leq p$. In this higher-dimensional setting, a convenient way to assess Granger causality is to estimate the VAR using methods that produce sparse estimates of the VAR coefficients. When we do this, we can draw conclusions about Granger causality by inspecting the pattern of zeros in the estimates.

One way to achieve this is to apply the LASSO to the problem of VAR estimation. So we estimate the VAR coefficients by solving a penalized least squares problem:

$$\hat{\mathbf{\Phi}}_T = \arg\min_{\mathbf{\Phi}} \left\{ \sum_{t=1}^{T} \left\| \mathbf{y}_t - \mathbf{a} - \sum_{l=1}^{p} \mathbf{\Phi}_l \mathbf{y}_{t-l} \right\|_2^2 + \lambda \sum_{i=1}^{n} \sum_{j=1}^{n} \sum_{l=1}^{p} \left| \phi_l^{(i,j)} \right| \right\}. \tag{8.14}$$

The addition of the $L_1$ penalty introduces the possibility that the estimate will contain exact zeros, and the extent of the sparsity is governed by the tuning parameter $\lambda$, which is usually selected via cross-validation. If $\lambda = 0$, then this reduces to the ordinary least squares (OLS) problem which will not generate parameter estimates with exact zeros. As $\lambda$ increases, the estimate will become more and more sparse.

The penalty in Eq. (8.14) is the simplest to write down, but there are many others explored in [38] and [39] that induce special structured forms of sparsity. These are implemented in the `BigVar` package. We illustrate implementation using Example Patient 4, which contains a simulated four-variate time-series of IEDs. If we wish to estimate functional connectivity between these electrodes using a dynamic dependency structure, we can use the following `R` code to load the dataset, tune $\lambda$ using rolling window cross-validation, and then return a sparse point estimate of the VAR coefficients:

```
# Load library
library(BigVAR)
# Load Example Patient 4
load('~/Example4.RData')
# Fit model
mymodel <- constructModel(as.matrix(Example4), p = 3, struct = "Basic",
                          cv = "Rolling", gran = c(150, 150))
```

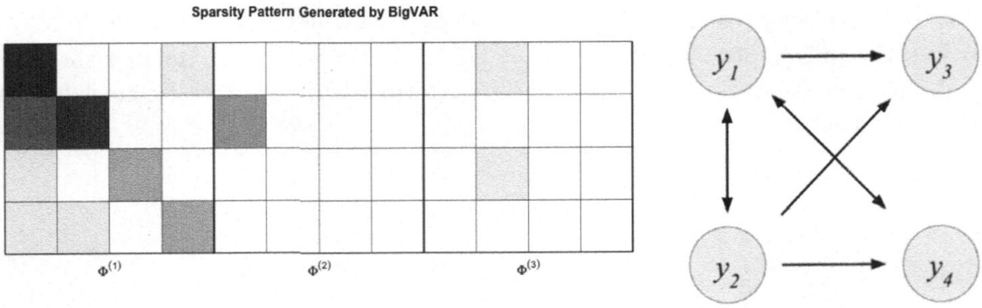


**FIGURE 8.5**
Pattern of zeros in (left panel) a sparse estimate of VAR coefficients and (right panel) the implied graph of Granger causality relationships. (Color version available in electronic supplement.)

```
results <- cv.BigVAR(mymodel)
SparsityPlot.BigVAR.results(results)
```

The sparsity pattern in these estimates is visualized in Figure 8.5. Based on these patterns, we can draw a graph that summarizes the dynamic dependency structure among the brain regions in $\mathbf{y}_t$. If we consider a graph with $n$ nodes corresponding to each of the $y_{i,t}$, we can draw a directed edge from node $i$ to node $j$ if variable $i$ Granger causes node $j$ (so at least one $\phi_l^{(j,i)} \neq 0$). The graph for this example is displayed in Figure 8.5. Estimating the graphical structure of dynamic dependencies is an important task in, for example, fMRI studies, where graphs encoding Granger causality can teach us about the functional connectivity among regions of the brain [8, 18, 19, 31], or for estimating the acute electrographic effects of responsive neurostimulation in rodents [58].

### 8.4.2 Vector Autoregressive Moving Average Models

Just as the VAR model generalizes the AR model to the multivariate setting, the vector autoregressive moving average (VARMA) model generalizes the ARMA to vector time-series. The VARMA$_n(p, q)$ model expresses an $n$-dimensional time-series $\mathbf{y}_t$ as a linear combination of both its $p$ most recent lagged values and the $q$ most recent lagged values of the error term $\boldsymbol{\varepsilon}_t$:

$$\mathbf{y}_t = \mathbf{a} + \sum_{l=1}^{p} \boldsymbol{\Phi}_l \mathbf{y}_{t-l} + \sum_{k=1}^{q} \boldsymbol{\Psi}_k \boldsymbol{\varepsilon}_{t-k} + \boldsymbol{\varepsilon}_t, \quad \boldsymbol{\varepsilon}_t \overset{\text{iid}}{\sim} \mathrm{N}_n(\mathbf{0}, \boldsymbol{\Sigma}). \tag{8.15}$$

As with the VAR, the VARMA model can be estimated using the method of maximum likelihood, and the lag orders $p$ and $q$ can be tuned by performing a grid search to optimize some chosen criteria.

**Example 8.4.1.** A VARMA model can be fit to the bilateral hippocampal IED counts for Example Patient 1 using the `MTS` package in `R`:

```
# Fit VARMA model
library(MTS)
> my_varma_model <- VARMA(Example1, p = 1, q = 1)

Estimates in matrix form:
Constant term:
Estimates:  0.03510274 -0.078094
```

$$\begin{array}{ccccccccccc} \mathbf{s}_0 & \rightarrow & \mathbf{s}_1 & \rightarrow & \mathbf{s}_2 & \rightarrow & \cdots & \rightarrow & \mathbf{s}_t & \rightarrow & \cdots \\ & & \downarrow & & \downarrow & & & & \downarrow & & \\ & & \mathbf{y}_1 & & \mathbf{y}_2 & & & & \mathbf{y}_t & & \end{array}$$

**FIGURE 8.6**
Graphical dependence structure of a general state space model.

```
AR coefficient matrix
AR( 1 )-matrix
          [,1]    [,2]
[1,] -0.00582 -0.0951
[2,] -0.08801 -0.4986
MA coefficient matrix
MA( 1 )-matrix
        [,1]   [,2]
[1,] -0.6110 -0.108
[2,] -0.0194 -0.957

Residuals cov-matrix:
          [,1]      [,2]
[1,] 0.7179340 0.0147859
[2,] 0.0147859 0.7760223
```

## 8.5 State-Space Models

The linear univariate and multivariate models discussed above are useful for time-series in which non-linear dynamics are not expected and interest is in modeling the observed time-series itself. In other applications in epilepsy, however, more complex non-linear and non-stationary phenomena may be at play, or the time-series of interest may be hidden and not directly observable. For example, in modeling dynamics of brain states, the problem of interest may be in characterizing the temporal dynamics of an unobservable quantity [11]. In this section, we discuss state-space models, which are a class of models that involve unobserved variables that describe the evolution of the underlying system. We cover basic foundations of state-space and hidden Markov models as well as an example of how these methods can accommodate non-linear dynamics via regime-switching models.

### 8.5.1 General State-Space Framework

In a state-space model [6, 13], the dynamics of an observed time series $\mathbf{y}_t$ (possibly multivariate) are driven by an unobserved (or latent) time series $\mathbf{s}_t$ (also possibly multivariate). The goal of inference is to use the time series we did observe to learn about the one that we did not. In general, the structure of a state-space model model is given by

$$\mathbf{y}_t \sim p(\mathbf{y}_t \,|\, \mathbf{s}_t, \, \boldsymbol{\phi}) \tag{8.16}$$

$$\mathbf{s}_t \sim p(\mathbf{s}_t \,|\, \mathbf{s}_{t-1}, \, \boldsymbol{\phi}) \tag{8.17}$$

$$\mathbf{s}_0 \sim p(\mathbf{s}_0 \,|\, \boldsymbol{\phi}). \tag{8.18}$$

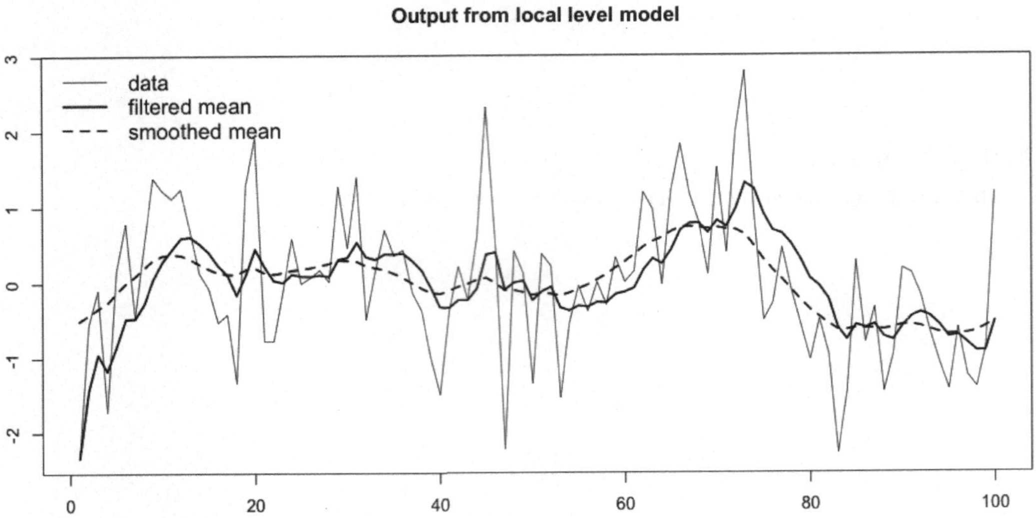


**FIGURE 8.7**
Posterior mean estimate of latent underlying signal in local level model.

Eq. (8.16) is called the *measurement*, *observation*, or *emission distribution*, and it describes how the observations $\mathbf{y}_t$ depend on the latent state $\mathbf{s}_t$. Eq. (8.17) is a first order Markov transition distribution called the *state transition distribution* or *law of motion*, and it describes our prior beliefs about how the unobserved state moves through time. The model is initialized by Eq. (8.18), and $\boldsymbol{\phi}$ is a vector of whatever static parameters govern the model. This is a graphical model, and the dependence structure is visualized in Figure 8.6.

The power of this general formulation is that it nests a wide range of important time series models that span several scientific fields:

**Example 8.5.1. (Local level model)** This is the canonical "signal-in-noise" model where we view the observed time-series $\mathbf{y}_t$ as a corrupted or noisy version of a latent underlying trend or signal $\boldsymbol{\theta}_t$ which follows a random walk:

$$\mathbf{y}_t = \boldsymbol{\theta}_t + \boldsymbol{\varepsilon}_t, \qquad \boldsymbol{\varepsilon}_t \overset{\text{iid}}{\sim} \mathrm{N}_n(\mathbf{0},\, \mathbf{V}) \tag{8.19}$$

$$\boldsymbol{\theta}_t = \boldsymbol{\theta}_{t-1} + \boldsymbol{\eta}_t, \qquad \boldsymbol{\eta}_t \overset{\text{iid}}{\sim} \mathrm{N}_n(\mathbf{0},\, \mathbf{W}) \tag{8.20}$$

$$\boldsymbol{\theta}_0 \sim \mathrm{N}_n(\overline{\boldsymbol{\theta}}_{0|0},\, \mathbf{P}_{0|0}). \tag{8.21}$$

In this case the static parameters are $\boldsymbol{\phi} = \{\mathbf{V},\, \mathbf{W}\}$. The goal of inference in this model is to "see through" the noise and extract the underlying signal. Figure 8.7 displays the posterior mean estimate of $\boldsymbol{\theta}_t$ when we apply this model (with $\mathbf{V} = 1$ and $\mathbf{W}$ estimated via MLE) to the left hippocampal time-series $y_t$ of Example Patient 1.

**Example 8.5.2. (Two-state switching Gaussian model)** In this model $y_t$ comes from one of two normal distributions, but *which* normal distribution is changing through time:

$$y_t \sim \mathrm{N}(\mu_{s_t},\, \sigma^2_{s_t}) \tag{8.22}$$

$$s_t \sim \mathrm{Bernoulli}(p_{s_{t-1}}) \tag{8.23}$$

$$s_0 \sim \mathrm{Bernoulli}(p_0). \tag{8.24}$$

In some periods $y_t$ comes from $\mathrm{N}(\mu_1, \sigma_1^2)$ and in other periods it comes from $\mathrm{N}(\mu_2, \sigma_2^2)$. The switching between these two distributions is determined by the value of $s_t$, which evolves through time according to a discrete-time, discrete state Markov chain. The static parameters in this case are $\phi = \{\mu_1, \mu_2, \sigma_1^2, \sigma_2^2, p_1, p_2\}$.

**Example 8.5.3. (Stochastic volatility model)** Section 8.3 described the (G)ARCH approach to incorporating heteroskedasticity into time-series models. An alternative approach is the stochastic volatility model, which is a state-space model where we treat the (log) variance of $y_t$ as a dynamic latent state that needs to be estimated:

$$y_t \sim \mathrm{N}(0, e^{h_t}) \tag{8.25}$$
$$h_t = \beta_0 + \beta_1 h_{t-1} + \eta_t, \quad \eta_t \sim \mathrm{N}(0, w) \tag{8.26}$$
$$h_0 \sim \mathrm{N}(\bar{h}_{0|0}, \tau_{0|0}^2). \tag{8.27}$$

In this case the static parameters are the AR parameters $\phi = \{\beta_0, \beta_1, w\}$ that govern the dynamics of the volatility process.

The first goal of inference in a state-space model is to estimate the unobserved states $\mathbf{s}_t$, and for this it is convenient to take a Bayesian approach. The measurement distribution implies a full data likelihood function

$$p(\mathbf{y}_{1:T} \,|\, \mathbf{s}_{0:T}, \phi) = \prod_{t=1}^{T} p(\mathbf{y}_t \,|\, \mathbf{s}_t, \phi), \tag{8.28}$$

and the state transition distribution together with the initial condition imply a prior distribution on the entire sequence of latent states

$$p(\mathbf{s}_{0:T} \,|\, \phi) = p(\mathbf{s}_0) \prod_{t=1}^{T} p(\mathbf{s}_t \,|\, \mathbf{s}_{t-1}, \phi). \tag{8.29}$$

Armed with these, the full posterior is given by Bayes' theorem

$$p(\mathbf{s}_{0:T} \,|\, \mathbf{y}_{1:T}, \phi) = \frac{p(\mathbf{y}_{1:T} \,|\, \mathbf{s}_{0:T}, \phi) p(\mathbf{s}_{0:T} \,|\, \phi)}{p(\mathbf{y}_{1:T} \,|\, \phi)}. \tag{8.30}$$

In general this distribution cannot be calculated exactly (the stochastic volatility model is a famous example of this), but we will review the important special cases of dynamic linear models (DLMs) and hidden Markov models (HMMs) where we can access the posterior analytically.

So far we have assumed that the static parameters $\phi$ are fixed and known, but in practice they often are not. One approach to inference is to place a prior $p(\phi)$ on them and try to access the full, joint posterior $p(\mathbf{s}_{0:T}, \phi \,|\, \mathbf{y}_{1:T})$ of the dynamic latent states and the system parameters. Alternatively, we can try to calculate the *integrated* likelihood in the denominator of Eq. (8.30) and then estimate the parameters via the method of maximum likelihood:

$$\hat{\phi}_T = \arg\max_{\phi} p(\mathbf{y}_{1:T} \,|\, \phi). \tag{8.31}$$

In the cases where the posterior Eq. (8.30) is analytically tractable, there are also convenient methods for calculating the MLE.

### 8.5.2 Dynamic Linear Models

Perhaps the most thoroughly studied example of a state-space model is the linear, Gaussian state-space model or dynamic linear model (DLM) [2, 41, 46, 57], which is given by

$$\mathbf{y}_t = \mathbf{F}_t \boldsymbol{\theta}_t + \boldsymbol{\varepsilon}_t, \qquad \boldsymbol{\varepsilon}_t \sim \mathrm{N}_n(\mathbf{0}, \mathbf{V}_t) \tag{8.32}$$

$$\boldsymbol{\theta}_t = \mathbf{G}_t \boldsymbol{\theta}_{t-1} + \boldsymbol{\eta}_t, \qquad \boldsymbol{\eta}_t \sim \mathrm{N}_p(\mathbf{0}, \mathbf{W}_t) \tag{8.33}$$

$$\boldsymbol{\theta}_0 \sim \mathrm{N}_p(\overline{\boldsymbol{\theta}}_{0|0}, \mathbf{P}_{0|0}). \tag{8.34}$$

This model treats an observed $n$-dimensional time-series $\mathbf{y}_t$ as a noisy linear transformation of some unobserved (or latent) $p$-dimensional time-series $\boldsymbol{\theta}_t$, which is called the *state*. That is, rather than observing the sequence of latent states $\boldsymbol{\theta}_t$, we observe the sequence of emitted observations $\mathbf{y}_t$, and we wish to infer the sequence of underlying states that gave rise to what we observed. As a starting point, we usually treat the sequences of system matrices $\mathbf{F}_t$, $\mathbf{V}_t$, $\mathbf{G}_t$, and $\mathbf{W}_t$ as fixed and known, and the goal of inference is to use the observed data to learn about the unobserved state of the system $\boldsymbol{\theta}_t$. It is also common to consider the *time-invariant* version of the model where the system matrices are constant for all $t$: $\mathbf{F}_t = \mathbf{F}$, $\mathbf{V}_t = \mathbf{V}$, $\mathbf{G}_t = \mathbf{G}$, and $\mathbf{W}_t = \mathbf{W}$.

The DLM nests several important models as special cases. The local level model in Example 8.5.1, for instance, is the time-invariant DLM with $p = n$ and $\mathbf{F} = \mathbf{G} = \mathbf{I}_n$. We can fit this model and others using the `R` packages `dlm` [40] and `KFAS` [22].

**Example 8.5.4.** If we observe a univariate response time-series $y_t \in \mathbb{R}$ and a covariate time-series $\mathbf{x}_t \in \mathbb{R}^p$, we can set $\mathbf{F}_t = \mathbf{x}_t^T$ and $\mathbf{V} = \sigma^2$, and the DLM becomes a multiple linear regression of $y_t$ on $\mathbf{x}_t$ with a vector of time-varying regression coefficients $\boldsymbol{\theta}_t$:

$$y_t = \mathbf{x}_t^T \boldsymbol{\theta}_t + \varepsilon_t, \quad \varepsilon_t \overset{\text{iid}}{\sim} \mathrm{N}(0, \sigma^2). \tag{8.35}$$

This allows us to model dynamic association between $\mathbf{x}_t$ and $y_t$ rather than the static association captured by the usual regression model.

**Example 8.5.5.** The ARMA model that we studied in Section 8.2.4 can be written as a special case of a DLM. If we set $r = \max\{p, q+1\}$, $\delta = 0$ (for convenience), $c_l = 0$ when $l > p$, and $d_l = 0$ when $l > q$, then the time-invariant DLM with $\boldsymbol{\theta}_t \in \mathbb{R}^r$, $\mathbf{F} = [1\,0 \ldots 0]$, $\mathbf{V} = 0$, $\mathbf{r} = [1\, d_1 \ldots d_{r-1}]^{\text{Trace}}$, $\mathbf{W} = \sigma^2 \mathbf{r}\mathbf{r}^{\text{Trace}}$, and

$$\mathbf{G} = \begin{bmatrix} c_1 & 1 & 0 & \cdots & 0 \\ c_2 & 0 & 1 & \cdots & 0 \\ \vdots & \vdots & & \ddots & \\ c_{r-1} & 0 & 0 & \cdots & 1 \\ c_r & 0 & 0 & \cdots & 0 \end{bmatrix}$$

is equivalent to the model in Eq. (8.5). By a similar construction, the VARMA model is also a special case of the DLM. This is useful because it allows us to apply the inferential tools developed for the DLM to these other models. For instance, rewriting a (V)ARMA model as a DLM is an important step in the process of estimating the AR and MA parameters via the method of maximum likelihood. The DLM representation provides a means of calculating the likelihood function, as we will see later.

**Filtering and Smoothing:** For notational convenience, collect all of the DLM system matrices into $\boldsymbol{\phi} = \{\mathbf{F}_{1:T}, \mathbf{V}_{1:T}, \mathbf{G}_{1:T}, \mathbf{W}_{1:T}\}$ and assume (for now) that they are all fixed and known. In general we wish to access the full posterior distribution of all the states

$p(\boldsymbol{\theta}_{0:T} \mid \mathbf{y}_{1:T}, \boldsymbol{\phi})$, and because the DLM is linear and Gaussian, this can be done exactly using the methods of [12] or [7]. In practice however, we focus special attention on particular marginal distributions of the full posterior. The *filtering distribution* is $p(\boldsymbol{\theta}_t \mid \mathbf{y}_{1:t}, \boldsymbol{\phi})$, the marginal posterior of the time $t$ state given all the data observed up to time $t$. This distribution describes what all of the data *so far* have to teach us about the *current* state of the system. It provides estimates of the state that are "one-sided" or "backward-looking" in the sense that the estimate only accounts for past data and ignores future data (because these data are not yet available). These estimates are the ones we want if we are interested in *tracking* the state of the system in real-time as new observations arrive one-after-another.

The *smoothing distribution* is $p(\boldsymbol{\theta}_t \mid \mathbf{y}_{1:T}, \boldsymbol{\phi})$ for some $t < T$, the marginal posterior of the time $t$ state given all of the data we have seen before *and after* time $t$. This distribution describes what the entire sample has to teach us about a past state of the system. It provides estimates of the state that are "two-sided" or "retrospective." If the filtering distribution was about tracking the current state of the system, then the smoothing distribution is about "looking back" at a past state after new data have arrived and learning what these subsequent observations have to teach us about it. So the filtering and smoothing distributions are posteriors for the same unobservable $\boldsymbol{\theta}_t$, but the smoothing distribution conditions on more data. As such, these distributions can generate different estimates. Indeed, we call it the smoothing distribution because the time-series of estimates tends to be "smoother" than the time-series of estimates from the filtering distribution. This is shown in Figure 8.7, where the solid line is the sequence of "filtered" means $\overline{\boldsymbol{\theta}}_{t|t} = E(\boldsymbol{\theta}_t \mid \mathbf{y}_{1:t}, \boldsymbol{\phi})$ and the dashed line is the sequence of "smoothed" means $\overline{\boldsymbol{\theta}}_{t|T} = E(\boldsymbol{\theta}_t \mid \mathbf{y}_{1:T}, \boldsymbol{\phi})$. We see that the dashed line is less jagged than the solid line.

Because the DLM is linear and Gaussian, the filtering and smoothing distributions can be calculated exactly. Indeed, all of the filtering and smoothing distributions are Gaussian:

$$\begin{aligned} \boldsymbol{\theta}_t \mid \mathbf{y}_{1:t}, \boldsymbol{\phi} &\sim \mathrm{N}_p\left(\overline{\boldsymbol{\theta}}_{t|t}, \mathbf{P}_{t|t}\right) \\ \boldsymbol{\theta}_t \mid \mathbf{y}_{1:T}, \boldsymbol{\phi} &\sim \mathrm{N}_p\left(\overline{\boldsymbol{\theta}}_{t|T}, \mathbf{P}_{t|T}\right). \end{aligned}$$

All that remains is to calculate their means and covariances. The *filtering problem* refers to the task of recursively calculating the mean and covariance of the filtering distribution as new observations arrive. That is, having calculated the filtering distribution $\mathrm{N}_p(\boldsymbol{\theta}_{t-1}; \overline{\boldsymbol{\theta}}_{t-1|t-1}, \mathbf{P}_{t-1|t-1})$ at the previous time point $t-1$, we observe $\mathbf{y}_t$ in period $t$ and wish to calculate the new mean $\overline{\boldsymbol{\theta}}_{t|t}$ and covariance $\mathbf{P}_{t|t}$ of the current filtering distribution:

$$\mathrm{N}_p(\overline{\boldsymbol{\theta}}_{0|0}, \mathbf{P}_{0|0}) \overset{\text{observe } \mathbf{y}_1}{\longrightarrow} \mathrm{N}_p(\overline{\boldsymbol{\theta}}_{1|1}, \mathbf{P}_{1|1}) \overset{\text{observe } \mathbf{y}_2}{\longrightarrow} \mathrm{N}_p(\overline{\boldsymbol{\theta}}_{2|2}, \mathbf{P}_{2|2}) \overset{\text{observe } \mathbf{y}_3}{\longrightarrow} \cdots$$

The solution to this problem is the famous *Kalman filter* [24].

The *smoothing problem* refers to the task of recursively calculating the smoothing distributions of past states backward through time. Having "filtered forward" and reached the last filtering distribution $\mathrm{N}_p(\overline{\boldsymbol{\theta}}_{T|T}, \mathbf{P}_{T|T})$ at the end of the current sample, we now wish to recursively "smooth backward" to characterize our updated beliefs about past states in the light of subsequent data:

$$\cdots \longleftarrow \mathrm{N}_p(\overline{\boldsymbol{\theta}}_{T-2|T}, \mathbf{P}_{T-2|T}) \longleftarrow \mathrm{N}_p(\overline{\boldsymbol{\theta}}_{T-1|T}, \mathbf{P}_{T-1|T}) \longleftarrow \mathrm{N}_p(\overline{\boldsymbol{\theta}}_{T|T}, \mathbf{P}_{T|T})$$

The solution to this problem is the *Rauch-Tung-Striebel fixed interval smoother*. See [46] for derivations of the filter and smoother.

The `dlm` package in `R` offers simple utilities for filtering and smoothing in the examples we have seen. We can specify a local level model with user-specified variances by running:

```
library(dlm)
my_dlm <- dlmModPoly(order = 1, dV = 1, dW = 1)
```

With this, it is straightforward to run the filter or the smoother. Here we apply the model to the left hippocampal time-series $y_t$ of Example 8.2.1:

```
dlm_data <- Example1$y
my_filter = dlmFilter(dlm_data, my_dlm)
my_smoother = dlmSmooth(dlm_data, my_dlm)

> head(my_filter$m)
[1]  0.0000000 -2.3350859 -1.1437702 -0.4871177 -1.2532278 -0.3779505
> head(my_smoother$s)
[1] -1.6341542 -1.6341544 -0.9332228 -0.6174015 -0.8258557 -0.1354853
```

To estimate a dynamic regression of $y_t$ on $x_t$ with a time-varying intercept and slope, we can run:

```
x <- Example1$x
y <- Example1$y
my_dynamic_reg = dlmModReg(x, addInt = TRUE, dV = 1, dW = 0.1 * c(1, 1))
my_reg_smoother = dlmSmooth(y, my_dynamic_reg)
```

**Parameter Estimation:** So far we have assumed that the system matrices $\mathbf{F}_t$, $\mathbf{V}_t$, $\mathbf{G}_t$, and $\mathbf{W}_t$ of the DLM are fixed and known, and conditional on them, we have studied inference for the dynamic latent states $\boldsymbol{\theta}_t$. In practice however, the system matrices are often unknown, and we wish to estimate them as well. In particular, the system matrices are usually determined by a small number of time-invariant parameters, and our goal is to estimate them. In the local level model for example, we still had the error covariance matrices $\boldsymbol{\phi} = \{\mathbf{V}, \mathbf{W}\}$ to deal with. In the dynamic regression model, there was still the error variance $\boldsymbol{\phi} = \sigma^2$ to specify. And in the rewritten ARMA model, $\mathbf{F}$ and $\mathbf{V}$ were fixed and known, but $\boldsymbol{\phi} = \{\mathbf{G}, \mathbf{W}\}$ is a function of the AR and MA parameters that we wish to estimate.

In order to estimate the parameters $\boldsymbol{\phi}$, we need to calculate the likelihood function $L(\boldsymbol{\phi}) = p(\mathbf{y}_{1:T} \mid \boldsymbol{\phi})$. Once we can do this, we can estimate $\boldsymbol{\phi}$ via the method of maximum likelihood. Fortunately, the Kalman filter allows us to do this. In order to calculate the filtering distributions $p(\boldsymbol{\theta}_t \mid \mathbf{y}_{1:t}, \boldsymbol{\phi})$, the Kalman filter also calculates the one-step-ahead predictive distributions $p(\mathbf{y}_t \mid \mathbf{y}_{1:t-1}, \boldsymbol{\phi})$ along the way. The product of these is the likelihood function for the parameters $\boldsymbol{\phi}$:

$$p(\mathbf{y}_{1:T} \mid \boldsymbol{\phi}) = p(\mathbf{y}_1 \mid \boldsymbol{\phi}) \prod_{t=2}^{T} p(\mathbf{y}_t \mid \mathbf{y}_{1:t-1}, \boldsymbol{\phi}). \tag{8.36}$$

Note that this is an *integrated likelihood* where the states $\boldsymbol{\theta}_t$ have been marginalized. From the point of view of static parameter inference, the states are nuisance parameters that we need to integrate out, and the Kalman filter provides us with a means of doing so exactly.

Armed with this insight, the `dlm` package provides routines for estimating the static parameters of a state-space model via the method of maximum likelihood. To reproduce Figure 8.7, we run:

```
dlm_build <- function(parm){
  dlmModPoly(order = 1, dV = 1, dW = exp(parm[1]))
}

mle = dlmMLE(dlm_data, parm = 0, build = dlm_build)
estimated_dlm = dlm_build(mle$par)
filter_output = dlmFilter(dlm_data, estimated_dlm)
smoother_output = dlmSmooth(dlm_data, estimated_dlm)
```

The `dlmMLE()` function takes data, an initial value for the optimization, and a user-defined function (called `dlm_build()` in this case) that takes in a vector of the parameters we are estimating and returns a DLM object, in this case a local level model. It then uses the built-in `optim()` function to numerically maximize the likelihood function, which is being evaluated using the Kalman filter. `dlmMLE()` returns the estimated vector of parameters, which we can then plug in to specify our model and proceed with filtering and smoothing conditional on the parameter estimates.

### 8.5.3 Hidden Markov Models

A hidden Markov model (HMM) is a state-space model where the latent state $s_t$ takes finitely many values $\{1, 2, ..., K\}$. In this case the transition distribution in Eq. (8.17) is a discrete-time, discrete-state Markov chain with transition probabilities $P(s_t = i \,|\, s_{t-1} = j) = q_{j,i}$. This framework captures a notion of dynamic "switching," as we saw in Example 8.5.2. The observed time series $\mathbf{y}_t$ can be governed by one of $K$ possible distributions, and which of these distributions prevails in a given period is determined by the value of the state $s_t$. HMMs have been used in epilepsy research, for example, as an approach to estimating seizure risk; by modeling seizure risk as a hidden state and clinical or electrographic seizures as a manifestation of the hidden state, various quantities of interest can be estimated, such as the probability of transitioning to a high- or low-seizure risk state in future time points, or the influence of responsive neurostimulation parameters on state-transitions [9, 11, 55].

As with the DLM, this is a rich class of models that encompasses many important special cases. For comprehensive introductions to HMMs, see [47, 59].

**Example 8.5.6. (Switching VAR)** To capture more complex autoregressive dynamics, authors such as [16, 50] consider the model:

$$\mathbf{y}_t = \sum_{l=1}^{p} \mathbf{\Phi}_l^{(s_t)} \mathbf{y}_{t-l} + \boldsymbol{\varepsilon}_t, \quad \boldsymbol{\varepsilon}_t \sim \mathrm{N}_n(\mathbf{0}, \mathbf{\Sigma}^{(s_t)}). \tag{8.37}$$

So $\mathbf{y}_t$ follows a VAR, but the VAR parameters are switching among one of $K$ values depending on the state $s_t$. The static parameters $\boldsymbol{\phi}$ in this model are all of the possible values of the VAR parameters $\mathbf{\Phi}_l^{(k)}$, as well as the state transition probabilities $\mathbf{Q}$.

**Parameter Estimation:** The unknown parameters of an HMM, including the transition probability matrix, emission probabilities, and initial state distribution can be estimated via maximum likelihood using the Baum-Welch algorithm. The Baum-Welch algorithm is a special case of the expectation-maximization (EM) algorithm, which alternates between the E-step (the forward-backward algorithm) and the M-step (parameter updates). Specifically, it first computes during the E-step the forward probabilities (probability of being in a specific state at a given time) and backward probabilities (probability of observing subsequent observations given being in a specific state at a given time). The M-step then updates the HMM parameters, including the transition probabilities, emission probability, and initial state distribution using the posterior probabilities from the E-step.

As an example, suppose that, rather than modeling the observed IED counts $y_t$ for Example Patient 1, we are interested in modeling fluctuations in the patient's seizure risk level, under a framework in which the brain generates IEDs with different probabilities according to whether the patient is in a high or low risk state. The two-state Gaussian HMM in Example 8.5.2 can be fit using the Baum-Welch algorithm to the $z$-transformed IED counts with the `depmix()` function from `depmixS4` package in `R` [53]:

```
# Fit two-state Gaussian HMM
library(depmixS4)
y <- Example1$y
hmm <- depmix(y ~ 1, nstates = 2, ntimes = length(y), family = gaussian())
fit_hmm <- fit(hmm)
```

The output of `fit_hmm` allows us to estimate the transitions between high and low risk states. Note that, if we had wished to fit an HMM with a Poisson emission distribution to the original count data, this could be done by specifying `family = Poission()` in the argument to `depmix`. Alternatively, MCMC procedures can be used to fit Bayesian hidden Markov models to count data using zero-inflated Poisson or zero-inflated negative binomial emission distributions that allow for additional complexity [11, 55]; these distributions may be of particular use in modeling events such as seizures due to the relative infrequency of these events.

**State inference:** Similar to the DLM, the posterior $p(s_{0:T} \,|\, \mathbf{y}_{1:T},\, \boldsymbol{\phi})$ of the latent states is analytically tractable, and samples can be drawn from it directly using a forward-backward algorithm that is similar to the Kalman filter and smoother. It is useful to summarize this distribution by calculating a point estimate of the states such as the *maximum a posteriori* (*MAP*) estimate, which is the sequence of states possessing the largest posterior probability:

$$\hat{s}_{0:T} = \arg\max_{s_{0:T}} p(s_{0:T} \,|\, \mathbf{y}_{1:T},\, \boldsymbol{\phi}). \tag{8.38}$$

The sequence of latent states can be decoded efficiently using the *Viterbi algorithm* [54], and the following `R` code performs this calculation:

```
# Viterbi decoding
viterbi(fit_hmm)
identical(viterbi(fit_hmm), fit_hmm@posterior)
```

### 8.5.4 Regime-Switching Models

A regime-switching (or Markov-switching) model is a state-space model that combines hidden Markov dynamics with other state-space model structure. In general, the model is formulated as

$$\mathbf{y}_t \sim p(\mathbf{y}_t \,|\, \boldsymbol{\theta}_t,\, \boldsymbol{\phi}^{(s_t)}) \tag{8.39}$$

$$\boldsymbol{\theta}_t \sim p(\boldsymbol{\theta}_t \,|\, \boldsymbol{\theta}_{t-1},\, \boldsymbol{\phi}^{(s_t)}), \tag{8.40}$$

where $\mathbf{y}_t$ is our observed time series governed by the measurement distribution in (8.39), $s_t \in \{1, 2, ..., K\}$ is a discrete latent state just as in Section 8.5.3, $\boldsymbol{\theta}_t \in \mathbb{R}^p$ is yet another latent state governed by the transition distribution in Eq. (8.39), and $\boldsymbol{\phi}$ is a vector of static parameters that determine the structure of the model. The distinguishing feature of this model is the coexistence of $s_t$ and $\boldsymbol{\theta}_t$, and the fact that the value of $s_t$ can alter both the measurement distribution and the state transition distribution. The graphical structure of this model is visualized in Figure 8.8, and [30] offer a textbook treatment.

**Example 8.5.7.** The switching dynamic linear model (SDLM) is given by

$$\mathbf{y}_t = \mathbf{F}^{(s_t)}\boldsymbol{\theta}_t + \boldsymbol{\varepsilon}_t, \qquad \boldsymbol{\varepsilon}_t \overset{\text{iid}}{\sim} \mathrm{N}_n(\mathbf{0},\, \mathbf{V}) \tag{8.41}$$

$$\boldsymbol{\theta}_t = \mathbf{G}^{(s_t)}\boldsymbol{\theta}_{t-1} + \boldsymbol{\eta}_t, \qquad \boldsymbol{\eta}_t \sim \mathrm{N}_p(\mathbf{0},\, \mathbf{W}^{(s_t)}). \tag{8.42}$$

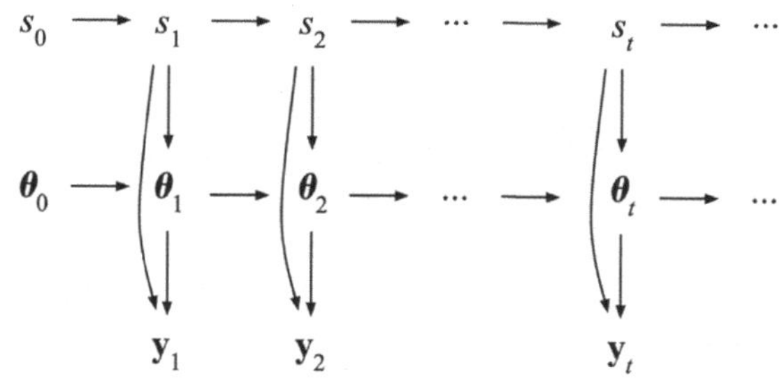


**FIGURE 8.8**
Graphical dependence structure of a regime-switching model.

This is a DLM where the system matrices governing the dynamics are switching between different values depending on the value of $s_t$. Filtering and smoothing for $\boldsymbol{\theta}_t$ are more challenging here than in the ordinary DLM, but [29] provides a solution.

**Example 8.5.8.** The switching model of [56] treats a patient's self-reported seizure counts $y_t$ as negative binomial, with parameters that depend on a vector of observed covariates $\mathbf{z}_t$ and two latent states $s_t \in \{1, 2\}$ and $\theta_t$:

$$y_t \sim \text{NB}(r_{s_t}, \psi_t). \tag{8.43}$$

$$\psi_t = \frac{1}{1 + \exp\left[-\left(\theta_t + \lambda_{s_t} + \mathbf{z}_t^{\text{trace}} \boldsymbol{\beta}_{s_t}\right)\right]} \tag{8.44}$$

$$\theta_t = \rho\theta_{t-1} + \nu_t, \qquad \nu_t \overset{\text{iid}}{\sim} \text{N}(0, \sigma^2). \tag{8.45}$$

Here, a mean parameter $\mu_t$ can be recovered from $\psi_t$ (see [55] for details) and is used by the authors to capture seizure risk as a continuous latent risk state evolving over time. Wang et al. propose use of this parameter as an estimator of the latent seizure-generating process, and show that spectral analysis of this hidden variable estimated from patient-reported clinical seizures recovers multidien periodicities similar to those identified from electrographic seizures [3, 26, 56].

## 8.6 Circular Data Analysis

Seizures, while conventionally thought to be unpredictable in their timing, are increasingly thought to exhibit cyclic rhythms in many individuals living with epilepsy [3, 26, 27]. An important area of investigation in epilepsy is whether or not seizures occur at specific phases of various cyclical physiological rhythms, such as heart rate, sleep cycles, or epileptiform discharges. That is, given a hypothesized cycle of some length in a physiological measure of interest, whether 24 hours, a week, or three months, when seizures occur, do they tend to occur at a particular phase of those physiological cycles? Approaches in *directional statistics*, otherwise known as *circular data analysis*, can be used to answer this question.

*Circular data* is defined as data that exhibits periodicity and takes values on a unit circle. Rather than following a linear progression, circular data has a cyclical structure and is often measured in angles between 0 and $2\pi$, rather than on a numerical scale. Examples of circular data include data that exhibits seasonal variability, such as temperature or daylight hours; time of day, which cycles over 24 hour periods; and biological rhythms such as cortisol secretion, which fluctuate with roughly 24-hour cycles. More recently, interictal epileptiform activity has also been found using chronic ambulatory EEG to exhibit periodic structure in a percentage of individuals with epilespy [3, 33].

Working with circular time-series data requires specialized statistical methods and visualizations designed for circular data, in the form of directional statistics. The field of directional statistics is vast and a comprehensive treatment of this subdiscipline of statistics can be found in resources such as [37]. Below, we provide several salient examples of methods in circular data analysis that have been used the field of epilepsy. The `circular` package in `R` provides routines for working with circular data [1], and can be applied to time-series data that are assumed to exhibit periodicity.

**Example 8.6.1. (Visualizing circular data).** Various circular plots can be used to explore circular time-series data, including *circular histograms* and *rose plots.*

Let us consider an example of seizure timestamps rescaled to the interval 0 to $2\pi$ provided in Example Patient 5. A circular histogram can be used to identify the distribution of seizure times relative to putative cycles. In particular, given a recording of seizure timestamps, we can partition the recording into adjacent bins of equal length reflecting the putative cycle period. We then record the position of each seizures in each sub-period as a point on the unit circle, or an angle between 0 and $2\pi$. For example, if a seizure occurs one-quarter of the way through the sub-period, this would have angle $\pi/2$; if it occurs halfway through the sub-period, this would have angle $\pi$ (Figure 8.9), and so forth.

A circular histogram of seizure times can be plotted using the `windrose()` function from the `circular` package in `R`. If there is a significant cyclical component to seizure timing, we would expect to observe the seizures clustering around the same phase of the cycle over time in a circular histogram:

```
# Load data
library(circular)
load('Example5.RData')

# Plot circular histogram
plot.circular(x, col = "red", main = "Circular datapoints")
windrose(x, rep(1, length(x)), main = "Circular histogram")
```

As shown in Figure 8.9, seizures for this patient tend to be concentrated betwen $\pi$ and $\frac{3\pi}{2}$, or in the third quarter of each cycle.

**Example 8.6.2. (Descriptive statistics for circular data and mean resultant vector).** Similar to descriptive statistics such as the mean, standard deviation, and correlation coefficient in linear data, analogous descriptive statistics can be used to summarize circular data, including the *circular mean*, *circular standard deviation*, and *circular correlation coefficient.* Another particularly useful statistic is the *mean resultant vector*, which measures the average direction of all the observations when they are plotted on the unit circle. The mean resultant vector ranges in magnitude from 0 to 1; the greater the magnitude, the more concentrated the circular distribution is around the mean, and the farther away it is from a uniform distribution. The magnitude of the mean resultant vector is also referred to as the *phase-locking value* [3]; in epilepsy research, the *phase-locking value* statistic has been used as a summary measure of how strongly seizures tend to occur at a specific phase of the cycle. Phase-locking value can be calculated by computing the magnitude of the mean resultant vector, using the `rho.circular()` function from the `circular` package:

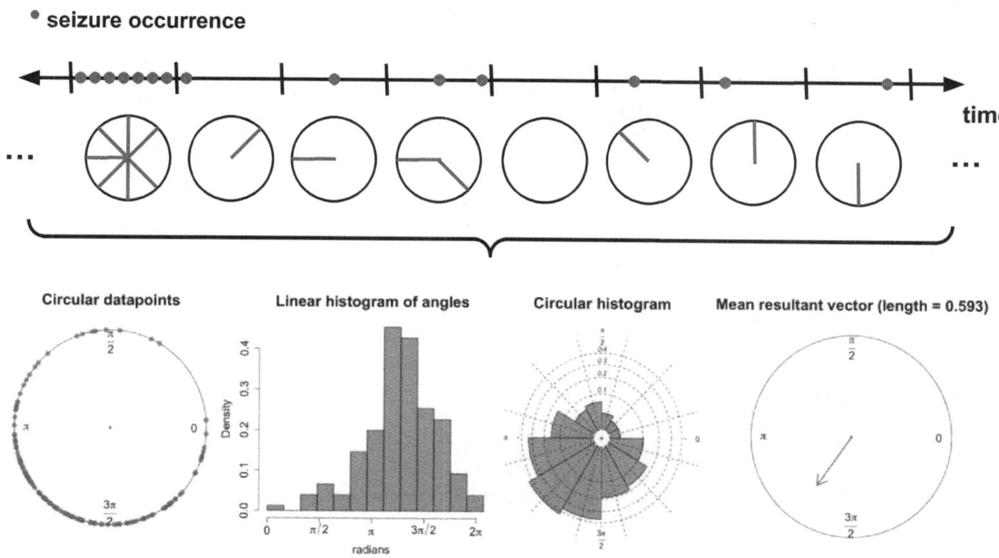


**FIGURE 8.9**
Data on seizure timing in relation to seizure cycles can be analyzed with circular data analysis. After partitioning the time period into bins of equal length, the timing of seizures within each bin (or "cycle") is recorded. (Bottom left panel) The timing of seizures within each cycle can then be plotted from 0 to $2\pi$. (Bottom middle panel) The distribution of seizure timing can be plotted on a linear scale using a linear histogram, or plotted on a circle using a circular histogram. (Bottom right panel) If seizures tend to occur at a specific phase, the distribution on the circle will be tightly concentrated around a mode (i.e. non-uniform), and the mean resultant length will be large. (Color version available in electronic supplement.)

```
# Calculate magnitude of mean resultant vector (phase-locking value)
> rho.circular(x)
[1] 0.5928573
```

**Example 8.6.3. (Testing for uniformity of a circular distribution).** An observation that the magnitude of the mean resultant vector is qualitatively large can be made rigorous with the *Rayleigh test*, where we test the null hypothesis that our data are uniformly distributed around the circle (i.e. no phase-locking), against the alternative that the data are concentrated around mean resultant vector. To perform the Rayleigh test in R, we use the function `rayleigh.test()` from the `circular` package:

```
# Rayleigh test of uniformity
> rayleigh.test(x)

       Rayleigh Test of Uniformity
       General Unimodal Alternative

Test Statistic:  0.5929
P-value:  0
```

The result of the test (small $p$-value) confirms that the distribution of the circular data is not uniform, as we saw in the circular histogram in Figure 8.9. This provides evidence that, when seizures occur, they tend to occur at a particular phase in the cycle. Alternatively, *Rao's spacing test of uniformity*, implemented through `rao.spacing.test()`, is another test for uniformity similar to Rayleigh's test. The choice between these two tests depends on the question under investigation, and many times are performed in conjunction. In general, Rayleigh's test may be particularly useful if the strength of concentration is of interest, while Rao's spacing test may be particularly useful if the specific clustering patterns of the data around the unit circle are of interest.

## 8.7 Summary

In summary, this chapter reviews the fundamental concepts behind several classical time-series modeling techniques that capture various aspects of time-series data. ARIMA models provide a flexible framework for modeling and forecasting univariate time-series, while conditional heteroskedasticity models enable the capture of volatility dynamics. Vector autoregressive models offer a multivariate approach to modeling interdependencies among variables, which may be used to estimate connectivity in neuroimaging or electroencephalography data. State-space models allow for flexible modeling of complex temporal patterns and inference on underlying hidden states, an increasing method used for seizure risk estimation and forecasting. Lastly, circular data analysis provides specialized methods that may be useful for exploring and understanding time-series data that is periodic in nature. By understanding and applying these methods to time-series data, epilepsy researchers may gain deeper insights into temporal phenomena in epilepsy.

## Bibliography

[1] Claudio Agostinelli and Ulric Lund. *R package `circular`: Circular Statistics (version 0.4-95).* CA: Department of Environmental Sciences, Informatics and Statistics, Ca' Foscari University, Venice, Italy. UL: Department of Statistics, California Polytechnic State University, San Luis Obispo, California, USA, 2022.

[2] Brian Anderson and John Moore. *Optimal Filtering.* Dover, 1979.

[3] Maxime Baud, Jonathan Kleen, Emily Mirro, Jason Andrechak, Edward Chang, and Vikram R. Rao. Multi-day rhythms modulate seizure risk in epilepsy. *Nature Communications*, 9(88):1–10, 2018.

[4] Lorenzo Bergomi. *Stochastic Volatility Modeling.* CRC Press, 2015.

[5] Tim Bollerslev. Generalized autoregressive conditional heteroskedasticity. *Journal of Econometrics*, 31(3):307–327, 1986.

[6] Olivier Cappé, Eric Moulines, and Tobias Rydén. *Inference in Hidden Markov Models.* Springer Series in Statistics. Springer, 2005.

[7] Joshua Chan and Ivan Jeliazkov. Efficient simulation and integrated likelihood estimation in state space models. *International Journal of Mathematical Modelling and Numerical Optimisation*, 1:101–120, 2009.

[8] Sharon Chiang, Michele Guindani, Hsiang Yeh, Zulfi Haneef, John Stern, and Marina Vannucci. Bayesian vector autoregressive model for multi-subject effective connectivity inference using multi-modal neuroimaging data. *Human Brain Mapping*, 38(3):1311–1332, March 2017.

[9] Sharon Chiang, Ankit N Khambhati, Emily T Wang, Marina Vannucci, Edward F Chang, and Vikram R Rao. Evidence of state-dependence in the effectiveness of responsive neurostimulation for seizure modulation. *Brain Stimulation*, 14(2):366–375, 2021.

[10] Sharon Chiang, Emilian R Vankov, Hsiang J Yeh, Michele Guindani, Marina Vannucci, Zulfi Haneef, and John M Stern. Temporal and spectral characteristics of dynamic functional connectivity between resting-state networks reveal information beyond static connectivity. *PLoS One*, 13(1):e0190220, 2018.

[11] Sharon Chiang, Marina Vannucci, Daniel Goldenholz, Robert Moss, and John Stern. Epilepsy as a dynamic disease: A Bayesian model for differentiating seizure risk from natural variability. *Epilepsia Open*, 3(2):236–246, 2018.

[12] James Durbin and Siem Jan Koopman. A simple and efficient simulation smoother for state space time series analysis. *Biometrika*, 89(3):603–616, August 2002.

[13] James Durbin and Siem Jan Koopman. *Time Series Analysis by State Space Methods*. Oxford University Press, 2012.

[14] Robert Engle. Autoregressive conditional heteroscedasticity with estimates of the variance of United Kingdom inflation. *Econometrica*, 50(4):987–1007, 1982.

[15] Jack L Follis and Dejian Lai. Modeling volatility characteristics of epileptic EEGs using GARCH models. *Signals*, 1(1):3, 2020.

[16] Emily Fox, Erik Sudderth, Michael I. Jordan, and Alan Willsky. Bayesian nonparametric inference of switching dynamic linear models. *IEEE Transactions on Signal Processing*, 59(4):1569–1585, April 2011.

[17] Domenico Giannone, Michele Lenza, and Giorgio Primiceri. Prior selection for vector autoregressions. *Review of Economics and Statistics*, 97(2):436–451, May 2015.

[18] Rainer Goebel, Alard Roebroeck, Dae-Shik Kim, and Elia Formisano. Investigating directed cortical interactions in time-resolved fMRI data using vector autoregressive modeling and Granger causality mapping. *Magnetic Resonance Imaging*, 21:1251–1261, 2003.

[19] Cristina Gorrostieta, Mark Fiecas, Hernando Ombao, Erin Burke, and Steven Cramer. Hierarchical vector auto-regressive models and their applications to multi-subject effective connectivity. *Frontiers in Computational Neuroscience*, 7:1–11, 2013.

[20] Clive Granger. Investigating causal relations by econometric models and cross-spectral methods. *Econometrica*, 37:424–438, 1969.

[21] Hossein Hassani and Mohammad Reza Yeganegi. Selecting optimal lag order in Ljung–Box test. *Physica A: Statistical Mechanics and its Applications*, 541:123700, 2020.

[22] Jouni Helske. KFAS: Exponential family state space models in R. *Journal of Statistical Software*, 78(10):1–39, June 2017.

[23] Rob J Hyndman and George Athanasopoulos. *Forecasting: Principles and Practice.* OTexts, 2018.

[24] Rudolf Kalman. A new approach to linear filtering and prediction problems. *Journal of Basic Engineering*, 81(1):35–45, March 1960.

[25] Sune Karlsson. Forecasting with Bayesian vector autoregression. In Graham Elliott and Allan Timmermann, editors, *Handbook of Economic Forecasting*, volume 2B, chapter 15, pages 791–897. North Holland, 2013.

[26] Philippa Karoly, Daniel Goldenholz, Dean Freestone, Robert Moss, David Grayden, William Theodore, and Mark Cook. Circadian and circaseptan rhythms in human epilepsy: A retrospective cohort study. *Lancet Neurology*, 17:977–985, 2018.

[27] Philippa J Karoly, Vikram R Rao, Nicholas M Gregg, Gregory A Worrell, Christophe Bernard, Mark J Cook, and Maxime O Baud. Cycles in epilepsy. *Nature Reviews Neurology*, 17(5):267–284, 2021.

[28] Shella D Keilholz, Wen-Ju Pan, Jacob Billings, Maysam Nezafati, and Sadia Shakil. Noise and non-neuronal contributions to the BOLD signal: Applications to and insights from animal studies. *Neuroimage*, 154:267–281, 2017.

[29] Chang-Jin Kim. Dynamic linear models with Markov-switching. *Journal of Econometrics*, 60(1-2):1–22, 1994.

[30] Chang-Jin Kim and Charles Nelson. *State-Space Models with Regime Switching: Classical and Gibbs-Sampling Approaches with Applications.* MIT Press, 2017.

[31] Jeong Hwan Kook, Kelly A Vaughn, Dana M DeMaster, Linda Ewing-Cobbs, and Marina Vannucci. BVAR-connect: A variational Bayes approach to multi-subject vector autoregressive models for inference on brain connectivity networks. *Neuroinformatics*, 19:39–56, 2021.

[32] Nikolas Kuschnig and Lukas Vashold. BVAR: Bayesian vector autoregressions with hierarchical prior selection in R. *Journal of Statistical Software*, 100(14):1–27, November 2021.

[33] Marc G Leguia, Ralph G Andrzejak, Christian Rummel, Joline M Fan, Emily A Mirro, Thomas K Tcheng, Vikram R Rao, and Maxime O Baud. Seizure cycles in focal epilepsy. *JAMA Neurology*, 78(4):454–463, 2021.

[34] Robert Litterman. A Bayesian procedure for forecasting with vector autoregression. MIT working paper, 1980.

[35] Greta M Ljung. Diagnostic testing of univariate time series models. *Biometrika*, 73(3):725–730, 1986.

[36] Helmut Lütkepohl. *New Introduction to Multiple Time Series Analysis.* Springer-Verlag, 2005.

[37] Kanti Mardia and Peter Jupp. *Directional Statistics.* Wiley Series in Probability and Statistics. Wiley, 1999.

[38] William Nicholson, David Matteson, and Jacob Bien. VARX-L: structured regularization for large vector autoregressions with exogenous variables. *International Journal of Forecasting*, 33(3):627–651, 2017.

[39] William Nicholson, Ines Wilms, Jacob Bien, and David Matteson. High dimensional forecasting via interpretable vector autoregression. *Journal of Machine Learning Research*, 21:1–52, 2020.

[40] Giovanni Petris. An R package for dynamic linear models. *Journal of Statistical Software*, 36(12):1–16, October 2010.

[41] Giovanni Petris, Sonia Petrone, and Patrizia Campagnoli. *Dynamic Linear Models with R*. Springer, 2009.

[42] Bernhard Pfaff. *Analysis of Integrated and Cointegrated Time Series with R*. Springer, New York, second edition, 2008. ISBN 0-387-27960-1.

[43] Bernhard Pfaff. VAR, SVAR and SVEC models: Implementation within R package `vars`. *Journal of Statistical Software*, 27(4):1–32, July 2008.

[44] Tung D Phan, Jessica A Wachter, Ethan A Solomon, and Michael J Kahana. Multivariate stochastic volatility modeling of neural data. *Elife*, 8:e42950, 2019.

[45] Vikram R Rao. Chronic electroencephalography in epilepsy with a responsive neurostimulation device: Current status and future prospects. *Expert Review of Medical Devices*, 18(11):1093–1105, 2021.

[46] Simo Särkkä. *Bayesian Filtering and Smoothing*. IMS Textbooks. Cambridge University Press, 2013.

[47] Steven Scott. Bayesian methods for hidden Markov models: recursive computing in the 21st century. *Journal of the American Statistical Association*, 97(457):337–351, March 2002.

[48] Ali Shojaie and Emily Fox. Granger causality: a review and recent advances. *Annual Review of Statistics and Its Applications*, 9:289–319, 2022.

[49] Robert Shumway and David Stoffer. *Time Series Analysis and Its Applications*, volume 3. Springer, 2000.

[50] Christopher Sims, Daniel Waggoner, and Tao Zha. Methods for inference in large multiple-equation Markov-switching models. *Journal of Econometrics*, 146(2):255–274, October 2008.

[51] Ruey Tsay. *Analysis of Financial Time Series*. Wiley, 2005.

[52] Ruey Tsay. *Multivariate Time Series Analysis: With R and Financial Applications*. Wiley, 2013.

[53] Ingmar Visser and Maarten Speekenbrink. `depmixS4`: an R package for hidden Markov models. *Journal of Statistical Software*, 36:1–21, 2010.

[54] Andrew Viterbi. Error bounds for convolutional codes and an asymptotically optimum decoding algorithm. *IEEE Transactions on Information Theory*, 13(2):260–269, 1967.

[55] Emily Wang, Sharon Chiang, Zulfi Haneef, Vikram Rao, Robert Moss, and Marina Vannucci. Bayesian non-homogeneous hidden Markov model with variable selection for investigating drivers of seizure risk cycling. *The Annals of Applied Statistics*, 17(1):333–356, 2023.

[56] Emily Wang, Marina Vannucci, Zulfi Haneef, Robert Moss, Vikram Rao, and Sharon Chiang. A Bayesian switching linear dynamical system for estimating seizure chronotypes. *Proceedings of the National Academy of Sciences*, 119(46):1–12, 2022.

[57] Mike West and Jeff Harrison. *Bayesian Forecasting and Dynamic Models.* Springer Series in Statistics. Springer, 1997.

[58] Fang Zhang, Yufang Yang, Yanjie Xin, Yuting Sun, Chang Wang, Junming Zhu, Tao Tang, Jianmin Zhang, and Kedi Xu. Efficacy of different strategies of responsive neurostimulation on seizure control and their association with acute neurophysiological effects in rats. *Epilepsy & Behavior*, 143:109212, 2023.

[59] Walter Zucchini, Iain MacDonald, and Roland Langrock. *Hidden Markov Models for Time Series: An Introduction Using R.* Monographs on Statistics and Applied Probability. CRC Press, 2016.

# 9

# *Spectral Analysis of Electrophysiological Data*

**Hernando Ombao**

*Statistics Program, King Abdullah University of Science & Technology (Saudi Arabia)*

**Marco Antonio Pinto-Orellana**

*Department of Biomedical Engineering, University of California, Irvine (USA)*

## CONTENTS



This chapter explores spectral analysis as a mathematical basis for modeling the oscillatory phenomena observed in electrical brain signals. These oscillations can reflect communication between multiple brain subsystems, and the spectral framework provides a unique perspective on the information they exhibit. We begin by analyzing the characteristics of a single-channel spectrum, discussing their significance, and describing several estimation techniques. We begin discussing an introduction of frequency filters, energy spectral density, and power spectrum density, stressing their characteristics and conceptual interpretations. Then, we look at signals where the spectrum changes over time and methods for extracting their features. Finally, we proceed to multivariate spectrum analysis, which enables us to extract spectral information from multiple channels. This multivariate framework provides a basis for investigating sophisticated models that go beyond describing the spectral properties of each channel, allowing us to define a variety of interactions across channels, including causality models. Examples are provided in the `R` programming language. Overall, this

DOI: 10.1201/9781003254515-9

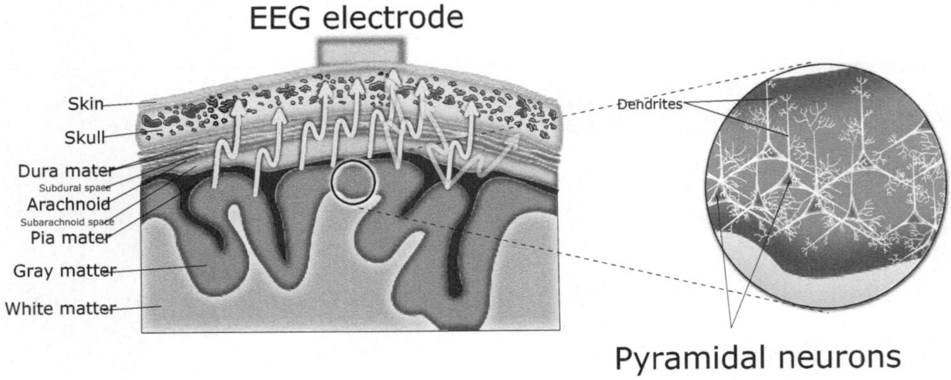


**FIGURE 9.1**
Electroencephalograms are electrical recordings of the synchronized activity of a large group of neurons (mainly pyramidal) after crossing the brain tissue and skull. (Color version available in electronic supplement.)

chapter offers a comprehensive overview of spectrum analysis and some of its possible uses in understanding brain signals.

## 9.1 Introduction

The relationship between the different functional systems inside the brain provides it with the ability to self-regulate and process sensory tasks. Information flows dynamically arise naturally to regulate these processes, and some of these signals have representative oscillatory patterns [60]. Research has been conducted to identify the fundamental mechanisms that link the brain's regulatory functions and observed measurement fluctuations. This line of research dates back to Mosso's pioneering work (1884) on fluctuations in blood flow [71], Pravdich-Neminsky (1925), and Berger (1930) on electrical signals [24, 36]. However, despite significant progress in the analysis of brain signals, not all of their physiological origins and consequences are well understood, as various research questions remain open for further study, such as the role of high-frequency oscillations in seizures [12], the effect of potential latent components on brain signal analysis [21] or the relationship between extreme values and epileptiform waves [33]. In this chapter, we will use spectral analysis as a mathematical basis for modeling oscillatory phenomena, which, in turn, can serve as a tool to get a deeper understanding of neurological processes.

## 9.2 Spectral-Encoded Information in EEG

Electroencephalograms (EEGs) are non-invasive biomedical signals obtained by measuring the difference in electrical potentials on the scalp [61, p.454]. As discussed in depth in Chapter 2, these signals result from synchronized electrical responses that travel through the gray matter to the skull, coming from groups of neurons, primarily pyramidal

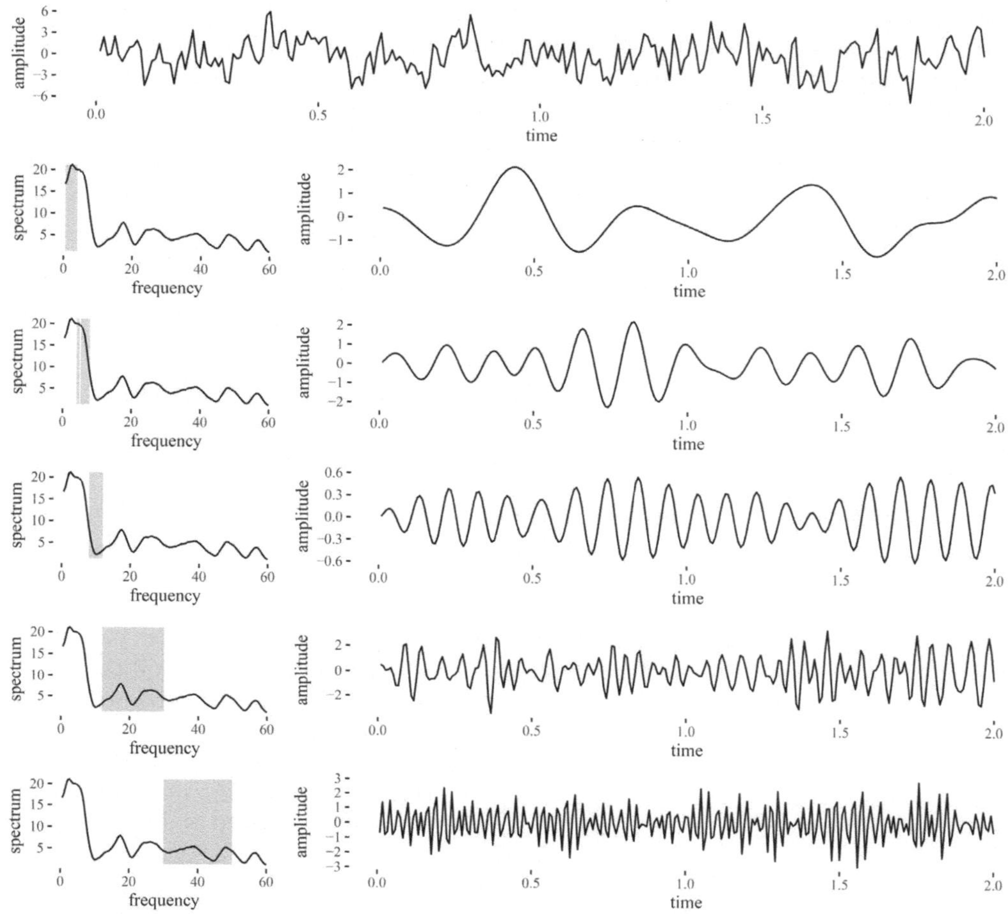


**FIGURE 9.2**
Five main oscillatory components (rhythms) of electroencephalograms: delta (0–4 Hz), theta (4–8 Hz), alpha (8–12 Hz), beta (12–30 Hz), and gamma (30+ Hz). At the left, the energy spectrum density is shown, while at the right the oscillations in the time domain are shown.

neurons, whose dendrites are perpendicular to the scalp (Figure 9.1). To provide a spatial/topological overview of electrical activity around the entire head, EEG is usually measured simultaneously from several locations (or channels) [54, p. 555], [61, p. 428].

The electrical properties of the brain tissue and the skull distort, and attenuate traveling waves. As a result, we cannot assume that EEG measurements originated exclusively from neuronal sources. Nonetheless, they can still capture the temporal dynamics of neuron activity [74, pp. 3, 19–22]. Despite these limitations, the portability and inexpensiveness of EEG make it possible to integrate it into clinical and realistic experimental conditions, which would not be possible to study with other biomedical imaging methods.

EEG waves are oscillations that occur in a wide frequency range, from 0 to 50 Hz. Classical EEG analysis divides the entire spectrum of oscillations into five main ranges: delta, theta, alpha, beta, and gamma rhythms based on specific frequency bands [41, pp. 47]. Each brain wave (or rhythm) in this scheme is associated with a particular set of psychophysiological characteristics (Figure 9.2):

- Delta waves (0–4 Hz) are the slowest observed signals in EEG. They are seen during NREM sleep, as well as during epileptic seizures and loss of consciousness [6]. There is also a relationship between these waves and a decrease in serum glucose concentration, and their abnormalities can result from encephalopathy [74].
- Theta waves (4–8 Hz) [74] are attributed to quiet concentration, cognitive processes including short-term memory tasks, memory retrieval, and mental imagery [6, 74]. Theta rhythm patterns can also be used to enhance emotion recognition [75].
- Alpha waves (8–12 Hz) are typically observed in the occipital region when the eyes are closed (the "Berger effect") [6, 75]. In addition, the absence of alpha waves in some individuals can be attributed to genetic diseases [74].
- Beta waves (12–30 Hz) are connected to alertness, normal waking consciousness, active thought, and focus [6, 72, 75]. Muscle artifacts can potentially contaminate these waves because their spectral responses lie in the same frequency range [74, 75].
- Gamma rhythms (>30 Hz) are an indicator of active information exchange between cortical and subcortical regions [6, 32]. They are used to detect event-related synchronization [72] and seem to be associated with cognitive performance [67].

This paradigm for classifying frequency can detect some unusual or pathological conditions. During hypoxic-ischemic encephalopathies, for instance, alpha and theta waves are significantly attenuated [1]. We refer to Stern et al. [74] for a detailed exploration of the time-domain patterns in brain rhythms and their clinical importance.

However, a five-band categorization may not provide enough detail for some experimental settings. For example, when depicting the effects of stimuli on brain waves in response to auditory stimuli, wide bands cannot provide sufficient detail [80]. Consequently, there is a growing trend toward more condition-specific (and narrow) analysis of frequency bands that may replace the current classification. In this direction, methods are being studied that make it possible to robustly identify the number of frequency peaks and their exact frequencies solely based on experimental data [30].

It is important to emphasize that the relationship between physiological mechanisms and fluctuation patterns is not exclusive to EEGs. This connection can be observed in other biological subsystems, such as the vagus nerve, which acts as a closed-system regulator of heart rate [60].

## 9.3 Deterministic and Nondeterministic Spectrum

There are two distinct ways to think about biomedical signals: as the output of fixed (deterministic) systems or as samples collected from stochastic systems. In a deterministic context, where the outputs can be precisely known if all inputs are given, the spectrum typically refers to the energy spectrum density (ESD), which is the squared modulus of the Fourier transform of the measurements [22].

Conversely, the current measurements cannot be considered the only possible value in a system with inherent randomness. Instead, they are viewed as a sample (also known as realization) of a stochastic process that describes the system. In this perspective, the spectrum is synonymous with the power spectrum density (PSD), which is the Fourier transform of the auto-covariance function of the time series.

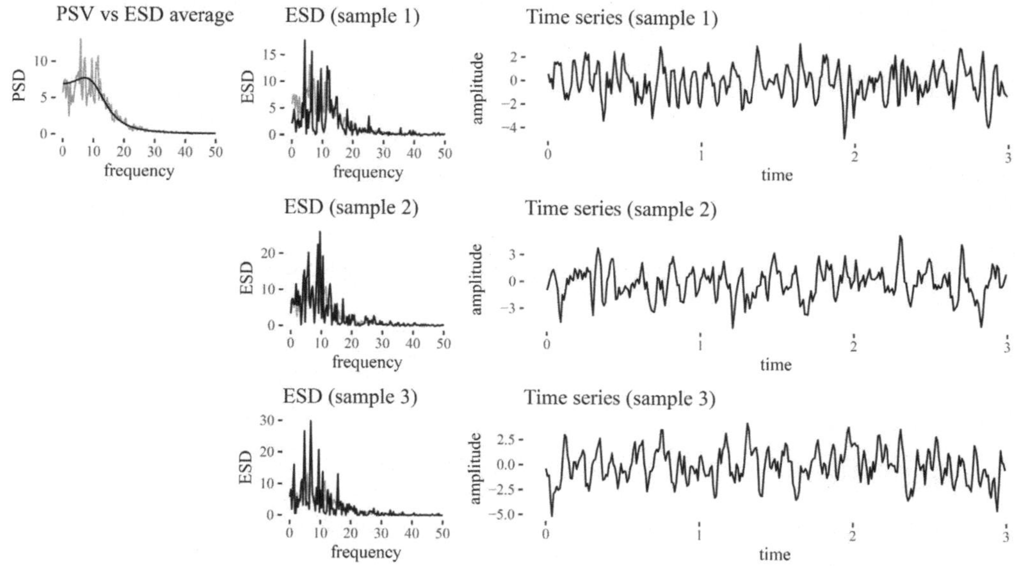


**FIGURE 9.3**
Energy spectrum density and power spectrum density of an oscillatory signal with central resonating frequency at 10 Hz.

Depending on the context, the term "spectrum" may refer to either ESD or PSD in the literature, even though they are not interchangeable. Unless explicitly stated otherwise, we will refer to PSD as the spectrum in the following sections.

**Example 9.3.1. (Deterministic and nondeterministic spectrum).** The ESD is not used in stochastic processes since the Fourier transform is only defined for deterministic values. Hence, we cannot calculate the ESD of a stochastic process itself, but we can compute the ESD of samples collected from the process [59]. The ensemble average of these ESDs will converge to the PSD after a large number of repetitions [44].

To illustrate this phenomenon, let us consider an EEG with a peak at 10 Hz (the alpha band) and suppose it can be described by the following dynamical system:

$$x(t) = 1.425\, x(t-1) - 0.776\, x(t-2) + \varepsilon(t)$$

where $\varepsilon(t)$ is a white noise process, $\varepsilon(t) \sim \mathcal{N}(0,1)$.

Suppose we observed and recorded this signal for four seconds in ten trials. Figure 9.3 shows the recordings of three of these trials and their associated ESD. Although all the ESD estimates capture the peak, note the difference in magnitude and significant volatility in their responses in the interval 0–20 Hz. The PSD (black line) is the same for all of them because they all come from the same process, and observe how the average of the ten ESD (left panel) is closer to the actual PSD.

### 9.3.1 Energy Spectrum Density

Under certain conditions, a deterministic signal can be expressed as a sum of sinusoids, i.e., it admits a discrete-time Fourier representation (DFT) [23]:

$$x(t) = \int_{\Omega_0} X(\omega)\, e^{j2\pi t\omega}\, d\omega$$

Here, $\Omega_0 = \left[-\frac{1}{2}, \frac{1}{2}\right]$ is the normalized frequency range, and $\omega$ is the normalized frequency.

As previously mentioned, the energy density spectrum (ESD) is the squared magnitude of the Fourier transform of the signal,

$$S_X(\omega) = |X(\omega)|^2$$

where $X(\omega)$ is the mapping of the signal in the frequency domain using the Fourier transform.

In some disciplines, the ESD has a direct physical interpretation. For instance, if the signal is the potential difference (measured in Volts) between EEG electrodes, the spectrum represents the energy in Watts that crosses a line with a resistance of 1 Ohm at frequency $\omega$.

## 9.4 Digital Linear Filters

As previously discussed, a signal can be viewed as a linear combination of oscillations. Consequently, frequency filters are necessary to isolate oscillatory components within a specific frequency range. A straightforward approach would be to take the Fourier transform of the signal, ignore the coefficients of irrelevant frequencies, and then apply the inverse Fourier transform. However, this method relies on DFT algorithms and has a time complexity of $\mathcal{O}(n^2)$, which means that for any input series of $n$ elements, its execution time grows with $n^2$. Although efficient implementations such as the Cooley-Tukey algorithm included in the widely used fast Fourier transform library FFTW [29] have a time complexity of $\mathcal{O}(n\log n)$, they can still be computationally prohibitively for large signal datasets.

An alternative to the Fourier transform is to use linear time-invariant frequency filters, which provide an efficient way to attenuate any frequency outside a specific range of interest. These filters only use a linear combination of past values of the input signal and previously filtered quantities [35]. They are typically classified as finite and infinite impulse response filters. Both types of filters have a linear time complexity of $\mathcal{O}(n)$.

Finite impulse response (FIR) filters use only current and past values, while infinite impulse response (IIR) filters use the feedback of previous states of the filter. FIR filters require more past values to filter signals in the same frequency range as their IIR counterparts, making them computationally more expensive. However, IIR filters require careful coefficient estimation to be stable in narrowband regions, and they may have a non-flat gain in the frequency range of interest [22].

For instance, for a signal with a sampling frequency `fs`, we can calculate the coefficients of a band-pass filter between 4 Hz and 8 Hz for a fourth-order Butterworth (IIR) filter:

```
# Load the 'signal' library
library(signal)
# Bandpass filter
filter_coeffs <- butter(4, c(4, 8)/(0.5 * fs), type="pass")
```

Alternatively, we can calculate the coefficients for a 100th FIR filter in the same frequency interval:

```
filter_coeffs <- signal::fir1(100, c(4, 8)/(0.5 * fs), type="pass")
```

These values then can be used to filter the signal:

```
 # One-sided filter
y_filtered <- as.numeric(filter(filter_coeffs, y))
# Two-sided filter
y_filtered <- as.numeric(filtfilt(filter_coeffs, y))
```

## 9.5 Univariate Stationary Spectrum

To provide neurological interpretations of the spectrum, we generally assume that analyzed signals have some "stability" or "stationarity" in their statistical properties. Preprocessing techniques can induce this stationarity if the assumption is not met due to artifacts [27]. Biological signals like EEG can typically be approximated as stationary signals during short time intervals [5, 27, 54]. As discussed in Chapter 8, a stochastic process $X(t)$ is strictly stationary if its joint probability distribution is identical for any possible sub-sample of the signal [34]. However, this kind of process is infrequent in real-world conditions, and we use a less strict definition of stationarity: wide-sense stationarity (WSS) [40]. A WSS process has a finite variance and a mean value that remains constant over time, while its correlation between any two points only depends on the time difference between them: $E\big[X(t)X(t+\tau)\big] = \text{corr}_{xx}(\tau) = \sigma_{xx}(\tau)$.

Typically, we define the PSD of a stationary process as the Fourier transform of the autocovariance function, which decomposes the signal variance across all frequencies (Parseval's theorem) [35, 51]. However, this definition does not intuitively interpret a signal's behavior in a specific frequency. Instead, we can use Cramér's representation as an alternative approach to defining the PSD. This representation states that a WSS signal in the time domain is a sum of complex oscillations modulated by zero-mean random coefficients. Then, the PSD is the variance of the coefficients associated with those complex oscillations. Although both PSD definitions are equivalent, both provide alternative perspectives about the characterization of spectrum in a stochastic signal. We refer to [55] for a more comprehensive and formal comparison of their properties.

In practice, we do not know the true stochastic process that produced the signal. Thus we must estimate the spectrum using limited sample data. The periodogram, the Fourier transform of the sampled signal squared magnitude, is a method to accomplish this. The periodogram is an asymptotically unbiased, but not consistent, PSD estimator since, for large samples, its expectation converges to the true spectrum, but its variance does not decrease [35]. Convergence properties are covered in depth in [45] and [35].

Several improvements to the algorithm have been proposed to overcome the aforementioned inherent limitations, such as the Bartlett and Welch approaches. The underlying idea in both is that – given that the signal is a WSS process and its mean and autocorrelation are not changing over time – the spectrum should remain constant under sub-sampling. Welch's approach separates the signal into overlapping segments (multiplied by a window function) and computes the periodogram for each segment. Then, in order to lower the estimator's variability, these periodograms are averaged. Similar to the periodogram, this estimator is also unbiased. Welch's spectrum estimate, in contrast, is consistent given that large repetitions bring its variance close to zero [45] and [35].

Under some circumstances, we can suppose that the sample data adhere to a recognized generating process and estimate the spectrum resulting from that process. Autoregressive (AR) models, discussed in the time domain in Chapter 8, are commonly used for this purpose because of their versatility [35] and generality in modeling [73]: "Any spectral density can be approximated, arbitrarily close by the spectrum of an AR process."

An AR($p$) model assumes that observations are the result of a linear combination of the previous p observations and an innovation component. The coefficients of this model can be estimated using methods such as the method of moments, least-square estimation [SMITH], and the Yule-Walker method [35]. Once estimated, these coefficients are then used to describe the signal's spectrum.

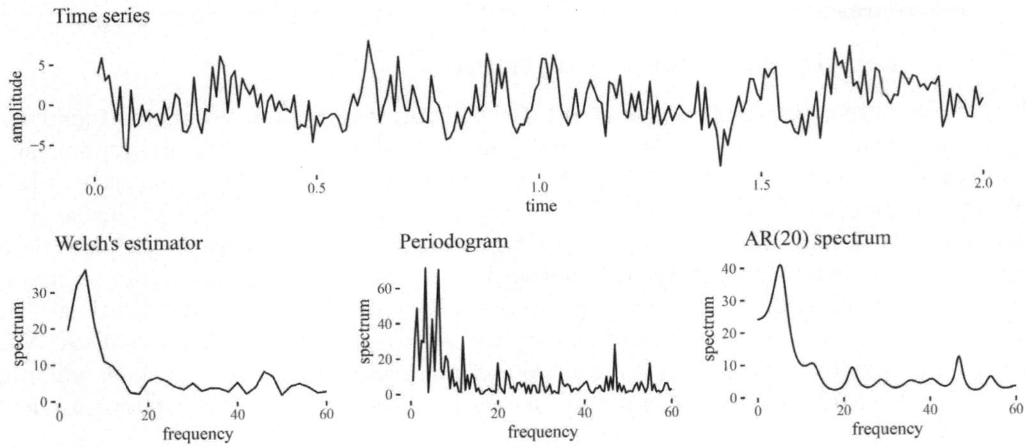


**FIGURE 9.4**
Comparison between spectrum estimations in EEG using Welch's method, a periodogram, and an AR(20) model.

**Example 9.5.1. (Comparison of spectrum estimators)** Let us simulate a 4-second segment of an EEG recording with a sample rate of 128 Hz:

```
fs <- 128
N <- fs * 4
y_sample_eeg <- simulate_EEG(N, fs)
```

We can compare the spectrum estimators obtained using a periodogram, Welch's method, and a 20th-order autoregressive model (Figure 9.4):

```
library(oce) # We will need this library to estimate Welch's spectrum

# AR(20) spectrum
spec_ar <- spectrum(y_sample_eeg, method = "ar", order = 20, plot = TRUE)

# Periodogram
spec_pgram <- spectrum(y_sample_eeg, method = "pgram", plot = TRUE)

# Welch's spectrum
spec_welch <- pwelch(y_sample_eeg, method = "pgram", plot = TRUE)
```

It is important to note that all three estimators accurately capture the low-pass behavior of the signal. However, there are differences in the magnitudes of the three approaches, with the autoregressive model being better suited to minimizing potential noisy artifacts. Conversely, the periodogram captures responses in the current measurements more effectively, but this comes at the cost of worse generalization. Interpreting these values would require careful consideration and depend on the experimental conditions.

### 9.5.1 AR(2) Processes

Second-order autoregressive, AR(2) or SAR, models are the simplest AR(p) process whose spectrum can be expressed with a unique peak frequency and spectral bandwidth. They also can approximate complicated spectrum responses by combining them as latent processes. A process $Z(t)$ is AR(2) if it can be represented as $x(t) - \phi_1 x(t-1) - \phi_2 x(t-2) = \epsilon(t)$, where $\epsilon(t)$ is a Gaussian white noise with zero mean and variance $\sigma_W^2$.

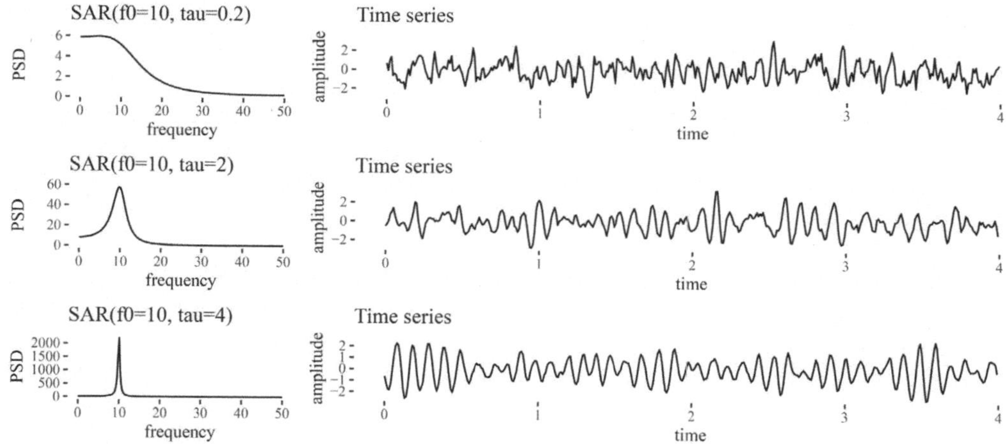


**FIGURE 9.5**
Comparison between three AR(2) processes with the same central frequency at 8 Hz and different bandwidths.

Here, we will focus on the subclass of $AR(2)$ models whose polynomial roots are non-real complex and conjugate. This category allows us to parametrize the coefficients of the autoregressive model as

$$\phi_1 = 2\left(1 + e^{-\tau}\right)\cos\left(2\pi f_0\right)$$
$$\phi_2 = -\left(1 + e^{-\tau}\right)$$

where $M = (1 + e^{-\tau})$ and $\tau > 0$ (to ensure $\left|z_1^{-1}\right|, \left|z_2^{-1}\right| > 1$).

In this parametrization, the spectrum of the modeled time series has a peak at $f_0$, and the bandwidth $\tau$ controls the spread of this peak. When the root magnitude $M$ is closed to 1 (or $\tau \to 0+$) then the bandwidth of the peak around $f_0$ becomes narrower. Conversely, the spread around $f_0$ increases with higher bandwidth (Figure 9.5).

**Example 9.5.2. (Spectral parametrization of AR(2) models).** To emphasize this new set of parameters, let us introduce the following notation for second-order autoregressive (SAR) models that $x(t)$:

$$x(t) \sim \text{SAR}\left(f_0, \tau, \sigma_W^2\right)$$

Suppose we have an AR(2) with a central frequency of 8 Hz and different bandwidths (Figure 9.5):

$$y(t) = 0.964y(t-1) - 0.302y(t-2) + \varepsilon(t) \Leftrightarrow SAR\left(f_0 = 8, \tau = 0.200, \sigma^2 = 1\right)$$
$$y(t) = 1.544y(t-1) - 0.776y(t-2) + \varepsilon(t) \Leftrightarrow SAR\left(f_0 = 8, \tau = 2.000, \sigma^2 = 1\right)$$
$$y(t) = 1.721y(t-1) - 0.964y(t-2) + \varepsilon(t) \Leftrightarrow SAR\left(f_0 = 8, \tau = 4.000, \sigma^2 = 1\right)$$

In those cases, the representation using the $SAR$ notation (and source code) is more compact to denote the spectral information about these processes:

```
N <- 1024
fs <- 128
y1 <- simulate_unstable_oscillator(N, f = 8, tau = 0.2, fs = fs, sigma = 1)
y2 <- simulate_unstable_oscillator(N, f = 8, tau = 2.0, fs = fs, sigma = 1)
y3 <- simulate_unstable_oscillator(N, f = 8, tau = 4.2, fs = fs, sigma = 1)
```

## 9.6 Univariate Nonstationary Spectrum

Most biomedical signals could exhibit some nonstationary characteristics such as trends and drifts caused by artifacts or stimuli-driven change-points [42]. Nevertheless, physiological signals can be accurately approximated as local-stationary in short time intervals because their parameters change smoothly [5, 27], as it is proposed in EEG [72] and fNIRS modeling [25].

A time-dependent generalization of the Cramér representation can be found in the Priestley-Dahlhaus model [19, 69]. This model suggests that the time series is a mixture of oscillations modulated by random coefficients $A_{xx}\left(\frac{t}{T},\omega\right)$ that changes over time. Time-varying spectrum is then estimated as the modulus-squared of these random coefficients. However, this time-varying coefficient $A_{xx}\left(\frac{t}{T},\omega\right)$ is defined for a rescaled time such that $0<\frac{t}{T}<1$. This has an interesting philosophical consequence in interpreting the time-varying spectrum: larger samples (larger $T$) do not imply getting more data but actually, improve the resolution of the time-varying spectrum.

As an alternative definition, the time-varying spectrum can be defined as the Fourier transform of the "ambiguity function" constructed from the conjugate covariant function. We refer to [50, 51] for details about the construction of this function.

### 9.6.1 Short-Time Fourier Transform Spectrogram

The short-time Fourier transform (STFT) expands the Fourier transform principle by adding a time-varying window function that detects changes in the spectral domain. STFT has been used to extract patterns that can be used to measure mental workload [4], predict seizures [70], or identify autism spectrum disorder [11]. The short-time Fourier transform (STFT) of a real-valued deterministic function $h(\cdot)$, with respect to a window function $g(\cdot)$, is defined as [31]:

$$V_g(\tau,\omega)=\int_{-\infty}^{\infty} h(t)\,\overline{g(t-\tau)}e^{-2j\pi t\omega}\,dt \tag{9.1}$$

Recall that $\bar{\cdot}$ is the complex conjugate operation.

In a deterministic context, the STFT spectrogram is given by the squared modulus of the STFT[31]:

$$S(\tau,\omega)\equiv|V_g(\tau,\omega)|^2 \tag{9.2}$$

It can be proved that the stochastic spectrogram (using Mallat's time-varying spectrum) is the expected value of the magnitude squared of the deterministic STFT spectrograms.

### 9.6.2 Wavelet Spectrum

A wavelet transform is defined as the linear transformation of a function $x(t)$ into a series of rescaled and shifted wavelet bases $\psi_{\tau,s}$[78] with respect to a time $\tau$ and a scale $s$:

$$W_X(\tau,s)=\int_{-\infty}^{\infty} x(t)\,\psi_{\tau,s}(t)\,dt \tag{9.3}$$

Each shifted and scaled $\phi_{\tau,s}$ is then obtained from a basis function $\psi(t)$, also known as mother wavelet:

$$\psi_{\tau,s}=\frac{1}{\sqrt{s}}\psi\left(\frac{t-\tau}{s}\right) \tag{9.4}$$

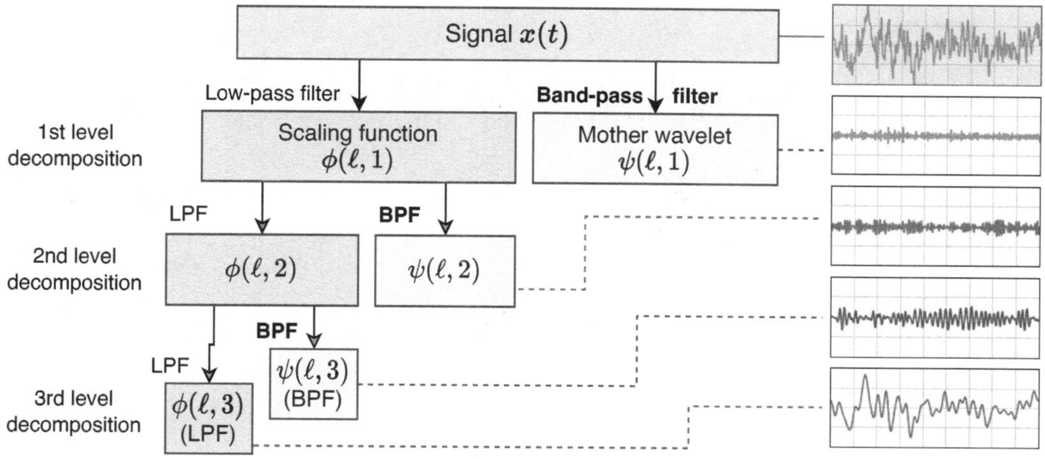


**FIGURE 9.6**
Multi-level dyadic decomposition with Daubechies 6 wavelets. (Color version available in electronic supplement.)

In contrast with the Fourier transform, the wavelet transform generalizes the idea of projecting a function $x(t)$ into any mother wavelet if it satisfies an admissibility and regularity condition. The admissibility property ensures that the Fourier transform of the mother-wavelet will be zero at the origin, and thus, it will behave as a band-pass filter. Regularity guarantees that the coefficients of the wavelet transform can be approximated with finite coefficients in a Taylor expansion [68].

The discrete wavelet representation extends Equation 9.4 to a discretized index time $l$ and scale $k$ ($l, k \in \mathbb{Z}$) with the introduction of a sampling time, or translation step $\tau_0$ and a dilation step $s_0 > 0$:

$$\psi_{l,k} = \frac{1}{\sqrt{s_0^k}} \psi \left( \frac{t - l\tau}{s_0^k} \right) \tag{9.5}$$

We should note that typically $s_0 = 2$ (dyadic sampling) and orthogonal mother wavelets are chosen:

$$\int \psi_{l,k}(t) \, \psi^*_{l',k'}(t) = \delta_{l,l'} \delta_{k,k'} \tag{9.6}$$

where $\delta_{a,b}$ is the Krockener delta, and $\psi^*$ is the complex conjugate of $\psi$.

Recall that for a signal $f(t)$ with a Fourier transform $F(\omega)$, scaling it in time $f(st)$ implies stretching its spectrum $\frac{1}{|s|} F\left(\frac{\omega}{s}\right)$. Therefore, a $k$-th dyadic scaling of the mother wavelet implies compressing its spectrum by a factor of $2^k$.

The dyadic spectrum dilation means that an infinite number of scales will be needed to cover the entire spectrum down to zero (Zeno's dichotomy paradox). Otherwise, a high reconstruction error could be introduced. To mitigate these issues, a scaling factor was introduced [49] that acts as a low-pass filter and to cover the remaining frequencies that the scaled mother wavelet, as a band-pass filter, does not reach.

We need to emphasize that there is not always a closed-form solution to relate a scale $k$ and a (Fourier) frequency $\omega$. Without such a relationship, we cannot take advantage of the spectrum interpretation of EEGs as it was discussed in Section 9.2. However, despite the lack of a direct expression $k \mapsto \omega$, an approximate pseudo-frequency $\omega^*$ can be calculated by:

$$\omega^* = \frac{\omega_0}{k} \tag{9.7}$$

where $\omega_0$ is the center frequency of the wavelet.

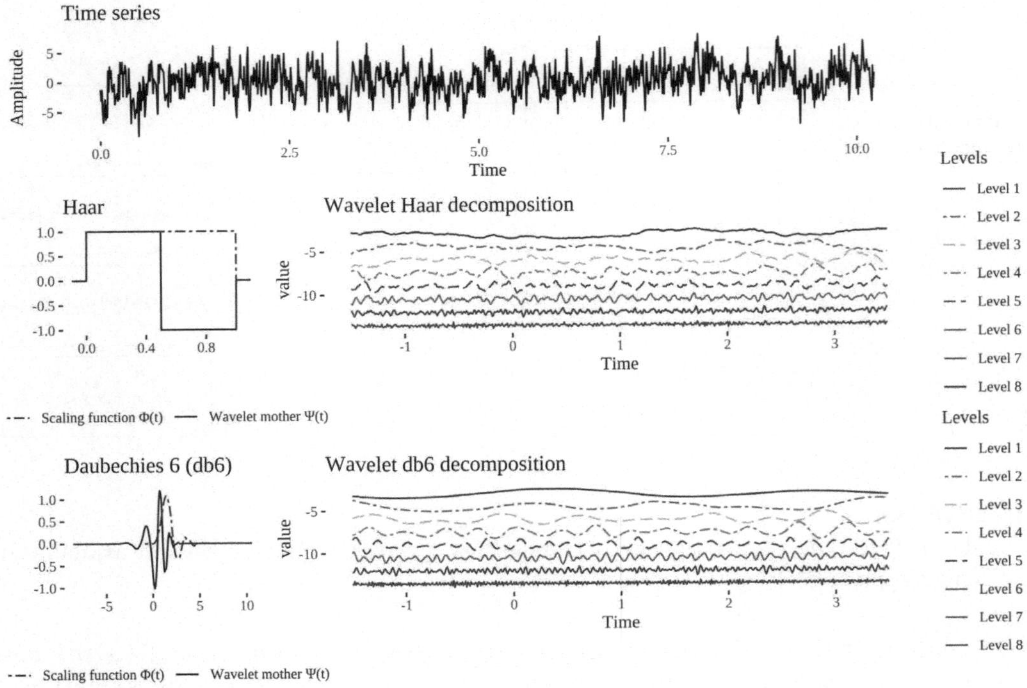


**FIGURE 9.7**
Comparison of wavelet families: Haar and Daubechies 6 (db6). (Color version available in electronic supplement.)

Wavelet research is exceptionally vast in diverse scenarios [9, 9, 38, 77], including EEG studies [10, 79]. However, there has been a tendency to focus on the analysis in the deterministic case (for instance, to obtain features for glucose measurement [46], pain assessment [47], artifact correction [15, 39], epilepsy classification [3], or cerebral autoregulation processes [2]).

For completeness, we need to emphasize that there is also a stochastic wavelet definition. Chiann et al. [14] defined the wavelet spectrum as a linear transformation of a wavelet autocorrelation function, constructed from shifted and scaled mother wavelets weighted by the signal autocorrelation [14, 78].

In the latter stochastic paradigm, we can also define a space-scale wavelet periodogram $\hat{\eta}_X(l, k)$ as an estimator for the stochastic wavelet as the squared-modulus of the deterministic wavelet of the sample. This estimator is asymptotically unbiased in large samples [14]. Suppose the EEG is weakly stationary. In that case, we can obtain an equivalent to the periodograms mentioned in the previous section: the wavelet scalogram that is the sum of the wavelet coefficients at time index $l$ [78].

**Example 9.6.1. (Effect of mother wavelets on wavelet coefficients).** The Haar wavelet is the simplest mother-wavelet, and it is defined by:

$$\psi(t) = \begin{cases} 1 & 0 \leq t < \frac{1}{2} \\ -1 & \frac{1}{2} \leq t < 1 \\ 0 & \text{otherwise} \end{cases} \tag{9.8}$$

Additionally, its scaling function $\varphi(t)$ (sometimes also named father-wavelet) is described by:

$$\varphi(t) = \begin{cases} 1 & 0 \leq t < 1 \\ 0 & \text{otherwise} \end{cases} \tag{9.9}$$

Another well-known wavelet family is the Daubechies orthonormal wavelets [20] which are well-localized in time and frequency. Although they do not have a closed-form solution, they have been applied in a large variety of engineering scenarios [17]. Typically, wavelets in this family are named db$L$ with $L$ as the order of the wavelet.

In Figure 9.7, we show how wavelets can influence the signal decomposition. In `R`, we can plot the mother wavelet and scaling function using the package `wavethresh`:

```
library(wavethresh)
# Sixth-order Daubechies wavelet
order = 6
family = "DaubExPhase"
# Plot the mother wavelet
draw.default(filter.number = order, family = family, scaling.function = FALSE)
# Plot the scaling function
draw.default(filter.number = order, family = family, scaling.function = TRUE)
```

### 9.6.3 Univariate SLEX Model

Wavelet offers a good scale-space estimation, but exact frequencies cannot be directly obtained. On the other hand, STFT functions are not orthogonal and cannot simultaneously ensure time and frequency localization (Balian-Low theorem [18]). However, it is possible to construct complex exponential basis orthogonal with both time and frequency localization, as was proved in [56]. This family of basis functions, the smooth localized complex exponential (SLEX) functions, are then also suited as generalizations of Fourier functions for nonstationary processes [55–57], and it has been used to capture time-frequency patterns in a variety of contexts EEGs from highly noisy wearable devices [52], epileptic pattern recognition [13] or lifecycle patterns in lithium batteries [37].

The SLEX waveforms $\phi_\omega(t)$ can be seen as time-localized versions of the Fourier waveforms and are constructed by applying window functions $\Psi_.(t)$ into the Fourier basis [56].

$$\phi_\omega(t) = \Psi_+(t)\, e^{j2\pi\omega t} \Psi_-(t)\, e^{-j2\pi\omega t} \tag{9.10}$$

where $\omega$ is a relative frequency $\omega \in \left[-\frac{1}{2}, \frac{1}{2}\right]$. Furthermore, the window functions have a domain in a compact interval $[\alpha_0 - \epsilon, \alpha_1 + \epsilon]$ where $\epsilon$ is the overlap allowed to exceed a parametrized interval $[\alpha_0, \alpha_1]$. The procedure of constructing the window functions is discussed in [16, 55–57]. Figure 9.8 shows an example of an SLEX basis $\phi_\omega(t)$ and its associated window functions $\Psi_+(t)$ and $\Psi_-(t)$.

Similarly to wavelet, a dyadic segmentation is defined for frequency identification in discrete domains. First, we can construct an SLEX library with a collection of basis defined on dyadic support on rescaled time. These bases are defined such that for a level $j$ a time series is divided into $2^j$ blocks with the same width.

An SLEX waveform with support on block $B(j, b)$ oscillating at frequency $\omega$ is denoted as $\Psi_{j,b,\omega}(t)$. A SLEX basis $\mathcal{B}(t)$ is defined as any combination of blocks $\{B(j_k, b_k)\}$ such that $\cup_k B(j_k, b_k)$ has a support of the time series.

The SLEX transformation allows defining of a time series as a sum of oscillations that exists only a particular time intervals (where the duration and location of such intervals are

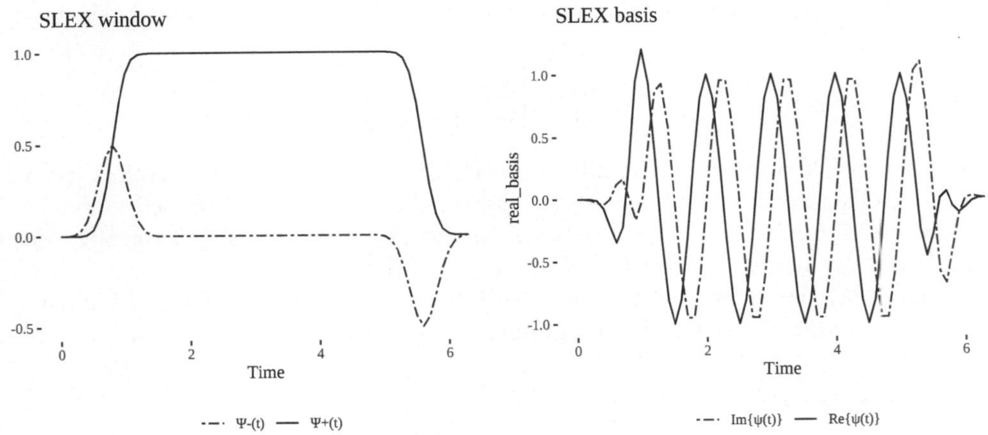


**FIGURE 9.8**
SLEX window functions $\Psi_+(t)$, $\Psi_-(t)$ for $a_0 = 32, a_1 = 64, \epsilon = 8$ and the SLEX basis $\psi_\omega(t)$ for $\omega = 0.1$. (Color version available in electronic supplement.)

defined by the basis family $\mathcal{B}$. Formally, this can be expressed as

$$X(t) = \sum_{(j,b)\in\mathcal{B}} \int_\omega \Theta_{j,b}(\omega)\psi_{j,b,\omega}(t)d\mathbf{Z}_{j,b}(\omega) \tag{9.11}$$

where $\Theta_{j,b}(\omega)$ is the SLEX transfer function defined on time block $B(j,b)$ and $\{dZ_{j,b}(\omega)\}$ is a random increment process that is orthonormal across time blocks $(j,b)$ and frequencies $\omega$.

Then, the time-dependent SLEX spectrum is defined as the squared magnitude of the block transfer functions similar to the classical Fourier approach. Note that each SLEX basis $\mathcal{B}$ is associated with a unique segmentation.

**Example 9.6.2. (SLEX basis).** Assume that a time series of length $T$ is divided into three levels. Then, the basis:

$$\begin{aligned}
\mathcal{B}_0 =& B(0,0)\\
\mathcal{B}_1 =& B(1,0) \cup B(1,1)\\
\mathcal{B}_2 =& B(1,0) \cup B(2,2) \cup B(2,3)\\
\mathcal{B}_3 =& B(2,0) \cup B(2,1) \cup B(1,1)B(2,0) \cup B(2,1) \cup B(2,2) \cup B(2,3)
\end{aligned}$$

Now, consider that the same time series is divided into four levels, as in Figure 9.9. There are 26 possible combinations for valid SLEX basis, one of which is displayed in the figure: $\mathcal{B}(t) = \{B(1,0) \cup B(3,4) \cup B(3,5) \cup B(2,3)\}$. Note that the number of possible combinations increases exponentially: 677 for five levels, 458330 for six levels, etc.

### 9.6.4 Dyadic Aggregated Autoregressive Model

As discussed in Section 9.5.1, AR(2) processes are the smallest autoregressive model whose spectrum can be expressed as a function of a central resonating frequency and a spectral bandwidth. This family of models provides a simple, robust, and smooth alternative

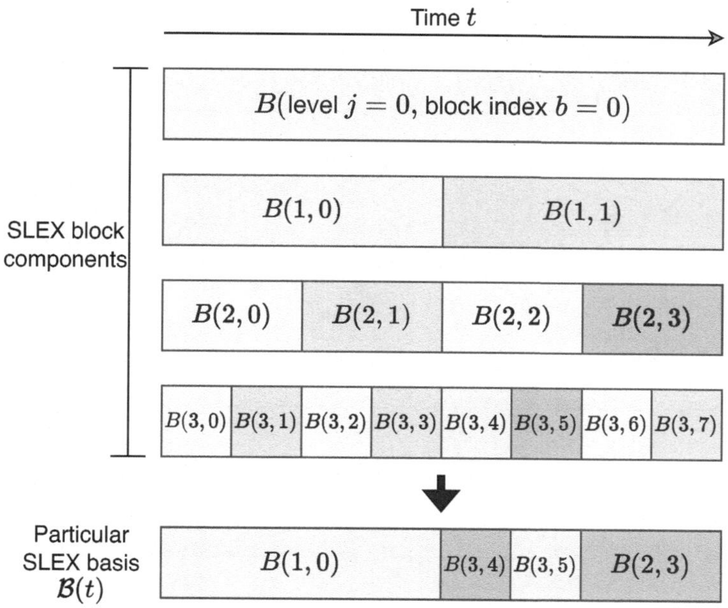


**FIGURE 9.9**
SLEX library and sample SLEX basis $\mathcal{B}(t) = \{B(1,0) \cup B(3,4) \cup B(3,5) \cup B(2,3)\}$.

to model periodically stationary processes. However, they are only capable of single-frequency localization while lacking time-localization as Fourier basis representations. These limitations were overcome by a dyadic division of the time domain (as it was also observed in wavelets and SLEX) through the dyadic aggregated autoregressive (DASAR) model introduced in [63, 65].

DASAR models the time-varying spectrum $S(t, \omega)$ as a weighted sum of several approximations based on $L$-level dyadic divisions. For each level $j$, the time support is split into $2^i$ segments with equal width, and a piece-wise local stationary spectrum is estimated for each division. The latter division's spectrum is modeled with an aggregated AR(2) autoregressive model, i.e., as the weighted sum of $k$ AR(2) models (stochastic oscillators) with different resonating frequencies and bandwidths.

To reduce the computationally cost of estimating DASAR models, an improved algorithm was introduced in [63] to narrow the latter de spectral space exploration to a specific frequency interval, not necessarily contiguous, but with biological interpretation or significance (spectrum region of interest, SROI).

**Example 9.6.3. (Comparison of STFT, wavelets, SLEX, and DASAR).**
Let $w(t)$ be a time-varying frequency:

$$w(t) = \begin{cases} 10t & t \in [0,4) \\ 4t & t \in [4,8) \\ 0.5t & t \in [8,12) \\ 2t & t \in [12,16) \end{cases}$$

Then, let $x(t)$ be a time series, with a sampling frequency of 16 Hz, described by

$$y(t) = \sin(2\pi w(t)\, t) + \varepsilon(t)$$

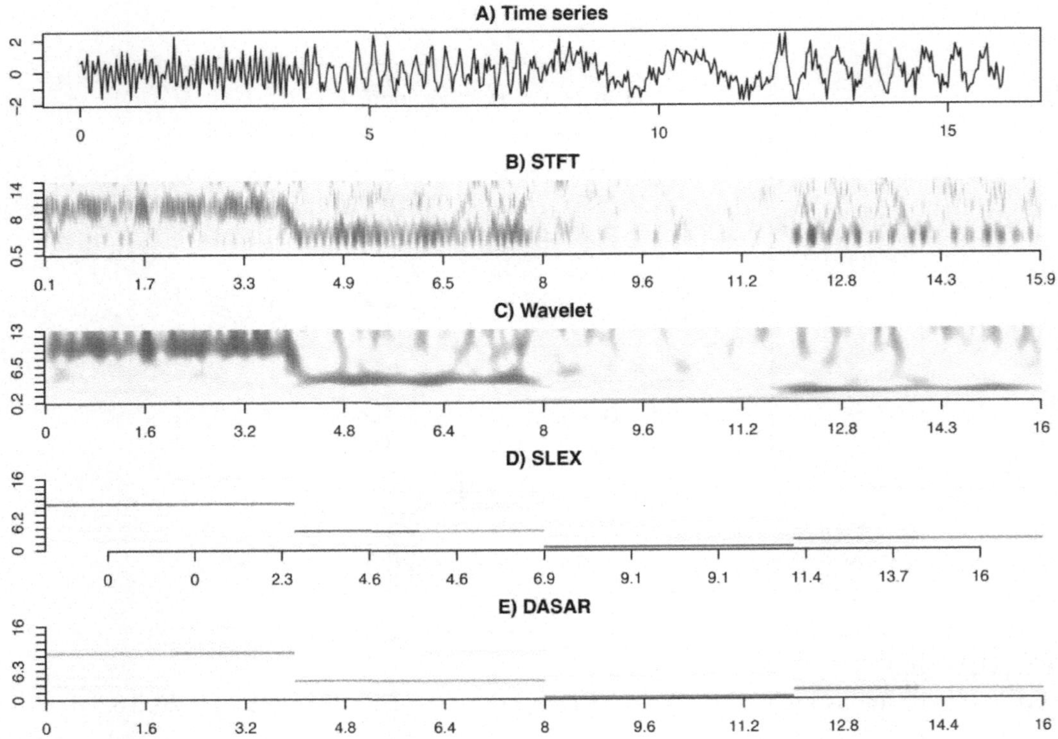


**FIGURE 9.10**
Comparison of time-varying spectrum estimation using STFT, wavelet, SLEX, and DASAR. (Color version available in electronic supplement.)

where $\varepsilon(t)$ is a white noise process with $\frac{1}{2}$ standard deviation:

```
fs = 32
N = 4*fs
frequencies = c(rep(10, length = N), rep(4, length = N), rep(0.5, length = N), rep
    (2, length = N))
y = sin(2 * pi * t * frequencies) + rnorm(16 * fs, sd = 0.5)
```

Figure 9.10 contrasts the time-varying spectrum estimation coefficients of $x(t)$ that can be found using the different methods discussed in this section:

```
stft_out <- evolfft(y, dt = 1 / fs , Nfft = 128, Ns = 128, Nov = 64, fl = 1, fh =
    fs/2)
plotevol(stft_out)
wavelet_out <- wlet.do(y, dt = 1/fs, noctave = 6, nvoice = 20, flip = TRUE)
slex_out <- slex_spectrogram(y, fs = fs, block_size = 64, plot = TRUE)
dasar_out <- dasar_spectrogram(y, fs, levels = 4, maximum_components = 5, plot =
    TRUE)
```

These commands depend on the library `RSEIS` and `R` packages from the repositories `git.sr.ht/~mpinto/slex-polyglot-implementation` and `git.sr.ht/~mpinto/dasar-polyglot-implementation` (also available from the repository accompanying this book).

## 9.7 Multivariate Stationary Spectrum

In a multivariate setting, a zero-mean, $P$-dimensional, weakly stationary process $\mathbf{X(t)}$ can be characterized by a sequence of covariance matrices at different lags. To ensure that the auto-correlation and cross-correlation decay sufficiently fast to zero, it is required that the sum of the absolute values of every element of the covariance matrix for each lag should be finite.

Similarly, as in the univariate case, we can define the spectrum based on the Fourier transform of the autocovariance matrix. This one-to-one relationship expresses that the spectral matrix $\mathbf{S}(\omega)$ is the Fourier transform of the covariance matrix. The single-spectrum of each channel, auto-spectrum, will be contained in the matrix diagonals.

The multivariate Cramér model denotes that a WSS time series can be seen as a random oscillation vector modulated by a transfer function matrix. Intuitively, the multivariate spectrum is the squared magnitude of this transfer function matrix.

We can use several methods to estimate the spectrum from real data. Intuitively, we can use a multivariate periodogram, which is asymptotically unbiased. Nevertheless, it is not consistent as it does not converge for large samples.

Alternatively, we can use a parametric approach by modeling the time series as a vector autoregressive (VAR) model (see also Chapter 8). A WSS process is said to be a $VAR(L)$ if it can be represented as a linear combination of the previous $L$ multivariate points:

$$\mathbf{X}(t) = \sum_{\ell=1}^{L} \mathbf{\Phi}_{\ell} \mathbf{X}(t-\ell) + \varepsilon(t) \tag{9.12}$$

where $\varepsilon$ is a multivariate zero-mean white noise with covariance $\Sigma_{\epsilon}$, and $\{\mathbf{\Phi}_1, \mathbf{\Phi}_2, \ldots, \mathbf{\Phi}_L\}$ of its VAR representation are coefficient matrices [48].

VAR models are a robust and versatile tool to study the spectrum of a system, given that the spectrum of a signal is entirely determined by the coefficients of its VAR representation. For completeness, the spectrum of a VAR model is given by

$$\mathbf{S}(\omega) = \left(I - \sum_{\ell=1}^{L} \mathbf{\Phi}_{\ell} e^{-j2\pi\omega\ell}\right)^{-1} \Sigma_{\epsilon} \left(\left(I - \sum_{\ell=1}^{L} \mathbf{\Phi}_{\ell} e^{-j2\pi\omega\ell}\right)^{-1}\right)^{*}$$

where $*$ is the complex conjugate operation.

### 9.7.1 Multivariate Granger Causality

Besides the robustness of VAR models, another benefit is that it allows for studying time causality. Granger, or time causality, establishes a cause-effect relationship between signals using the notion of linear predictability. According to this framework, a time series $x_A(t)$ is Granger-causing a signal $x_B(t)$ (alternatively, $x_A(t)$ is "causing" another channel $x_B(t)$ in Granger's sense) when the mean squared error of the $h$-step ahead forecast of $x_B(t)$ is reduced after adding $x_A(\tau), \tau < n$ in the predictive model $x_B(t)$[48].

It is relevant to emphasize that the direct definition of GC implies testing $(M^3 - M^2)$ linear models that consider every possible channel combination. A VAR model allows us to efficiently estimate the Granger causality in a multivariate setting using a single model (assuming no multicollinearity in the channels). As Lutkep ohl denoted, $x_i(t)$ Granger-causes $x_j(t)$ if there is a non-zero coefficient $\phi_{i,j}^{\ell} \neq 0$ for some lag $\ell = 1, \ldots, p$ [48]. Then, a causality link $x_i \mapsto x_j$ can be assessed by checking the statistical significance of an estimate $\hat{\phi}^{\ell}_{i,j}$. Several methods for estimating significance are introduced in [48].

VAR coefficients allow us to provide several layers of interpretation: quantifying undirected cross-channel interactions (functional connectivity), directed impacts from one channel into another (specific connectivity) and identifying the maximum delay when these interactions occur [55, 64, 66] Due to these directed and undirected properties, these coefficients can be used to describe brain dynamic networks in a spectral domain using linear features. A detailed explanation of non-linear network structures and features is depicted in Chapter 7.

### 9.7.2 Cross-Coherence

Let us recall that correlation measures the linear dependence or similarity between two time series. Correlation between two components, $X_p$ and $X_q$, can also be calculated when a time lag h shifts the first signal $h$: y $r_{p,q}(h) = \mathrm{Cor}\left(X_p\left(t+h\right), X_q\left(t\right)\right)$. Correlation is a metric always in the interval $[-1, 1]$ reaching its extremes when one of the signals is proportional to the other. This simplicity of interpretation and calculation allows correlation $r_{p,q}(h)$ to be one of the simplest methods to quantify the linear dependence at a specific lag $h$ between a pair of time series.

In a similar manner to the correlation, in the time domain, we can define another measure that quantifies the similarity between the simultaneous spectral response of two signals, $X_p$ and $X_q$. This metric, coherency, measures the cross-frequency response between the two time series normalized by the frequency response of each signal independently.

Its square magnitude is known as cross-coherence, or simply, coherence:

$$\rho_{pq}\left(\omega\right) = \left|\tau_{pq}\left(\omega\right)\right|^2 = \frac{\left|f_{pq}\left(\omega\right)\right|^2}{f_{pp}\left(\omega\right) f_{qq}\left(\omega\right)} \tag{9.13}$$

Cross-coherence measures dependencies in the interval $[0, 1]$, and it will achieve its maximum value only when both compared time series have a proportional cross-frequency response.

In practical EEG analysis, coherence between channels is defined and estimated at some frequency bands (such as the rhythms discussed in a previous section) instead of isolated resonating oscillations.

Coherence is unambiguously defined for a single frequency $\omega$. Nevertheless, we have two alternative coherence definitions for a frequency set $\Omega$: as the total normalized cross-spectra in the frequency set, or as the average coherence in the frequency set [55]. This ambiguity was also raised and discussed by [43]. However, in this chapter, we will rely on the first definition – which was also applied in other EEG research [76].

While correlation has a straightforward interpretation as a method to measure the level of synchrony of a signal, coherence would represent a challenge to interpret. However, under the Cramér representation, it has a linear-filtering interpretation in the time domain: coherence is the maximum squared cross-correlation between filtered signals in a desired frequency set $\Omega$ [54, 58]:

$$\widehat{\rho}_{p,q}\left(\Omega\right) = \max_{\ell}\left|\widehat{\mathrm{Cor}}\left[X_{p,\Omega}\left(t\right), X_{q,\Omega}\left(t-\ell\right)\right]\right|^2$$

For a comprehensive and formal comparison for coherence using several spectrum definitions, and the ambiguity in the definition between frequency intervals is explored in [55]. The proof of the equivalency between coherency and frequency was developed in [53].

### 9.7.3 Partial Coherence

Let us assume an experiment when three distinct EEG channels $p$, $q$, and $r$ are recorded where the signal $r$ is a 35 Hz-epileptiform wave that is being propagated to channels $p$ and $q$. In the time domain, a standard approach is to measure, exclusively, the relationship between $q$ and $p$ using partial correlation [28]. Partial correlation is essentially the cross-correlation between $X_p$ and $X_q$ after removing the linear effect of $X_c$. However, this likely will not isolate the 35 Hz frequency effect.

The linear-filtering interpretation of coherence allows us to introduce an equivalent to partial correlation in the frequency domain: partial coherence, to measure the "partial" dependence in specific frequency ranges.

There are several methods to calculate partial coherence. The straightforward method is to invert the spectral matrix $S(\omega)$, and normalize it by a pre and post-multiplication with a diagonal matrix with the auto-spectra of each signal as diagonal [26]. Note that this method allows calculating partial coherence across all channels simultaneously. Nevertheless, the quality of its estimations relies enormously on the quality of the spectrum matrix and its inverse.

A second method is to analyze the mutual linear effect between the signals after filtering. Partial coherence is the correlation between filtered signal components not attributable to the effects of other channels in the system with the same frequency. For simplicity, let us consider the $\omega$-oscillations for the three channels $p$, $q$ and $c$, which we denote as $X_{p,\omega}$, $X_{q,\omega}$ and $X_{c,\omega}$, respectively. We can obtain these components by applying a frequency filter. Then, we can regress $X_{p,\omega}(t)$ against $X_{c,\omega}(t)$ and extract the residuals $(R_{p\dot{c},\omega}(t))$ and also remove the effect of $X_{c,\omega}(t)$ from $X_{q,\omega}(t)$ through another linear regression and extract the residuals $(R_{q\dot{c},\omega}(t))$. Finally, the zero-phase partial coherence between $X_p$ and $X_q$ at frequency $\omega$ is described by

$$\rho_{pq\dot{c}}(\omega) = |\text{Cor}\left[R_{p\dot{c},\omega}, R_{q\dot{c},\omega}\right]|^2 .$$

This filtering approach requires $\mathcal{O}(P^2)$ linear regressions to check all possible signal dependence links. However, it offers a more flexible framework to examine the effects on frequency bands rather than frequency singletons.

### 9.7.4 Partial Directed Coherence

The different coherence metrics mentioned up to this point exclude directionality. As previously noted, VAR models can give information in the time domain within a Granger-causality framework. Partial directed coherence (PDC), introduced in [8] and [7], introduces a method that extrapolates the causality framework to the spectral domain. Then, PDC measures the information flow between two channels at a specific frequency $\omega$ using a VAR model as a modeling basis.

Recall the transfer function matrix of a VAR model $\Psi_x\left(e^{-j2\pi\omega}\right)$ with elements $\Psi_{i,j}\left(e^{-j2\pi\omega}\right)$ are the $(p,q)$ elements of the matrix. Then, the PDC from a channel $X_q$ to $X_p$ at frequency $\omega$ is

$$\pi_{pq}\left(\omega\right) = \frac{\left|\Psi_{pq}\left(e^{-j2\pi\omega}\right)\right|^2}{\sum_r \left|\Psi_{rq}\left(e^{-j2\pi\omega}\right)\right|^2}.$$

Item $\pi_{p,q}(\omega)$ in the PDC matrix has the domain $[0,1]$ and measures the amount of information flow at frequency $\omega$ from component $X_q$ to $X_p$. This item considers the amount of flow from $X_q$ to all components. Note that $\pi_{pq}(\omega)$ is close to 1, then most of the $\omega$-information flow from $X_q$ goes directly to component $X_p$.

Under this framework, we can estimate PDC fitting a VAR($P$) model to the data $\mathbf{X}(t), t = \{1, \ldots, T\}$ where the optimal order $P$ can be selected using some objective criterion like the Akaike information criterion (AIC) or the Bayesian-Schwartz information criterion (BIC).

### 9.7.5 Spectral Causality

There are limitations to PDC as a measure of dependence. For instance, it does not capture phase or lag effects between oscillatory components. While it is useful to know the direction $X_q \Longrightarrow X_p$ at frequency $\omega$, it would be crucial to identify the time lag $\tau_{pq,\omega}$ via some relationship, such as

$$X_{p,\omega}(t) = A_{pq,\omega} X_{q,\omega}(t - \tau_{pq,\omega}) + \epsilon_{p,\omega}(t)$$

for some coefficient $A_{pq,\omega}$ and time lag $\tau_{pq,\omega}$.

In addition, PDC only captures directionality only for the same frequency (or frequency bands). It only models how the past $\omega$-oscillations in channel $X_q$ could impact the future $\omega$-oscillations in channel $X_p$. It would be more desirable to capture between-frequencies directionality as in the dual-frequency setting, for example,

$$X_{p,\omega_1}(t) = A_{pq,\omega_1} X_{a,\omega_1}(t - \tau_{pq,\omega_1}) + A_{pq,\omega_2} X_{a,\omega_2}(t - \tau_{pq,\omega_2}) + \epsilon_{p,\omega_1}(t).$$

Consider the situation where we want to investigate the potential causality from channel $X_q$ at a frequency band $\omega_1$ to the $\omega_2$-oscillations of channel $X_p$:

$$X_{q,\omega_q}(t) \mapsto X_{p,\omega_p}(t - \ell)$$

where $\Omega = \{\delta, \theta, \alpha, \beta, \gamma\}$ and $C_{\omega_k}$ is a one-sided filters.

This approach was explored in [62] to propose a method, the spectral causality (SCAU) model, to overcome these limitations based on dependence analysis on amplitude demodulated signals. SCAU can capture information flows that can take place among the channels and the frequencies. In addition, it also covered modulated spectral relationships that a typical VAR model could not have recognized.

To carry out its purpose, SCAU begins by filtering the signal into distinct interpretable frequency ranges. Then, these channel-frequency components are translated into an intermediate frequency (for numerical stability reasons), and finally, a VAR model is used to study their linear interactions. Thus, it is possible to examine the dependencies in the EEG channels at three levels: spatial, time, and frequency.

## 9.8 Summary

EEG signals exhibit a distinctive characteristic in which physiological phenomena are inherently associated with their oscillatory nature. In this chapter, we delve into a statistical framework to formally represent this information. A crucial assumption in this framework is local stationarity, which refers to the ability of biomedical signals to maintain their statistical characteristics over short periods. When this condition is satisfied, we can estimate the power spectrum density, which allows for the decomposition of the signal variance across all frequencies. However, we additionally explore additional techniques that can help us analyze a time-varying spectrum when local stationarity cannot be ensured: short-time Fourier transform spectrograms, wavelet transform, SLEX spectrograms, or dyadic autoregressive models. These spectral methods can also be extended to a multivariate setting that may provide a more comprehensive overview of EEG signals, which are commonly recorded in multiple channels. We explore the methods that allow us to analyze spectral interactions between channels: multivariate spectrum, correlation, coherence, and partial coherence. In addition, we discuss briefly the connection between these multivariate models and time causality. These diverse methods serve as valuable tools to improve understanding of brain dynamics and alterations in epilepsy by studying the changes in its oscillatory characteristics.

## Bibliography

[1] Bassel Abou-Khalil and Karl E Misulis. *Atlas of EEG & Seizure Semiology.* Butterworth Heinnemann: Elsevier, Philadelphia, 2006.

[2] Paul S. Addison. A review of wavelet transform time frequency methods for NIRS-based analysis of cerebral autoregulation. *IEEE Reviews in Biomedical Engineering*, 8:78–85, 2015.

[3] Hojjat Adeli, Ziqin Zhou, and Nahid Dadmehr. Analysis of EEG records in an epileptic patient using wavelet transform. *Journal of Neuroscience Methods*, 123(1):69–87, February 2003.

[4] Haleh Aghajani, Marc Garbey, and Ahmet Omurtag. Measuring mental workload with EEG+fNIRS. *Frontiers in Human Neuroscience*, 11, July 2017.

[5] Michael A. Arbib, editor. *The Handbook of Brain Theory and Neural Networks.* MIT Press, Cambridge, Mass, 2nd edition, 2003.

[6] Bernard J. Baars, editor. *Cognition, Brain, and Consciousness: Introduction to Cognitive Neuroscience.* Elsevier, Acad. Press, Amsterdam, 1. ed., reprinted edition, 2007.

[7] L. A. Baccalá, C. S. N. de Brito, D. Y. Takahashi, and K. Sameshima. Unified asymptotic theory for all partial directed coherence forms. *Philosophical Transactions of the Royal Society A: Mathematical, Physical and Engineering Sciences*, 371(1997):20120158, August 2013.

[8] Luiz A Baccalá and Koichi Sameshima. Partial directed coherence: A new concept in neural structure determination. *Biological Cybernetics*, 84(6):463–474, 2001.

[9] George Bachman, Lawrence Narici, and Edward Beckenstein. *Fourier and Wavelet Analysis.* Universitext. Springer New York, New York, NY, 2000.

[10] Hanieh Bakhshayesh, Sean P. Fitzgibbon, Azin S. Janani, Tyler S. Grummett, and Kenneth J. Pope. Detecting synchrony in EEG: A comparative study of functional connectivity measures. *Computers in Biology and Medicine*, 105:1–15, February 2019.

[11] Hamid Behnam, Ali Sheikhani, Mohammad Reza Mohammadi, Maryam Noroozian, and Pari Golabi. Analyses of EEG background activity in Autism disorders with fast Fourier transform and short time Fourier measure. In *2007 International Conference on Intelligent and Advanced Systems.* IEEE, November 2007.

[12] Krit Charupanit, Indranil Sen-Gupta, Jack J. Lin, and Beth A. Lopour. Amplitude of high frequency oscillations as a biomarker of the seizure onset zone. *Clinical Neurophysiology*, 131(11):2542–2550, November 2020.

[13] Joris Chau and Rainer von Sachs. Time-varying spectral matrix estimation via intrinsic wavelet regression for surfaces of Hermitian positive definite matrices. *Computational Statistics & Data Analysis*, 174:107477, October 2022.

[14] Chang Chiann and Pedro A. Morettin. A wavelet analysis for time series. *Journal of Nonparametric Statistics*, 10(1):1–46, January 1998.

[15] Antonio M. Chiarelli, Edward L. Maclin, Monica Fabiani, and Gabriele Gratton. A kurtosis-based wavelet algorithm for motion artifact correction of fNIRS data. *NeuroImage*, 112:128–137, May 2015.

[16] Ronald R. Coifman and M. Victor Wickerhauser. *Wavelets and Adapted Waveform Analysis*, first edition, pages 399–423. CRC Press, Boca Raton, 1994.

[17] Solymar Ayala Cortez, Laxman Bokati, Aaron Velasco, and Vladik Kreinovich. Why Daubechies wavelets are so successful. *Journal of Intelligent & Fuzzy Systems*, pages 1–6, August 2022.

[18] Wojciech Czaja and Alexander M. Powell. Recent Developments in the Balian-Low Theorem. In Christopher Heil, editor, *Harmonic Analysis and Applications*, pages 79–100. Birkhäuser Boston, Boston, MA, 2006.

[19] R Dahlhaus. Fitting time series models to nonstationary processes. *The Annals of Statistics*, 25(1):1–37, 1997.

[20] Ingrid Daubechies. Orthonormal bases of compactly supported wavelets. *Communications on Pure and Applied Mathematics*, 41(7):909–996, October 1988.

[21] David Degras, Chee-Ming Ting, and Hernando Ombao. Markov-switching state-space models with applications to neuroimaging. *Computational Statistics & Data Analysis*, 174:107525, October 2022.

[22] Vinay K. Ingle Dimitris G. Manolakis. *Applied Digital Signal Processing: Theory and Practice.* Cambridge University Press, New York, 2011.

[23] Douglas F. Elliott, editor. *Handbook of Digital Signal Processing: Engineering Applications.* Academic Press, San Diego, 1987.

[24] Jacob Empson. *Human Brainwaves The Psychological Significance of the Electroencephalogram.* 1986.

[25] Tomer Fekete, Denis Rubin, Joshua M. Carlson, and Lilianne R. Mujica-Parodi. The NIRS analysis package: Noise reduction and statistical inference. *PLoS ONE*, 6(9):e24322, September 2011.

[26] Mark Fiecas and Hernando Ombao. The generalized shrinkage estimator for the analysis of functional connectivity of brain signals. *The Annals of Applied Statistics*, 5(2A):1102–1125, June 2011.

[27] Frank A. Fishburn, Ruth S. Ludlum, Chandan J. Vaidya, and Andrei V. Medvedev. Temporal Derivative Distribution Repair (TDDR): A motion correction method for fNIRS. *NeuroImage*, 184:171–179, January 2019.

[28] Roland Fried, Vanessa Didelez, and Vivian Lanius. Partial Correlation Graphs and Dynamic Latent Variables for Physiological Time Series. In Daniel Baier and Klaus-Dieter Wernecke, editors, *Innovations in Classification, Data Science, and Information Systems*, pages 259–266. Springer-Verlag, Berlin/Heidelberg, 2005.

[29] M. Frigo and S.G. Johnson. FFTW: An adaptive software architecture for the FFT. In *Proceedings of the 1998 IEEE International Conference on Acoustics, Speech and Signal Processing, ICASSP '98 (Cat. No.98CH36181)*, volume 3, pages 1381–1384, IEEE Seattle, WA, USA, 1998.

[30] Guilllermo Granados-Garcia, Mark Fiecas, Shahbaba Babak, Norbert J. Fortin, and Hernando Ombao. Brain waves analysis via a non-parametric Bayesian mixture of autoregressive kernels. *Computational Statistics & Data Analysis*, 174:107409, October 2022.

[31] Karlheinz Grochenig. *Foundations of Time-Frequency Analysis*. Birkhauser, Boston, 2001.

[32] Yameng Gu, Lucas E. Sainburg, Sizhe Kuang, Feng Han, Jack W. Williams, Yikang Liu, Nanyin Zhang, Xiang Zhang, David A. Leopold, and Xiao Liu. Brain activity fluctuations propagate as waves traversing the cortical hierarchy. Preprint, Neuroscience, August 2020. Please see https://pubmed.ncbi.nlm.nih.gov/33822908/ for information.

[33] Matheus B. Guerrero, Raphaël Huser, and Hernando Ombao. Conex-Connect: Learning Patterns in Extremal Brain Connectivity From Multi-Channel EEG Data. *arXiv:2101.09352 [q-bio, stat]*, January 2021.

[34] Bruce Hajek. *Random Processes for Engineers*. Cambridge University Press, first edition, March 2015.

[35] M. H. Hayes. *Statistical Digital Signal Processing and Modeling*. John Wiley and Sons, New York, 1996.

[36] Christoph S. Herrmann, Daniel Strüber, Randolph F. Helfrich, and Andreas K. Engel. EEG oscillations: From correlation to causality. *International Journal of Psychophysiology*, 103:12–21, May 2016.

[37] Zhelin Huang and Fangfang Yang. Quality classification of lithium battery in microgrid networks based on smooth localized complex exponential model. *Complexity*, 2021:1–10, January 2021.

[38] A. Jensen and A. La Cour-Harbo. *Ripples in Mathematics: The Discrete Wavelet Transform*. Springer, Berlin; New York, 2001.

[39] Carrie A. Joyce, Irina F. Gorodnitsky, and Marta Kutas. Automatic removal of eye movement and blink artifacts from EEG data using blind component separation. *Psychophysiology*, 41(2):313–325, March 2004.

[40] Steven M. Kay. *Intuitive Probability and Random Processes Using MATLAB*. Springer, New York, 2006.

[41] Bassel Khalil. *Atlas of EEG and Seizure Semiology*. Butterworth-Heinemann/Elsevier, Philadelphia, 2006.

[42] Truong Quang Dang Khoa and Masahiro Nakagawa. Recognizing brain activities by functional near-infrared spectroscope signal analysis. *Nonlinear Biomedical Physics*, 2(1):3, December 2008.

[43] A. P. Kulaichev. The informativeness of coherence analysis in EEG studies. *Neuroscience and Behavioral Physiology*, 41(3):321–328, March 2011.

[44] Alberto Leon-Garcia and Alberto Leon-Garcia. *Probability, Statistics, and Random Processes for Electrical Engineering.* Pearson/Prentice Hall, Upper Saddle River, NJ, 3rd edition, 2008.

[45] Ta-Hsin Li. *Time Series with Mixed Spectra.* CRC Press/Chapman & Hall, Boca Raton, Fla., 2014.

[46] Xiaoli Li and Chengwei Li. Study on the application of wavelet transform to non-invasive glucose concentration measurement by NIRS. In *2015 Fifth International Conference on Instrumentation and Measurement, Computer, Communication and Control (IMCCC).* IEEE, September 2015.

[47] Daniel Lopez-Martinez, Ke Peng, Arielle Lee, David Borsook, and Rosalind Picard. Pain detection with fNIRS-measured brain signals: A personalized machine learning approach using the wavelet transform and Bayesian hierarchical modeling with Dirichlet process priors. In *2019 8th International Conference on Affective Computing and Intelligent Interaction Workshops and Demos (ACIIW).* IEEE, September 2019.

[48] Helmut Lutkepohl. *New Introduction to Multiple Time Series Analysis.* New York Springer, Berlin, 2005.

[49] S. G. Mallat. *A Wavelet Tour of Signal Processing: The Sparse Way.* Elsevier/Academic Press, Amsterdam; Boston, 3rd edition, 2009.

[50] Stéphane Mallat, George Papanicolaou, and Zhifeng Zhang. Adaptive covariance estimation of locally stationary processes. *The Annals of Statistics*, 26(1):1–47, February 1998.

[51] Antonio Napolitano. *Generalizations of Cyclostationary Signal Processing: Spectral Analysis and Applications.* John Wiley & Sons, Ltd, Chichester, UK, September 2012.

[52] Praveena Nuthakki, J Manju, R. Geetha, Suguna M, and A. Sheik Abdullah. A Smart wearable motion sensor and acoustic signal processing based on vocabulary for monitoring children's wellbeing using Big Data. In *2022 International Conference on Advanced Computing Technologies and Applications (ICACTA)*, pages 1–9, IEEE, Coimbatore, India, March 2022.

[53] Hernando Ombao and Sébastien Van Bellegem. Coherence analysis of nonstationary time series: A linear filtering point of view. *IEEE Transactions on Signal Processing* 56 (2006): 2259–2266.

[54] Hernando Ombao, Martin Lindquist, Wesley Thompson, and John Aston. *Handbook of Neuroimaging Data Analysis.* 2017.

[55] Hernando Ombao and Marco Pinto. Spectral dependence. *arXiv:2103.17240 [stat]*, March 2021.

[56] Hernando Ombao, Rainer von Sachs, and Wensheng Guo. SLEX analysis of multivariate nonstationary time series. *Journal of the American Statistical Association*, 100(470):519–531, June 2005.

[57] Hernando C Ombao, Jonathan A Raz, Rainer von Sachs, and Beth A Malow. Automatic statistical analysis of bivariate nonstationary time series. *Journal of the American Statistical Association*, 96(454):543–560, June 2001.

[58] Ombao, H. and Van Bellegem. S. Coherence analysis of nonstationary time series: a linear filtering point of view. *IEEE Trans on Signal Proc*, 56(6):2259–2266, 2008.

[59] Alan Oppenheim. *Signals, Systems & Inference*. Pearson, Boston, 2016.

[60] Gianfranco Parati, J. Philip Saul, Marco Di Rienzo, and Giuseppe Mancia. Spectral analysis of blood pressure and heart rate variability in evaluating cardiovascular regulation: A critical appraisal. *Hypertension*, 25(6):1276–1286, June 1995.

[61] Sudip Paul, editor. *Biomedical Engineering and Its Applications in Healthcare*. Springer Singapore, Singapore, 2019.

[62] Marco Pinto, Peyman Mirtaheri, and Hugo Hammer. SCAU: Modeling spectral causality for multivariate time series with applications to electroencephalograms, 2021.

[63] Marco A. Pinto-Orellana, Habib Sherkat, Peyman Mirtaheri, and Hugo L. Hammer. Dyadic aggregated autoregressive (DASAR) model for time-frequency representation of biomedical signals. *arXiv:2105.10406 [physics, stat]*, May 2021.

[64] Marco Antonio Pinto-Orellana and Hugo L. Hammer. Analysis of optical brain signals using connectivity graph networks. *Machine Learning and Knowledge Extraction*, 12279:485–497, 2020.

[65] Marco Antonio Pinto-Orellana and Hugo Lewi Hammer. Dyadic Aggregated Autoregressive Model (DASAR) for Automatic Modulation Classification. *IEEE Access*, 8:156096–156103, 2020.

[66] Marco Antonio Pinto-Orellana, Peyman Mirtaheri, Hugo L. Hammer, and Hernando Ombao. SCAU: Modeling spectral causality for multivariate time series with applications to electroencephalograms. *arXiv:2105.06418 [q-bio, stat]*, May 2021.

[67] Hugo F. Posada-Quintero, Natasa Reljin, Jeffrey B. Bolkhovsky, Alvaro D. Orjuela-Cañón, and Ki H. Chon. Brain activity correlates with cognitive performance deterioration during sleep deprivation. *Frontiers in Neuroscience*, 13, September 2019.

[68] Alexander D. Poularikas. *Handbook of Formulas and Tables for Signal Processing*. The Electrical Engineering Handbook Series. CRC Press, Boca Raton, 2019.

[69] MB Priestley. Evolutionary spectra and non-stationary processes. *Journal of the Royal Statistical Society Series B. (Methodological)*, 27(2):204–237, 1965.

[70] Kaveh Samiee, Peter Kovacs, and Moncef Gabbouj. Epileptic seizure classification of EEG time-series using rational discrete short-time Fourier transform. *IEEE Transactions on Biomedical Engineering*, 62(2):541–552, February 2015.

[71] Stefano Sandrone, Marco Bacigaluppi, Marco R. Galloni, Stefano F. Cappa, Andrea Moro, Marco Catani, Massimo Filippi, Martin M. Monti, Daniela Perani, and Gianvito Martino. Weighing brain activity with the balance: Angelo Mosso's original manuscripts come to light. *Brain: A Journal of Neurology*, 137(Pt 2):621–633, February 2014.

[72] Saeid Sanei and Jonathon Chambers. *EEG Signal Processing*. John Wiley & Sons, Chichester, England; Hoboken, NJ, 2007.

[73] Robert H. Shumway and David S. Stoffer. *Time Series Analysis and Its Applications*. Springer Texts in Statistics. Springer New York, New York, NY, 2011.

[74] John Stern. *Atlas of EEG Patterns.* Wolters Kluwer/Lippincott Williams & Wilkins Health, Philadelphia, 2013.

[75] William Tatum. *Handbook of EEG Interpretation.* Demos Medical Pub, New York, 2008.

[76] Robert W Thatcher. Neuropsychiatry and quantitative EEG in the 21st Century. *Neuropsychiatry*, 1(5):495–514, October 2011.

[77] Wim van Drongelen. *Signal Processing for Neuroscientists: Introduction to the Analysis of Physiological Signals.* Elsevier/Academic Press, Amsterdam; Burlington, MA, 2007.

[78] Brani Vidakovic. *Statistical Modeling by Wavelets.* John Wiley and Sons, 2009.

[79] Dominik Wetzel, Nico Spahn, Martin Heilemann, Marcus M. Loffler, Markus Seidel, Silke Kolbig, and Dirk Winkler. Evaluation of electroencephalography analysis methods. In *2019 41st Annual International Conference of the IEEE Engineering in Medicine and Biology Society (EMBC)*, pages 767–773, IEEE, Berlin, Germany, July 2019.

[80] Nathaniel J. Zuk, Jeremy W. Murphy, Richard B. Reilly, and Edmund C. Lalor. Envelope reconstruction of speech and music highlights stronger tracking of speech at low frequencies. *PLOS Computational Biology*, 17(9):e1009358, September 2021.

# 10

## *Spatial Modeling of Imaging and Electrophysiological Data*

**Rongke Lyu**

*Department of Statistics, Rice University (USA)*

**Michele Guindani**

*Department of Biostatistics, University of California, Los Angeles (USA)*

**Marina Vannucci**

*Department of Statistics, Rice University (USA)*

### CONTENTS



In this chapter, we review advanced methods that use spatial information to improve the study of epilepsy using imaging and electrophysiological data, with an emphasis on Bayesian methodologies. We first focus on methods for the analysis of functional MRI data – a technology often used to map the proximity of seizure foci to brain areas associated with specific functions. We also discuss how to use a scalar-on-image regression approach to link a clinical outcome to the images. We then consider models for the analysis of positron emission tomography, MRI, and electrophysiological data. We provide an illustration of these approaches using a publicly available dataset of patients with epilepsy undergoing electrical stimulation during functional MRI (es-fMRI). We also briefly report on available open-source software for implementing spatial models in SPM and FSL.

DOI: 10.1201/9781003254515-10 

## 10.1 Introduction

Imaging and electrophysiological data are frequently employed in the evaluation of epilepsy. By measuring data such as electrophysiological activity via electroencephalography (EEG), blood-oxygen-level-dependent signal via functional magnetic resonance imaging (fMRI), metabolic activity via positron emission tomography (PET), or signal abnormality using MRI, it is possible to map the regions and networks involved in seizure generation [27, 55, 58]. Thanks to their high spatial resolution, fMRI can also be used to study cortical activation during epileptic activity, conduct pre-surgical assessment of drug-resistant epilepsy, and identify areas where cognitive function has been reorganized as a consequence of long-term epileptic activity. Furthermore, computed tomography (CT), PET, and structural MRI scans can be used to detect focal areas of increased/decreased perfusion and metabolic activity. Therefore, statistical approaches that take into account the spatial distribution and association of brain measurements are becoming increasingly important for investigating which brain regions may be involved in the generation of seizure precursors and for identifying targets of therapeutic interventions that aim at preventing seizure generation [54].

In this chapter, we provide a review of recent statistical methods that investigate spatial associations for a range of neuroimaging technologies. The methods we present have been often borrowed from the analysis of spatial data in statistics, where the data are assumed as the realization of a process which is spatially organized. In our context, we discuss the use of spatially informed models – such as Gaussian processes, Gaussian Markov random fields, and conditional autoregressive models – to improve accuracy of the inference and the power of the tests by taking explicitly into account the spatial organization of the data. We place particular emphasis on Bayesian methodologies. Indeed, when the interest is in taking advantage of the information provided by the spatial resolution of each technology, the Bayesian framework allows a natural encoding of the existing spatial information via the use of prior distributions. The prior information is used together with the information from the data, encoded in the likelihood, to provide an updated (posterior) state of knowledge about the parameters of interest. We also discuss scalar-on-image regression, which aims at finding an association between a clinical outcome and the values observed in the imaging data, assumed as covariates. The findings might be utilized to identify imaging-based signatures (biomarkers) of subgroups in epilepsy or associated changes in cognitive function, with the ultimate objective of developing targeted therapies for treatment.

In our review of statistical models that account for the spatial distribution of different neuroimaging data types, we focus particularly on several models developed for the analysis of fMRI data (Section 10.2). We then discuss models for MRI (Section 10.3), PET data (Section 10.4) and electrophysiological data (Section 10.5). We conclude by briefly mentioning approaches for multi-type and/or multi-study data (Section 10.6) and existing open-source software for the spatial analysis of neuroimaging data (Section 10.7).

## 10.2 Spatial Models for fMRI Data

Functional magnetic resonance imaging (fMRI) is a non-invasive neuroimaging method that measures brain activity by detecting changes associated with blood flow as blood-oxygen level-dependent (BOLD) signals. When an area of the brain is active, more oxygen-rich blood flows to the active area. This causes a relative increase in oxyhemogloblin in activated brain areas and a relative decrease in deoxyhemoglobin. BOLD signals measure the difference between oxyhemogloblin and deoxyhemoglobin levels in local blood flow. In this section we first review spatio-temporal models for activation detection, including single-subject modeling, multi-subject modeling, detection methods for pre-surgical planning and models for cortical surface fMRI. We then describe regression models where imaging features are employed as covariates, for the prediction of a clinical outcome of interest.

### 10.2.1 Spatio-Temporal Models for Activation Detection

The Gaussian linear model, known as general linear model (GLM), as first proposed by Friston [14], is widely used to model time series of BOLD responses. This approach simply models the observed fMRI signal as the underlying BOLD response plus a noise component.

**Single-Subject Modeling:** Let $Y_v$ be the $T \times 1$ response vector of time-series data for voxel $v$, for $v = 1, \dots, V$, with $T$ indicating the number of time points and $V$ the number of voxels. Let $X_v$ be the $T \times p$ design matrix, with $p$ the number of experimental tasks or input stimuli. We write the voxel-wise GLM as

$$Y_v = X_v \beta_v + \varepsilon_v, \tag{10.1}$$

where $\beta_v = (\beta_{v,1}, \dots, \beta_{v,p})^T$ is a $p \times 1$ vector of regression coefficients and $\varepsilon_v$ is a $T \times 1$ error vector. The error component captures random noise and various nuisance components due to hardware and subject-related physiological noise, while the underlying BOLD response component $X_v\beta_v$ captures the relationship between the vascular response and the stimuli. When measuring the change in the metabolism of the BOLD response due to an outside stimulus, the MR signal gets delayed hemodynamically [3]. This is taken into account by introducing an hemodynamic response function (HRF) in model (10.1) and modeling each column (task or input stimulus) of $X_v$ as

$$\int_0^t x(s)\, h_v(t-s)\, ds, \tag{10.2}$$

where $x(s)$ is the external time-dependent stimulus function for that particular task, and $h_v(t)$ is the HRF. Several models have been proposed for the HRF, for example Poisson functions [14], Gaussian functions [13], Gamma functions [35], and many others [12, 40]. Additionally, a significant amount of work has gone toward capturing temporal correlation via the choice of the noise structure. One strategy is to prewhiten the data by obtaining an estimate of the autocorrelation structure based on the data and then removing this structure by data transformation [14]. Another strategy is to model the error term in model (10.1) directly, for example as an auto-regressive (AR) structure of order $q$ [36, 51, 52, 66, 77]. Teng et al. [66], for example, assume spatially varying AR orders across neighboring voxels and allow the data to determine the order of the AR process at each voxel. Alternatively, Zhang et al. [82] assume a long-memory error structure and apply discrete wavelet transforms (DWT) to model (10.1), to decorrelate the data, performing inference on the transformed data.

Spatial correlation is expected in a voxel-level analysis of fMRI data, since the response observed at a voxel is likely to be similar across neighboring voxels. Distant voxels can also be correlated, for example if they belong to symmetric areas of the brain across the two hemispheres. In statistical modeling, Bayesian approaches are often used as a flexible way to capture spatial correlation between brain voxels. In a Bayesian model, correlation is captured by imposing spatial priors on model parameters. For example, a Gaussian Markov random field (GMRF) prior [21, 53] can be imposed on the $j$th regression coefficient vector $\beta_{(j)} = (\beta_{1,j}, ..., \beta_{V,j})^T$ as

$$p\left(\beta_{(j)} \mid \lambda\right) \propto \exp\left(-\frac{1}{2}\lambda\beta_{(j)}^T\mathbf{Q}\beta_{(j)}\right), \tag{10.3}$$

where the precision matrix $Q$ has elements

$$\mathbf{Q}_{v,k} = \begin{cases} n_v, & v = k \\ -1, & v \sim k \\ 0, & \text{otherwise}, \end{cases} \tag{10.4}$$

with $n_v$ the number of neighbors of voxel $v$, and with $v \sim k$ denoting that $v$ and $k$ are neighbors. Similarly, Penny et al. [52] considered a spatial prior on $\beta_{(j)}$ of the type

$$\begin{aligned} \beta_{(j)} &\sim N\left(0, \alpha_j^{-1}\left(\mathbf{S}^T\mathbf{S}\right)^{-1}\right) \\ \alpha_j &\sim Ga(a, b), \end{aligned} \tag{10.5}$$

with $\mathbf{S}$ a $V \times V$ spatial kernel matrix equal to the Laplacian operator $L$. Other examples of spatial priors on regression coefficients include the diffusion-based spatial priors of Harrison et al. [24], the conditional autoregressive (CAR) priors of Harrison and Green [23] and the sparse spatial basis function (SSBF) priors on wavelet-based regression coefficients of Flandin and Penny [11].

Alternative modeling approaches look at the task of selecting activated voxels as a variable selection problem, which amounts to identify the nonzero $\beta_{v,i}$ in model (10.1) [59, 60, 82]. Those approaches assume *spike-and-slab* priors on the regression coefficients of the type

$$\beta_{v,j} \sim \gamma_{v,j} N\left(0, \tau_{v,j}\right) + \left(1 - \gamma_{v,j}\right) I\left(\beta_{v,j} = 0\right), \tag{10.6}$$

with $\gamma_v = (\gamma_{v,1}, \ldots, \gamma_{v,p})$ a set of binary indicators such that $\beta_{v,j} = 0$ if $\gamma_{v,j} = 0$ and $\beta_{v,j} \neq 0$ if $\gamma_{v,j} = 1$. Furthermore, a Markov Random Field (MRF) prior, also called Ising prior, is assumed on the binary indicators $\gamma_{v,j}$ as

$$P\left(\gamma_{\nu,j} \mid d, e, \gamma_{k,j}, k \in N_\nu\right) \propto \exp\left(\gamma_{\nu,j}\left(d + e\sum_{k\in N_\nu}\gamma_{k,j}\right)\right), \tag{10.7}$$

with $N_v$ the set of neighbors of voxel $v$, $d$ a parameter that controls sparsity and $e > 0$ a smoothing parameter. According to prior (10.7), the probability that a voxel is activated increases as the number of activated neighboring voxels increases.

For posterior inference, the major goal is to generate a spatial mapping of the activated brain regions. This can be achieved via inference on the regression parameters $\beta_v$'s in model (10.1) [15, 16]. Specifically, for Bayesian approaches, activations can be detected by constructing posterior probability maps (PPMs) obtained by thresholding the conditional posterior probabilities at a specified confidence level. In particular, at each voxel the conditional posterior probability that a particular effect, specified by a contrast weight vector $\mathbf{w}$, exceeds some threshold $\kappa$ is calculated as

$$p = 1 - \Phi\left(\frac{\kappa - \mathbf{w}^T\mathbf{M}_{\beta_v|\mathbf{Y}}}{\sqrt{\mathbf{w}^T\mathbf{C}_{\beta_v|\mathbf{Y}}\mathbf{w}}}\right), \tag{10.8}$$

with $\mathbf{M}_{\beta_v|\mathbf{Y}}$ and $\mathbf{C}_{\beta_v|\mathbf{Y}}$ the posterior mean and covariance of the parameter $\beta_v$, respectively. PPMs can also be obtained directly by thresholding the activation probabilities $p\left(\gamma_{v,j} = 1 \mid \mathbf{Y}\right)$ when a spike and slab prior (10.6) is employed. Specifically, an individual voxel can be classified as active if $p\left(\gamma_{v,j} = 1 \mid \mathbf{Y}\right) > \mathcal{Q}$, and as inactive otherwise [19, 59, 60]. Kalus et al. [29] suggested choosing the threshold based on the Bayesian false discovery rate (FDR). The decision on the optimal threshold can also be formulated in a compound decision theoretic framework by minimizing a loss function defined as a linear combination of false positive and false negative counts [48]. Sun et al. [63] have shown that procedures thresholding posterior probability maps allow to control also the frequentist FDR in large-scale spatial multiple testing.

**Multi-Subject Modeling:** Model (10.1) can be extended to multiple subjects as

$$\mathbf{Y}_{iv} = \mathbf{X}_{iv}\,\beta_{iv} + \mathbf{E}_{iv}, \tag{10.9}$$

with $\mathbf{Y}_{i\nu} = (Y_{i\nu 1}, ..., Y_{i\nu T})^T$ the BOLD response data at voxel $\nu$ for subject $i$, $\mathbf{X}_{i\nu}$ the $T \times P$ covariate matrix, and $\beta_{iv} = (\beta_{iv1}, \ldots \beta_{ivp})$ with $\beta_{ivk}$ the effect corresponding to condition $k$ on voxel $v$ for subject $i$, for $i = 1, ..., N$ and $\nu = 1, ..., V$. The error term in model (10.9) follow a multivariate normal distribution with mean zero and covariance $\sum_{i\nu}$.

The computation challenges of the multi-subject formulation (10.9) have motivated researchers to adopt approaches where voxels are grouped into regions of interest (ROIs) and 'summary statistics' are calculated for each ROI, so that inference at the group level is based on the summary statistics from the lower level. One Bayesian approach that uses this two-stage modeling was proposed by Bowman et al. [2]. At the first stage, a voxel-wise GLM is fitted for each subject, where errors are assumed serially correlated and the HRF is pre-specified. At the second stage, the authors consider an anatomical parcellation of the brain consisting of $G$ ROIs and define a contrast fMRI BOLD response vector associated with stimulus $j$ as $\beta_{igj} = (\beta_{ig(1)j}, ..., \beta_{ig(V_g)j})^T$, with $V_g$ the number of voxels in $g = 1, ..., G$. Then they fit a Bayesian hierarchical model

$$\begin{aligned}
\beta_{igj} \mid \mu_{gj}, \alpha_{igj}, \sigma^2_{gj} &\sim \text{Normal}\left(\mu_{gj} + 1\alpha_{igj}, \sigma^2_{gj}\mathrm{I}\right)\\
\boldsymbol{\mu}_{gj} \mid \lambda^2_{gj} &\sim \text{Normal}\left(1\mu_{0gj}, \lambda^2_{gj}\mathbf{I}\right)\\
\sigma^{-2}_{gj} &\sim \text{Gamma}\left(a_0, b_0\right)\\
\alpha_{ij} \mid \boldsymbol{\Gamma}_j &\sim \text{Normal}\left(0, \boldsymbol{\Gamma}_j\right)\\
\lambda^{-2}_{gj} &\sim \text{Gamma}\left(c_0, d_0\right)\\
\boldsymbol{\Gamma}^{-1}_j &\sim \text{ Wishart }\left(\left(h_0\mathbf{H}_{0j}\right)^{-1}, h_0\right),
\end{aligned} \tag{10.10}$$

with $\boldsymbol{\mu}_{gj} = \left(\mu_{g(1)j}, \ldots, \mu_{g(V_g)j}\right)^T$ and $\boldsymbol{\alpha}_{ij} = \left(\alpha_{i1j}, \ldots, \alpha_{g(V_g)j}\right)^T$. Sanyal and Ferreira [57] proposed a different two-stage approach. The authors consider a GLM of type (10.9) where errors are assumed independent and regressors $X_{iv}$ are a convolution of the stimulus function with an empirically derived subject-specific HRF. They first estimate regression coefficients by an empirical Bayesian method and then apply DWT with spike and slab priors imposed on the wavelet coefficients. Bayesian mixture models have also been successfully applied as second stage models. For example, Xu et al. [79] assume that each subject data are fit with an intra-subject fMRI signal model, producing scalar t-images, and then model the intra-subject variability in activation location by using Gaussian mixtures to infer what proportion of subjects had a significant activity in a given region. Also, Thirion et al. [67] model the spatial positions of brain regions via infinite mixtures in a Bayesian nonparametric framework. Furthermore, Johnson et al. [28] proposed a Bayesian non-parametric Potts model by assuming that the z-score image from a patient can be segmented into activated, deactivated, and null classes, or states, and imposing mixtures of Dirichlet process priors.

As an alternative to two-stage analyses, Zhang et al. [81] extended spike-and-slab priors of the type (10.6) to a non-parametric construction for a single-stage analysis of multi-subject fMRI data. The authors consider the general linear model (10.9) with a Poisson HRF and auto-correlated errors and define a multi-subject non-parametric variable selection prior on $\beta_{i\nu}$ where the slab distribution is a hierarchical Dirichlet Process (HDP) as

$$\begin{aligned} \beta_{iv} \mid \gamma_{iv}, G_i &\sim \gamma_{iv} G_i + (1-\gamma_{iv})\, I(\beta_{iv}=0) \\ G_i \mid \eta_1, G_0 &\sim \mathrm{DP}\,(\eta_1, G_0) \\ G_0 \mid \eta_2, P_0 &\sim \mathrm{DP}\,(\eta_2, P_0) \\ P_0 &= N(0,\tau), \end{aligned} \tag{10.11}$$

where $\tau$ is fixed, $\eta_1$, $\eta_2$ are the mass parameter, and $P_0$ is the base measure. The nonparametric HDP prior allows within-subject clustering of activated voxels as well as clustering of the subjects according to common activation patterns. An Ising prior of type (10.7) is placed on the selection indicators $\gamma_{i,v}$.

A major challenge for spatial models and the Bayesian approach for inference is the required computations. Thus, mean-field variational Bayes (VB) approximations are common for Bayesian inference. This is the strategy adopted by Kook et al. [34] in their *NPBayes fMRI*, a MATLAB GUI that implements the spatiotemporal general linear regression models of Zhang et al. [81]. The GUI consists of two parts: model fitting and visualization of the results. The VB algorithm is run within model fitting. The user can specify number of subjects, type of analysis (single 2D slice or a 3D whole-brain parcellation), and model parameters. For visualization of the results, the GUI is able to produce three types of output: activation maps by subject, activation maps by clusters, and contrast maps by subject. Also, Teng et al. [65] considered a model including spatially-varying coefficients and explored the performances of VB approximation and Hamiltonian Monte Carlo (HMC). The authors reported that the computation time for VB is less than for HMC, as expected. In settings with high or moderate signal-to-noise ratio (SNR) the authors found that two approaches produced very similar results, while with low SNR notable differences were found. This type of exploration can suggest circumstances where VB approximations are accurate or have limitations.

**Pre-surgical planning:** There has been a growing interest in using fMRI for pre-surgical planning as a less invasive tool to map out functionally relevant brain regions as a reference for direct electrical stimulation mapping (ESM) during surgery. In pre-surgical planning, false negatives are of greater concern than false positives since damage to false negative regions of the brain may lead to irreversible deficits in function. Additionally, spatial resolution plays an important role as the signal-to-noise ratio in fMRI increases linearly with voxel volume.

Liu et al. [42] proposed a spatially adaptive CAR model for a single patient pre-surgical fMRI data. Let $\mathbf{Y} = (Y_1, \ldots, Y_N)$ represent the unsmoothed 3-dimensional Z-statistic intensities at $N$ voxels. The authors assume $Y_i \sim N(\mu_i, \sigma_i^2)$, with $\mu_i$ the smoothed Z-statistic intensity at the $i$-th voxel, and impose spatially adaptive CAR priors on the model parameters with hyperparameters that vary across voxels. A novel loss function is constructed to explicitly control false negatives and false positives. Furthermore, Liu et al. [41] propose a statistical method for pre-surgical fMRI analysis with two fMRI scans at two different spatial resolutions (referred to as "standard" and "high" resolution). To address the "change of support" problem arisen by using data collected at different spatial resolutions, the authors coregister the motion- and distortion-corrected standard resolution functional image space and the corresponding fMRI data recorded at high spatial resolution to an unbiased within-subject high-resolution template space. Thus, each voxel in the high spatial resolution image has a corresponding voxel in the standard resolution image using nearest-neighbor interpolation. The interpolated image of the fMRI data at standard resolution is referred as the interpolated standard resolution image. Let $X_i$ and $Y_i$ denote the Z-statistic intensity at the $i$-th voxel in the interpolated standard resolution image and the high resolution image, respectively. Assuming $Y_i \sim N(\mu_i, \tau^2)$, the authors relate the mean $\mu_i$ to $X_i$ as $\mu_i = \beta_0 + (\beta_1 + b_{1i})X_i$. The slope $b_{1i}$ captures the associations between images in the two different resolutions, which the authors assume to vary spatially via imposing a CAR prior on $\mathbf{b}_1 = (b_{11}, \ldots, b_{1N})^T$. Finally, Whiteman et al. [74] proposed a more flexible approach where the image data collected at the two spatial resolutions, $h$ and $s$, are assumed to be realizations from a unifying generative process,

$$\begin{aligned} Y_h(v_h) &\sim N(\mu(v_h), \sigma_h^2), \quad v_h \in B_h \\ Y_s(v_s) &\sim N(\mu(v_s), \sigma_s^2), \quad v_s \in B_s, \end{aligned}$$

with $B$ a generic brain image space. The authors assign a weakly informative prior for noise variance with restriction $\sigma_h^2 > \sigma_s^2$ and a mean zero Gaussian process prior on the mean, $\mu(v) \sim GP(0, K(v, v'))$, that captures correlation between voxels across the two images, with a non-stationary covariance function $K(v, v')$ to map between data sets.

**Cortical surface fMRI:** Cortical surface fMRI (cs-fMRI) has gained popularity in recently years [10, 18]. This type of data is transformed from volumetric fMRI by applying a triangular mesh to the internal boundary of the cortical gray matter ribbon in order to form a 2-dimensional manifold surface representation. Mejia et al. [45] proposed a Bayesian GLM of the type (10.1) for single-subject cs-fMRI data and then extended it to multi-subject analysis. Differently from the classical GLM, which is based on a massive univariate approach, Mejia et al. leverage spatial dependencies among neighboring cortical vertices to generate more accurate estimates and areas of functional activation. Integrated nested Laplacian approximation (INLA), as an alternative to MCMC, is utilized for approximating inference. Under the same framework, Spencer et al. [62] assessed the reliability and power of the individual and group average measures of task activation. The results show that this framework produces highly reliable activations in individual subjects and is powerful to detect trait-like functional topologies. It also enhances the reliability of group-level analysis, has high power even in small samples and is computationally efficient. Mejia et al. [44] further extended the previous framework by proposing a longitudinal model to leverage information across visits.

### 10.2.2 Scalar-on-Image Regression Models

Regression models where the response variable is the clinical outcome of interest and where the predictors include imaging features are referred to as *scalar-on-image* (SI) regression models. Performing variable selection and identifying the imaging features that help predicting the outcome are often the goals of the inference in such models.

Variable screening methods have been widely used in many applications in order to accommodate ultrahigh-dimensional data. Those methods seek to exclude a large amount of predictors that are not associated with the response variable, thus reducing dimensionality [26]. The overarching goal is to identify the active set of regression coefficients

$$\mathcal{S}_0 = \{j : \beta_j \neq 0, j = 1, \ldots, p\}. \tag{10.12}$$

SURE independence screening [9], for example, selects all variables having high correlation with the response,

$$\widehat{\mathcal{S}}_{\text{SIS}}(\gamma) = \left\{ j : \left| \widehat{\text{Corr}}\,(\mathbf{y}, \mathbf{x}_j) \right| > \gamma \right\}, \tag{10.13}$$

while the high-dimensional ordinary-least squares projection (HOLP) [73] method uses

$$\widehat{\mathcal{S}}_{\text{HOLP}}(\gamma) = \{ j : |\tilde{\beta}_j| > \gamma \}, \tag{10.14}$$

with $\widetilde{\beta}_j = \tilde{\boldsymbol{\beta}} = \mathbf{X}^T(\mathbf{X}\mathbf{X}^T)^{-1}\mathbf{y}$ the projected OLS estimate of $\beta_j$. Partition-based screening (PartS) [30] leverages prior information to group predictors and calculates OLS estimates as $\widehat{\boldsymbol{\beta}}_g^T = \left(\widetilde{\mathbf{X}}_g^T \widetilde{\mathbf{X}}_g\right)^{-1} \widetilde{\mathbf{X}}_g^T \mathbf{y}$, for variables belonging to group $g$. Covariance-insured screening (CIS) [25] compartmentalizes covariates into blocks so that variables from distinct blocks are less correlated and uses partial correlations to determine the importance of the predictors.

In the Bayesian framework, spatial information can be incorporated into scalar-on-image modeling via the choice of the prior distribution on $\beta$. Li et al. [37] proposed a joint Ising and Dirichlet Process (Ising-DP) prior within the framework of Bayesian stochastic search variable selection for selecting brain voxels in high-dimensional SI regressions. Goldsmith et al. [20] developed a scalar-on-image regression model for images which uses registered multidimensional manifolds to estimate the image coefficients. The authors formulate the scalar-on-image regression model as $y_i = \boldsymbol{w}_i^T \boldsymbol{\alpha} + \boldsymbol{X}_i \cdot \boldsymbol{\beta} + \varepsilon_i$, where $\alpha$ is a fixed effects vector, $\beta$ is a collection of regression coefficients defined on the same lattice as the image predictors. A Gaussian MRF prior is proposed for the regression coefficients:

$$[\beta_l \mid \gamma_l = 1, \boldsymbol{\beta}_{-l}, \gamma_{-l}] \sim \text{N}\left[\bar{\beta}_{\delta_l}, \sigma^2_{\boldsymbol{\beta}}/d_l\right] \tag{10.15}$$

with an Ising prior on the binary indicators and where $\bar{\beta}_{\delta_l} = \frac{\sum^{\beta}_{l' \in \delta_l} {l'}^{\gamma'_l}}{d_l}$ is the average taken over the neighboring regression coefficients and $d_l$ is the number of elements in $\delta_l$.

Kang et al. [33] proposed a novel class of Bayesian nonparametric models via a soft-thresholded Gaussian process, which provides large prior support over the class of piecewise-smooth, sparse and continuous spatially varying regression coefficient functions. By assuming a set of locations $S = \{s_j\}_{j=1}^{p_n}$ as a fixed subset of a compact closed region $\mathcal{B} \subseteq \mathbb{R}^d$, the authors consider a scalar-on-image regression model with spatially varying coefficient functions $\beta(\cdot)$ defined on $\mathcal{B}$. The authors assume that many locations have $\beta(s_j) = 0$, that the sites with nonzero coefficients cluster spatially, and that the coefficients vary smoothly in clusters of nonzero coefficients. Thus, $\beta(\cdot)$ is represented as a transformation of a Gaussian process $\beta(s) = g_\lambda\{\tilde{\beta}(s)\}$ and

$$g_\lambda(x) = \left\{ \begin{array}{cl} 0, & |x| \leqslant \lambda \\ \text{sgn}(x)(|x| - \lambda), & |x| > \lambda \end{array} \right. \tag{10.16}$$

This soft-thresholded Gaussian process prior is denoted by $\beta \sim \text{STGP}(\lambda, \kappa)$. Additionally, under regularity conditions, this soft-thresholded Gaussian process prior leads to posterior consistency for parameter estimation and variable selection, even when the number of predictors is larger than the sample size.

Finally, we briefly mention Morris et al. [47], who developed a scalar on network regression model where the response variable is scalar and the predictors are network data, typically represented as adjacent matrices or weighted adjacent matrices. The authors develop a new boosting method for model fitting with sub-network markers selection.

## 10.3 Spatial Models for MRI Data

MRI, discussed in Chapter 3, plays an important role in studying various neurological disorders. Ge et al. [17] presented a Bayesian spatial model for MRI via spatially varying coefficients to model binary lesion maps and to determine whether there is spatial dependence between lesion location and subject specific covariates. The authors proposed a spatial probit mixed-effects model:

$$\Phi^{-1}\left\{\Pr\left[Y_i\left(s_j\right)=1 \mid \eta_i\left(s_j\right)\right]\right\}=\mathbf{x}_i^{\mathrm{T}}\left[\boldsymbol{\alpha}+\boldsymbol{\beta}\left(s_j\right)\right]+w\left(s_j\right)\gamma, \tag{10.17}$$

with $s_j$ denoting the $j$th voxel within the brain, $Y_i(s_j)$ denoting a binary variable where $[Y_i(s_j)=1]$ indicates the presence and $[Y_i(s_j)=0]$ indicates the absence of a lesion, and with $\boldsymbol{\beta}(s_j)$ denoting spatially varying random effects.

Taschler et al. [64] considered methods for classification of multiple sclerosis disease subtypes and proposed two spatially informed models: a Bayesian Spatial Generalized Linear Mixed Model (BSGLMM), where the prior distribution of coefficients can be expressed as

$$\pi[\boldsymbol{\beta} \mid \boldsymbol{\Sigma}] \propto \exp\left\{-1/2 \sum_{s_i \sim s_j}\left[\boldsymbol{\beta}\left(s_i\right)-\boldsymbol{\beta}\left(s_j\right)\right]^T \boldsymbol{\Sigma}^{-1}\left[\boldsymbol{\beta}\left(s_i\right)-\boldsymbol{\beta}\left(s_j\right)\right]\right\}, \tag{10.18}$$

with $s_i \sim s_j$ indicating two neighboring voxels, and a Log Gaussian Cox Process (LGCP) model, which takes into account the random spatial variation in lesion location.

Dai et al. [6] considered longitudinal structural MRI data and investigated the relationship between the temporally changing spatial topography of cortical thickness and disease stages from mild cognitive impairment to Alzheimer's disease (AD). The authors developed a novel Bayesian latent spatial model that captures the spatial information underlying the thickness effects across the cortical surface. In the frequentist setting, [50] proposed a permutation-based approach to inference for the identification of non-null spatial clusters of vertices in longitudinal MRI data.

## 10.4 Spatial Models for PET Data

PET is a type of *in vivo* nuclear medicine imaging. Based on detecting two time-coincident high-energy photons from the emission of a positron emitting radioisotope, it uses radioactive substances known as radiotracers to visualize and measure changes in metabolic processes.

Vardi et al. [69] first considered various estimation methods, such as the maximum likelihood method, the method of moments, and least squares methods, to estimate the emission density. Vizza et al. [71] defined an automatic classification tool using topological relations among ROIs and used it in AutoSPET, a plugin in SPM (Statistical Parametric Mapping), a software widely used by physicians for ROI identification and imaging analysis based on PET data. Veronese et al. [70] showed that covariance statistics can be applied to PET neuroimaging data to investigate the topological characteristics of the tracer kinetics and its related targets.

Among Bayesian approaches, Chiang et al. [5] proposed a hierarchical Bayesian modeling framework that identifies individual pathological brain states. Let $\boldsymbol{X}_i$ be the $R \times 1$ vector of

**TABLE 10.1**
Brain regions with highest marginal posterior probabilities of inclusion (PPI) for relevance in predicting seizure laterality.

| Region | PPI |
|---|---|
| Right temporal pole | 1 |
| Right entorhinal cortex | 0.858 |
| Left temporal pole | 0.403 |
| Left parahippocampal gyrus | 0.400 |

normalized PET image predictors on $R$ brain regions of interest(ROIs), for subject i, and let $Y_i$ be the corresponding post-surgical outcome. The authors factorize the joint distribution of $\mathbf{Z}_i = \{Y_i, \mathbf{X}_i\}_{i=1}^n$ as $f(\mathbf{Z} \mid \boldsymbol{\eta}) = \prod_{i=1}^n f(Y_i \mid \eta_i) f(\mathbf{X}_i \mid \eta_i)$, with $\eta_i$ a latent pathological state of subject $i$, out of $K$ possible pathological states. The authors considered a finite Gaussian mixture model to estimate the latent states with spatially informed selection priors on the mean components where the slab is specified as an intrinsic conditional autoregressive (ICAR) prior

$$p(\mu_{k,j} \mid \gamma_j, \boldsymbol{\mu}_{k,j}) = \gamma_j \mathbf{N}\left(\frac{\sum_{j'=1}^R s_{j,j'}\mu_{k,j'}}{\sum_{j'=1}^R s_{j,j'}}, \frac{c_k}{\sum_{j'=1}^R S_{j,j'}}\right) + (1-\gamma_j)\, I(\mu_{k,j}=0), \quad (10.19)$$

with an Ising prior on the binary indicators as $p(\gamma) \propto \exp\left\{e\mathbf{1}_R^T\gamma + f\gamma^T S\gamma\right\}$. Conditional on the latent states, the authors specify $f(\mathbf{Y} \mid \boldsymbol{\eta})$ as a generalized linear model. Among other Bayesian approaches, Li et al. [39] considered image-on-scalar regression and investigated the spatial variability of covariate effects on imaging responses via a partially linear spatially varying coefficient model. Considering available estimates of a similar quantity from multiple data sources, Yao et al. [80] proposed a bivariate hierarchical Bayesian model that incorporates correlation.

### 10.4.1 Data Application

To demonstrate one of these methods, we implemented the model by Chiang et al. [5] using publicly available data from 26 patients with drug-resistant epilepsy who had elected to undergo neurosurgical treatment for their epilepsy [68], a treatment with often high clinical success rates assuming that the focus can be accurately localized. In order to facilitate localization of the epileptogenic zone, concurrent electrical stimulation and 3T fMRI in awake patients with implanted depth electrodes was perfomed [68]. Pre-processed data are available where the brain surfaces have been reconstructed using `recon-all` (FreeSurfer 6.0.1) [7].

For this analysis, we restricted our attention to the subset of patients with seizure onset zones located in the temporal lobes. Thus, we selected $n = 13$ patients and further extracted measurements of cortical thickness from $R = 68$ region of interests (ROIs), both in the left and the right hemispheres, to use as imaging predictors, $\mathbf{X}_i$, $i = 1, \ldots, 13$. The binary outcome variable is the laterality of the seizure focus of the patient (left hemispheric or right hemispheric). We considered several choices for the number of components of the Gaussian mixture model, $K$, namely $K = 2, ..., 6$, and eventually chose $K = 2$ based on the deviance information criterion (DIC). We assumed spike-and-slab priors with Normal slabs on the mean components of the mixture and further set the sparsity and smoothness parameters of the Ising prior on the binary indicators to $e = -0.1$ and $f = 0.05$, respectively. We set the hyperparameter of the Dirichlet prior on the mixing probabilities to $\alpha_k = 9$, $k = 1, \ldots, K$.

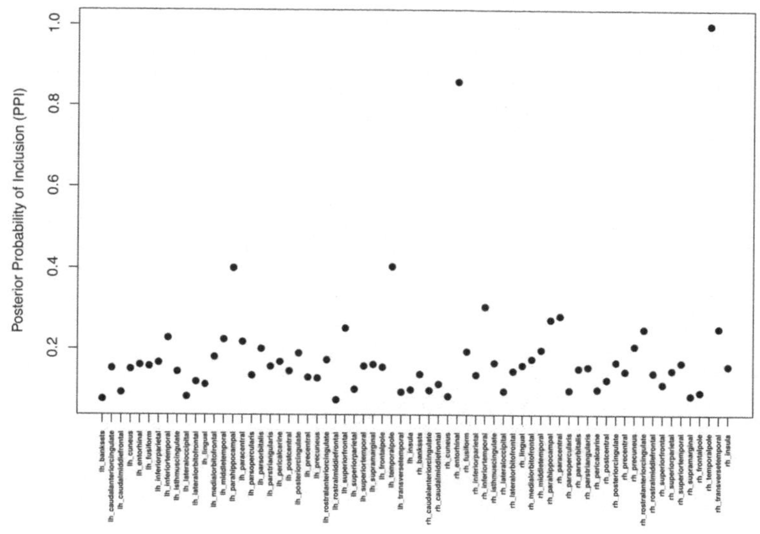


**FIGURE 10.1**
Marginal posterior probabilities of inclusion of brain regions in predicting seizure laterality.

**TABLE 10.2**
(a) Posterior mean; (b) 95% credible interval; (c) posterior probability of odds ratio > 1.

| | (a) | (b) | (c) |
|---|---|---|---|
| $\beta_0$ | −0.162 | [−1.275 , 0.917] | 0.384 |
| $\beta_1$ | 0.295 | [−2.014 , 2.748] | 0.591 |

The remaining parameters were chosen as in [5]. Figure 10.1 reports the marginal posterior probabilities of inclusions (PPIs) for the 68 ROIs. The four regions with highest PPIs are listed in Table 10.1. Conditional on the two latent states, the logistic portion of the model returned posterior inference on $\beta$ as reported in Table 10.2 where $\beta_1 \equiv$ Cluster 1 (vs. Cluster 2).

## 10.5 Spatial Models for Measurements of Electrophysiological Activity

Scalp EEG is a non-invasive technique that records the brain's spontaneous electrical activity over a period of time, as recorded from multiple electrodes placed on the scalp. Electrocorticography (ECoG), or intracranial EEG, involves invasive electrodes and records signal on a different scale of activity than the brain activity recorded from scalp EEG. Low voltage, high frequency components that cannot be seen easily (or at all) in scalp EEG can often be seen quite clearly in ECoG. Magnetoencephalography (MEG) is another non-invasive technique complementary to EEG that measures changes in magnetic fields generated by neural activity (see Chapter 2). These electrophysiological techniques are widely used in epilepsy work-up and presurgical evaluation.

Diagnostic applications based on EEG/ECoG data often focus either on event-related potentials, obtained by time locking potential fluctuations to an event, such as "stimulus onset" or "button press," or on the spectral content of EEG, to analyse neural oscillations in the frequency domain. A few statistical approaches exist that incorporate spatial aspects in the modeling of such data. For example, Zhang et al. [83] proposed a modular and indicator-based dynamic directional model (MIDDM) to model the effective connectivity in ECoG data, and Li et al. [38] developed a state-space multivariate autoregression (SSMAR) to model the directional connectivity in iEEG data.

Estimating the location of the signal based on data measured outside of the head via EEG/MEG techniques leads to an *inverse problem*, which is proved to have infinite solutions. Daunizeau and Friston [8] proposed a mesostate space model for EEG and MEG inverse problem under the assumption of independent mixture allocation variables. Inspired by this model, Song et al. [61] developed a Potts-mixture spatio-temporal joint model of the two modalities. Let $\mathbf{M}(t) = (M_1(t), M_2(t), \ldots, M_{n_M}(t))'$ and $\boldsymbol{E}(t) = (E_1(t), E_2(t), \ldots, E_{n_E}(t))'$ be the MEG and EEG data, respectively, with $n_M$ and $n_E$ the number of sensors. Specifically,

$$\boldsymbol{M}(t) = \boldsymbol{X}_M \boldsymbol{S}(t) + \boldsymbol{\epsilon}_M(t), \quad \boldsymbol{\epsilon}_M(t) \mid \sigma_M^2 \overset{iid}{\sim} \text{MVN}\left(\mathbf{0}, \sigma_M^2 \boldsymbol{H}_M\right), \quad t = 1, \ldots, T, \tag{10.20}$$

$$\boldsymbol{E}(t) = \boldsymbol{X}_E \boldsymbol{S}(t) + \boldsymbol{\epsilon}_E(t), \quad \boldsymbol{\epsilon}_E(t) \mid \sigma_E^2 \overset{iid}{\sim} \text{MVN}\left(\mathbf{0}, \sigma_E^2 \boldsymbol{H}_E\right), \quad t = 1, \ldots, T, \tag{10.21}$$

with $\boldsymbol{S}(t) = (S_1(t), \ldots S_P(t))'$ the unknown neural activity at the same time point. Assuming latent Gaussian mixture on $S_j(t)$, the authors relaxed the assumption of independent mixture allocation variables and adopted the Potts model of spatial dependence. Let $\mathbf{Z} = \left(\mathbf{Z}_1', \mathbf{Z}_2', \ldots, \mathbf{Z}_{N_v}'\right)'$ be a labelling process defined over the grid of voxels, then

$$P(\mathbf{Z} \mid \beta) = \frac{\exp\left\{\beta \sum_{h \sim j} \delta\left(\mathbf{Z}_{\boldsymbol{j}}, \boldsymbol{Z}_{\boldsymbol{h}}\right)\right\}}{G(\beta)}, \quad \delta\left(\mathbf{Z}_{\boldsymbol{j}}, \mathbf{Z}_{\boldsymbol{h}}\right) = 2\mathbf{Z}_j' \mathbf{Z}_h - 1, \tag{10.22}$$

where $h \sim j$ means $h$ and $j$ are neighbors. The Iterated Conditional Modes (ICM) algorithm of [1] was implemented for simultaneous point estimation and model selection. However, the convergence of the ICM is sensitive to the starting value. Motivated by this issue, Opoku et al. [49] further implemented Ant Colony System (ACS) optimization with ICM.

Ma et al. [43] studied EEG-based brain-computer interface (BCI) – a system that translates brain activity into commands to operate technology. The P300 event-related potential (ERP) is elicited in the process of decision making by the rare occurrence of target stimuli among common nontarget stimuli, and it is commonly used in EEG BCI. The authors proposed a novel Bayesian approach to multi-channel real EEG signals under the P300 ERP-BCI design, with the goal of identifying relevant spatial temporal differences of the neural activity, which provides statistical evidence of P300 ERP responses and helps design individually efficient and accurate BCIs. Suppose $X_{l,i,e}(t)$ are the observed EEG signals where $l = 1, \ldots, L$ indicates the target character, $i = 1, \ldots, I$ is the sequence index, and $e = 1, \ldots, E$ is the channel index. The authors considered the following model:

$$\begin{aligned} X_{l,i,e}(t) &= M_{l,i,e}(t) + \epsilon_{l,i,e}(t), \quad \tau_{l,i,j} = t - (W_{l,i,j} - 1)\, d \\ M_{l,i,e}(t) &= \sum_{j=1}^{J} \left[\beta_{1,e}\left(\tau_{l,i,j}\right) Y_{l,j} + \beta_{0,e}\left(\tau_{l,i,j}\right)\left(1 - Y_{l,j}\right)\right] \mathbb{I}_{[0,T_z]}\left(\tau_{l,i,j}\right), \end{aligned} \tag{10.23}$$

where $Y_l$ is the given stimulus-type indicators, $W_{l,i}$ is the stimulus occurring times, and $M_{l,i,e}(t)$ indicates the expected EEG signals. The error term is dependent spatially and temporally as

$$\begin{aligned}\epsilon_{l,i,e}(t) &= \zeta_{l,i,e} + \varepsilon_{l,i}(t)\\ \zeta_{l,i} &= (\zeta_{l,i,1}, \ldots, \zeta_{l,i,E})^{\top} \sim \mathcal{N}(0, C_s)\\ \varepsilon_{l,i}(t) &= \rho_{t,0} + \sum_{m=1}^{q} \rho_{t,m}\varepsilon_{l,i}(t - md) + \varepsilon_{l,i,0}(t)\\ \varepsilon_{l,i,0}(t) &\sim \mathcal{N}\left(0, \sigma_x^2\right),\end{aligned}$$

where $\zeta_{l,i,e}$ is the spatial random effect, and $\varepsilon_{l,i}(t) \sim AR(q)$ is the temporal random effect. A split and merge Gaussian prior (SMGP) is proposed for $\beta_{0,e}$ and $\beta_{1,e}$.

## 10.6 Approaches for Multi-Type and/or Multi-Study Data

Several of the methods presented above incorporate multi-modal information, i.e., data from multiple modalities. These modalities typically measure different aspects of brain function and structure. By combining the different types of information contained in several data sources, it is possible to obtain a more thorough understanding of brain processes, and their association with clinical and behavioral outcomes of interest. Multi-modal approaches allow overcoming the limitations of single modalities and can lead to more accurate estimates and outcome predictions. For example, the model by Daunizeau and Friston [8] simultaneously processes EEG and MEG data, whereas the model for PET data by Chiang et al [5] integrates information from resting-state fMRI data into the prior construction. An additional example of integrative model that leads to improved estimation of latent source signals is that by Wu et al. [78]. They propose a Distribution Independent Component Analysis (DICA) two-stage framework that performs spatial source separation and identifies functional networks by decomposing the images obtained using different imaging modalities (e.g. fMRI and DTI data) via Bayesian mixture models. Zhao, Wu and Kang [85] recently presented a unified Bayesian prior model that identifies main effect features and intermodality interactions simultaneously within the same inference platform, taking into account both the data structure and the brain anatomical architecture.

We conclude by briefly mentioning a few related approaches devised for meta-analysis, i.e. the synthetic review of multiple independently conducted studies to establish the foundation of wider clinical evidence on the basis of appropriate statistical methods. In particular, Samartsidis et al. [56] present an overview of two types of existing meta-analysis methods for fMRI studies: kernel-based methods and model-based methods. Kang et al. [31] proposed a Bayesian hierarchical marked spatial independent cluster process. Kang et al. [32] further implemented a nonparametric Bayesian approach for meta analysis data from multiple classes or types of studies, named Hierarchical Poisson/Gamma Random Fields model (HPGRF). Alternatively, Wagor et al. [72] presented a Bayesian Spatial Point Process (BSPP) model for identifying the number and locations of activation. Furthermore, Montagna et al. [46] developed a spatial Bayesian latent factor regression for coordinate-based meta-analysis data (CBMA).

## 10.7 Spatial Models in SPM and FSL

Last, we describe a few resources with open-source software that may be used for analysis of neuroimaging and electrophysiological data, including Statistical Parametric Mapping (SPM) (`https://www.fil.ion.ucl.ac.uk/spm/`) and FMRIB Software Library (FSL) (`https://fsl.fmrib.ox.ac.uk/fsl/fslwiki/`).

SPM incorporates Bayesian estimation procedures for fMRI models. The underlying method is based on the GLM model as in Eq. (10.1). The user-specific choices include spatial priors for regression coefficients, such as Unweighted Graph Laplacian (UGL), Gaussian Markov Random Field (GMRF) as in Eq. (10.3), Low resolution Tomography Prior (LRTP) and Weighted Graph Laplacian (WGL). Additionally, they include regularized voxel-wise auto-regressive (AR) models for the error term. Posterior inference is achieved via Variational Bayes (VB).

Several FSL tools provide Bayesian methods for different neuroimaging data:

- **FAST [84]:** This is an automated segmentation tool for structural MRI images which is based on hidden Markov random field (HMRF) models and Expectation-Maximization (EM) algorithms for correction of spatial intensity variations.
- **BASIL [4, 22]:** This is a Bayesian inference tool for Arterial Spin Labeling (ASL) MRI. The underlying method is based on the voxelwise model $\boldsymbol{y}_v = \mathbf{g}(\boldsymbol{w}_v) + \boldsymbol{e}_v$, where $\boldsymbol{y}_v$ is a $T \times 1$ vector of time series data for voxel $v$, $g(\cdot)$ is a generative predictor function, and $\boldsymbol{w}_v$ is a $K \times 1$ vector of parameter values. The spatial prior of Penny et al. [52], defined as in equation (10.5) can be specified on $\boldsymbol{w}_v$, to account for spatial homogeneity among voxels.
- **FABBER [4, 22, 75]:** This is a tool for approximate Bayesian inference for ASL MRI data using Variational Bayes. Similar to BASIL, it implements the spatial prior of Penny et al. [52] for spatial smoothing.
- **MM [76]:** Referred to as Mixture Modeling, this is an inference-based method that explicitly models the null part and the activation part. The user may choose to use the implemented spatial enhancement that uses spatial Markov Random Field (MRF) priors on the class labels of the voxel/region spatial locations. The labelling of the voxels is then smoothed to null, activated and deactivated.

## 10.8 Summary

In this chapter, we have presented modern approaches for the analysis of neuroimaging and electrophysiological modalities that takes into account the spatial organization of the data. Many of the methods we have presented allow for the investigation of inter- and intra-subjects variability across spatially oriented measures of brain activity. They also often incorporate the selection of relevant imaging biomarkers that are associated to individual behavioral or clinical outcomes, with the goal of identifying the seizure onset zoner or epileptogenic zone to improve the treatment of epilepsy.

From a computational perspective, successful implementation of Bayesian models for the analysis of high-dimensional complex neuroimaging and electrophysiological data requires scalable computational routines. Optimization-based methods, such as variational Bayes approaches, may provide scalability, although at the expense of uncertainty quantification. Alternatively, expert-informed dimension-reduction procedures ma be considered to focus the analysis on specific regions of interest and their association. Ultimately, the quantification of spatial variability and uncertainty in neuroimaging and electrophysiological data is still an active area or research, and has the potential to strengthen the understanding of functional specialization and local organization of neural activity.

## Bibliography

[1] Julian Besag. On the statistical analysis of dirty pictures. *Journal of the Royal Statistical Society: Series B (Methodological)*, 48(3):259–279, 1986.

[2] Fredrick DuBois Bowman, Brian Caffo, Susan Spear Bassett, and Clinton Kilts. A Bayesian hierarchical framework for spatial modeling of fMRI data. *NeuroImage*, 39(1):146–156, 2008.

[3] Richard B Buxton and Lawrence R Frank. A model for the coupling between cerebral blood flow and oxygen metabolism during neural stimulation. *Journal of Cerebral Blood Flow & Metabolism*, 17(1):64–72, 1997.

[4] Michael A Chappell, Adrian R Groves, Brandon Whitcher, and Mark W Woolrich. Variational Bayesian inference for a nonlinear forward model. *IEEE Transactions on Signal Processing*, 57(1):223–236, 2008.

[5] Sharon Chiang, Michele Guindani, Hsiang J Yeh, Sandra Dewar, Zulfi Haneef, John M Stern, and Marina Vannucci. A hierarchical Bayesian model for the identification of PET markers associated to the prediction of surgical outcome after anterior temporal lobe resection. *Frontiers in Neuroscience*, 11:669, 2017.

[6] Ning Dai, Hakmook Kang, Galin L Jones, and Mark B Fiecas. A Bayesian latent spatial model for mapping the cortical signature of progression to Alzheimer's disease. *Canadian Journal of Statistics*, 49(1):46–62, 2021.

[7] Anders M Dale, Bruce Fischl, and Martin I Sereno. Cortical surface-based analysis: I. segmentation and surface reconstruction. *Neuroimage*, 9(2):179–194, 1999.

[8] Jean Daunizeau and Karl J Friston. A mesostate-space model for EEG and MEG. *NeuroImage*, 38(1):67–81, 2007.

[9] Jianqing Fan and Jinchi Lv. Sure independence screening for ultrahigh dimensional feature space. *Journal of the Royal Statistical Society: Series B (Statistical Methodology)*, 70(5):849–911, 2008.

[10] Bruce Fischl. Freesurfer. *Neuroimage*, 62(2):774–781, 2012.

[11] Guillaume Flandin and William D Penny. Bayesian fMRI data analysis with sparse spatial basis function priors. *NeuroImage*, 34(3):1108–1125, 2007.

[12] Karl J Friston, P Fletcher, Oliver Josephs, ANDREW Holmes, MD Rugg, and Robert Turner. Event-related fMRI: Characterizing differential responses. *Neuroimage*, 7(1):30–40, 1998.

[13] Karl J Friston, Andrew P Holmes, JB Poline, PJ Grasby, SCR Williams, Richard SJ Frackowiak, and Robert Turner. Analysis of fMRI time-series revisited. *Neuroimage*, 2(1):45–53, 1995.

[14] Karl J Friston, Peter Jezzard, and Robert Turner. Analysis of functional MRI time-series. *Human Brain Mapping*, 1(2):153–171, 1994.

[15] Karl J Friston and W Penny. Posterior probability maps and SPMs. *NeuroImage*, 19(3):1240–1249, 2003.

[16] Karl J Friston, William Penny, Christophe Phillips, S Kiebel, G Hinton, and John Ashburner. Classical and Bayesian inference in neuroimaging: Theory. *NeuroImage*, 16(2):465–483, 2002.

[17] Tian Ge, Nicole Müller-Lenke, Kerstin Bendfeldt, Thomas E Nichols, and Timothy D Johnson. Analysis of multiple sclerosis lesions via spatially varying coefficients. *The Annals of Applied Statistics*, 8(2):1095, 2014.

[18] Matthew F Glasser, Stamatios N Sotiropoulos, J Anthony Wilson, Timothy S Coalson, Bruce Fischl, Jesper L Andersson, Junqian Xu, Saad Jbabdi, Matthew Webster, Jonathan R Polimeni, et al. The minimal preprocessing pipelines for the human connectome project. *NeuroImage*, 80:105–124, 2013.

[19] Rainer Goebel, Alard Roebroeck, Dae-Shik Kim, and Elia Formisano. Investigating directed cortical interactions in time-resolved fMRI data using vector autoregressive modeling and Granger causality mapping. *Magnetic Resonance Imaging*, 21(10):1251–1261, 2003.

[20] Jeff Goldsmith, Lei Huang, and Ciprian M Crainiceanu. Smooth scalar-on-image regression via spatial Bayesian variable selection. *Journal of Computational and Graphical Statistics*, 23(1):46–64, 2014.

[21] Christoff Gössl, Dorothee P Auer, and Ludwig Fahrmeir. Bayesian spatiotemporal inference in functional magnetic resonance imaging. *Biometrics*, 57(2):554–562, 2001.

[22] Adrian R Groves, Michael A Chappell, and Mark W Woolrich. Combined spatial and non-spatial prior for inference on MRI time-series. *Neuroimage*, 45(3):795–809, 2009.

[23] Lee M Harrison and Gary GR Green. A Bayesian spatiotemporal model for very large data sets. *NeuroImage*, 50(3):1126–1141, 2010.

[24] Lee M Harrison, W Penny, Jean Daunizeau, and Karl J Friston. Diffusion-based spatial priors for functional magnetic resonance images. *NeuroImage*, 41(2):408–423, 2008.

[25] Kevin He, Jian Kang, Hyokyoung G Hong, Ji Zhu, Yanming Li, Huazhen Lin, Han Xu, and Yi Li. Covariance-insured screening. *Computational Statistics & Data Analysis*, 132:100–114, 2019.

[26] Kevin He, Han Xu, and Jian Kang. A selective overview of feature screening methods with applications to neuroimaging data. *Wiley Interdisciplinary Reviews: Computational Statistics*, 11(2):e1454, 2019.

[27] Rasoul Hekmati, Robert Azencott, Wei Zhang, Zili D. Chu, and Michael J. Paldino. Localization of epileptic seizure focus by computerized analysis of fMRI recordings. *Brain Informatics*, 7(1):13, 2020.

[28] Timothy D Johnson, Zhuqing Liu, Andreas J Bartsch, and Thomas E Nichols. A Bayesian non-parametric Potts model with application to pre-surgical fMRI data. *Statistical Methods in Medical Research*, 22(4):364–381, 2013.

[29] Stefanie Kalus, Philipp G Sämann, and Ludwig Fahrmeir. Classification of brain activation via spatial Bayesian variable selection in fMRI regression. *Advances in Data Analysis and Classification*, 8(1):63–83, 2014.

[30] Jian Kang, Hyokyoung G Hong, and Yi Li. Partition-based ultrahigh-dimensional variable screening. *Biometrika*, 104(4):785–800, 2017.

[31] Jian Kang, Timothy D Johnson, Thomas E Nichols, and Tor D Wager. Meta analysis of functional neuroimaging data via Bayesian spatial point processes. *Journal of the American Statistical Association*, 106(493):124–134, 2011.

[32] Jian Kang, Thomas E Nichols, Tor D Wager, and Timothy D Johnson. A Bayesian hierarchical spatial point process model for multi-type neuroimaging meta-analysis. *The Annals of Applied Statistics*, 8(3):1800, 2014.

[33] Jian Kang, Brian J Reich, and Ana-Maria Staicu. Scalar-on-image regression via the soft-thresholded Gaussian process. *Biometrika*, 105(1):165–184, 2018.

[34] Jeong Hwan Kook, Kelly Vaughn, Dana DeMaster, Linda Ewing-Cobbs, and Marina Vannucci. BVAR-connect: A variational Bayes approach to multi-subject vector autoregressive models for inference on brain connectivity networks. *Neuroinformatics*, 19:39–56, 2021.

[35] Nicholas Lange and Scott L Zeger. Non-linear Fourier time series analysis for human brain mapping by functional magnetic resonance imaging. *Journal of the Royal Statistical Society: Series C (Applied Statistics)*, 46(1):1–29, 1997.

[36] Kuo-Jung Lee, Galin L Jones, Brian S Caffo, and Susan Spear Bassett. Spatial Bayesian variable selection models on functional magnetic resonance imaging time-series data. *Bayesian Analysis (Online)*, 9(3):699, 2014.

[37] Fan Li, Tingting Zhang, Quanli Wang, Marlen Z Gonzalez, Erin L Maresh, and James A Coan. Spatial Bayesian variable selection and grouping for high-dimensional scalar-on-image regression. *The Annals of Applied Statistics*, 9(2):687–713, 2015.

[38] Huazhang Li, Yaotian Wang, Guofen Yan, Yinge Sun, Seiji Tanabe, Chang-Chia Liu, Mark S Quigg, and Tingting Zhang. A Bayesian state-space approach to mapping directional brain networks. *Journal of the American Statistical Association*, 116(536):1637–1647, 2021.

[39] Xinyi Li, Li Wang, Huixia Judy Wang, and Alzheimer's Disease Neuroimaging Initiative. Sparse learning and structure identification for ultrahigh-dimensional image-on-scalar regression. *Journal of the American Statistical Association*, 116(536):1994–2008, 2021.

[40] Martin A Lindquist and Tor D Wager. Validity and power in hemodynamic response modeling: a comparison study and a new approach. *Human Brain Mapping*, 28(8):764–784, 2007.

[41] Zhuqing Liu, Andreas J Bartsch, Veronica J Berrocal, and Timothy D Johnson. A mixed-effects, spatially varying coefficients model with application to multi-resolution functional magnetic resonance imaging data. *Statistical Methods in Medical Research*, 28(4):1203–1215, 2019.

[42] Zhuqing Liu, Veronica J Berrocal, Andreas J Bartsch, and Timothy D Johnson. Pre-surgical fMRI data analysis using a spatially adaptive conditionally autoregressive model. *Bayesian Analysis (Online)*, 11(2):599, 2016.

[43] Tianwen Ma, Yang Li, Jane E Huggins, Ji Zhu, and Jian Kang. Bayesian inferences on neural activity in EEG-based brain-computer interface. *Journal of the American Statistical Association*, pages 1–12, 2022.

[44] Amanda F Mejia, Vincent Koppelmans, Laura Jelsone-Swain, Sanjay Kalra, and Robert C Welsh. Longitudinal surface-based spatial Bayesian GLM reveals complex trajectories of motor neurodegeneration in ALS. *NeuroImage*, page 119180, 2022.

[45] Amanda F Mejia, Yu Yue, David Bolin, Finn Lindgren, and Martin A Lindquist. A Bayesian general linear modeling approach to cortical surface fMRI data analysis. *Journal of the American Statistical Association*, 115(530):501–520, 2020.

[46] Silvia Montagna, Tor Wager, Lisa Feldman Barrett, Timothy D Johnson, and Thomas E Nichols. Spatial Bayesian latent factor regression modeling of coordinate-based meta-analysis data. *Biometrics*, 74(1):342–353, 2018.

[47] Emily L Morris, Kevin He, and Jian Kang. Scalar on network regression via boosting. *Annals of Applied Statistics*, 2022.

[48] Peter Muller, Giovanni Parmigiani, and Kenneth Rice. FDR and Bayesian multiple comparisons rules. *Proc. Valencia/ISBA 8th World Meeting on Bayesian Statistics*, 2006.

[49] Eugene A Opoku, Syed Ejaz Ahmed, Yin Song, and Farouk S Nathoo. Ant colony system optimization for spatiotemporal modelling of combined EEG and MEG data. *Entropy*, 23(3):329, 2021.

[50] Jun Young Park, Mark Fiecas, Alzheimer's Disease Neuroimaging Initiative, et al. Permutation-based inference for spatially localized signals in longitudinal MRI data. *NeuroImage*, 239:118312, 2021.

[51] Will Penny, Stefan Kiebel, and Karl Friston. Variational Bayesian inference for fMRI time series. *NeuroImage*, 19(3):727–741, 2003.

[52] William D Penny, Nelson J Trujillo-Barreto, and Karl J Friston. Bayesian fMRI time series analysis with spatial priors. *NeuroImage*, 24(2):350–362, 2005.

[53] Alicia Quirós, Raquel Montes Diez, and Dani Gamerman. Bayesian spatiotemporal model of fMRI data. *NeuroImage*, 49(1):442–456, 2010.

[54] Thorsten Rings, Randi von Wrede, and Klaus Lehnertz. Precursors of seizures due to specific spatial-temporal modifications of evolving large-scale epileptic brain networks. *Scientific Reports*, 9(1):10623, 2019.

[55] Seyyed Mostafa Sadjadi, Elias Ebrahimzadeh, and Hamid Soltanian-Zadeh. fMRI functional connectivity analysis for localizing epileptic focus. In *2022 30th International Conference on Electrical Engineering (ICEE)*, pages 660–664, 2022.

[56] Pantelis Samartsidis, Silvia Montagna, Thomas E Nichols, and Timothy D Johnson. The coordinate-based meta-analysis of neuroimaging data. *Statistical Science: A Review Journal of the Institute of Mathematical Statistics*, 32(4):580, 2017.

[57] Nilotpal Sanyal and Marco AR Ferreira. Bayesian hierarchical multi-subject multiscale analysis of functional MRI data. *NeuroImage*, 63(3):1519–1531, 2012.

[58] Yue Shi, Xin Zhang, Chunlan Yang, Jiechuan Ren, Zhimei Li, and Qun Wang. A review on epileptic foci localization using resting-state functional magnetic resonance imaging. *Mathematical Biosciences and Engineering*, 17(3):2496–2515, 2020.

[59] Michael Smith and Ludwig Fahrmeir. Spatial Bayesian variable selection with application to functional magnetic resonance imaging. *Journal of the American Statistical Association*, 102(478):417–431, 2007.

[60] Michael Smith, Benno Pütz, Dorothee Auer, and Ludwig Fahrmeir. Assessing brain activity through spatial Bayesian variable selection. *NeuroImage*, 20(2):802–815, 2003.

[61] Yin Song, Farouk Nathoo, and Arif Babul. A Potts-mixture spatiotemporal joint model for combined magnetoencephalography and electroencephalography data. *Canadian Journal of Statistics*, 47(4):688–711, 2019.

[62] Daniel Spencer, Yu Ryan Yue, David Bolin, Sarah Ryan, and Amanda F Mejia. Spatial Bayesian GLM on the cortical surface produces reliable task activations in individuals and groups. *NeuroImage*, page 118908, 2022.

[63] Wenguang Sun, Brian J Reich, T Tony Cai, Michele Guindani, and Armin Schwartzman. False discovery control in large-scale spatial multiple testing. *Journal of the Royal Statistical Society: Series B (Statistical Methodology)*, 77(1):59–83, 2015.

[64] Bernd Taschler, Tian Ge, Kerstin Bendfeldt, Nicole Müller-Lenke, Timothy D Johnson, and Thomas E Nichols. Spatial modeling of multiple sclerosis for disease subtype prediction. In *International Conference on Medical Image Computing and Computer-Assisted Intervention*, pages 797–804. Springer, 2014.

[65] Ming Teng, Timothy D Johnson, and Farouk S Nathoo. Time series analysis of fMRI data: Spatial modelling and Bayesian computation. *Statistics in Medicine*, 37(18):2753–2770, 2018.

[66] Ming Teng, Farouk S Nathoo, and Timothy D Johnson. Bayesian analysis of functional magnetic resonance imaging data with spatially varying auto-regressive orders. *Journal of the Royal Statistical Society: Series C (Applied Statistics)*, 68(3):521–541, 2019.

[67] Bertrand Thirion, Alan Tucholka, Merlin Keller, Philippe Pinel, Alexis Roche, Jean-Franccois Mangin, and Jean-Baptiste Poline. High level group analysis of fMRI data based on Dirichlet process mixture models. In *Biennial International Conference on Information Processing in Medical Imaging*, pages 482–494. Springer, 2007.

[68] William H. Thompson, Remya Nair, Hiroyuki Oya, Oscar Esteban, James Shine, Christopher Petkov, Russell Poldrack, Matthew A. Howard, and Ralph Adolphs. A data resource from concurrent intracranial stimulation and functional MRI of the human brain. *Scientific Data*, 7(1):1–13, 2020.

[69] Yehuda Vardi, Larry A Shepp, and Linda Kaufman. A statistical model for positron emission tomography. *Journal of the American Statistical Association*, 80(389):8–20, 1985.

[70] Mattia Veronese, Lucia Moro, Marco Arcolin, Ottavia Dipasquale, Gaia Rizzo, Paul Expert, Wasim Khan, Patrick M Fisher, Claus Svarer, Alessandra Bertoldo, et al. Covariance statistics and network analysis of brain PET imaging studies. *Scientific Reports*, 9(1):1–15, 2019.

[71] Patrizia Vizza, Giuseppe Tradigo, Demetrio Messina, Giuseppe Lucio Cascini, and Pierangelo Veltri. Methodologies for the analysis and classification of PET neuroimages. *Network Modeling Analysis in Health Informatics and Bioinformatics*, 2(4):191–208, 2013.

[72] Tor D Wager, Jian Kang, Timothy D Johnson, Thomas E Nichols, Ajay B Satpute, and Lisa Feldman Barrett. A Bayesian model of category-specific emotional brain responses. *PLoS Computational Biology*, 11(4):e1004066, 2015.

[73] Xiangyu Wang and Chenlei Leng. High dimensional ordinary least squares projection for screening variables. *Journal of the Royal Statistical Society: Series B (Statistical Methodology)*, 78(3):589–611, 2016.

[74] Andrew S Whiteman, Andreas J Bartsch, Jian Kang, and Timothy D Johnson. Bayesian inference for brain activity from functional magnetic resonance imaging collected at two spatial resolutions. *arXiv preprint arXiv:2103.13131*, 2021.

[75] Mark W Woolrich, Peter Chiarelli, Daniel Gallichan, Joanna Perthen, and Thomas T Liu. Bayesian inference of hemodynamic changes in functional arterial spin labeling data. *Magnetic Resonance in Medicine: An Official Journal of the International Society for Magnetic Resonance in Medicine*, 56(4):891–906, 2006.

[76] Mark William Woolrich, Timothy Edward John Behrens, Christian F Beckmann, and Stephen M Smith. Mixture models with adaptive spatial regularization for segmentation with an application to fMRI data. *IEEE Transactions on Medical Imaging*, 24(1):1–11, 2005.

[77] Mark William Woolrich, Mark Jenkinson, J Michael Brady, and Stephen M Smith. Fully Bayesian spatio-temporal modeling of fMRI data. *IEEE Transactions on Medical Imaging*, 23(2):213–231, 2004.

[78] Ben Wu, Subhadip Pal, Jian Kang, and Ying Guo. Distributional independent component analysis for diverse neuroimaging modalities. *Biometrics*, 2021.

[79] Lei Xu, Timothy D Johnson, Thomas E Nichols, and Derek E Nee. Modeling inter-subject variability in fMRI activation location: A Bayesian hierarchical spatial model. *Biometrics*, 65(4):1041–1051, 2009.

[80] Yujing Yao, R Todd Ogden, Chubing Zeng, and Qixuan Chen. Bivariate hierarchical Bayesian model for combining summary measures and their uncertainties from multiple sources. *arXiv preprint arXiv:2109.07560*, 2021.

[81] Linlin Zhang, Michele Guindani, Francesco Versace, Jeffrey M. Engelmann, and Marina Vannucci. A spatio-temporal nonparametric Bayesian model of multi-subject fMRI data. *Annals of Applied Statistics*, 10(2):638–666, 2016.

[82] Linlin Zhang, Michele Guindani, Francesco Versace, and Marina Vannucci. A spatio-temporal nonparametric Bayesian variable selection model of fMRI data for clustering correlated time courses. *NeuroImage*, 95:162–175, 2014.

[83] Tingting Zhang, Qiannan Yin, Brian Caffo, Yinge Sun, and Dana Boatman-Reich. Bayesian inference of high-dimensional, cluster-structured ordinary differential equation models with applications to brain connectivity studies. *The Annals of Applied Statistics*, 11(2):868–897, 2017.

[84] Yongyue Zhang, Michael Brady, and Stephen Smith. Segmentation of brain MR images through a hidden markov random field model and the expectation-maximization algorithm. *IEEE Transactions on Medical Imaging*, 20(1):45–57, 2001.

[85] Yize Zhao, Ben Wu, and Jian Kang. Bayesian interaction selection model for multimodal neuroimaging data analysis. *Biometrics*, 2022.

# Part III

# Machine Learning Methods

# 11

# *Unsupervised Learning*

**Giuseppe Vinci**

*Department of Applied and Computational Mathematics & Statistics, University of Notre Dame (USA)*

## CONTENTS



Unsupervised learning methods are powerful tools for the exploration and the analysis of complex and high-dimensional data. Several classes of unsupervised learning methods are widely used in the analysis of epilepsy data, including dimension reduction, clustering, and matrix completion. Unsupervised learning methods are pivotal in the analysis of massive neural electrophysiological and imaging data, especially for the rapid and accurate detection of epileptic seizures, source separation of EEG signals, and the analysis of other complex data, such as partially observed survey data. In this chapter, classical and most advanced techniques and key algorithms of unsupervised learning implemented in `R` are presented together with real data applications. Clinicians and neuroscientists engaged in quantitative research with epilepsy data will benefit from the application of the methodologies presented in this chapter.

DOI: 10.1201/9781003254515-11

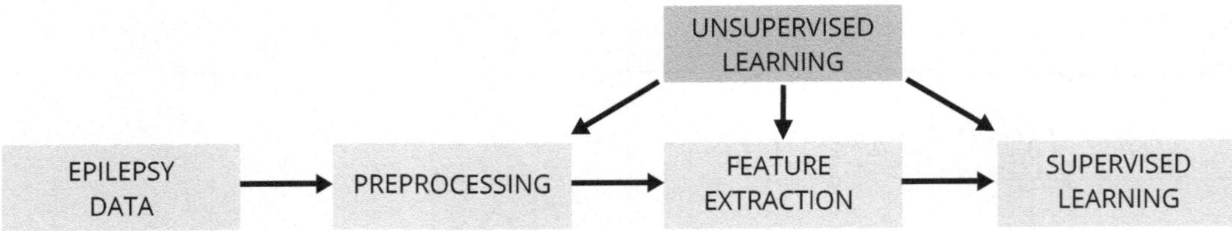


**FIGURE 11.1**
Unsupervised learning can be auxiliary to the preprocessing of epilepsy data, feature extraction, and supervised learning. (Color version available in electronic supplement.)

## 11.1 Introduction

Unsupervised learning methods are useful for the exploration and the analysis of complex and massive datasets, which are difficult to analyse using standard methods that are suitable for low-dimensional data. Unsupervised learning methods let us find meaningful structures in the data without the "supervision" of response variables or labels, as opposed to supervised learning. Unsupervised methods can be used at various stages of data analysis, including exploratory data analysis, hypothesis formulation, and visualization of final results. Unsupervised learning methods are pivotal in the analysis of massive neural electrophysiological and imaging data, especially for the rapid and accurate detection of epileptic seizures, source separation of EEG signals, and the analysis of other complex data, such as partially observed survey data. Unsupervised learning can be auxiliary to preprocessing of epilepsy data, feature extraction, and supervised learning (Figure 11.1).

Several classes of unsupervised learning methods are widely used in the analysis of epilepsy data. These include dimension reduction, clustering, and matrix completion. *Dimension reduction* techniques let us project multivariate data onto a lower dimensional space, allowing us to visualize the multivariate data on a 2D or 3D space, to reduce artifact effects, and to perform a source separation or blind selection of features to be used in subsequent supervised learning analyses. *Clustering* techniques allow us to identify groups of data points such that points within the same group are similar, while points in different groups are substantially dissimilar. For an individual patient, clustering is useful to localize portions of the EEG waveforms that have similar pattern, especially those that are characterized by seizures; for multiple patients, clustering may be used to identify groups of patients with similar brain seizure activity patterns. *Matrix completion* techniques allow us to reconstruct data matrices that contain missing entries. A typical example is survey data, where survey respondents may voluntarily or involuntarily omit some answers, thereby producing incomplete data that cannot be readily analysed in the same way as complete data.

In this chapter, we present classical and most advanced techniques, and key algorithms of unsupervised learning implemented in R together with real data applications. In Section 11.2, we describe six dimension reduction techniques (principal components analysis, multi-dimensional scaling, isometric feature mapping, t-distributed stochastic neighbor embedding, uniform manifold approximation and projection, and independent components analysis) and their applications to the analysis of EEG data. In Section 11.3, we present two clustering techniques ($K$-means and hierarchical clustering) and their applications to the analysis of preictal and interictal periods from EEG data. In Section 11.4, we present two approaches (KNN completion and Low-Rank completion) for the completion of survey data matrices and the recovery of corrupted electrophysiological recordings. In Section 11.5, we present the R code for the implementation of the methods presented throughout this chapter. Finally, in Section 11.6, we provide some final remarks, briefly discussing the relationship between unsupervised and supervised methods and other existing unsupervised learning methods.

## 11.2 Dimension Reduction

Let $\mathbf{X} \in \mathbb{R}^{n \times p}$ be a data matrix with $n$ samples and $p$ features. In epilepsy studies based on EEG recordings, $p$ is typically in the order of hundreds of dimensions, due to multiplicity of EEG channels, experimental stimuli, and the particular feature extraction approach used. There may be various reasons to compress $\mathbf{X}$ into a lower dimensional object $\mathbf{Z} \in \mathbb{R}^{n \times q}$ ($q << p$) that retains most of the useful information contained in $\mathbf{X}$. These reasons include data visualization ($q \leq 3$), implicit or blind feature selection that could be useful for supervised learning, source separation, and artifact removal.

In this section we present five dimension reduction techniques: principal components analysis, multi-dimensional scaling, isometric feature mapping, t-distributed stochastic neighbor embedding, uniform manifold approximation and projection, and independent components analysis. We further provide examples of their applications to the analysis of epilepsy data. In Section 11.5.2 we show how all these methods can be implemented with the user-friendly function `reduction()` of the R package `unSuper`.

### 11.2.1 Principal Component Analysis

Principal component analysis (PCA) has the goal of "centering" and "rotating" the $n$ data points in $\mathbf{X} \in \mathbb{R}^{n \times p}$ to obtain a new data matrix $\mathbf{P} \in \mathbb{R}^{n \times p}$ containing $p$ new feature vectors called *principal components* that are *uncorrelated* and arranged in decreasing order according to their variances. In many situations, we may find that the first $q < p$ principal components contain almost all of the information contained in $\mathbf{X}$, and so the matrix $\mathbf{Z} \in \mathbb{R}^{n \times q}$ consisting of the first $q$ columns of $\mathbf{P}$ is a valuable lower dimensional approximation of $\mathbf{X}$.

**Algorithm 1** PCA

INPUT: Data matrix $\mathbf{X} \in \mathbb{R}^{n \times p}$; integer $q \leq p$.

1. Center the data: $\tilde{\mathbf{X}} = [\tilde{x}_{ij}] \in \mathbb{R}^{n \times p}$, where $\tilde{x}_{ij} = x_{ij} - \bar{x}_j$ and $\bar{x}_j = \frac{1}{n}\sum_{i=1}^{n} x_{ij}$ is the sample mean of the $j$-th feature vector.
2. Compute sample covariance matrix: $\hat{\Sigma} = \frac{1}{n}\tilde{\mathbf{X}}^T\tilde{\mathbf{X}}$.
3. Spectral decomposition: $\hat{\Sigma} = V \Lambda V^T$, where $\Lambda = \text{diag}(\lambda_1, ...., \lambda_p)$, $\lambda_1 \geq \lambda_2 \geq ... \geq \lambda_p$ are the eigenvalues, and $V \in \mathbb{R}^{p \times p}$ is the matrix of eigenvectors.
4. Principal component vectors: $P_i = V^T \tilde{\mathbf{x}}_i$, for $i = 1, ..., n$

OUTPUT: Matrix $\mathbf{Z} \in \mathbb{R}^{n \times q}$, with row $\mathbf{z}_i = (P_{i1}, ..., P_{iq})$, for $i = 1, ..., n$.

Transforming $\mathbf{X}$ into $\mathbf{P}$ may sound like a hard task, but it can actually be implemented by using standard matrix algebra operations, as outlined in Algorithm 1, where (1) we first center the data, so that each variable vector has zero mean*; (2) we compute the sample

*If the feature vectors are measured on quite different scales or units, a variant of step 1 might be

covariance matrix $\hat{\Sigma}$ of the standardized variables; (3) we extract the eigenvectors and eigenvalues of the sample covariance matrix $\hat{\Sigma}$; and (4) we use the eigenvectors to obtain the $p$ principal components of the data. It can be shown that the empirical variance of the $i$-th principal component $P_i$ is equal to the $i$-th largest eigenvalue $\lambda_i$ of $\hat{\Sigma}$, and that $P_i$ and $P_j$ are nearly uncorrelated, for any $i \neq j$. Since $\lambda_1 \geq \lambda_2 \geq ... \geq \lambda_p$, the $i$-th principal component $P_i$ should be considered as more important than any other component $P_j$, if $j > i$. Ideally, we would like to retain as few principal components as possible for our analyses, and it is wise to retain the first $q$ components. But how do we pick the number $q$? A simple criterion is to find the smallest $q$ such that the cumulative proportion of variance explained $\text{CPVE}_q := \frac{\sum_{i=1}^{q} \lambda_i}{\sum_{i=k}^{p} \lambda_k}$ is larger than some threshold, e.g. 90%.

In Figure 11.2A we show a 60-sec portion of 19 EEG waveforms recorded for more than four hours from a subject diagnosed with epilepsy. In Figure 11.2B we show the $n \times p$ matrix of extracted spectral features, where $n = 1600$ is the number of 10sec time bins, and $p = 114$ is the total number of spectral features (six frequency bands: 0–4 Hz, 4–8 Hz, 8–16 Hz, 16–32 Hz, 32–64 Hz, 64–128 Hz, for each EEG waveform). We implement PCA and find that just the first $q = 6$ out of $p = 114$ principal components carry more than 90% of the variability in the feature space (Figure 11.2C). In Figure 11.2D we plot the first two principal components. In addition, we plot the trajectories of three known seizure events. It is interesting to note that the three trajectories follow a similar pattern in the reduced 2-dim space.

### 11.2.2 Multi-Dimensional Scaling

Multi-Dimensional Scaling (MDS) lets us find a lower-dimensional representation $\mathbf{Z} \in \mathbb{R}^{n \times q}$ of the data matrix $\mathbf{X} \in \mathbb{R}^{n \times p}$, where the $n$ points in $\mathbf{Z}$ preserve the pairwise distances between the $n$ points in $\mathbf{X}$ as best as possible. The MDS Algorithm 2 proceeds as follows: (1) we first compute all distances between all pairs of observed data points $\mathbf{x}_1, ..., \mathbf{x}_n$; then (2) we find the lower $q$-dimensional objects $\mathbf{z}_1, ..., \mathbf{z}_n$ by minimizing the *stress function* $S(\mathbf{z}_1, ..., \mathbf{z}_n) = \sum_{i \neq j} h(d_{ij}, g_q(\mathbf{z}_i, \mathbf{z}_j))$, which assesses the difference between the distances computed in the $p$-dimensional space with the ones computed between pairs of $\mathbf{z}_1, ..., \mathbf{z}_n$ in the $q$-dimensional space.

---

**Algorithm 2** MDS

---

INPUT: $\mathbf{x}_1, ..., \mathbf{x}_n \in \mathbb{R}^p$; integer $q \leq p$; distance functions $g_m : \mathbb{R}^m \times \mathbb{R}^m \to \mathbb{R}_+$ and $h : \mathbb{R}^2 \to \mathbb{R}_+$.

1. Compute the distance matrix $\mathbf{D} \in \mathbb{R}^{n \times n}$, where $d_{ij} = g_p(\mathbf{x}_i, \mathbf{x}_j)$.
2. Find $\mathbf{z}_1, ..., \mathbf{z}_n \in \mathbb{R}^q$ that minimize the *stress function*

$$S(\mathbf{z}_1, ..., \mathbf{z}_n) = \sum_{i \neq j} h(d_{ij}, g_q(\mathbf{z}_i, \mathbf{z}_j))$$

OUTPUT: $\mathbf{z}_1, ..., \mathbf{z}_n \in \mathbb{R}^q$.

---

Common choices of the distance functions used in Algorithm 2 are the Euclidean distance $g_m(x, y) = \sqrt{\sum_{i=1}^{m} (x_i - y_i)^2}$, for $x, y \in \mathbb{R}^m$, and $h(x, y) = (x - y)^2$, for $x, y \in \mathbb{R}$. This setting is usually called Kruscal-Shephard scaling; other settings are classical scaling, Sammon mapping, and Shephard-Kruskal nonmetric scaling [11]. In Figure 11.3 we show the MDS

desirable, in which the data are also rescaled, i.e. we set $\tilde{x}_{ij} = (x_{ij} - \bar{x}_j)/s_j$, where $s_j^2 = \frac{1}{n} \sum_{i=1}^{n} x_{ij}^2 - (\bar{x}_j)^2$ is the empirical variance of the $j$-th feature vector.

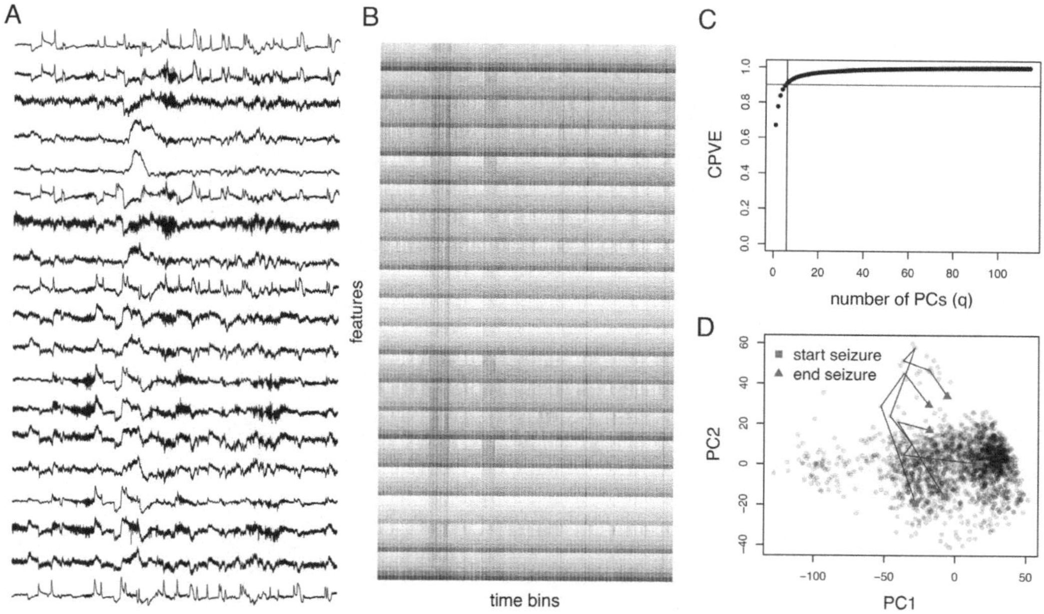


**FIGURE 11.2**
(A) A 60-sec sample of 19 EEG waveforms recorded from one patient diagnosed with epilepsy. (B) Spectral features (10-sec bins, 6 frequency bands for each waveform; total 114 features) extracted from the full recording session (1600 10-sec time bins). (C) Cumulative proportion of variance explained versus number of principal components of the matrix in (B). The first $q = 6$ principal components explain at least 90% of the variability. (D) Scatterplot of the first two principal components, with trajectories of three seizure events. (Color version available in electronic supplement.)

vectors (classical scaling) obtained from the feature matrix in Figure 11.2B. We can see that the embedding is equivalent to PCA (Figure 11.2D) up to sign flips (a property of classical scaling [11]) and, indeed, so are the trajectories of three seizure events. The use of non-Euclidean distances, such as Manhattan, Minkowski, tangent distance, and geodesic distances on manifolds (see next section) may yield quite different data compressions.

### 11.2.3 Isometric Feature Mapping

Isometric feature mapping (ISOMAP) is a *nonlinear dimension reduction* approach based on MDS. ISOMAP assumes the observed $p$-dimensional data to lie on a lower-dimensional *manifold*, i.e. a subset of $\mathbb{R}^p$ that has intrinsic dimensionality smaller than $p$. For instance, the set of points $\{(x_1, x_2) \in \mathbb{R}^2 : x_2 = 2 - 3x_1\}$ is a subset of $\mathbb{R}^2$, but it is also just a straight line which is a 1-dimensional object (indeed, the pair $(x_1, x_2)$ can be identified by each $x_1$ or $x_2$ alone via the equation $x_2 = 2 - 3x_1$). Similarly the hyperplane $\{x \in \mathbb{R}^p : x^T\beta + \beta_0 = 0\}$ is a $(p-1)$-dimensional manifold embedded in $\mathbb{R}^p$; infinitely many other types of manifolds, linear and nonlinear, can be identified with various linear and nonlinear constraints. If the data lie on a lower dimensional manifold, in order to learn the data structure, it is more reasonable to compute the *geodesic distance* between points over the manifold, i.e. the length of the shortest curve on the manifold connecting the two points, rather than the Euclidean distance in the full $p$-dimensional space. The ISOMAP Algorithm 3 is implemented as

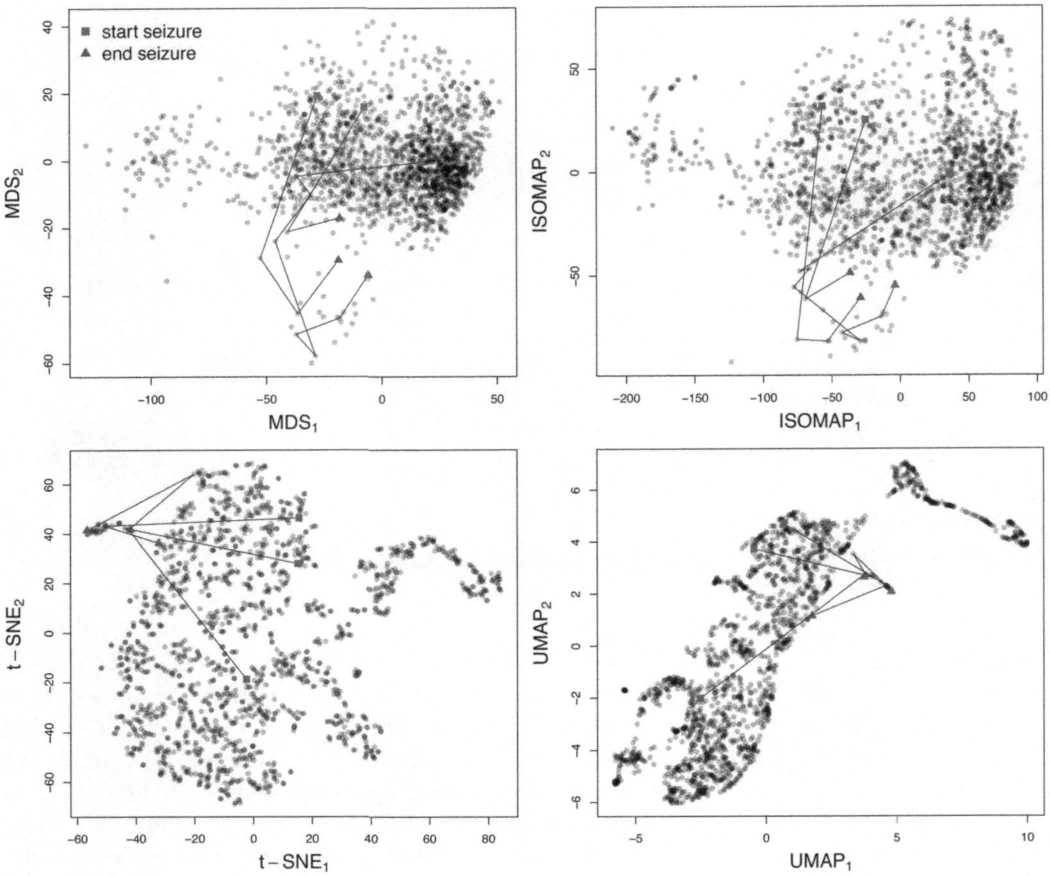


**FIGURE 11.3**
MDS, ISOMAP, t-SNE, and UMAP 2-dimensional representations of the feature matrix in Figure 11.2B. In addition, the trajectories of three known seizure events are plotted. (Color version available in electronic supplement.)

follows: (1) we approximate the manifold with a graph where the nodes are the data points and an edge connects a pair of points $(\mathbf{x}_i, \mathbf{x}_j)$ if $\mathbf{x}_j$ is one of the $K$-nearest neighbors of $\mathbf{x}_i$, for some prespecified integer $K \geq 1$; (2) we approximate the geodesic distance between any two points on the manifold by the shortest path connecting them on the graph; and finally (3) we apply MDS on the matrix of distances to obtain lower dimensional vectors. In Figure 11.3 we show the ISOMAP vectors obtained from the feature matrix in Figure 11.2B, using $K = 10$ neighbors. Also in this ISOMAP reduced space, as in PCA and MDS, the trajectories of three seizure events follow similar patterns.

### 11.2.4 t-distributed Stochastic Neighbor Embedding

The t-distributed Stochastic Neighbor Embedding (t-SNE) is a *nonlinear dimension reduction* method whose main application is *data visualization*, so the desired reduced number of dimensions is typically $q = 2$ or $q = 3$. The t-SNE algorithm is implemented as follows: (1) we first estimate a pairwise joint probability distribution for each pair of data points $(\mathbf{x}_i, \mathbf{x}_j)$ such that the probability is larger whenever $\mathbf{x}_i$ and $\mathbf{x}_j$ are close, and vice versa; (2) then, we specify pairwise joint probabilities on lower dimensional variables

**Algorithm 3** ISOMAP

INPUT: $\mathbf{x}_1, ..., \mathbf{x}_n \in \mathbb{R}^p$; integer $q \leq p$; number of neighbors $K \geq 1$.

1. Connect each data point with its $K$ nearest neighbors to create a graph where the nodes are the data points.
2. Compute the geodesic (shortest path) distance $d_{ij}$ between each pair $(x_i, x_j)$ of data points over the graph.
3. Implement step 2 of the MDS Algorithm 2 using the $n \times n$ matrix of geodesic distances $\mathbf{D} = [d_{ij}]$, to find lower dimensional points $\mathbf{z}_1, ..., \mathbf{z}_n \in \mathbb{R}^q$.

OUTPUT: $\mathbf{z}_1, ..., \mathbf{z}_n \in \mathbb{R}^q$.

$(\mathbf{z}_i, \mathbf{z}_j)$; and finally (3) we find $\mathbf{z}_1, ..., \mathbf{z}_n$ as the minimizers of the *Kullback–Leibler divergence* between the two sets of distributions. We refer to [25] for more details on the algorithm. An important parameter of the t-SNE algorithm is the *perplexity*, which can be interpreted as a continuous version of the number of neighbors in ISOMAP.

In Figure 11.3 we show the t-SNE 2-dimensional representations of the feature matrix in Figure 11.2B, using perplexity equal to 10. Also in this reduced space, as in the previously presented approaches, the trajectories of three seizure events follow similar patterns.

### 11.2.5 Uniform Manifold Approximation and Projection

Uniform Manifold Approximation and Projection (UMAP) can be seen as a substantial improvement to t-SNE. While t-SNE is designed to primarily preserve local structures, UMAP can well balance both local and global structures. UMAP assumes that the data are uniformly distributed on a Riemaniann manifold, the Riemaniann metric is approximately locally constant, and that the manifold is locally connected. The UMAP algorithm follows steps similar to t-SNE, with the main difference of minimizing the *cross-entropy* rather than the Kullback-Leibler divergence. This different objective function lets UMAP yield embeddings that preserve both short and long distances of the original space. The UMAP algorithm has two main parameters: *number of neighbors* and *minimum distance*. The first parameter acts in a similar way to the perplexity parameter of t-SNE. The second one instead is the minimum distance between any two points in the reduced space; this allows to avoid the so-called *clumping problem*, i.e. the case where many points in the reduced space are too close together. We refer to [18] for more details on the algorithm.

In Figure 11.3 we show the UMAP 2-dimensional representations of the feature matrix in Figure 11.2B, using number of neighbors equal to 10 and minimum distance equal to 0.1. Also in this reduced space, as in the previously presented approaches, the trajectories of three seizure events follow similar patterns.

### 11.2.6 Independent Components Analysis

Independent Components Analysis (ICA) is a statistical technique that allows us to decompose the observed multivariate signals into a number of "source signals" that are mutually statistically independent. Let $\mathbf{x}_t \in \mathbb{R}^p$ be the observed vector of neuronal signals (e.g. EEG or ECoG) at time $t$. The goal of ICA is to find a $q \times p$ matrix $U$, where $q \leq p$, such that the components of the lower dimensional vector $\mathbf{s}_t = U\mathbf{x}_t \in \mathbb{R}^q$, are statistically as independent as possible. Thus, ICA is similar to PCA, but ICA requires the components to be *independent*, not just uncorrelated. For the identification of $U$, no more than one of the components of $s_t$ is allowed to be Gaussian distributed. ICA can be implemented efficiently

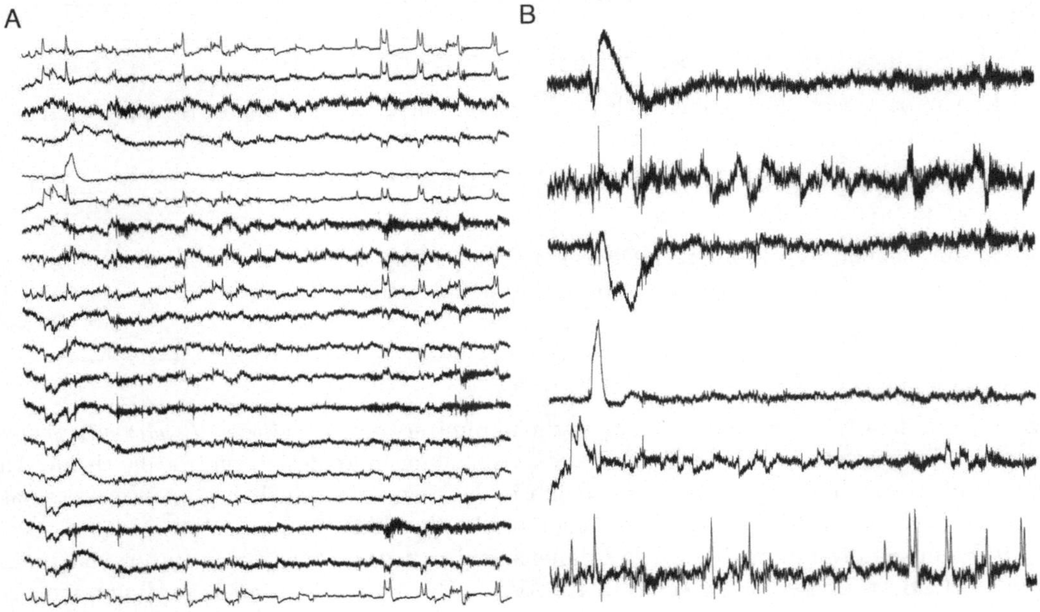


**FIGURE 11.4**
(A) A 60-sec portion of 19 EEG waveforms recorded from a patient diagnosed with epilepsy. (B) Plot of the six ICA components.

via the FastICA algorithm, which recovers the vectors $\{s_t\}$ by minimizing their mutual information, an information theoretical measure of multivariate dependence. We refer to [12] for details on the algorithm.

In the analysis of epilepsy data, ICA can be used for *blind source separation*. In Figure 11.4A we show a 60-sec portion of 19 EEG waveforms (same data as in Figure 11.2), and in Figure 11.4B we show six (independent) extracted source signals using ICA. The ICA features can then be used in subsequent analyses, for example as features for supervised learning tasks, including regression and classification.

## 11.3 Clustering

Clustering is an unsupervised approach that allows us to partition a set of data points into groups called *clusters* such that points within the same group are similar, while points belonging to different groups are substantially dissimilar. There are at least two possible uses of clustering in the study of epilepsy: (a) to identify different classes of patterns in the neural recordings of a patient; (b) to identify different groups of patients either based on their dissimilar neural activity under same experimental conditions, or based on their answers to surveys. Case (a) is of particular interest because clustering can help identify candidate *preictal, seizure, interictal periods* or other abnormal activity patterns in an automated way, without the use of training data, as opposed to classification (i.e., supervised), which requires labeled data. In case (b), clustering may be used to better understand common factors characterizing groups of patients. In this chapter we will focus on two widely applied clustering methods, $K$-means and hierarchical clustering, and their application to the analysis of epilepsy data. In Section 11.5.2 we show how these two methods can be implemented with the user-friendly function `clustering()` of the `R` package `unSuper`.

### 11.3.1 K-means Clustering

Given $n$ data points $\mathbf{x}_1, ..., \mathbf{x}_n \in \mathbb{R}^p$, we want to find a *partition* $C_1, ..., C_K$ of the data index set $\{1, ..., n\}$ (i.e. a collection $C_1, ..., C_K$ such that $\cup_{k=1}^{K} C_k = \{1, ..., n\}$ and $C_i \cap C_j = \emptyset$ if $i \neq j$) that minimizes the *objective dissimilarity*

$$W(C_1, ..., C_K) = \sum_{k=1}^{K} V(C_k) \tag{11.1}$$

where

$$V(C_k) = \frac{1}{|C_k|} \sum_{i,j \in C_k} \text{diss}(\mathbf{x}_i, \mathbf{x}_j) \tag{11.2}$$

is the *within-cluster variation*, and $\text{diss}(\mathbf{x}_i, \mathbf{x}_j)$ is a *dissimilarity* measure.

---

**Algorithm 4** $K$-MEANS CLUSTERING

INPUT: $\mathbf{x}_1, ..., \mathbf{x}_n \in \mathbb{R}^p$; number of clusters $K$; random partition $C_1, ..., C_K$.

1. Compute centroids $\hat{\mu}_1, ..., \hat{\mu}_K$.
2. Compute dissimilarity matrix $D \in \mathbb{R}^{n \times K}$, where $D_{ik} = \text{diss}(\mathbf{x}_i, \hat{\mu}_k)$.
3. Update clusters: for $k = 1, ..., K$

$$C_k := \left\{ i \in \{1, ..., n\} : \operatorname*{arg\,min}_{1 \leq j \leq K} D_{ij} = k \right\}$$

4. Repeat steps 1–3 until clusters do not change.

OUTPUT: Clusters $C_1, ..., C_K$.

---

A widely used clustering approach is *K-means clustering*, which finds $K$ clusters that minimize the objective dissimilarity $W(C_1, ..., C_K)$ in Equation (11.1), using the dissimilarity measure $\text{diss}(\mathbf{x}_i, \mathbf{x}_j) = \|\mathbf{x}_i - \mathbf{x}_j\|_2^2$. It can be shown that in this case Equation (11.1) reduces to

$$W(C_1, ..., C_K) = 2 \sum_{k=1}^{K} \sum_{i \in C_k} \sum_{j=1}^{p} (x_{ij} - \hat{\mu}_{kj})^2 \tag{11.3}$$

where $\hat{\mu}_k = (\hat{\mu}_{k1}, ..., \hat{\mu}_{kp}) = \frac{1}{|C_k|} \sum_{i \in C_k} \mathbf{x}_i$ is the *centroid* of cluster $C_k$. Algorithm 4, based on the alternative formulation of the objective dissimilarity, implements $K$-means clustering efficiently: starting from an initial random partition $C_1, ..., C_K$ of the $n$ data points $\mathbf{x}_1, ..., \mathbf{x}_n$, (1) we find the centroids $\hat{\mu}_1, ..., \hat{\mu}_K$; (2) we compute the distances of all data points from the $K$ centroids; (3) we update the clusters by assigning each data point to the cluster with closest centroid; and (4) we repeat the procedure multiple times until the clusters do not change. *Warning*: there may exist multiple local minimizers of the objective dissimilarity, and it is wise to run Algorithm 4 multiple times with different initial random partitions, and then select the output with the smallest objective dissimilarity. The number $K$ may be picked based on prior knowledge about how many groups of data we expect to find. However,

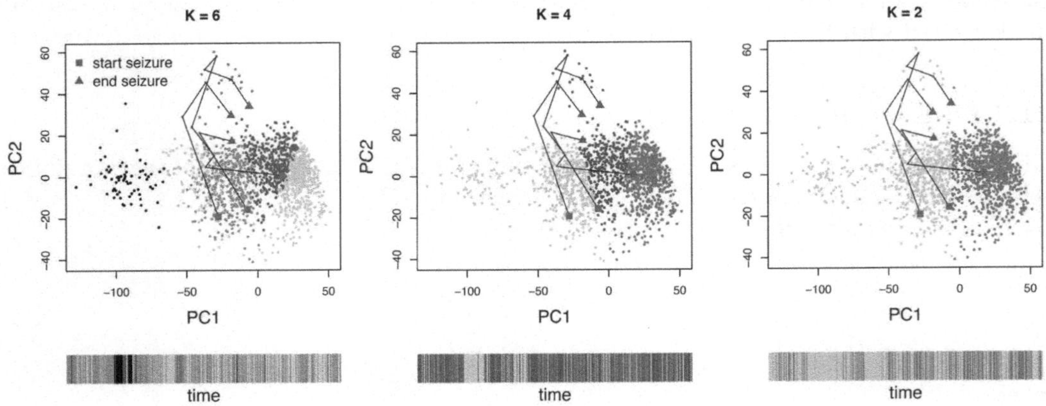


**FIGURE 11.5**
Clusters identified by $K$-means clustering, for three values of $K$. On the top, we plot the first two principal components with colors corresponding to different cluster assignments. On the bottom, we show how the spectral features (Figure 11.2B) are assigned to different clusters over the time. The start and end of the three seizure events fall within different clusters in most cases. (Color version available in electronic supplement.)

there exist various criteria to choose the number of clusters automatically, including the GAP statistic [23], the Silhouette method [19], and the Elbow method [22].

In Figure 11.5 we show the $K$-means cluster assignments for the 1600 114-dim data points (spectral features) displayed in Figure 11.2B, for various numbers of $K$ (GAP statistic suggested 4 clusters). We use PCA for visualizing the data on a 2-dimensional space. In most cases, the start and end of the three seizure events fall within different clusters.

### 11.3.2 Hierarchical Clustering

Hierarchical clustering is another widely used clustering approach. The main component of hierarchical clustering is the *dendrogram*, a tree structure that summarizes the evolution of cluster assignments for a varying allowed level of *between-cluster dissimilarity.* In Figure 11.6A we show a dendrogram for the extracted features displayed in Figure 11.2B. For a sufficiently small allowed between-cluster dissimilarity, every data point is a cluster. This corresponds to "cutting" the dendrogram on the bottom, yielding $n$ clusters consisting of the individual $n$ data points. For an increasing allowed between-cluster dissimilarity, clusters fuse into larger clusters. In Figure 11.6B we show three cluster assignments corresponding to different levels of allowed between-cluster dissimilarity (height of the dendrogram). The fusion of two leaves is straightforward, while the fusion of two clusters (multiple points) requires the computation of a *linkage*, a summary of the dissimilarities between the points belonging to different clusters; in other words, the linkage measures the dissimilarity between two clusters. Given a dissimilarity metric diss : $\mathbb{R}^p \times \mathbb{R}^p \to \mathbb{R}_+$ (e.g. $\text{diss}(x_i, x_j) = \|x_i - x_j\|_2^2$ or $\text{diss}(x_i, x_j) = -\text{cor}(x_i, x_j)$ (dimension-wise)) we can define various types of linkage between two clusters $A, B \subseteq \{1, ..., n\}$ with centroids $\hat{\mu}_A$ and $\hat{\mu}_B$, respectively:

1. *Complete* linkage: $d_{\text{complete}}(A, B) = \max_{i \in A, j \in B} \text{diss}(\mathbf{x}_i, \mathbf{x}_j)$
2. *Single* linkage: $d_{\text{single}}(A, B) = \min_{i \in A, j \in B} \text{diss}(\mathbf{x}_i, \mathbf{x}_j)$

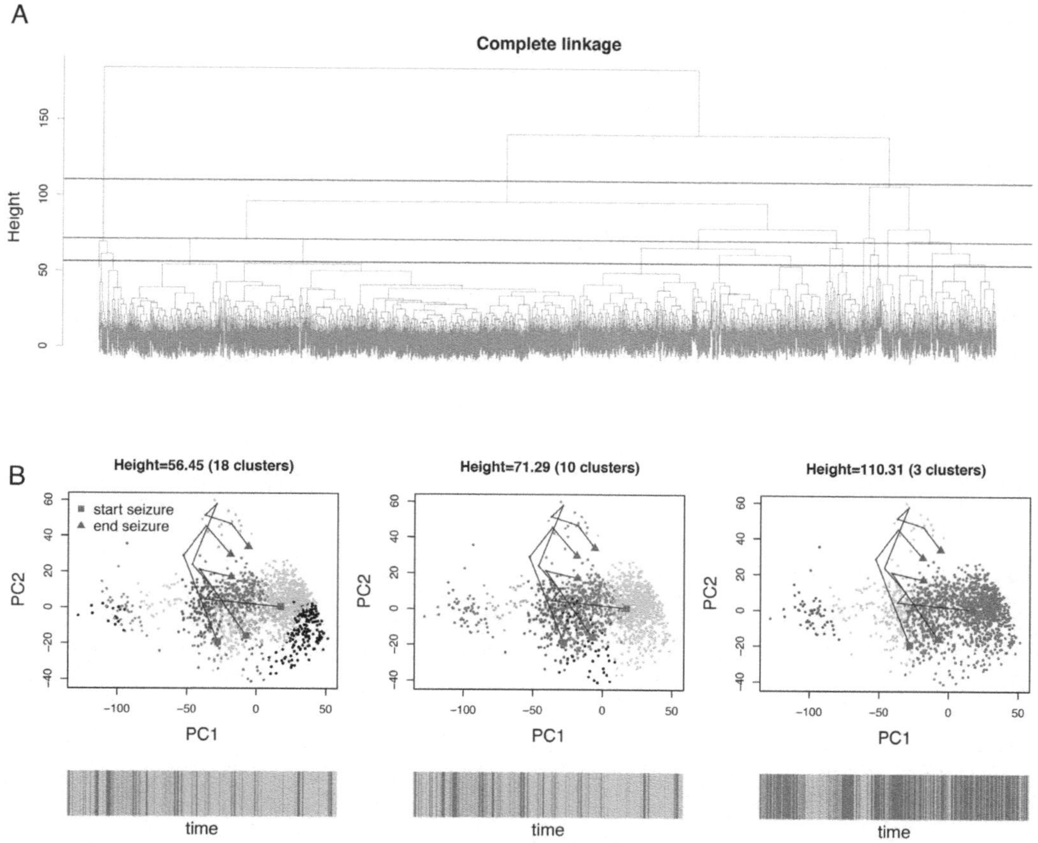


**FIGURE 11.6**
(A) Dendrogram for the extracted features displayed in Figure 11.2B. Each leaf corresponds to one of the 1600 time bins. For larger allowed levels of between-cluster dissimilarity (height), leaves merge into clusters, and clusters merge into larger clusters according to their complete linkage. (B) Cluster assignments corresponding to the three heights (between-cluster dissimilarity) highlighted in (A). In the bottom, we show the cluster assignments of the spectral features over time. (Color version available in electronic supplement.)

3. *Average* linkage: $d_{\text{ave}}(A, B) = \frac{1}{|A||B|} \sum_{i \in A, j \in B} \text{diss}(\mathbf{x}_i, \mathbf{x}_j)$
4. *Centroid* linkage: $d_{\text{centroid}}(A, B) = \text{diss}(\hat{\mu}_A, \hat{\mu}_B)$

With complete linkage, we look for the largest of the pairwise dissimilarities between a point in cluster $A$ and a point in cluster $B$; single linkage finds instead the smallest of all such dissimilarities. Average linkage is simply the average of all dissimilarities, while centroid linkage computes the dissimilarity between the centroids of the two clusters. The dendrogram shape strongly depends on the dissimilarity measure and linkage. Complete and average linkage are the most widely used because they usually produce more balanced clusters; centroid linkage often generates inversions, where a cluster may split into two clusters for larger allowed dissimilarities, rather than merging with another cluster. Algorithm 5 outlines the steps to produce the dendrogram.

**Algorithm 5** HIERARCHICAL CLUSTERING (DENDROGRAM)

INPUT: $\mathbf{x}_1, ..., \mathbf{x}_n \in \mathbb{R}^p$; $h = 0$; linkage function $d(*, *)$.

1. $K = n$ clusters given by $C_1 = \mathbf{x}_1, ..., C_n = \mathbf{x}_n$.
2. For $K = n, ..., 2$,
   (a) Compute $\mathbf{D} = [d_{ij}] \in \mathbb{R}^{K \times K}$, where $d_{ij} = d(C_i, C_j)$.
   (b) Merge the two clusters $C_i, C_j$ that have smallest $d_{ij} = d^*$. Update cluster indices $C_1, ..., C_K$, where $K = n - 1$, and $h := (h, d^*)$.
   (c) Define $\mathcal{C}_K := \{C_1, ..., C_K\}$.

OUTPUT: Sequence of cluster sets $\mathcal{C}_1, ..., \mathcal{C}_n$, and height of merging site $h$.

## 11.4 Matrix Completion

In epilepsy studies, we may encounter datasets that are *incomplete.* A typical example is survey data, where several entries are *missing* because survey respondents may have, voluntarily or involuntarily, omitted to provide some answers, thereby producing incomplete data that cannot be readily analysed in the same way as complete data. Moreover, electrophysiological recordings, such as EEG and ECoG, may be affected by artifacts and other measurement errors that strongly corrupt time portions of the recordings, which ultimately need to be discarded and treated as missing data. Similarly, in MRI and fMRI, various causes of artifacts may cause data missingness, such as, incomplete imaging of the brain regions of interest. Finally, data collected via wearable machines is often incomplete because the patient may perform some sudden movements or just temporarily take off the device. *Matrix completion* techniques allow us to reconstruct data matrices that contain missing entries. In this section, we will focus on two approaches: *K-nearest neighbor completion* and *low-rank completion.* In Section 11.5.2 we show how these two methods can be implemented with the user-friendly function `completion` of the `R` package `unSuper`.

### 11.4.1 K-Nearest Neighbors Matrix Completion

Suppose that we cannot observe the data matrix $\mathbf{X} \in \mathbb{R}^{n \times p}$ fully, but only a portion $\mathbf{X}_O = (X_{ij})_{(i,j) \in O}$, where $O \subset \{1, ..., n\} \times \{1, ..., p\}$. Can we try to guess the values $\mathbf{X}_{O^c}$? The *K-nearest neighbors* (KNN) matrix completion is probably the most straightforward approach for filling in the missing entries of a data matrix. According to the KNN approach, a missing entry $(i, j)$ of an $n \times p$ matrix $\mathbf{X}$ is filled in by a value that is an appropriate *summary* of the $j$-th feature values found on the other $K$ rows that appear to be most similar to row $i$. Specifically, the KNN Algorithm 6 proceeds as follows: for every partially observed data vector $\mathbf{x}_{i.}$, (1) we compute some suitable distance from $\mathbf{x}_{i.}$ to all other $n - 1$ data vectors, and (2) for every unobserved feature value $x_{ij}$ on row $i$, (a) we find the $K$-nearest neighbor data vectors that contain an observation for feature $j$, and then (b) we combine such $K$ values to obtain a guess for the missing entry $x_{ij}$.

KNN can be used with various types of data, including *numerical* and *categorical.* Indeed, KNN is especially appropriate for survey data, because surveys may involve questions that require categorical answers (sex, seizure types, epilepsy etiology) and numerical answers, either *continuous* (age, time since last seizure) or *discrete* (number of antiseizure medicines,

**Algorithm 6** KNN Matrix Completion

Input: $\mathbf{X}_O$; integer $K > 0$; distance function dist(, ); summary functions $g_1(\omega), ..., g_p(\omega)$.

For each $i \in \{h : \exists j, (h, j) \notin O\}$

1. Compute $D_{ik} = \text{dist}(\mathbf{x}_{i.}, \mathbf{x}_{k.})$, for $k = 1, ..., n$.
2. For all $j$ such that $(i, j) \notin O$,
   (a) Find $\mathcal{N}_K(i; j) = \{k \in O_j : D_{ik} \leq d_{ijK}\}$, where $O_j = \{k : x_{kj} \text{ is observed}\}$, and $d_{ijK}$ is such that $|\mathcal{N}_K(i; j)| = K$.
   (b) Update $x_{ij} := g_j\left((x_{kj})_{k \in \mathcal{N}_K(i;j)}\right)$.

Output: Complete data matrix $\mathbf{X}$.

seizure frequency). Depending on the type of data that is missing, appropriate data *summary functions* should be used. For instance, the *mean* is appropriate for continuous data; the *median* is reasonable for continuous and discrete data; the *mode* is appropriate for discrete and categorical data. Moreover, the distance between data vectors should be based only on the jointly observed features. For example, given two partially observed 4-dimensional data vectors $x = (x_1, x_2, \star, x_4)$ and $y = (\star, y_2, y_3, y_4)$, where "$\star$" denotes a missing entry, the distance between $x$ and $y$ should be replaced by the distance between the restricted 2-dimensional vectors $\tilde{x} = (x_2, x_4)$ and $\tilde{y} = (y_2, y_4)$, since only features 2 and 4 have observations in both data vectors $x$ and $y$. If the Euclidean distance was used, then we would have $\text{dist}(x, y) = \sqrt{(x_2 - y_2)^2 + (x_4 - y_4)^2}$.

The number $K$ can be picked with various criteria. A simple one requires to apply KNN on a more incomplete version of $\mathbf{X}$, obtained by randomly removing data entries that were actually observed, and then evaluating the reconstruction performance of the algorithm for various values of $K$. Algorithm 6 can also accommodate cases where the data matrix $\mathbf{X}$ contains continuous data together with discrete and/or categorical variables. All we need is to define a distance function that appropriately combines for distances between points in a Euclidean space (e.g. Euclidean distance or Manhattan distance) and class discrepancies (e.g. Hamming distance); alternatively, we may simply compute distances based only on the continuous features or only on the discrete or the categorical ones.

In Figure 11.7 we show the performance of KNN at reconstructing incomplete survey data. In Figure 11.7A we show the ground truth survey (simulated) data with $n = 200$ survey responses about 4 categorical variables (two binary, one with 3 levels, and one with 4 levels) and 16 numerical variables. In Figure 11.7B we show an incomplete version of the data matrix in A. We applied KNN to recover the matrix in A from the matrix in B. We used the mean summary function to complete the missing continuous variable entries, and the mode summary function to complete the missing categorical variable entries. The distance function to identify neighbors was defined as the Euclidean distance between only the continuous variables. In Figure 11.7C we display the completion risk obtained as the average loss (Euclidean distance) between reconstructed values and true values of an additional 10% of data entries that we randomly dropped from the observed set $\mathbf{X}_O$. We find optimal $K = 21$. In Figure 11.7D we show the reconstructed matrix obtained by applying KNN to the matrix in Figure 11.7B. In Figure 11.7E and F we summarize the performance of the recovery of the 4 categorical survey answers, and the performance at recovering the missing observations about the 16 continuous quantities. KNN appears to perform well.

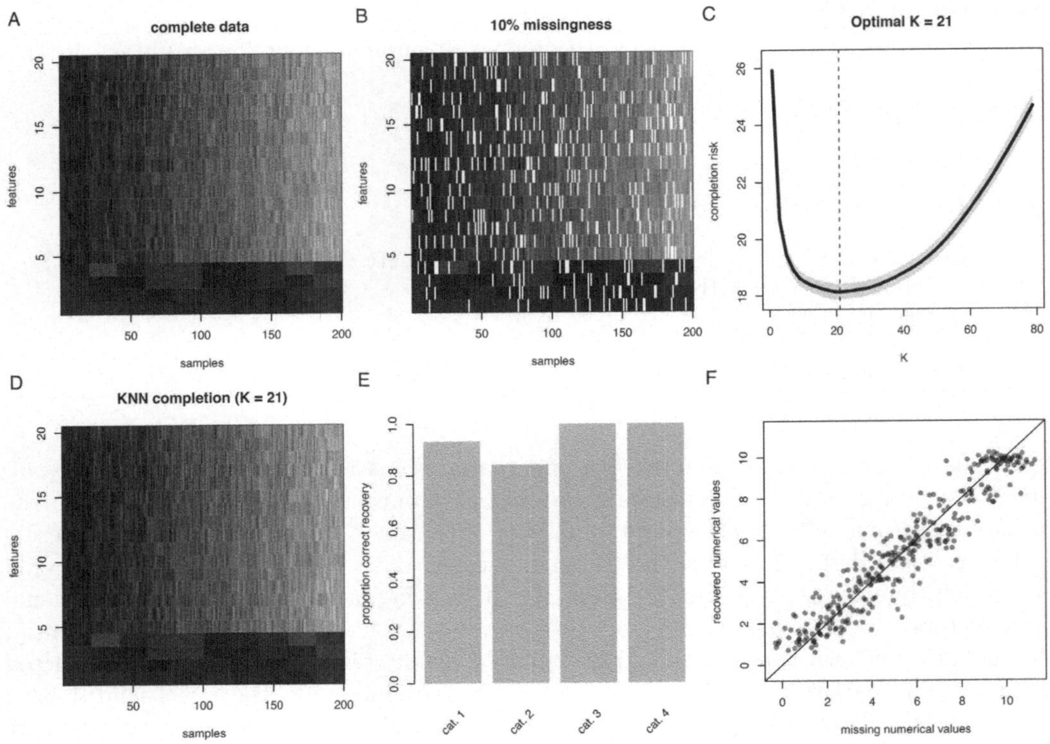


**FIGURE 11.7**
(A) Heatmap of complete (simulated) survey data with $n = 200$ survey responses about 4 categorical variables and 16 numerical variables. (B) Incomplete version of the data matrix in (A) (10% missing values). (C) Completion risk and the optimal $K$. (D) Reconstructed matrix obtained by applying KNN to the incomplete matrix in (B) using the optimal $K = 21$. (E) Recovery accuracy of the missing categorical survey answers. (F) Recovery accuracy of the missing numerical survey answers.

### 11.4.2 Low-Rank Completion

Another approach to matrix completion, when the entries are numerical, is *low-rank completion*. The complete data matrix $\mathbf{X} \in \mathbb{R}^{n \times p}$ has rank $q := \text{rank}(\mathbf{X}) \leq \min\{n, p\}$ if it can be written as

$$\mathbf{X} = \sum_{k=1}^{q} \sigma_k \mathbf{u}_k \mathbf{v}_k^T$$

where $\sigma_1, ..., \sigma_q$ are nonzero *singular values*, and $\mathbf{u}_k \in \mathbb{R}^n$ and $\mathbf{v}_k \in \mathbb{R}^p$ are orthonormal vectors; $\mathbf{X}$ is low-rank if $q < \min\{n, p\}$. Under some conditions [5], a general optimization problem for the exact recovery of a low-rank matrix $\mathbf{X}$ based on a set of observed entries $\mathbf{X}_O = (x_{ij})_{(i,j)\in O}$ is

$$\begin{aligned} &\min_{\mathbf{Z}} \ \text{rank}(\mathbf{Z}) \\ &\text{s.t. } z_{ij} = x_{ij}, \ (i,j) \in O \end{aligned} \tag{11.4}$$

where the portion $\mathbf{Z}_{O^c}$ of the solution $\mathbf{Z}$ recovers $\mathbf{X}_{O^c}$. However, this problem is non-convex, and alternative more efficient approaches have been proposed. One approach [5] replaces $\text{rank}(\mathbf{Z})$ with the nuclear norm $\|\mathbf{X}\|_* := \sum_{k=1}^{\min\{n,p\}} \sigma_k$, making the problem solvable via semidefinite programming. Another efficient approach, which we discuss here more in depth, is based on PCA [13, 17], and we outline it in Algorithm 7, where we *impute* the missing values $\mathbf{X}_{O^c}$ by iteratively recovering a low rank matrix approximation of the full data matrix based on the observed data. Specifically, (1) we first create a simple complete data matrix $\mathbf{Z}$, which equals $\mathbf{X}$ over the entry set $O$, and approximate the values in $O^c$ as the column-wise averages based on the available observed data. Then, (2) we obtain the low-rank approximation $\mathbf{Z} \approx A \times B$, where $A \in \mathbb{R}^{n \times q}$ and $B \in \mathbb{R}^{q \times p}$, with $q << p$; the matrices $A$ and $B$ are simply given by the first $q$ vectors of principal components of $\mathbf{Z}$ and the first $q$ corresponding eigenvectors. Then, (3) we update the values $\mathbf{Z}_{O^c}$ with $(A \times B)_{O^c}$; we repeat the operations in steps 2–3 until we observe no substantial changes in the low-rank recovery of $\mathbf{Z}_O$.

**Algorithm 7** PCA Low-rank Matrix Completion

INPUT: $\mathbf{X}_O$; integer $q \leq p$.

1. Obtain $\mathbf{Z} \in \mathbb{R}^{n \times p}$, where $\mathbf{Z}_O = \mathbf{X}_O$, and $z_{ij} = \frac{1}{|O_j|} \sum_{k \in O_j} x_{kj}$, where $O_j = \{k : (k, j) \in O\}$ for $(i, j) \notin O$.
2. Solve
$$(A, B) = \underset{A \in \mathbb{R}^{n \times q}, B \in \mathbb{R}^{q \times p}}{\arg\min} \sum_{i=1}^{n} \sum_{j=1}^{p} (z_{ij} - A_{i.} B_{.j})^2$$
via PCA applied to the matrix $\mathbf{Z}$.
3. Update $z_{ij} = A_i B_j$, for all $(i, j) \notin O$.
4. Repeat 2–3 until $\sum_{(i,j) \in O} (z_{ij} - A_{i.} B_{.j})^2$ stops decreasing.

OUTPUT: Complete data matrix $\mathbf{Z}$.

The low-rank completion approach is most appropriate with data entries that are numerical continuous variables. If the variables are discrete, then the algorithm could be adjusted by applying an appropriate thresholding or rounding operation on the approximated entry values. If the incomplete data contains categorical features, then other matrix completion approaches should be pursued, such as KNN (Section 11.4.1).

In Figure 11.8 we show the performance of the PCA low-rank completion Algorithm 7 at recovering the spectral features of EEG recordings. In Figure 11.8A we display the complete data (200 time bins, 114 features; this is a subset of the data used in Figure 11.2), while in Figure 11.8B we present an incomplete version of the data, where we randomly dropped 10% of the data values. In Figure 11.8C we compute the completion risk by dropping additional entries and evaluating the recovery accuracy of those known entries; we find that rank $q = 17$ is optimal. In Figure 11.8D we show the completed data matrix based on the PCA completion Algorithm 7, and in Figure 11.8E we compare the recovered values with the true missing values. Finally, in Figure 11.8F we compare the recovered values with those recovered by using the theoretically more accurate but more computationally expensive nuclear norm minimization [5]: the recovered values yielded by the two methods appear to be reasonably close.

## 11.5 R Code

The R package `unSuper` can be used to implement the unsupervised learning methods presented in this chapter and is available at the repository accompanying this book and

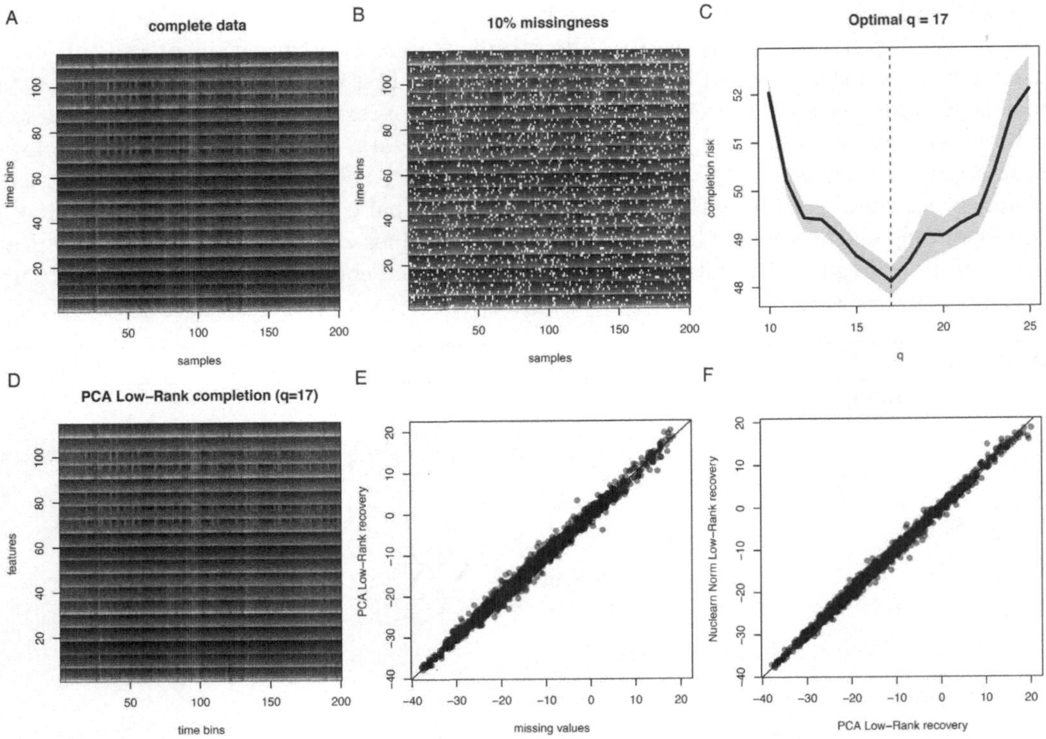


**FIGURE 11.8**
(A) A portion of EEG spectral densities as in Figure 11.2. (B) Incomplete version of the data matrix in (A) (10% missing values). (C) Completion risk and the optimal rank $q$. (D) Reconstructed matrix by applying the PCA completion Algorithm 7 to the incomplete data in (B). (E) Recovery accuracy for the missing values. (F) Comparison of values recovered via PCA completion versus values obtained via nuclear norm minimization: the values appear to be reasonably similar.

`https://github.com/gvincistat/unSuper`. Example EEG data (`EEG.Rdata`) and survey data (`SURVEY.Rdata`) are available in the book repository and `https://github.com/gvincistat/UnsupEpilepsy`.

### 11.5.1 Datasets

The file `EEG.Rdata` contains EEG data extracted from the file `PN10-4.5.6.edf` that is publicly available in the repository https://physionet.org/content/siena-scalp-eeg/1.0.0/PN10/#files-panel. The EEG signals were recorded from one patient for 4 hours and 37 minutes, during which 3 seizures happened, with sampling rate 512Hz using electrodes arranged on the basis of the international 10-20 System (19 channels). Inside `EEG.Rdata` there are four objects: `RAW`, `X`, `seizures`, and `sRate`. The matrix `RAW` contains EEG signals relative to the first five minutes of the experiment (300sec $\times$ 512 = 153600 rows, 19 columns). The matrix `X` contains power densities extracted from the whole EEG dataset at the six frequency bands 0–4 Hz, 4–8 Hz, 8–16 Hz, 16–32 Hz, 32–64 Hz, and 64–128 Hz, over time bins of 10 sec length. The matrix `X` has $n = 1600$ rows (time bins) and $p = 114$ columns (6 spectral features for each of the 19 EEG channels). Finally, the list `seizures` contains the time bins of the three seizures, and `sRate=512` is the EEG sampling rate. The file `SURVEY.Rdata` contains the matrix `SURVEY`, a simulated matrix of survey data with 20 columns, corresponding to 20 hypothetical questions of which four are categorical and 16 are numerical.

### 11.5.2 The R Package "unSuper"

This package contains three functions: `reduction()`, `clustering()`, and `completion()`. The package contains its own tutorial with basic examples, but here we present other examples for the analysis of epilepsy data. The package can be loaded with the command:

```
library(unSuper)
```

**Dimension reduction:** The function `reduction()` has five main arguments: `X`, an $n \times p$ matrix where $n$ is the number of samples and $p$ is the number of features; `q`, the desired number of dimensions of the reduced space; `method`, the name of the dimension reduction method to use (`"pca"`, `"mds"`, `"isomap"`, `"tsne"`, `"umap"`, or `"ica"`); `rescale`, which asks whether we want to rescale the data (default is `FALSE`); and `Plot`, which asks whether we want an output plot of the results. Additional arguments can be used given different `method`.

We now present some examples of use of the function. First, let us load the data (make sure the file `EEG.Rdata` is in the working directory of `R`):

```
load(file = "EEG.Rdata")
X <- EEG$X
RAW <- EEG$RAW[1:(60*512), ]
```

The following code implements PCA on the matrix `X`, and will return various objects, including a matrix `Z` containing the first $q = 2$ principal components vectors:

```
PCA <- reduction(X = X, method = "pca", q = 2, cpve = 0.9, Plot = TRUE)
```

The option `Plot=TRUE` will also yield a figure containing the plot of cumulative proportion of variance explained (CPVE) versus the number of principal components, and the scatterplot of the first two principal components. Moreover, it will print the proportion of variance explained by the first q=2 principal components and how many components would be required to explain at least a proportion of variance `cpve=0.9`. The PCA computation is based on the function `prcomp` of the R-package `stats`. The full output of the `prcomp()` function is in the output object `full`. Additional arguments of the `prcomp()` function can be input as argument of `reduction()` (type `?prcomp` for more details). All other methods can be implemented in a similar fashion as follows (however, note that ICA is applied on the matrix `RAW` of EEG signals rather than the power densities):

```
MDS <- reduction(X = X, method = "mds", q = 2)
ISOMAP <- reduction(X = X, method = "isomap", q = 2, neighbors = 10)
set.seed(123)
TSNE <- reduction(X = X, method = "tsne", q = 2, neighbors = 10, max_iter = 5000)
set.seed(123)
UMAP <- reduction(X = X, method = "umap", q = 2, neighbors = 10, min_dist = 0.1)
set.seed(123)
ICA <- reduction(X = RAW, method = "ica", q = 6, tol = 10e-8, maxit = 200)
```

By adding the argument `Plot=TRUE` a visual output similar to the one presented in this chapter will be produced from each of the commands above.

**Clustering:** The function `clustering()` has six main arguments: `X`, an $n \times p$ matrix where $n$ is the number of samples and $p$ is the number of features; `K`, the desired number of clusters; `method`, the name of the clustering method to use (`"kmeans"` or `"hierarchical"`); `linkage`, the type of linkage to use if `method="hierarchical"`; `rescale`, which asks whether we want to rescale the data (default is `FALSE`); and `Plot`, which asks whether we want an output plot of the results. Additional arguments can be used given different `method`.

We now present some examples of use of the function. First, let us load the data (make sure the file `EEG.Rdata` is in the working directory of `R`):

```
load(file = "EEG.Rdata")
X <- EEG$X
```

The following code implements K-means clustering and Hierarchical clustering on the matrix `X`, and will return various objects, including: a vector `cluster` of indices identifying the cluster number for each data point; a $K \times p$ matrix `centroids` containing the coordinates of the $K$ cluster centroids; and `full`, which is the full output of the clustering function used (either `kmeans()` or `hclust()` from the `R` package `stats`).

```
KMEANS <- clustering(X, K = 4, method = "kmeans", iter.max = 10000, nstart = 500,
    Plot = TRUE)
HCLUST <- clustering(X, K = 3, method = "hierarchical", linkage = "complete", Plot
    = TRUE)
```

The optional argument `gap.boot` is the number of bootstrap samples for the computation of the GAP statistic if `method = "kmeans"` is used; if `gap.boot = 0`, then it is not computed. To learn more about optional arguments, type `?kmeans` for K-means and `?hclust` for hierarchical clustering.

**Matrix completion:** The function `completion()` has nine arguments: `XO`, an $n \times p$ matrix where $n$ is the number of samples and $p$ is the number of features, and missing entries are equal to `NA`; `method`, the matrix completion method to be used (`"knn"` or `"lowrank"`); `notquant`, a vector of column numbers of the categorical features; `neighbors`, the number of neighbors $K$ to use in the KNN algorithm, or a vector of values of $K$ from which one will be automatically selected; `q`, the rank of the low-rank completion, or a vector of values from which one will be automatically selected; `reps`, the number of iterations for the selection of optimal parameter (number of neighbors $K$ if `method="KNN"`, and $q$ if `method="lowrank"`); `max.iters`, the maximum number of iterations for low-rank completion; `tol`, tolerance parameter for convergence accuracy of low-rank completion; `Plot`, which asks whether we want an output plot of the results.

*KNN matrix completion*

We now present an example of use of the function `completion()` with `method = "KNN"`. First let us load the data (make sure the file `SURVEY.Rdata` is in the working directory of `R`) and create an incomplete version of it for illustration:

```
load(file = "SURVEY.Rdata")
X <- SURVEY
set.seed(123)
propmiss <- 0.1
n <- nrow(X)
p <- ncol(X)
XO <- X
XO[sample(1:(n*p), size = round(propmiss*n*p))] <- NA
```

The following code implements the KNN matrix completion on the incomplete matrix XO, and will return various objects, including a $n \times p$ matrix Z, which is a completed version of XO. Other components of the output are about the completion performance at each of the values of $K$ provided in the input vector neighbors:

```
COMPL.KNN <- completion(XO, method = "KNN", notquant = 1:4, neighbors = seq(1, 80,
     2), reps = 50, Plot = TRUE)
```

*Low-Rank matrix completion*

We now present an example of use of the function completion() with method = "lowrank". First let us load the data (make sure the file EEG.Rdata is in the working directory of R) and create an incomplete version of it for illustration:

```
load(file = "EEG.Rdata")
X <- EEG$X[1:200,]
set.seed(123)
propmiss <- 0.1
n <- nrow(X); p <- ncol(X)
XO <- X
XO[sample(1:(n*p), size = round(propmiss*n*p))] <- NA
```

The following code implements the low-rank matrix completion on the incomplete matrix XO, and will return various objects, including a $n \times p$ matrix Z, which is a completed version of XO. Other components of the output are about the approximate completion performance at each of the values of $q$ provided in the input vector q:

```
COMPL.LR <- completion(XO = XO, method = "lowrank", q = 10:25, max.iters = 1000,
     tol = 10^-7, reps = 50, Plot = TRUE)
```

## 11.6 Summary

In this chapter, we discussed several powerful unsupervised learning methods, including dimension reduction, clustering, and matrix completion, and demonstrate their application to complex and high-dimensional data in epilepsy.

Compared with supervised learning methods, unsupervised learning allows us discover meaningful structures in the data without the "supervision" of response variables or labels. However, unsupervised learning can be auxiliary to supervised learning. For instance, the principal components of a large set of predictor variables can be used as features for regression or classification, while clustering may be used to identify new meaningful distinct classes of EEG patterns that may become the object of a subsequent classification performed on future datasets. Dimension reduction approaches can also reduce the noise in feature spaces, ultimately improving the performance of supervised learning applications. Matrix completion approaches are essential to implement supervised learning when regression or classification involve incomplete data matrices. Dimension reduction and clustering techniques can also be used simply for visualization, in any step of the data analysis pipeline, whenever we want to visualize outputs that have dimension larger than three.

Beyond the material presented in this chapter, the field of unsupervised learning is extensive, and many other methods may be of use to researchers in epilepsy. For example, the PCA algorithm discussed in Algorithm 1 performs well when $n$ is larger than $p$, and the relationships between variables are linear. Otherwise, alternative approaches should be considered, including sparse PCA [11], kernel PCA [6], and robust PCA [3]. Other useful dimension reduction methods include functional PCA [9], linear discriminant analysis, self-organizing maps [16], principal curves [10], local linear embedding [20], and local MDS [26]. Similarly, $K$-means clustering and hierarchical clustering are only two possible clustering methods; others include $K$-medoids [14], Gaussian mixture model [2, 21], and spectral clustering [27], as well as many others. For more literature on matrix completion, we refer the readers to [1, 4, 7, 8, 15, 17, 24].

## Bibliography

[1] Rebecca R Andridge and Roderick JA Little. A review of hot deck imputation for survey non-response. *International Statistical Review*, 78(1):40–64, 2010.

[2] Javad Birjandtalab, Maziyar Baran Pouyan, and Mehrdad Nourani. Unsupervised EEG analysis for automated epileptic seizure detection. In *First International Workshop on Pattern Recognition*, volume 10011, pages 124–128. SPIE, 2016.

[3] Thierry Bouwmans and El Hadi Zahzah. Robust PCA via principal component pursuit: A review for a comparative evaluation in video surveillance. *Computer Vision and Image Understanding*, 122:22–34, 2014.

[4] Jian-Feng Cai, Emmanuel J Candès, and Zuowei Shen. A singular value thresholding algorithm for matrix completion. *SIAM Journal on Optimization*, 20(4):1956–1982, 2010.

[5] Emmanuel J Candès and Benjamin Recht. Exact matrix completion via convex optimization. *Foundations of Computational Mathematics*, 9(6):717, 2009.

[6] LJ Cao, Kok Seng Chua, WK Chong, HP Lee, and QM Gu. A comparison of PCA, KPCA and ICA for dimensionality reduction in support vector machine. *Neurocomputing*, 55(1-2):321–336, 2003.

[7] Sourav Chatterjee. Matrix estimation by universal singular value thresholding. *The Annals of Statistics*, 43(1):177–214, 2015.

[8] Andrew Gelman and Jennifer Hill. *Data Analysis Using Regression and Multilevel/Hierarchical Models.* Cambridge University Press, 2006.

[9] Peter Hall, Hans-Georg Müller, and Jane-Ling Wang. Properties of principal component methods for functional and longitudinal data analysis. *The Annals of Statistics*, 34(3):1493–1517, 2006.

[10] Trevor Hastie and Werner Stuetzle. Principal curves. *Journal of the American Statistical Association*, 84(406):502–516, 1989.

[11] Trevor Hastie, Robert Tibshirani, and Jerome H Friedman. *The Elements of Statistical Learning: Data Mining, Inference, and Prediction*, volume 2. Springer, 2009.

[12] Aapo Hyvarinen. Fast and robust fixed-point algorithms for independent component analysis. *IEEE Transactions on Neural Networks*, 10(3):626–634, 1999.

[13] Gareth James, Daniela Witten, Trevor Hastie, and Robert Tibshirani. An introduction to statistical learning, second edition. New York: Springer, 2021.

[14] Leonard Kaufman and Peter J Rousseeuw. Partitioning around medoids (program PAM). *Finding Groups in Data: An Introduction to Cluster Analysis*, 344:68–125, 1990.

[15] Raghunandan H Keshavan, Andrea Montanari, and Sewoong Oh. Matrix completion from a few entries. *IEEE Transactions on Information Theory*, 56(6):2980–2998, 2010.

[16] Teuvo Kohonen. Self-organized formation of topologically correct feature maps. *Biological Cybernetics*, 43(1):59–69, 1982.

[17] Rahul Mazumder, Trevor Hastie, and Robert Tibshirani. Spectral regularization algorithms for learning large incomplete matrices. *The Journal of Machine Learning Research*, 11:2287–2322, 2010.

[18] Leland McInnes, John Healy, and James Melville. UMAP: Uniform manifold approximation and projection for dimension reduction. *arXiv preprint arXiv:1802.03426*, 2018.

[19] Peter J Rousseeuw. Silhouettes: a graphical aid to the interpretation and validation of cluster analysis. *Journal of Computational and Applied Mathematics*, 20:53–65, 1987.

[20] Sam T Roweis and Lawrence K Saul. Nonlinear dimensionality reduction by locally linear embedding. *Science*, 290(5500):2323–2326, 2000.

[21] Abdulhamit Subasi. Eeg signal classification using wavelet feature extraction and a mixture of expert model. *Expert Systems with Applications*, 32(4):1084–1093, 2007.

[22] Robert Thorndike. Who belongs in the family? *Psychometrika*, 18(4):267–276, 1953.

[23] Robert Tibshirani, Guenther Walther, and Trevor Hastie. Estimating the number of clusters in a data set via the gap statistic. *Journal of the Royal Statistical Society: Series B (Statistical Methodology)*, 63(2):411–423, 2001.

[24] Olga Troyanskaya, Michael Cantor, Gavin Sherlock, Pat Brown, Trevor Hastie, Robert Tibshirani, David Botstein, and Russ B Altman. Missing value estimation methods for dna microarrays. *Bioinformatics*, 17(6):520–525, 2001.

[25] Laurens Van der Maaten and Geoffrey Hinton. Visualizing data using t-SNE. *Journal of Machine Learning Research*, 9(11), 2008.

[26] Jarkko Venna and Samuel Kaski. Local multidimensional scaling. *Neural Networks*, 19(6-7):889–899, 2006.

[27] Yair Weiss. Segmentation using eigenvectors: a unifying view. In *Proceedings of the Seventh IEEE International Conference on Computer Vision*, volume 2, pages 975–982. IEEE, 1999.

# 12

## *Supervised Learning*

**Emilian R. Vankov**
*Wayfair (USA)*

**Kais Gadhoumi**
*Duke University (USA)*

### CONTENTS



Supervised learning is a class of machine learning and artificial intelligence used across a large spectrum of disciplines to solve prediction, classification, and regression problems. This class of algorithms feed on pre-labelled data to learn input-to-output mapping functions. Many clinical and experimental applications in epilepsy use supervised learning approaches. Examples include automatic seizure detection and prediction, EEG and imaging analysis, surgical planning, and prediction of surgical outcome. This chapter reviews a selection of important methods of supervised learning and illustrates their application to seizure detection and classification through worked examples in Python using a public real-world EEG dataset. The chapter discusses important topics in supervised learning such as statistical fit, data imbalance, and performance evaluation.

DOI: 10.1201/9781003254515-12

## 12.1 Introduction

Supervised learning algorithms are a widely studied class of algorithms in the field of machine learning that aim to infer or predict an outcome, given a set of features (also called predictors) that can be used to explain the variability in the outcome. More specifically, given pairs of observations $(y_i, X_i)$, where $i = 1, \ldots, n$ are $n$ observations, $y_i$ is the outcome, and $X_i \in \mathbf{R}^d$ is a $d$-dimensional vector for each observation $i$, interest lies in performing inference or prediction on $y_i$ given the observed features $X_i$. Supervised problems are typically divided into classification and regression. Classification refers to a set of problems for which the outcome is a label, which may be binary or multi-class. For example, predicting whether a particular EEG segment reflects an ictal state (i.e., seizure) or an interictal state (i.e., between seizures) is a binary classification problem. Predicting what type of seizure is associated with an EEG signal can be formulated as a multi-class classification problem, assuming recordings of more than two seizure types. Alternatively, when the outcome is a quantity, which may be discrete or continuous, the problem is a regression. For example, predicting the number of seizures in the next one hour or the time until the next seizure given a set of EEG data can be considered a regression problem. In this chapter, we illustrate the use of supervised approaches through two classification problems in epilepsy; seizure detection and seizure classification. The algorithms presented have straightforward extensions to a regression setting.

The first three sections introduce fundamental algorithms in supervised learning: logistic regression (Section 12.2), k-nearest neighbors (Section 12.3), and trees and ensembles (Section 12.4). Methods and measures for model training and evaluation are then described (Section 12.5). A demonstration of how these approaches and concepts are applied to seizure detection and seizure classification is presented in Section 12.6. Using a publicly available EEG dataset, we provide implementation examples in Python of these algorithms as well as of the data preprocessing, data arrangement, and feature extraction procedures that typically precede the modeling task. We discuss the performance of these algorithms and their suitability for the seizure detection and classification problems.

## 12.2 Logistic Regression and Regularization

Logistic regression, also discussed in Chapter 5, is a fundamental supervised learning algorithm used for binary classification. It is most appropriate in situations where the prediction outcome of interest, $y_i$, is binary (i.e., 1 or 0, yes or no). To motivate logistic regression, consider the following binary classification problem: Suppose for a given EEG signal, one defines $Y_i = 1$ if the EEG signal corresponds to a seizure and 0 otherwise, for $i = 1, \ldots, n$ samples. One way to predict whether a future EEG signal corresponds to a seizure is to model the probability of observing a seizure given the historical EEG. If the probability is high, then the EEG signal may be associated with a seizure. In prediction, one is interested in $P(Y_i = 1|f(X_i))$, where $f(X_i)$ is a function of the EEG signal and its derived features. EEG features are generally calculated from the EEG time series or from its transforms, and can range from simple statistical descriptors to complex non-linear measures. The logistic regression model assumes that the function $f(X_i)$ is a linear combination of the features $X\theta$, where $\theta$ is a $d$-dimensional vector of parameters. Given the outcome variable $Y$, also referred to as a label in classification tasks, and the EEG signal $X$, the goal is to find the parameter set $\theta$ to not only best fit the data, but to also generalize to unseen data. To accomplish the former, one can maximize the probability of $P(Y_i = 1|X_i\theta)$ with respect to the parameters $\theta$. Once the optimal set of $\theta$ is found, predicting new samples is accomplished by applying the model with the new sample features and returning the probability of the output being 1. If the probability is high (more specifically, above a selected threshold), the sample is classified as 1, otherwise as 0. Since $y_i$ can take only two values in a binary classification problem, a natural choice for modeling its probability is the Bernoulli distribution with parameter $X_i$. Thus, one is interested in maximizing the quantity:

$$\max_{\theta} P(Y_i = 1|X_i\theta) = \max X_i y_i (1 - X_i)(1 - y_i) \tag{12.1}$$

$$\max_{\theta} \log(P(Y_i = 1|X_i\theta)) = \max y_i \log(X_i\theta) + (1 - y_i)\log(1 - X_i) \tag{12.2}$$

$$\min_{\theta}(-\log(P(Y = 1|X\theta))) = \min \frac{1}{n}\sum_{i=1}^{n}(-y_i\log(X_i\theta) - (1 - y_i)\log(1 - X_i\theta)) \tag{12.3}$$

for every $i = 1, \ldots, n$. The second equality comes from taking the natural logarithm on both sides and using properties of log to simplify. The first two equations above are equivalent when maximizing over $\theta$ as the log function is a monotonically non-decreasing transformation of the probability function. It is often more convenient to find the minimum of a function. Moreover, adding a constant to the objective function does not change the value that maximizes/minimizes it. Therefore, the maximum value of $\theta$ from Eq. (12.2) corresponds to the minimum value of $\theta$ in Eq. (12.3). Note that in this equation, all $n$ samples are combined in vector form and $y^T$ stands for the transpose of the vector $y$. The minimization problem presented in Eq. (12.3) does not have an analytical solution for finding the value of $\theta$ and numerical procedures must be used. Some examples include coordinate gradient descent [8] and the Limited Broyden–Fletcher–Goldfarb–Shanno algorithm (LBFGS) [15].

To find the values for $\theta$, one needs the number of samples, $n$, to exceed the number of features, $d$ ($n \gg d$). If the feature set is large relative to the sample size ($n<d$), then one may need to reduce the dimension of the feature set to be able to learn. One way to achieve this is through *regularized logistic regression*, which rewrites Eq. (12.3) as follows:

$$\min_{\theta} \log(P(Y = 1|X\theta)) = \min \frac{1}{n}\left(-y^T\log(X\theta) - (1 - y)^T\log(1 - X\theta)\right) + \frac{\lambda}{n}\|\theta\|_{\gamma}, \tag{12.4}$$

where $\lambda$ is the penalty parameter and $\gamma$ is the selected penalty norm which is typically the L1 (absolute) or L2 (Euclidean) norm. Adding an L1 penalty is referred to as *LASSO regression*, while adding L2 penalty is referred to as *ridge regression* [12]. A linear combination of the L1 and L2 parameters can also be used, known as Elastic Net [24]. Both penalty parameters are typically learned from the data. Thus, the penalty parameters can force some values of $\theta$ to be close to zero hence reducing the dimensionality of the feature set. An additional benefit of the loss function in Eq. (12.4) is that it can help automatically reduce overfitting, as we discuss with more details in later sections, by reducing the model complexity and selecting a smaller and more impactful subset of features.

While the intuitive interpretation of the relationship between a unit change in the feature set $X$ and the labels $Y$ may not be directly clear from Eq. (12.1), it is possible to think of the logistic regression problem in terms of the log-odds, defined as:

$$\log\frac{P(Y_i = 1|X_i\theta)}{P(Y_i = 0|X_i\theta)} = \log\frac{P(Y_i = 1|X_i\theta)}{(1 - P(Y_i = 1|X_i\theta))} = \log(\exp(X\theta)) = X\theta. \tag{12.5}$$

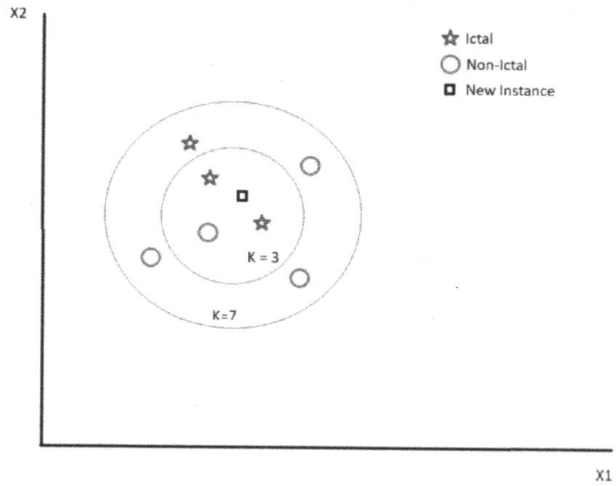


**FIGURE 12.1**
K-Nearest Neighbors: The unknown sample (black square) is assigned to class "star" when $k = 3$ neighbors are used and to class "circle" when $k = 7$ neighbors are used. (Color version available in electronic supplement.)

Writing the log-odds as in Eq. (12.5) indicates that there is a linear relationship between the log-odds of the label $Y$ and the feature set $X$. This means that an increase of 1% in a feature results in the corresponding percent increase in the log-odds of $Y$.

## 12.3 K-Nearest Neighbors

**k-Nearest Neighbors (kNN)** is another common supervised learning algorithm used for classification. The kNN algorithm estimates the outcome of a particular sample based on the outcomes of its neighbors. Suppose, for instance, that one is interested in estimating the label of the black square in Figure 12.1. A natural way to estimate the label of a point of interest is to look at the labels of nearby points and take a majority vote. Two important decisions that need to be made in kNN are the *distance metric* used to determine neighbors, and the *number of neighbors* ($k$) to include in the prediction of the unknown sample. For example, using Euclidean distance and $k = 3$ neighbors leads to a prediction of the unknown square sample as belonging to the star class (there are two stars and one circle within the neighborhood of the square). If, on the other hand, we increase the neighborhood to include the closest seven neighbors ($k = 7$), however, then a majority vote will predict that the square sample belongs to the circle class (there are four circles and three stars within the neighborhood of the square). Practical recommendations for selecting these values are discussed in Section 12.6.6.

In kNN, the probability of a new sample belonging to a given class is given by:

$$P(Y_i = c|X_i = x_{\text{new}}) = \frac{1}{k} \sum_{j \in N_i} I(y_j = c), \tag{12.6}$$

where $c$ denotes each individual class, $x_{\text{new}}$ denotes the sample to classify, $k$ denotes the number of neighbors to use, and $N$ denotes the set of closest data points to $x_{\text{new}}$. The probability for a sample belonging to a given class is estimated according to Eq. (12.6) and the sample is assigned to the class with the highest probability.

One important difference between kNN and many other machine learning algorithms is that kNN does not learn a model using training data (see Section 12.5). In contrast, for example, in Section 12.2, we saw that in logistic regression, we learn a set of parameters $\theta_{\text{train}}$ from a set of training data. We proceed to retrieve these parameters when new observations become available and use them to predict the probability $P(Y_i = 1|X_i = x_{\text{new}}, \theta_{\text{train}})$. In contrast, kNN does not learn parameters from a training data set. To predict the class of a new sample $x_{\text{new}}$, it only stores the training sample values and retrieves the neighbors of $x_{\text{new}}$ using the provided distance metric to calculate the probabilities of belonging to each class, according to Eq. (12.6), assigning $x_{\text{new}}$ to the class with the highest probability.

## 12.4 Trees and Ensembles

Decision trees are hierarchical models that recursively partition the data based on decision rules following a tree-like model and are another class of supervised learning methods used for binary and multi-class classification as well as regression problems.

### 12.4.1 Binary Decision Trees

Logistic regression and regularized regression methods discussed in Section 12.2 employ a linear combination of feature values to predict the labels. To account for interaction effects in logistic regression, they must be explicitly created. Moreover, higher order effects are more difficult to account for. Tree-based methods, in contrast, are top-down greedy algorithms that recursively partition the feature space with the objective of separating the samples into homogenous subsets with respect to the features. By construction, they allow for non-linearity and higher order effects in the model. A top-down greedy tree algorithm starts at the root (top) of the tree and grows the tree downward. At each node, the best split for that node only is selected, that is, without considering consequences for nodes further down the tree.

Figure 12.2 illustrates the structure of a binary tree. Here, a tree is called binary when each parent node has two child nodes. To illustrate the idea behind a decision tree, let us use the *Iris* dataset as an example [7]. The *Iris* dataset contains 150 observations of three species of *Iris* flower – *setosa*, *versicolor*, and *virginica*. There are four features in the dataset – sepal length, sepal width, petal length, and petal width. The binary decision tree uses the four features to partition the data with the aim of reducing heterogeneity with respect to the three classes. Even though all features are available at each step of the process, at most one is used to split the parent node into two child nodes. The decision tree keeps on growing (splitting on a feature) until there are no more splits available, or if it has reached some predefined criteria.

The binary decision tree in Figure 12.2 displays the distribution of petal length with respect to the three classes. The *setosa* class (yellow) is clearly separated from the other two classes (blue and green) as all of the samples in the *setosa* class have petal length less than 2.45 cm. Splitting the node based on that value leads to two child nodes. The left child node contains only the fifty *setosa* samples present in the data (the yellow circle), also referred to as a pure node. It has no heterogeneity with respect to the classes, i.e. all samples are of a single class, and therefore, there is no need to split this node any further. This node is declared a terminal node. If a new sample is presented to the algorithm which has petal length less than 2.45, the decision tree will classify it as *setosa*. The right child node contains the remainder of the samples, which are a mix of *virginica* and *versicolor*. The binary tree indicates that the largest heterogeneity with respect to all features at that node is with respect to petal width. In particular, the best split, which reduces the heterogeneity in the data the most, occurs at petal width of 1.75 cm. Since this partitioning does not result in pure nodes, further partitioning is possible. The right child node has predominantly *virginica*. In particular, for petal length greater than 4.85 cm, the tree reaches another pure node consisting of 43 *virginica* samples. Samples satisfying the condition in that node are the samples with petal length 2.45, petal width 1.75, and petal length 4.85. The first and third conditions can be combined into petal length 4.85, as they are based on the same feature. Any new sample that satisfies these conditions will be classified as *virginica*. Tracking the samples via the tree in such a manner illustrates how decision tree algorithms naturally enable nonlinear combinations of features and feature interactions.

The binary decision tree is grown until all nodes are pure nodes. While this procedure allows for a perfect segmentation of the data into the three classes, in certain situations, it may not be desirable. In particular, several of the terminal nodes at the bottom of the tree contain between 1 and 3 samples. If a new sample is to reach one of these nodes, it will be classified using the label attributed to a pure node based only on 1 to 3 samples. This, in turn, can lead to prediction error. An alternative strategy is to grow the tree until some minimum number of samples is reached within a node. Note that this may not lead to pure terminal nodes as in the example considered here. However, new samples reaching these nodes can be classified via a majority vote rule rather than assigning the single pure class in a terminal node, potentially reducing the prediction error within each node.

More concretely, consider the two terminal child nodes at the very left of Figure 12.2. The left child node contains 47 samples of the *versicolor* class, and the right child node contains one sample from the *virginica* class. The parent node was split based on a petal width of 1.65 cm. Since the parent node has a total of 48 samples and only one is *virginica*, it is possible that this is due to chance. If another 1000 new samples make it to the parent node at this part of the tree, a sizable number of these samples will have petal width greater than 1.65 cm without necessarily belonging to the *virginica* class, and the child node will no longer be pure. If one sets the minimum samples required for a node to be 48, then the parent node will never be further partitioned, and the tree will terminate at the parent node containing 47 samples of *versicolor* and one *virginica*. Taking a majority vote for predicting the correct class in that node will result in predicting the *versicolor* class. The resultant prediction accuracy will be 47 out of 48 on the training data. While this does not lead to 100% accuracy as in the original tree, the modified tree still maintains high classification accuracy within the node but reduces the impact of misclassifying new data due to using a single sample from the training data to classify all future unseen data points.

As mentioned earlier, binary decision trees are built greedily, considering only the information available at the current node. Therefore, at each node, there is a chance that the algorithm makes a sub-optimal decision on how to split the data with respect to the global objective of finding homogeneous subsets of the data with respect to each class. To improve the overall performance of the tree, one can use tree pruning, a technique that operates on the tree in a bottom-up fashion. Pruning tracks the splits at each node, from terminal nodes to the root, and assesses whether the splits along the tree are optimal with respect to the global objective. The splits that are found to be unnecessary are merged back together to recover the parent node.

**Recursively Partitioning the Feature Space:** So far, we have discussed how a binary decision tree is built. We noted that at each node, the tree needs to decide whether a split is necessary and, if so, what feature to use to make the split. Here, we provide details on the various measures used for selecting the optimal split at each node of the tree.

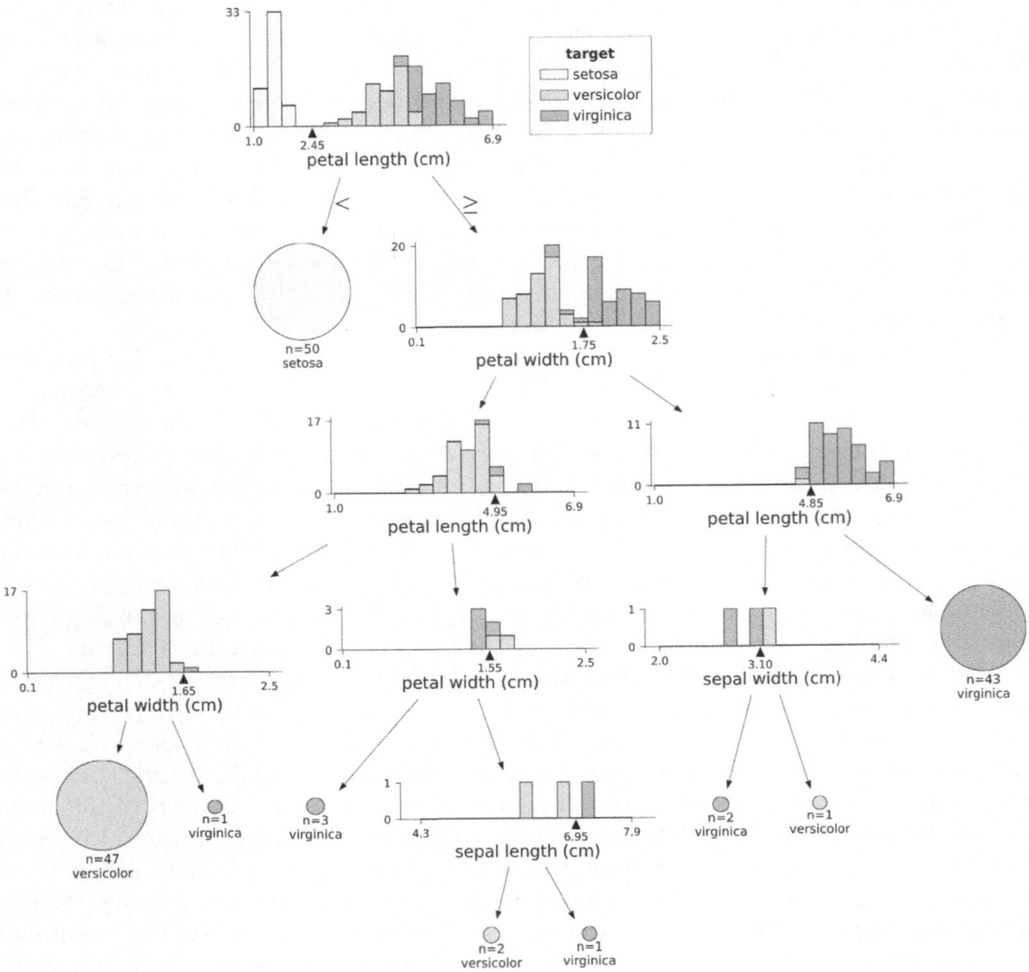


**FIGURE 12.2**
Binary decision tree for the *Iris* dataset. Circles indicate terminal nodes. Histograms represent the distribution of each feature used for partitioning the data at each node. The value of the feature used for partitioning is displayed on the $x$-axis of the histogram (triangle). Figure generated using the dtreeviz library in Python [22]. (Color version available in electronic supplement.)

One metric used in recursively partitioning the feature space is entropy. Entropy is a measure used in information theory to describe the heterogeneity in a system. Given a collection of labels $Y$, the entropy is defined as:

$$\text{Entropy}(Y) = \sum_{i=1}^{c} -p_i \log_2(p_i), \tag{12.7}$$

where $p_i$ is the proportion of positive labels in $Y$ and $c$ is the number of classes. The entropy, as defined in Eq. (12.7), takes values between 0 and 1. An entropy of 0 indicates a homogeneous collection of labels in $Y$ where all labels are of the same class and an entropy of 1 indicates an equal number of positive and negative labels in the set.

One can define a measure for determining whether partitioning a node based on one of the available features will result in a decrease in the overall value of the entropy in the child nodes relative to the parent node. One such measure is information gain $\text{IG}(Y, X_j)$, where $X_j$ represents feature $j$. Let $R_1 = \{X_j \mid X_j < t\}$ and $R_2 = \{X_j \mid X_j \geq t\}$ define two disjoint regions based on a threshold value $t$. Then the information gain is defined as:

$$\text{IG}(Y, X_j) = \text{Entropy}(Y) - \sum_{x_{ij} \in R_1} |yx_{ij}| \, \text{Entropy}(YX_{ij}) - \sum_{x_{ij} \in R_2} |yx_{ij}| \, \text{Entropy}(YX_{ij}), \tag{12.8}$$

where $x_{ij}$ are all possible values that feature $X_j$ can take within each of the non-overlapping regions and $|y|$ represents the cardinality of the set $y$. The information gain looks at the difference in entropy present in the parent node from the sum of the entropies present in both child nodes weighted by the number of samples within each child node. To find the best split, one can greedily test over all possible values of $t$ for all $X_j$, $j = 1, \ldots, p$ and select the one with the largest information gain. In the example above, at the root node, the maximum information gain was achieved for petal length and the cutoff $t = 2.45$ with regions $R_1 = \{X_j = \text{petal length} \mid t < 2.45\}$ and $R_2 = \{X_j = \text{petal length} \mid t \geq 2.45\}$. Pseudocode for building a binary decision tree is provided in Algorithm 8.

**Algorithm 8** Decision Tree

1: **procedure** DecisionTree($X \in \mathbf{R}^{n \times d}$, $y \in \{0, 1\}$ or $y \in \mathbf{R}$)
2:     **if** feature space is empty **then**
3:         **return** majority vote over all labels in the training set and terminate
4:     **end if**
5:     **if** entropy over all samples is 0 **then**
6:         **return** single label over the training data
7:     **end if**
8:     **if** minimum predetermined criteria for current node is reached **then**
9:         **return** majority label
10:     **else**
11:         calculate information gain over all $X_j$ for all $t$ and all possible regions $R_1$
12:         and $R_2$ for the current node using Eq. (12.8)
13:         Select $X_j$ and $t$ that return the highest information gain
14:         Create two child nodes based on $R_1$ and $R_2$
15:         For each child node, repeat steps 8–11
16:     **end if**
      **Outputs:** $f : \mathbf{R}^{n \times d} \rightarrow \{0, 1\}$ (or $\mathbf{R}$ in case of continuous label)
17: **end procedure**

**Practical and Bias Considerations for Decision Trees:** Binary decision trees, as given by Algorithm 8, exhibit bias with respect to preference for shorter over longer trees and placing features with higher information gain toward the top of the tree. For additional in-depth consideration of bias issues within decision trees, we refer the reader to [17].

A practical consideration when building decision trees is handling continuous features. In particular, in Algorithm 8, the pseudocode requires that all possible split values that each feature can take are considered. While this is feasible for binary and categorical features, it may be computationally expensive for continuous features with a large number of distinct values. One practical approach is to build a histogram for the distribution of each feature, as shown in Figure 12.2, and to use the midpoint of the bins as cutoff values when creating the regions for each feature. In such a way, a smaller feature space must be explored, which can yield significant computational gains. However, this may give rise to another type of bias, in that the information gain measure is biased toward the selection of features with a higher number of distinct categories. This occurs because such features can better discriminate between classes within the training data. The training data can be separated by the features into very small subsets that give much higher information gain than features that are perhaps preferable but have a lower number of unique values. To help overcome this bias, other metrics are available for creating data splits. Examples of such metrics include the gain ratio [17] and the Gini index, calculated as $\text{Gini}(Y) = 1 - \sum_{i=1}^{c} p_i^2$.

### 12.4.2 Ensembles of Trees

Binary trees are a great choice for modeling non-linear relationships and providing a good visual representation of them. However, they are seldom used in practice for prediction tasks. Due to the greedy fashion in which a decision tree is built, considering only the information at a given node, decision trees can be sensitive to the training data and exhibit high variance in prediction error. In particular, changing the training data slightly can result in construction of a different tree and therefore predictions. In the example of Figure 12.2, if one were to collect ten more samples on *setosa* that had petal length greater than 5 cm, it is possible that the first split would no longer be based on petal length being smaller than 2.4 cm. Since this split occurs at the root node, the entire tree may completely change, leading to different predictions. In the following subsections, we introduce two algorithms that are widely used in practice for mitigating the high prediction variance present in decision trees: random forest and gradient boosting.

**Random Forest:** One way of reducing the variance of estimators is through bootstrapping. Bootstrapping is a method of data resampling with replacement. Bootstrap-based estimators reduce variance by averaging the values across all generated datasets. Consider identically and independently distributed (i.i.d.) random samples $X_1, X_2, ..., X_T$ from a distribution with a given variance $\sigma^2$. By randomly resampling the realizations of these random variables and averaging across the resulting datasets, new random variables $X_1, ..., X_m$ are obtained, where $m$ is the number of bootstrapped samples, from a distribution with variance $\sigma^2/T$.

In the context of decision trees, bootstrapping can be used to build trees based on resampled training sets. These trees are then aggregated so that the prediction estimates will have lower variance compared to a single decision tree. The label of a new sample can then be predicted by obtaining an individual prediction from each tree and aggregating the results over all trees to produce one final prediction. More formally, to generate the classification for a given sample $X$ from $T$ trees, we use:

$$RF_{\text{pred}} = \arg\max_{i} \sum_{j=1}^{T} w_j I(f_j(X) = i) \tag{12.9}$$

where $i$ is the class, $f_j(X)$ is the prediction from tree $j$, $w_j$ is the weight assigned to each tree, $I$ is the indicator function defined as $I(X = x) = 1$ if $X = x$ and 0 otherwise. For example, if 50 trees are generated based on 50 bootstrapped samples of the data, and 40 trees predicted the sample to be of class 1, while 10 trees predicted the sample to be of class 0, then the final prediction for the sample will be class 1.

When building trees based on bootstrapped samples of the data, the resulting trees tend to be correlated with each other, due to the random samples not being independent across different training data sets. One way to reduce this correlation and further reduce the variance in the final estimated predictions is to use only a proportion of all samples and features available at each node of each tree [4]. More specifically, one can randomly sample a proportion of the features to be used when evaluating a split. Combining this strategy with bootstrapping to generate different training sets is known as a Random Forest. A Random Forest algorithm builds a forest of trees by randomly sampling the rows (observations) and columns (features) of a dataset. It has been shown that Random Forest algorithms generally improve predictive performance over decision trees [4]. Pseudocode for building a Random Forest is given in Algorithm 9.

**Algorithm 9** Random Forest

```
procedure RandomForest(X ∈ R^{n×d}, y ∈ {0,1} or y ∈ R, T ∈ N, m ∈ N, k ∈ N)
    for t = 1 to T do
        Sample k observations with replacement from the dataset X.
        Grow a tree using Algorithm 8 considering only m features for each
        split (randomly sampled).
    end for
    Calculate the final output for each sample across all trees T by using majority vote.
     Outputs: f : R^{n×d} → {0,1} (or R in case of continuous label)
end procedure
```

Note that the parameters $T$, $m$ and $n$ are application-specific and are typically selected based on available data. A downside of using a Random Forest over a single decision tree is reduced explainability and ability to look at the individual splits at each step of the tree. A method to quantify the importance of each feature for predicting the outcome consists of summing the decrease in Gini index or Entropy when splitting on a feature within each tree and averaging across all trees. High values of feature importance indicate that the feature has resulted in large decreases in the splitting criteria and is important in explaining the observed predictions.

**Gradient Boosting:** An alternative approach of combining estimators, such as trees, is boosting. Like Random Forest, boosting relies on combining many trees in order to improve the predictive ability of the algorithm. The boosting paradigm can work with general function estimators and not just trees (e.g., linear functions). Boosting is based on the idea that a model can progressively improve by learning from errors. Rather than building trees independently of each other based on bootstrapped samples of the data, trees can instead be built sequentially by improving the predictions from previous trees. Boosting achieves this by fitting a binary tree algorithm on the residuals of the previous tree and updating the residuals every time a new tree is built. The final prediction is the sum of the predictions from each tree. Motivated by gradient descent, gradient boosting aims to minimize a specific loss function by updating the residuals, using the data, at each step in the direction that provides the biggest improvements. Pseudocode for a general boosting algorithm for classification is provided in Algorithm 10.

The learning rate is used to ensure that the algorithm takes smaller steps toward the target. This has been shown to achieve faster convergence in practice and helps prevent overshooting as the predicted probabilities approach the observed data. Calculating $F_{\text{new}}$ in line 8 of the algorithm is needed to ensure that the update step in line 9 is valid and the quantities being added are in the same space. In fact, one can show that the numerator represents the derivative of the loss function with respect to the log-odds, and the denominator is the second derivative. The derivation of the exact form of the update in line 8 is beyond the scope of this book, and we refer the reader to [10] for an in-depth discussion.

An interesting observation is that in line 7 of Algorithm 10, the decision tree that is fit is a regression tree rather than the classification tree from Algorithm 8. This is due to the

**Algorithm 10** Gradient Boosting

1: **procedure** GradientBoosting($X \in \mathbf{R}^{n \times d}$, $y \in \{0,1\}$, $T \in \mathbf{N}$, $\alpha \in [0, \infty)$, $m \in \mathbf{N}$, $k \in \mathbf{N}$)
2: Initialize learning rate $\alpha$, number of boosting iterations $T$
3: $F_0 = \log(\text{odds}) = \log\left(\frac{\text{class Positive}}{\text{class Negative}}\right)$
4: $P_0(y_i = 1) = \frac{exp(F_0)}{1+\exp(F_0)}$ for all samples $i$
5: $resid_i = y_i - P_0(y_i = 1)$ for all samples $i$
6: **for** $t = 1$ to $T$ **do**
7: Fit a regression decision tree on the training data $(X_i, resid_i)$ for all samples $i$
8: Update the outputs at each terminal leaf of the tree to be the new log(odds) for every $i$ via:

$$F_{\text{new}} = \frac{\sum_{i=1}^{\text{nleaf}} \text{resid}_i}{\sum_{i=1}^{\text{nleaf}} P_{t-1}(y_i = 1) \times (1 - P_{t-1}(y_i = 1))}$$

9: Update $F_t = F_{t-1} + \alpha \times F_{\text{new}}$
10: Update $P_t(y_i = 1) = \frac{exp(F_t)}{1+\exp(F_t)}$ for every sample $i$
11: Update $resid_i = y_i - P_t(y_i = 1)$ for all samples $i$
12: **end for**
**Outputs:** $f : \mathbf{R}^{n \times d} \to \{0, 1\}$
13: **end procedure**

residuals serving as the target rather than the original classes; the residuals, as calculated in line 11 of Algorithm 10, are no longer binary, and hence a regression tree is needed. To build such a regression tree, the entropy just need to be replaced with any deviance that supports continuous-valued outcomes, such as mean squared error.

An important extension of the gradient boosting algorithm is the Extreme Gradient Boosting (XGBoost) [5]. XGBoost introduces an algorithm for parallel tree learning, offering a significant reduction in the training time over gradient boosting.

## 12.5 Model Training and Evaluation

In Sections 12.2–12.4, we discussed several common supervised learning algorithms. When applying these algorithms in practice, interest often lies in estimating predictive performance. To quantify the ability of model predictions to generalize to new observations, one needs to (1) apply model predictions to unseen future data, and (2) quantify the performance of these predictions on the unseen future data. We discuss each of these points in turn.

### 12.5.1 Model Validation Approaches

When it is not possible to directly assess the performance of a machine learning algorithm on new unobserved data, one alternative is to use hold-out validation. Hold-out validation refers to splitting the observed dataset into two subsets: the first for fitting the supervised learning algorithm (training data); and the second for testing the performance of the algorithm (test data). A typical split is 80% for training and 20% for testing. In larger data and compute resource settings, it is advisable to include a third set of data, validation data. Inclusion of a third validation set allows us to fine tune the algorithm parameters without inducing bias in the reported performance results on the test data. An example split in these situations is 70%/15%/15% for training/validation/test, respectively. The test data represents future unobserved data and should follow two assumptions: (1) the test data and future unobserved data must have the same distribution; and (2) the sample size of the test data needs to be large enough that any evaluation that is conducted is generalizable to the population of unseen samples. Note that, while the first assumption may not generally hold true over long intervals of time, it is reasonable over shorter periods. Thus, by retraining the models frequently using the new data, we can get close to satisfying this assumption.

The second assumption is harder to satisfy and is application-specific. For some industries such as e-commerce, where petabytes of data are available, it is easily satisfied. This also holds true for the seizure detection and classification examples considered in this chapter. Yet in other applications, collecting large datasets may be prohibitive. In these cases, another technique known as $k$-fold cross-validation is often employed. When the observational data is small, to generate a better generalization of the unseen data, this method splits the data into $k$ folds, using $k-1$ folds to train the algorithm and the $k$-th fold for testing. The procedure is repeated with each fold serving as the test data. The final evaluation is obtained by averaging the results on each test fold. As before, it is possible to include a validation fold for fine-tuning the algorithm. The choice of $k$ can affect the evaluation procedure. If one chooses $k = 1$, also known as leave-one-out cross-validation, then the model will be fitted $n-1$ times, using each observation as a test set. This induces a large computational cost, especially when the dataset is large. Moreover, there exists a variance-bias trade-off in the choice of $k$. In this context, bias refers to providing good estimates for the test error and variance refers to the test error variance.

The relationship between training/test misclassification errors and model complexity is depicted in the left panel of Figure 12.3. As the model complexity increases, the training error generally decreases, approaching zero. Similarly, the test error decreases, but at a certain point it can start increasing again. This is typically indicative of the model overfitting on the training data and memorizing it, which results in poor ability of the model to generalize to unseen data. To balance the trade-off between the training and test error, in practice, the parameter complexity is learned from the data so that the test error is minimized.

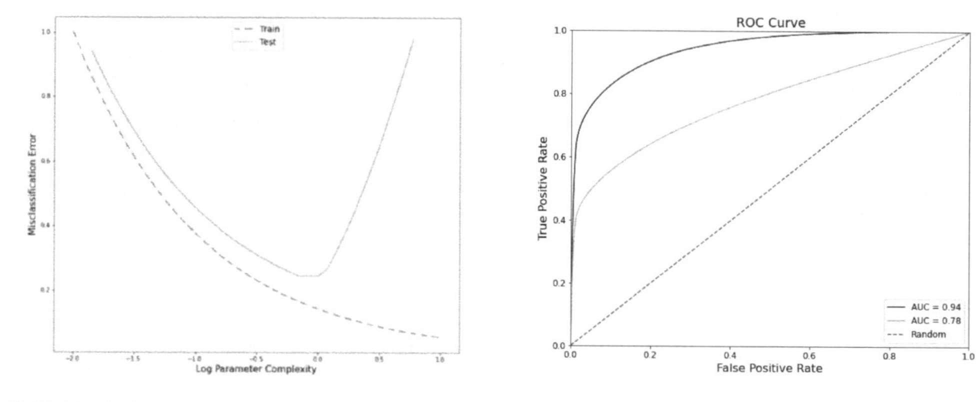


**FIGURE 12.3**
(Left panel) Misclassification training (blue) and test (orange) errors as a function of the model parameter complexity on a log scale. (Right panel) Receiver operating characteristic curve. (Color version available in electronic supplement.)

### 12.5.2 Performance Metrics

To quantify the performance of an algorithm on the test data, we need metrics that can be used to determine how well an algorithm generalizes its performance to unseen data. There are various performance metrics used widely for supervised learning, which may be split into two classes, depending on whether the application is regression or classification. In this section, we focus on introducing classification performance metrics; we briefly mention several regression performance metrics and provide references to external resources for further reading.

When evaluating the performance of a binary classification algorithm, where we refer to labels of 1 as a positive and labels of 0 as negative, there are four possible outcomes. We can (1) predict 1 when the correct label is 1, referred to as true positive (TP); (2) predict 0 when the correct label is 0, referred to as true negative (TN); (3) predict 1 when the correct label is 0, referred to as false positive (FP); or (4) predict 0 when the correct label is 1, referred to as false negative (FN). An intuitive metric following these definitions is the notion of *accuracy*, which measures the total number of correct predictions out of all the samples. Accuracy is defined as:

$$\text{Accuracy} = \frac{TP + TN}{TP + TN + FP + FN}.$$

Accuracy, bounded by 0 and 1, is one of the most commonly used metrics for classification. However, to understand one pitfall of relying solely on accuracy across all datasets, consider a dataset consisting of 100 segments of EEG that are either labeled as 1 (representing seizure) and 0 (representing non-seizure). Since most of the EEG recording is non-seizure data, we can imagine a situation in which 95 EEG segments are labeled as non-seizure and 5 segments are labeled as seizure. In this imbalanced dataset, an algorithm can attain high accuracy by predicting all segments as belonging to the non-seizure class. In that case, the accuracy of the algorithm, by always predicting non-seizure, will yield 0.95. While achieving high accuracy, an algorithm that always predicts EEG segments to be non-seizure may not be useful, because we are interested in the correct prediction of EEG segments with seizure activity. *Recall* (a.k.a. *sensitivity*), with support on $[0, 1]$, is defined as:

$$\text{Recall} = \frac{TP}{TP + FN}.$$

This measure provides an answer to the question of how many of the seizures were classified correctly as seizures. In the above example, if we predict every EEG data point to be non-seizure, the value of recall will be 0. However, use of the recall metric in isolation has a similar issue: if we were to predict all segments as seizure, then the recall value will be 1. This would similarly not be useful as it would suggest that performance is maximized by predicting all EEG segments to be seizure, which is not desirable. The drawback of the recall metric can be addressed by consideration of *precision* (a.k.a. *positive predictive value*), defined as:

$$\text{Precision} = \frac{TP}{TP + FP} \tag{12.10}$$

The metric quantifies the proportion of the EEG segments that were correctly classified as seizure. The difference between precision and recall is in the denominator, which now penalizes incorrect predictions for seizures. Returning to our running example, if all segments are naively predicted as the majority class (non-seizure), the precision will still be 0, but now if all segments are predicted as seizure, then the precision will be 0.05.

While precision provides better insight into the performance of naive classifiers that predict a single class, it alone is also not sufficient, because it does not tell us how many of the seizures we missed. Rather, precision tells us how well we did every time we predicted a segment to be seizure. Moreover, recall and precision typically are inversely related and improving an algorithm with respect to one will reduce the performance with respect to the other. To address this, recall and precision can be combined into a single metric called the *F1 score*, which is defined as:

$$\text{F1 score} = 2\frac{\text{Precision} * \text{Rrecall}}{\text{Precision} + \text{Rrecall}}$$

The F1 score, ranging between 0 and 1, represents the harmonic mean between the precision and the recall values, with higher indicating better performance. Extensions of the F1 score are also available that allow for differential weighting of precision and recall, based on the application at hand [19].

Last, we discuss one more commonly used performance metric, the area under the receiver operating characteristic curve (ROC-AUC or AUROC; right panel of Figure 12.3). Many machine learning classification algorithms output a numeric value between 0 and 1 (can be a proper probability or otherwise) rather than a dichotomous label. The criterion used to select the optimum cut-off point to map the numeric output to a binary label may then be chosen in several ways. Commonly used thresholds include Youden's index [23] or the use of 0.5 as the threshold, where outcomes are classified as 1 if the output is greater than 0.5, and 0 otherwise. The ROC-AUC metric approaches the problem of model evaluation by building a probability curve which plots the true positive rate (TPR) against false positive rate (FPR) for varying values of the classification threshold and calculating the area under that curve. The TPR rate is equivalent to the recall metric discussed earlier; FPR is defined as:

$$\text{FPR} = \frac{\text{FP}}{\text{FP} + \text{TN}}$$

The metrics provided above serve for evaluating binary classification problems. Many of them can be extended and are used in practice for evaluating multi-class classification problems. The multi-class classification problem can be viewed as an extension of the binary case. Two generally used methods are one-vs-all and one-vs-one. One-vs-all fits one binary classifier to each class, using the class as a positive label and any of the other classes as a negative example. Thus, this method involves fitting as many binary classifiers as classes present in the data. One-vs-one, on the other hand, is an approach that fits one binary classifier for each pair of labels. This implies that a much larger set of binary classifiers is needed. The final prediction is obtained by taking a majority vote across all binary classifiers. This results in a higher computational cost than one-vs-all, especially when the number of classes is large. There are also direct methods for performing multi-class classification. For example, in deep learning, the final layer of the network in a multi-class setting is represented by one neuron for each class and the softmax function defined as:

$$\text{softmax}(y_i) = \frac{\exp y_i}{\sum_{k=1}^{K} \exp y_k}$$

where $k = 1, \cdots, K$ are the number of distinct classes. The softmax function generates a probability distribution over the classes. The class selected for the given sample is $\text{argmax}_i\, \text{softmax}(y_i)$.

Natural extensions from the binary to the multi-class classification problem exist. Recall, precision and F1 score can all be calculated on the global or local level followed by global aggregation. As an example, extending Eq. (12.10) on the global level is possible by calculating the total number of true and false positives over all classes, regardless of which of the three methods above is used to fit the multi-class classifier. Eq. (12.10) can then be applied directly. This is usually referred to as "micro" precision. Similarly, micro recall and F1 score can be calculated. An alternative way is to calculate each metric for each class, as if it were a binary class, and then average the results across all classes to obtain the final metric value. This approach is referred to as "macro." From the definitions of the "micro" and "macro" metrics, one can see that the "micro" metric calculation will tend to be more biased toward the larger classes, while the "macro" metrics will assign equal contribution of each metric to the final result.

Last, we briefly touch on regression performance metrics. One common performance metric used is regression is *absolute mean error (AME)*:

$$\mathrm{AME} = \frac{1}{n}\sum_{i=1}^{n} |y_i - \hat{y}_i|,$$

where $\hat{y}_i$ stands for the predicted target from the supervised learning model. The absolute value sign is needed to ensure that negative and positive errors do not cancel out. The lower the values of AME, the better the model. Another common regression performance metric is *mean squared error (MSE)*:

$$\mathrm{MSE} = \frac{1}{n}\sum_{i=1}^{n} (y_i - \hat{y}_i)^2.$$

Compared to AME, MSE replaces the absolute difference with squared differences between the observed and estimated values, resulting in penalization of larger errors. A related metric is the *root mean squared error (RMSE)*, calculated as the square root of the MSE. For more extensive treatment of these and other regression performance metrics, we refer the readers to [12].

## 12.6 Seizure Detection and Classification

Epileptic seizures have long been thought to occur randomly. Seizures are characterized by their type and by the time and location of the EEG changes marking the beginning of the seizure. Accurate recognition of seizures is essential in epilepsy diagnosis and treatment guidance. The emergence of automatic seizure detection and classification tools has helped alleviate the burden of manual review of EEG recordings and enabled novel applications in epilepsy monitoring, diagnosis, and treatment.

Seizure detection and classification systems recognize seizures by analyzing biological signals, typically but not exclusively EEG, and applying a decision rule or an algorithm to the signal or to features extracted from the signal, generally in a sliding window fashion. Many of these algorithms assign the extracted data or features to a class (for example, "seizure" or "non-seizure"). When a seizure is detected, an algorithm can then be applied to determine the seizure type. Seizures can either be flagged as soon as a window is assigned a "seizure" label, or a latent time period can also be applied to confirm the persistence of a seizure state (a.k.a. ictal state). While the use of latent time periods reduces the chances of false detections, it may delay detection of the first electrographic change signaling the beginning of a seizure, known as the seizure onset time.

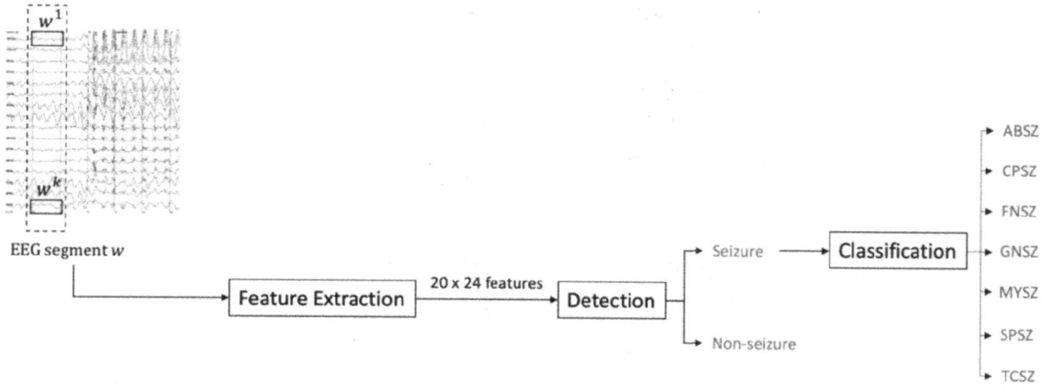


**FIGURE 12.4**
Schematic of sliding window analysis, feature extraction, and input into seizure detection and classification algorithms in illustrative example. (Color version available in electronic supplement.)

In this section, we demonstrate application of the supervised machine learning algorithms discussed in Sections 12.2–12.4 to seizure detection and seizure classification, using EEG data from the Temple University Hospital EEG corpus [18]. The TUH Seizure Corpus is a set of multi-channel EEG recordings annotated by neurologists for seizure presence and seizure type. It is a publicly available dataset and can be downloaded at `https://isip.piconepress.com/projects/tuh_eeg/downloads/tuh_eeg_seizure/` (Credentials are required to access the datasets and can be requested from the administrators of the site). For each seizure, the start time, end time, and seizure type are recorded. The EEG data files (.EDF) are provided with their corresponding annotation files (.TSE and .LBL).

A simplified seizure detection problem can be formulated as a task of binary classification of EEG data, where an EEG signal is partitioned into consecutive equal-size data segments that are each classified as "seizure" or as "non-seizure." The identification of the seizure type can be formulated as a multi-class classification problem. Version v1.4.0 of the TUH Seizure Corpus has 30 annotated events, including 11 types of seizures (focal nonspecific seizure (FNSZ), generalized seizure (GNSZ), simple partial seizure (SPSZ), complex partial seizure (CPSZ), absence seizure (ABSZ), tonic seizure (TNSZ), clonic seizure (CNSZ), tonic-clonic seizure (TCSZ), atonic seizure (ATSZ), myoclonic seizure (MYSZ), and non-epileptic seizure (NESZ)). Four of the 11 seizure types were relatively infrequent in the TUH seizure corpus. To develop a robust seizure classification system, seizure data from the seven seizure types with sufficient samples are retained in this illustrative example. These seizures are "ABSZ," "CPSZ," "FNSZ," "GNSZ," "SPSZ," "TCSZ," and "MYSZ."

Each EEG data file in the TUH Seizure Corpus contains $N$ EEG signals (channels). We segment the signal in the $N$ channels into $n$ overlapping windows of size $w$, where the size of the window can be in seconds or or number of samples. Features are then extracted from each window in each EEG channel, which can range from simple statistical descriptors to complex non-linear measures, and aggregated into an input vector for each $N$-channel EEG segment. Here, we derive a set of spectral features using the Fast Fourier Transform (FFT) of the EEG signal (Chapter 9) [20]. This input vector is then used to classify each EEG segment either as "seizure" or "non-seizure" using a binary classifier. EEG segments classified as "seizure" are subsequently classified into various seizure types using a multi-class classification algorithm (Figure 12.4). Full Python code to replicate this example and preprocessed data derived from version 1.4.0 of the TUH Seizure Corpus are provided in the repository accompanying the book. It is important to note that this example does not replicate the functionalities of a fully operational seizure detection and classification system; such systems require typically advanced data preprocessing (e.g., artifact rejection and noise removal; see Chapter 2), post-processing (reduction of false detections), and an alarm-triggering protocol.

### 12.6.1 Feature Extraction

Each EEG recording in the TUH Seizure Corpus is composed of $N = 20$ channels. Each channel is sampled at 250 Hz, with relatively fewer channels sampled at 256 Hz, 400 Hz, or 512 Hz. To apply FFT, the EEG channels need to have a uniform sampling rate. Resampling the channels at a rate that allows recovery of seizure frequencies is required. Since seizures are typically below 50 Hz [11], the EEG channels are downsampled to 200 Hz, which is more than adequate to resolve frequencies up to the Nyquist frequency.

Each resampled EEG channel is segmented into $k$ overlapping windows. We set the length of windows to $w = 1s$ (i.e., 200 data points per window) and the overlap between windows to 0.5 (i.e., 50% overlap). A 200-point FFT is then applied to each window. Each window is represented with a 24-dimensional feature vector by extracting the magnitudes of the frequencies between 1 and 24 Hz and applying a $\log_{10}$ transform to each value.

### 12.6.2 Data Arrangement

To train machine learning algorithms, input data are typically shaped into a matrix of observations and features. For this example, we shape the input data into a matrix where each row is a sliding window from teh $N$ EEG signals, and each column is a feature extracted from the time-aligned windows of all 20 channels (Figure 12.5). Using data from the training set, the resulting matrix is used as an input to train the algorithms. A matrix of the same dimensions is similarly constructed from the testing set.

To follow along with this example, the preprocessed data can be downloaded from the repository accompanying the book. After downloading the data, the paths should be set to match the directory where the files are downloaded:

```
# Set the directory where the seizure detection and seizure classification data
    are stored. #Please change the folder structure to match your own
path_detect = './User/downloaded_data_folder/'
path_classify = './User/downloaded_data_folder/'

# Load seizure detection data
X_detect = pickle.load(open(path_detect + 'X.pkl', 'rb'))
y_detect = pickle.load(open(path_detect + 'y.pkl', 'rb'))

# Load seizure classification data and the seizure labels
X_classify = pickle.load(open(path_classify + 'X.pkl', 'rb'))
y_classify = pickle.load(open(path_classify + 'y.pkl', 'rb'))

# Labels for classification
label_names = ['ABSZ', 'CPSZ', 'FNSZ', 'GNSZ', 'MYSZ', 'SPSZ', 'TCSZ']
```

The data is then split into training, validation, and test sets as described in Section 12.5.

```
# Sample the training, validation and test sets for detection and classification
train_size = 0.7

# Split the data 70/30 where 30 is the test set; set the state of the random split
     for reproducibility.
X_detect, X_detect_test, y_detect, y_detect_test = train_test_split(X_detect,
    y_detect, random_state=42, train_size = train_size)
```

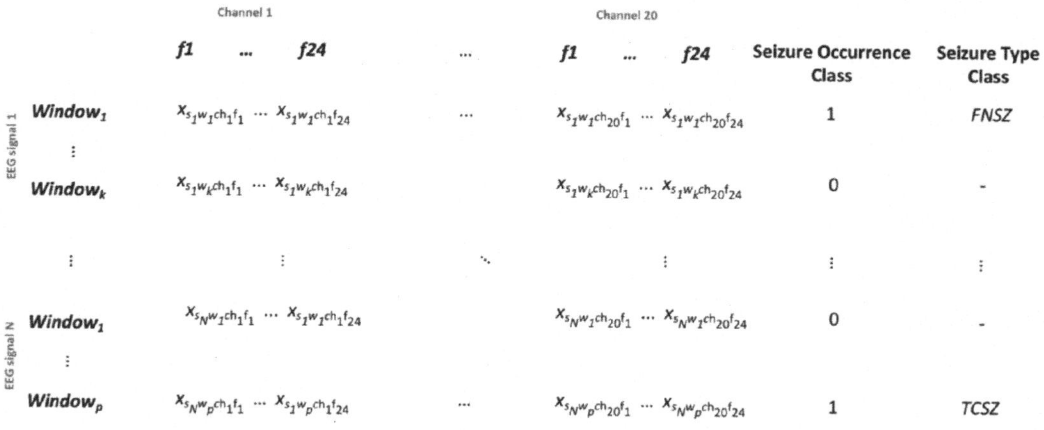


**FIGURE 12.5**
Features extracted from the $N$ EEG signals are arranged into a matrix, where each row is a sliding window from the $N$ EEG signals, and each column is a feature. Here, $X$ denotes the value of each feature, where $s$ indexes the order of the signal, $w$ indexes the sliding windows, $ch$ indexes the EEG channels, and $f$ indexes the frequency. Each sliding window is labeled with a binary label (0 or 1) in the seizure detection problem, where 1 indicates "seizure" and 0 indicates "non-seizure," and with one of seven seizure types (ABSZ, CPSZ, FNSZ, GNSZ, MYSZ, SPSZ, and TCSZ) used in the seizure classification problem.

```
# Split the data non test data 70/30 where 70 is the training set and 30 is the
    validation set.
X_detect_train, X_detect_val, y_detect_train, y_detect_val = train_test_split(
    X_detect, y_detect, random_state=42, train_size = train_size)

# Repeat for the classification case.
X_classify, X_classify_test, y_classify, y_classify_test = train_test_split(
    X_classify, y_classify, random_state=42, train_size = train_size)
X_classify_train, X_classify_val, y_classify_train, y_classify_val =
    train_test_split(X_classify, y_classify, random_state=42, train_size =
    train_size)
```

## 12.6.3 Data Balancing

A good (and mandatory) practice is to evaluate how balanced class labels are in the dataset prior to applying classification algorithms. Class imbalance often leads to bias toward classes with the highest number of samples (majority classes), which in turn may result in a high misclassification rate for the classes with the lowest number of samples (minority classes). Therefore, class imbalance is important to evaluate, particularly in healthcare application where the adverse event has generally low prevalence, as in the case of seizures in EEG recordings, with the interictal state typically dominating the electrographic signature of the EEG.

Examining the class distribution in the TUH Seizure Corpus v1.4.0 indeed reveals a class imbalance, both in the seizure occurrence and the seizure type classes. In the training dataset, the ratio of seizure to non-seizure sample segments is 0.11 (i.e., one seizure sample for every ten non-seizure samples; Figure 12.6, left panel) and the distribution of seizure types shows a dominance of three types: "CPSZ," "FNSZ," and "GNSZ" (Figure 12.6, right panel).

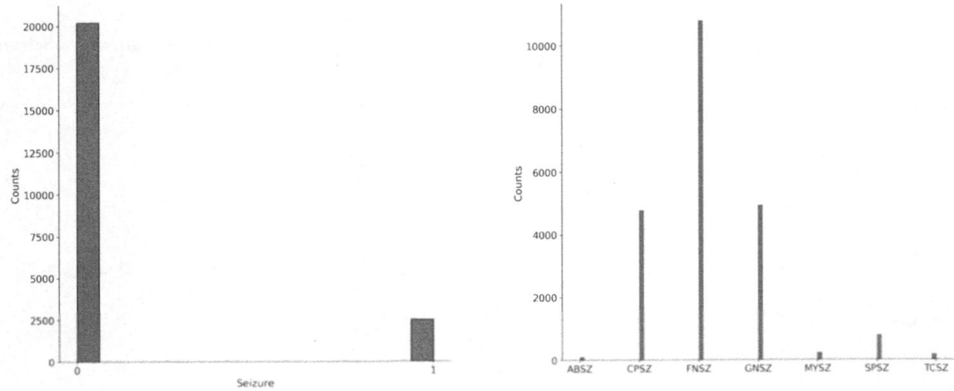


**FIGURE 12.6**
Distributions of (left panel) seizure occurrences and (right panel) seizure type in the training dataset. (Color version available in electronic supplement.)

```
# Plot the distribution of seizures vs non-seizure EEG
sns.displot(y_detect_train)
print('Ratio of seizure samples in the training data = {}'
      .format(round(y_detect_train.sum()/ len(y_detect_train), 4)))

# Plot the distribution of seizures of types
# Label distributions
plt.rcParams['figure.dpi'] = 100
sns.displot(y_classify_train)
plt.xticks(range(len(label_names)), labels=label_names);
```

To correct for data imbalance, weights inversely proportional to the frequencies of the class can be applied to the samples of the training set when evaluating the loss function. This is provided through an input argument to the `LogisticRegression()` function in Python (see code in Section 12.2). Other data balancing techniques exist, including techniques that augment the minority class by generating new samples. Examples of such techniques are SMOTE (Synthetic Minority Oversampling Technique)[3] and ADASYN (Adaptive Synthetic Sampling) [13].

### 12.6.4 Feature Scaling

A common issue encountered in practice is variability across the ranges of different features. Feature scaling brings all features to the same scale, which is important because it allows for proportioned treatment of variables regardless of their value ranges.

There are two main types of feature scaling: normalization and standardization. Data normalization typically rescales the values to fall into the range [0, 1], whereas data standardization transforms the data such that all variables have a zero mean and unit standard deviation. Normalization may be performed through min-max normalization, in which the minimum value of each feature is transformed to 0 and the maximum value of each feature is transformed to 1:

$$X_{normalized} = \frac{X - X_{min}}{X_{max} - X_{min}},$$

whereas standardization is commonly performed through a $z$-transformation:

$$X_{standardized} = \frac{X - E[X]}{\sqrt{Var[X]}}$$

where $E[X]$ is the mean of $X$ and $Var[X]$ is the variance of $X$. Normalization is typically used when the data does not have a Gaussian distribution. Normalization is highly sensitive to outliers; therefore, it is recommended that outliers be treated through methods such as trimming/removing, capping, or imputation of values prior to normalization. Standardization is typically used when the data distribution is reasonably assumed to be Gaussian. In contrast to normalization, standardization is generally not affected by outliers since the range of transformed features is unbounded.

The following Python code uses the `scikit-learn` class function `StandardScaler()` of the `preprocessing` library to standardize the data:

```
# Apply the standard scaler to training, validation and testing data

# Seizure detection data
scaler = StandardScaler().fit(X_detect_train)
X_detect_train = scaler.transform(X_detect_train)
X_detect_val = scaler.transform(X_detect_val)
X_detect_test = scaler.transform(X_detect_test)

# Seizure classification data
scaler = StandardScaler().fit(X_classify_train)
X_classify_train = scaler.transform(X_classify_train)
X_classify_val = scaler.transform(X_classify_val)
X_classify_test = scaler.transform(X_classify_test)
```

To normalize rather than standardize the data, the function `MinMaxScaler()` can be used.

### 12.6.5 Logistic Regression Application

To fit a logistic regression model in Python, we use the `scikit-learn` function `LogisticRegression()`. The main arguments to the function are the type of regularization (`penalty`, which can take values of no regularization, L1 penalty, L2 penalty, or combined L1 and L2 penalties); a regularization parameter dictating the inverse of the strength of regularization (`C`, where smaller values denote stronger regularization); the optimization algorithm (`solver`); the number of iterations for the optimization algorithm to converge (`max_iter`); and the weights associated with the classes (`class_weight`; setting this last argument to `"balanced"` automatically adjusts the weights inversely proportional to class frequencies in the training data). Other arguments to the `LogisticRegression()` class in `scikit-learn` can be found on the documentation page of the `scikit-learn` package.

Selecting the right parameters is a learning exercise and part of the optimization/training process. In our seizure detection example, we evaluate the performance of different logistic regression models by varying the type and the strength of regularization in the function `LogisticRegression()` and ultimately measuring the F1 score on the test to evaluate the end performance. Setting input parameter `multi_class='multinomial'` allows the use of a multi-class version of logistic regression, called multinomial logistic regression, or softmax regression. Multinomial logistic regression predicts the probability of class membership such that the sum of membership probabilities for all classes is equal to 1.

```
# Set ranges for the parameters to vary
pen_param = np.logspace(-3, 1.5, 15)
pen_type = ['l1', 'l2']
df_cols = ['penalty', 'param', 'f1_score']
f1_detect_df = pd.DataFrame(columns = df_cols)
f1_classify_df = pd.DataFrame(columns = df_cols)
for pen in pen_type:
```

```
    for c in pen_param:
        print('Current penalty parameter is = {}'.format(pen))
        print('Current penalty value is = {}'.format(c))

       # Seizure Detection
       # Initialize a logistic regression model
        lr_detect = LogisticRegression(C = c, penalty = pen, fit_intercept = True,
     solver = 'saga', max_iter = 500, class_weight = 'balanced', verbose = 0,
    random_state = 42, n_jobs = -1)
       # Fit the model
        lr_detect_fit = lr_detect.fit(X_detect_train, y_detect_train)
        # Classify
        y_detect_pred = lr_detect_fit.predict(X_detect_val)
        f1_detect = f1_score(y_detect_val, y_detect_pred)
        f1_detect_df = pd.concat([f1_detect_df, pd.DataFrame([[pen, np.log10(c),
    f1_detect]], columns = df_cols)])
                # Seizure Classification
        lr_classify = LogisticRegression(C = c, penalty = pen, fit_intercept =
    True, multi_class = 'multinomial', solver = 'saga', max_iter = 500,
    class_weight ='balanced', verbose = 0, random_state = 42, n_jobs = -1)
        lr_classify_fit = lr_classify.fit(X_classify_train, y_classify_train)
        y_classify_pred = lr_classify_fit.predict(X_classify_val)
        # Calculate the unweighted average f1 score (use average='macro')
        f1_classify = f1_score(y_classify_val, y_classify_pred, average = 'macro')
        f1_classify_df = pd.concat([f1_classify_df, pd.DataFrame([[pen, np.log10(c
    ), f1_classify]], columns. = df_cols)])

f1_detect_df.reset_index(inplace = True)
f1_classify_df.reset_index(inplace = True)

# plot the curve f1_score @ c for L1 and L2 regularization
plt.figure(figsize = (10,8))
sns.lineplot(data = f1_detect_df.reset_index(), x = 'param', y = 'f1_score', hue =
    'penalty')
plt.title('Seizure Detection')

plt.figure(figsize = (10,8))
sns.lineplot(data = f1_classify_df.reset_index(), x = 'param', y =. 'f1_score',
    hue = 'penalty')
plt.title('Seizure Classification')
```

The F1 score validation curve is obtained by plotting F1 score against the regularization strength parameter $c$, with smaller values of $c$ indicating greater regularization of model parameters. Figure 12.7 shows how the performance varies differently for L1 and L2 penalties. With L1 regularization, small values of $c$ result in heavy regularization and low F1 scores. Compared with L1 regularization, L2 regularization achieves a higher F1 score for both seizure detection and classification, though for different levels of regularization strength ($c = 10^{-3}$ and $c = 10^{-1}$, respectively). This indicates that some features may have a detrimental effect if left "unpenalized" in the seizure detection model, while a moderate penalty works best in the seizure classification model.

### 12.6.6 K-Nearest Neighbors Application

Next, we fit a kNN model for the tasks of seizure detection and classification. kNN is best used with normalized data because it relies on the distance between samples to optimize prediction. To fit a kNN model in Python, we use the `scikit-learn` function `KNeighborsClassifier()`. The main parameters to set are the number of neighbors (`n_neighbors`), the distance metric (`metric`), and the algorithm used to compute the nearest neighbors (ball tree, k-d Tree, brute force, or automatic selection of the best

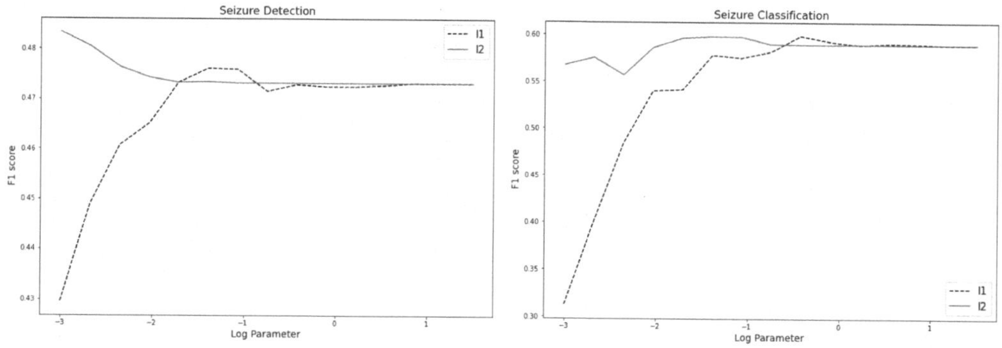


**FIGURE 12.7**
F1 score of penalized logistic regression as a function of penalty type and regularization strength, for (left panel) seizure detection and (right panel) seizure classification. The performance of the penalized logistic regression varies with the selected penalty type (L1 and L2) and the strength of regularization $c$, shown on the $x$-axis. Using the validation dataset, the highest F1 score is achieved using L2 penalty and a strength $c = 10^{-3}$ for the seizure detection and $c = 10^{-1}$ for the seizure classification.

algorithm). For a complete list of parameters, please refer to the package's documentation page. The code below initializes a kNN classifier with a different number of neighbors, weight functions, and nearest neighbor computation algorithms while setting the distance metric to Euclidean distance:

```
n_neighbors = np.linspace(1, 50, 5).astype('int')
weights = ['uniform', 'distance']
df_cols = ['weights', 'n_neighbors', 'f1_score']
f1_df_knn_detect = pd.DataFrame(columns = df_cols)
f1_df_knn_classify = pd.DataFrame(columns = df_cols)
for w in weights:
    for k in n_neighbors:
        print('Current weight parameter is = {}'.format(w))
        print('Current #neighbors value is = {}'.format(k))

        # Initialize a KNN classifier for seizure detection
        knn_detect = KNeighborsClassifier(n_neighbors=k, weights = w, algorithm='
    auto', p = 2, n_jobs = -1)
        knn_detect_fit = knn_detect.fit(X_detect_train, y_detect_train)
        y_detect_pred = knn_detect_fit.predict(X_detect_val)
        f1 = f1_score(y_detect_val, y_detect_pred)
        f1_df_knn_detect = pd.concat([f1_df_knn_detect, pd.DataFrame([[w, k, f1]],
     columns = df_cols)])

        # Initialize a KNN classifier for seizure classification
        knn_classify = KNeighborsClassifier(n_neighbors = k, weights = w,
    algorithm = 'auto', p=2, n_jobs = -1)
        knn_classify_fit = knn_classify.fit(X_classify_train, y_classify_train)
        y_classify_pred = knn_classify_fit.predict(X_classify_val)
        f1 = f1_score(y_classify_val, y_classify_pred, average = 'macro')
        f1_df_knn_classify = pd.concat([f1_df_knn_classify, pd.DataFrame([[w, k,
    f1]], columns = df_cols)])

f1_df_knn_detect.reset_index(inplace = True)
f1_df_knn_classify.reset_index(inplace = True)
plt.figure(figsize=(10,8))

#Plot the curve f1_score @ 'n_neighbors'
```

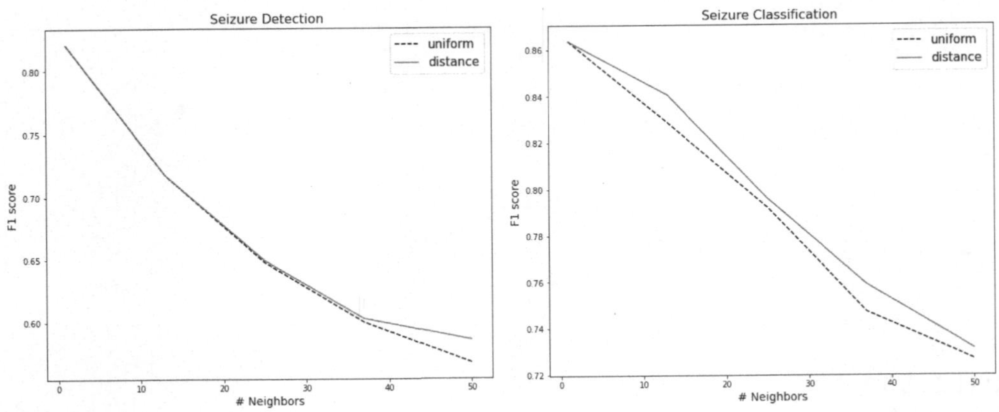


**FIGURE 12.8**
Performance of k-nearest neighbors (kNN) classifier evaluated using F1 score for different numbers of neighbors ($k$) and different weights. For both (left panel) seizure detection and (right panel) seizure classification tasks, the performance drops quasi-linearly with the number of neighbors. $k = 1$ leads to the highest F1 score. In practice, increasing the number of neighbors at the cost of a small drop in performance is recommended because it leads to improved generalization and robustness to outliers.

```
sns.lineplot(data = f1_df_knn_detect, x = 'n_neighbors', y = 'f1_score', hue = '
    weights')
sns.lineplot(data = f1_df_knn_classify, x = 'n_neighbors', y = 'f1_score', hue = '
    weights')
```

As shown in Figure 12.8, the performance of the kNN classifier decreases linearly with the number of neighbors $k$. With $k$=1, an F1 score of about 0.8 can be achieved for both seizure detection and classification tasks. While this choice of $k$ leads to a good validation performance, it may not be the best choice. Using only one neighbor is problematic because estimating the class probability based on a single sample is sensitive to outliers and mislabeled data. Moreover, with $k$=1, a kNN tends generally to overfit the training data and poorly generalize its overoptimistic performance over an independent test set. Using more neighbors is often warranted for robust classification with kNN.

### 12.6.7 Random Forest Application

To fit a Random Forest in Python, we use the `RandomForestClassifier()` function from `scikit-learn`. Fitting a Random Forest requires the optimization of many parameters. As discussed in Section 12.4.2, two parameters are particularly important to explore when fitting a Random Forest because they fundamentally shape how the model fits the data: the number of trees in the forest and the number of features considered at each split of the tree. More parameters can be used to fine-tune the fitting process. We encourage the reader to check `scikit-learn` documentation for more information. The code below initializes a Random Forest algorithm with a combination of a number of trees and a number of features considered at each split node. The F1 score evaluates the performance of the algorithm for each combination:

```
ntrees = np.linspace(100, 2000, 15).astype('int')
nfeatures = X_train.shape[1]
features = [nfeatures, int(np.sqrt(nfeatures)), int(nfeatures**(1/3))]
df_cols = ['features', 'trees', 'f1_score']
```

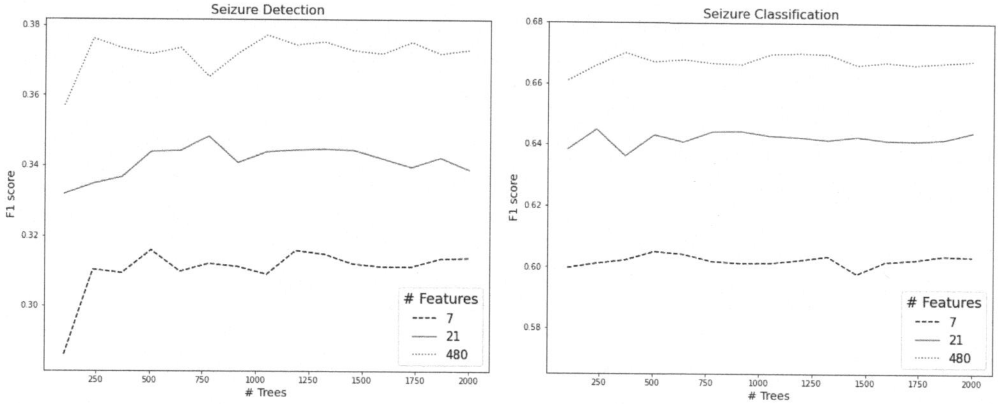


**FIGURE 12.9**
F1 score performance of Random Forest classifier as a function of the number of trees and number of features evaluated at each split, for (left panel) seizure detection and (right panel) seizure classification. The F1 score improves significantly when the number of features is increased, but not when the number of trees (shown on the $x$-axis) is increased. (Color version available in electronic supplement.)

```
f1_df_rf_detect = pd.DataFrame(columns = df_cols)
f1_df_rf_classify = pd.DataFrame(columns = df_cols)
for tree in ntrees:
    for f in features:
        print('Current feature parameter is = {}'.format(f))
        print('Current #trees value is = {}'.format(tree))

        # Initialize a Random Forest classifier for seizure detection
        rf_detect = RandomForestClassifier(n_estimators = tree, max_features = f,
    random_state = 42, class_weight = 'balanced', verbose = 0, n_jobs = -1)
        rf_fit_detect = rf_detect.fit(X_detect_train, y_detect_train)
        y_detect_pred = rf_fit_detect.predict(X_detect_val)
        f1 = f1_score(y_detect_val, y_detect_pred)
        f1_df_rf_detect = pd.concat([f1_df_rf_detect, pd.DataFrame([[f, tree, f1
    ]], columns = df_cols)])

        # Initialize a Random Forest classifier for seizure classification
        rf_classify = RandomForestClassifier(n_estimators = tree, max_features = f
    , random_state = 42, class_weight = 'balanced', verbose = 0, n_jobs = -1)
        rf_fit_classify = rf_classify.fit(X_classify_train, y_classify_train)
        y_classify_pred = rf_fit_classify.predict(X_classify_val)
        f1 = f1_score(y_classify_val, y_classify_pred, average = 'macro')
        f1_df_rf_classify = pd.concat([f1_df_rf_classify, pd.DataFrame([[f, tree,
    f1]], columns = df_cols)])

f1_df_rf_classify.reset_index(inplace = True)
f1_df_rf_detect.reset_index(inplace = True)
```

Figure 12.9 shows the performance of a Random Forest classifier for seizure detection and classification, evaluated for different numbers of trees and features at each split. Even though the F1 score increases when more features are used, the Random Forest algorithm does not achieve acceptable levels of F1 score in either task. This is not an unexpected result. The Random Forest algorithm is generally not suited for time-series data, as the non-tabular structure of time-series cannot easily be partitioned. However, other ensemble machine learning algorithms are known to work well in time-series classification problems and can be explored. Examples of these algorithms include the Hierarchical

Vote Collective of Transformation-based Ensembles (HIVE-COTE), a heterogeneous meta ensemble algorithm that captures different sources of possible discriminatory features in time series [2, 14, 16]. Another ensemble method tailored for time series classification is the Time Series Combination of Heterogeneous and Integrated Embedding Forest (TS-CHIEF), which uses forest classifiers and efficient time-series embedding to achieve high classification accuracy while being more computationally efficient than HIVE-COTE [21]. Other algorithms with remarkable performance for time-series classification tasks that are not ensemble methods include the Random Convolutional Kernel Transform (ROCKET) [6] and the deep learning based approach InceptionTime [9].

### 12.6.8 XGBoost Application

XGBoost is a powerful distributed gradient-boosted decision tree machine learning library. In Python, it is implemented under the module `xgboost` and it is initialized using the function `XGBClassifier()`. Two of the many tunable input parameters of `XGBClassifier()` are the number of boosting rounds (i.e., the number of trees to build, `n_estimator`) and the learning rate (step-size shrinkage to prevent overfitting, `learning_rate`). The code below shows an example of XGBoost implementation. It iterates through multiple values of the number of boosting rounds and the learning rate and evaluates the performance of the XGBoost classifier for each combination. For a complete description of all the input parameters for XGBoost, the reader is referred to the official library XGBoost documentation.

```
Lrs = [0.001, 0.01, 0.1]
nboost = np.linspace(50, 2000, 10).astype(int)
scale_pos_weight = (len(y_train) - sum(y_train))/ sum(y_train)
# Create balanced class weights for the multi-class classification problem
sample_weights = compute_sample_weight(class_weight =. 'balanced', y = y_train)
df_cols = ['lr', 'trees', 'f1_score']
f1_df_xgb_detect = pd.DataFrame(columns = df_cols)
for boost in nboost:
    for lr in lrs:
        print('Current learning rate is = {}'.format(lr))
        print('Current #boosters value is = {}'.format(boost))

        # Initialize an XGBoost classifier for seizure detection
        xgb_detect = xgb.XGBClassifier(n_estimators = boost,
                                       learning_rate = lr,
                                       objective = 'binary:logistic',
                                       random_state = 42, scale_pos_weight =
    scale_pos_weight,n_jobs = -1)
        xgb_fit_detect = xgb_detect.fit(X_detect_train, y_detect_train)
        y_detect_pred = xgb_fit_detect.predict(X_detect_val)
        f1 = f1_score(y_detect_val, y_detect_pred)
        f1_df_xgb_detect = pd.concat([f1_df_xgb_detect, pd.DataFrame([[lr, boost,
    f1]], columns = df_cols)])


        # Initialize an XGBoost classifier for seizure classification
        xgb_classify = xgb.XGBClassifier(n_estimators = boost,
                                         learning_rate = lr,
                                         objective = 'multi:softmax',
                                         random_state = 42,
                                         n_jobs = -1)
        xgb_fit_classify = xgb_classify.fit(X_classify_train, y_classify_train,
    sample_weight=sample_weights)
        y_classify_pred = xgb_fit_classify.predict(X_classify_val)
        f1 = f1_score(y_classify_val, y_classify_pred, average = 'macro')
```

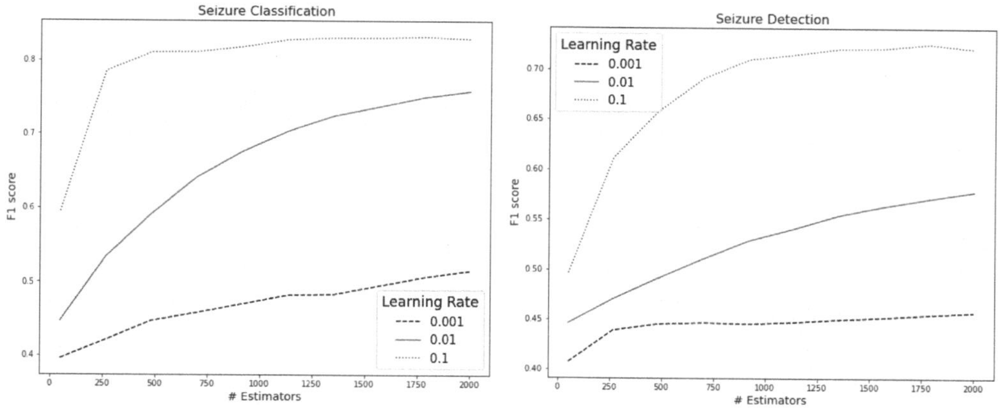


**FIGURE 12.10**
F1 score performance of XGBoost as a function of the number of trees and learning rate, for (left panel) seizure detection and (right panel) seizure classification. In both tasks, the performance of the classifier improves significantly when the number of trees and the learning rate are increased. Beyond 1500 trees, the increase in performance is marginal. (Color version available in electronic supplement.)

```
        f1_df_xgb_classify = pd.concat([f1_df_xgb_classify, pd.DataFrame([[lr,
    boost, f1]], columns = df_cols)])


f1_df_xgb_detect.reset_index(inplace = True)
f1_df_xgb_classify.reset_index(inplace = True)


# Performance plots
plt.figure(figsize = (10,8))
sns.lineplot(data = f1_df_xgb_detect, x = 'trees', y = 'f1_score', hue = 'lr',
    palette = ['r', 'b', 'g'])
plt.figure(figsize = (10,8))
sns.lineplot(data = f1_df_xgb_classify, x = 'trees', y = 'f1_score', hue = 'lr',
    palette = ['r', 'b', 'g'])
```

Figure 12.10 shows the F1 score using XGBoost for seizure detection (left panel) and seizure classification (right panel) as a function of the number of trees (boosting rounds) for three learning rate values. There is a clear trend of performance improvement as the number of trees is increased. However, improvement becomes marginal as more trees are added beyond 1000 trees for both seizure detection and classification tasks. With a learning rate of 0.1 and 1750 trees, XGboost achieves an F1 score of 0.73 in seizure detection. A slightly higher F1 score of 0.81 is achieved in seizure classification when setting the learning rate to 0.1 and the number of trees to 1500.

Next, we explore whether widening the range of parameters can lead to further improvement in F1 score. The following code evaluates the F1 score as a measure of training performance over a larger set of parameters, for both the learning rate and the number of trees, using a random search over the parameter set with a 20-fold cross-validation. Note that in a random search, a fixed number of parameter combinations is selected. These combinations are picked randomly; therefore, not every combination is evaluated.

```
param_grid = {'n_estimators': np.linspace(50, 2000, 20).astype(int),
              'learning_rate': [0.1],
              'gamma': np.linspace(0., 5., 10), # range(0,infty)
```

```
                'max_depth': np.linspace(3, 30).astype(int), # range(0, infty)
                'min_child_weight': np.linspace(3., 50., 10).astype(int), # range
    (0, infty)
                'subsample': np.linspace(0.51, 1, 10), # range (0, 1]
                'colsample_bytree': np.linspace(0.7, 1, 5),
                'reg_lambda': np.logspace(-2, 2, 15),
                'reg_alpha': np.logspace(-2, 2, 15)
                }
xgb_estimator = xgb.XGBClassifier(objective = 'binary:logistic',
random_state = 42, scale_pos_weight=scale_pos_weight, n_jobs = -1)

split_index = [-1] * X_detect_train.shape[0] + [0] * X_detect_val.shape[0]
cross_validation_type = PredefinedSplit(test_fold=split_index)
xgb_rs = RandomizedSearchCV(estimator = xgb_estimator, param_distributions =
    param_grid, cv = cross_validation_type, scoring = 'f1', n_iter = 20, refit =
    True)
X = np.concatenate((X_detect_train, X_detect_val))
y = np.concatenate((y_detect_train, y_detect_val))

xgb_cv_fit = xgb_rs.fit(X,y)
```

The random search over the parameter spaces for learning rate and number of trees using cross-validation leads to a maximum F1 score of 0.74 for seizure detection. Although this yields only moderate improvement, it encourages the investigation of further combinations of parameters that may have been missed in a random search. Compared to a random search, a grid search tests all combinations of parameters, which may potentially lead to identification of parameters yielding better performance than random search. However, full grid search is a computationally expensive procedure. An alternative procedure is to conduct a random search followed by a grid subsearch near the optimum parameters found in the random search.

To estimate the ultimate performance of XGBoost for seizure detection, the F1 score is calculated on the test set, using the optimized parameters identified from a grid search on the training set:

```
# Test performance using the test dataset
y_pred = xgb_cv_fit_detect.predict(X_detect_test)
f1 = f1_score(y_detect_test, y_pred)
```

This results in an F1 score of 0.76 for the seizure detection task.

Table 12.1 shows the confusion matrix for XGBoost applied to the seizure detection task, which is a matrix showing the number of correctly and incorrectly classified seizure and non-seizure segments. We observe that XGBoost misclassifies twice as many "seizure" segments as "non-seizure," compared to "non-seizure" segments that were misclassified as "seizure." This reflects a seizure detection system with a higher specificity than sensitivity. In clinical applications where the cost of false detection is high (e.g., a system that triggers a therapeutic intervention when a seizure is detected), the seizure detection system may be tuned such that the specificity is maximized (lowest false detection rate) while tolerating few missed seizures (lower sensitivity).

**TABLE 12.1**
Confusion matrix for seizure detection using XGBoost.

| | | Actual Class | |
|---|---|---|---|
| | | Non-Seizure | Seizure |
| Predicted | Non-Seizure | 12148 (87%) | 215 (1%) |
| | Seizure | 456 (3%) | 1101 (8%) |

For the seizure classification task, a random grid search over the parameters on the training data leads to a near-perfect best F1 score of 0.99 using the training data, an F1 score of 0.83 using the validation data, and an F1 score of 0.83 using the test data.

Table 12.2 shows the confusion matrix applied to the seizure type classification task. It is important to examine the confusion matrix to identify seizure types that are more often misclassified than others. While most seizure types have a relatively small number of misclassifications, seizure types "FNSZ" (focal nonspecific seizures), "GNSZ" (generalized seizures), and "CPSZ" (complex partial seizures) have a sizable number of misclassifications, possibly due to similarity of electrographic signatures shared by the three seizure types, particularly between "FNSZ" and "CPSZ," as many of the focal nonspecific seizures could indeed be elusive complex partial seizures.

**TABLE 12.2**
Confusion matrix for seizure classification using XGBoost.

| | | Actual Class | | | | | |
|---|---|---|---|---|---|---|---|
| | | ABSZ | CPSZ | FNSZ | GNSZ | MYSZ | SPSZ |
| Predicted | ABSZ | 66 (0.49%) | 1 (0.01%) | 0 (0%) | 4 (0.03%) | 1 (0.01%) | 1 (0.01%) |
| | CPSZ | 6 (0.04%) | 2378 (17.77%) | 474 (3.54%) | 67 (0.50%) | 3 (0.02%) | 18 (0.13%) |
| | FNSZ | 3 (0.02%) | 339 (2.53%) | 5890 (44.02%) | 236 (1.76%) | 5 (0.04%) | 15 (0.11%) |
| | GNSZ | 2 (0.01%) | 68 (0.51%) | 407 (3.04%) | 2590 (19.36%) | 2 (0.01%) | 27 (0.20%) |
| | MYSZ | 1 (0.01%) | 2 (0.01%) | 16 (0.12%) | 2 (0.01%) | 128 (0.96%) | 1 (0.01%) |
| | SPSZ | 3 (0.02%) | 5 (0.04%) | 40 (0.30%) | 33 (0.25%) | 2 (0.01%) | 403 (3.01%) |
| | TCSZ | 0 (0%) | 21 (0.16%) | 33 (0.25%) | 1 (0.01%) | 0 (0%) | 2 (0.01%) |

## 12.7 Summary

In this chapter, we present fundamental concepts of supervised learning to demonstrate how supervised machine learning approaches may be applied to classification problems in epilepsy research, including tasks such as seizure detection and classification. Here, we focus on three popular supervised machine learning algorithms and illustrate their implementation; other popular algorithms, such as support vector machines, naive Bayes classifiers, and linear discriminant analysis, may be suitable depending on the data. Artificial neural networks are another field of machine learning which have successfully been applied in different fields of epilepsy research, including seizure detection and prediction, image analysis, and medical and surgical management of epilepsy [1] and are discussed in Chapter 13. The principles and examples covered in this chapter are intended to familiarize the reader with basic concepts in carrying out supervised learning as well as several popular algorithms that may be encountered, and to illustrate practical problems that researchers may anticipate when applying supervised learning algorithms to eal-world data in epilepsy. As multimodal and large scale data continues to be collected in epilepsy with interest in prediction and classification, supervised learning applications will continue to comprise a dominant field in epilepsy research.

## Bibliography

[1] Bardia Abbasi and Daniel M. Goldenholz. Machine learning applications in epilepsy. *Epilepsia*, 60(10):2037–2047, 2019.

[2] Anthony Bagnall, Michael Flynn, James Large, Jason Lines, and Matthew Middlehurst. A tale of two toolkits, report the third: on the usage and performance of HIVE-COTE v1.0, 2020.

[3] Kevin W. Bowyer, Nitesh V. Chawla, Lawrence O. Hall, and W. Philip Kegelmeyer. SMOTE: Synthetic Minority Over-sampling Technique. *CoRR*, abs/1106.1813, 2011.

[4] Leo Breiman. Random forests. *Machine Learning*, 45(1):5–32, 2001.

[5] Tianqi Chen and Carlos Guestrin. XGBoost: A scalable tree boosting system. In *Proceedings of the 22nd ACM SIGKDD International Conference on Knowledge Discovery and Data Mining*, KDD '16, page 785–794, New York, NY, USA, 2016. Association for Computing Machinery.

[6] Angus Dempster, Franccois Petitjean, and Geoffrey I. Webb. ROCKET: Exceptionally fast and accurate time series classification using random convolutional kernels. *Data Mining and Knowledge Discovery*, 34(5):1454–1495, jul 2020.

[7] Dheeru Dua and Casey Graff. UCI machine learning repository, 2017.

[8] Rong-En Fan, Kai-Wei Chang, Cho-Jui Hsieh, Xiang-Rui Wang, and Chih-Jen Lin. Liblinear: A library for large linear classification. *Journal of Machine Learning Research*, 9(Aug):1871–1874, 2008.

[9] Hassan Ismail Fawaz, Benjamin Lucas, Germain Forestier, Charlotte Pelletier, Daniel F. Schmidt, Jonathan Weber, Geoffrey I. Webb, Lhassane Idoumghar, Pierre-Alain Muller, and Francois Petitjean. InceptionTime: Finding AlexNet for time series classification. *Data Mining and Knowledge Discovery*, 34(6):1936–1962, sep 2020.

[10] Jerome H. Friedman. Greedy function approximation: A gradient boosting machine. *The Annals of Statistics*, 29(5):1189–1232, 2001.

[11] Sukhi Grewal and Jean Gotman. An automatic warning system for epileptic seizures recorded on intracerebral EEGs. *Clinical Neurophysiology*, 116(10):2460–2472, 2005.

[12] Trevor Hastie, Robert Tibshirani, and Jerome Friedman. *The Elements of Statistical Learning: Data Mining, Inference and Prediction.* Springer, 2nd edition, 2009.

[13] Haibo He, Yang Bai, Edwardo A. Garcia, and Shutao Li. ADASYN: Adaptive synthetic sampling approach for imbalanced learning. In *2008 IEEE International Joint Conference on Neural Networks (IEEE World Congress on Computational Intelligence)*, pages 1322–1328, 2008.

[14] Jason Lines, Sarah Taylor, and Anthony Bagnall. Time series classification with hive-cote: The hierarchical vote collective of transformation-based ensembles. *ACM Transactions on Knowledge Discovery from Data*, 12(5), jul 2018.

[15] Dong C. Liu and Jorge Nocedal. On the limited memory BFGS method for large scale optimization. *Mathematical Programming*, 45(1–3):503–528, aug 1989.

[16] Matthew Middlehurst, James Large, Michael Flynn, Jason Lines, Aaron Bostrom, and Anthony Bagnall. HIVE-COTE 2.0: a new meta ensemble for time series classification, 2021.

[17] Tom M Mitchell. *Machine Learning*, volume 1. McGraw-Hill, New York, 1997.

[18] Iyad Obeid and Joseph Picone. The temple university hospital EEG data corpus. *Frontiers in Neuroscience*, 10, 2016.

[19] C. J. Van Rijsbergen. *Information Retrieval.* Butterworth-Heinemann, 2nd edition, 1979.

[20] Stephanie Roy, Umar Asif, J. Tang, and Stefan Harrer. Seizure type classification using eeg signals and machine learning: Setting a benchmark. *2020 IEEE Signal Processing in Medicine and Biology Symposium (SPMB)*, pages 1–6, 2020.

[21] Ahmed Shifaz, Charlotte Pelletier, Franccois Petitjean, and Geoffrey I. Webb. TS-CHIEF: A scalable and accurate forest algorithm for time series classification. *Data Mining and Knowledge Discovery*, 34(3):742–775, mar 2020.

[22] Prince Grover Terrence Parr, Tudor Lapusan. dtreeviz: Decision tree visualization. GitHub repository, 2021. Accessed: April 23, 2023.

[23] W. J. Youden. Index for rating diagnostic tests. *Cancer*, 3(1):32–35, 1950.

[24] Hui Zou and Trevor Hastie. Regularization and variable selection via the elastic net. *Journal of the Royal Statistical Society. Series B (Statistical Methodology)*, 67(2):301–320, 2005.

# 13

# *Natural Language Processing*

**Christfried H. Focke**
*AppFolio (USA)*

**Rob M. Sylvester**
*Reltio Inc. (USA)*

## CONTENTS



In this chapter, we introduce modern natural language processing (NLP) libraries, techniques and their applications. This chapter focuses on deep learning methods and less on computational linguistics that require nuanced knowledge of linguistics. We explore what it means to represent words and sequences of words with rich numeric representations that are better-suited toward modern computational tasks. We aim to capture some of these modern fine-tuned representations that are specially catered toward a semantic lexicon for

DOI: 10.1201/9781003254515-13

medical language. First, we provide an introduction to fundamental NLP concepts, followed by review of deep learning in NLP. We provide a discussion of embeddings and medical text representations and discuss general use case patterns of NLP techniques in epilepsy. We end with a discussion of modern generative NLP models. Epilepsy-specific examples of these topics are provided in Python. This chapter is intended to endow the reader with a general knowledge of the building blocks of state-of-the-art NLP models, and an understanding of how these pieces fit together into a model such as GPT4.

## 13.1 Introduction

Natural language processing (NLP) is a field of computer science that deals with the extraction, processing, and understanding of human language. It is known as the field of computer linguistics and is a subfield of artificial intelligence. Common NLP tasks include sentence segmentation, tokenization, part-of-speech tagging, named-entity recognition, parsing, question answering, summarization and classification.

How can we teach a computer to perform these tasks? The first challenge is that computers, at their core, only understand numbers. So first we need to think about how words, or more generally text, can be represented with numbers such that we can perform calculations on them. The numbers should allow the computer to assign meaning to words and their context of surrounding words.

There is no perfect way to represent language in this numeric fashion. The best we can do is to capture representations that we feel capture the *syntactic* features of text, as well as *semantic* features of text. Syntactic information refers to grammatical constructs and the way that words are put together in a language. Semantic information refers to the meaning of this body of text. Such distinctions are fundamental concepts in computer science and date back to the very foundations of information theory [16]. Much of this chapter, as well as much of the current work in the field of computational linguistics is centered around finding better and better representations that capture both types of this information.

How do we begin to choose these representations? Do we choose to represent words, or perhaps individual letters? Do we choose all the words? What do we do with punctuation and numbers?

### 13.1.1 Vocabularies and Words

In NLP, the set of unique words in a corpus is called a *vocabulary*. While *the* is the most common word in the English language, it is only one entry in a very large vocabulary table. A rare word like *hemispherectomy* is also one entry in this table. Both *apple* and *apples* might be separate entries in our vocabulary table. Generally the first step in many NLP systems is defining this vocabulary and the rules behind which words are in this table and which words are not.

The process of splitting text into separate smaller units, in this case words, is known as *tokenization*. When we run many NLP tasks, we almost always preprocess our text by putting it into one of these tokenizers. The output tokens, in this case words, are the indexes in our lookup table to different numeric representations that can be understood by a machine. There are a number of great tokenization libraries that are open source, and these should always be used rather than implementing on one's own.

**Example 13.1.1.** (Spacy tokenization using medical words).

```
import spacy
sample = "After a temporal lobe resection, the " \
         "atonic and clonic seizure frequency " \
         "fell by 50%."

nlp = spacy.load("en_core_web_sm")
english_vocab = set(nlp.vocab.strings)
spacy_document = nlp(sample)

for token in spacy_document:
    found = token.text in english_vocab
    print("{}: {}".format(token.text, found))
```

The discrete numeric entities created in Example 13.1.1 are the indexes for our representations. The tokenizer system did much of the magic under the hood, lowercasing and standardizing text and creating special tokens for punctuation and numbers.

When we build a vocabulary $V$, we define a preset vocabulary size $|V|$. There is a tradeoff in your choice of $|V|$. If a number is chosen that is too small, then the system will only recognize a few words and lose a lot of important task-specific vocabulary. However, if the entire English language is included, the system will be slow, expensive, and will not perform as well. Commonly this number is set around 20,000–40,000 words in English, though it can be much larger.

Often a vocabulary will include special tokens that make our lives easier when working with NLP tasks. Common special tokens include:

- `[EOS]` – An end of sentence/input marker.
- `[PAD]` – Special inputs to ignore, usually following an EOS marker.
- `[SEP]` – A separator, which can be used in inputs that contain multiple sentences or samples.
- `[OOV]` – Out of vocabulary, also commonly represented as [UNK] (unknown), which is used when we come across a word that does not exist in our vocabulary.

The out-of-vocabulary token is of particular importance in medicine. If we load a vocabulary with 30,000 words, often these are roughly the most common 30,000 words in the English language. We will still have a few [OOV] tokens for rare words. However, just because a general system chooses its vocabulary based on word frequency does not mean that this is the best choice of vocabulary for the task at hand. Medical corpora have a very different word frequency distribution than non-medical corpora, particulary because of nuanced vocabulary that is crucial.

In Example 1 above, notice the importance of the words that have been thrown away. If this sentence were to be loaded into a machine as is, we might be losing far too much information because we have to replace nearly all of the relevant terminology with OOV tokens. We will address this issue in the ensuing sections. For now, suffice it to say that we should make sure our vocabularies are catered toward our task at hand or are built in such a way that they can still extract signal from these tokens. Furthermore, we should always sanity check our sample token outputs against our raw text inputs.

### 13.1.2 Word Representations

Given that we have defined a vocabulary $V$ of words, these are the keys to our lookup table of numeric representations. But what do we store in that table as the value?

A simple way to achieve this representation for $V$ is to assign each word a unique integer $i$. The word is then represented as a vector $w$ of length $|V|$ with all zeros and a one at index $i$, otherwise known as one-hot encoding.

```
have = [1, 0, 0, 0, 0, 0, ... 0]
a    = [0, 1, 0, 0, 0, 0, ... 0]
good = [0, 0, 1, 0, 0, 0, ... 0]
day  = [0, 0, 0, 1, 0, 0, ... 0]
...
```

We could now represent a sentence as the sum of the word vectors $S = \sum_j w_j$. This representation is suitable as input for any classification algorithm (such as logistic regression or decision trees; see Chapter 12), to make a prediction about our target variable, e.g. whether the sentence is relevant to our epilepsy task. This simple representation fulfills our requirements but comes with some drawbacks:

1. We implicitly assume that each word in the sentence is equally important.
2. Each word is equally similar to every other word (e.g. by taking the Euclidean distance between word vectors).
3. The representation is invariant to a reordering of the words.

The first point is a problem, because as we add more word vectors together, the sentence representation will converge to the global average and drown out any signal relevant to the specific sentence at hand. To address this, we can instead write a weighted sum $S = \sum_j \lambda_j w_j$, where each word vector is weighted by its importance $\lambda_j$. There are statistical methods we can use to compute an importance value, such as the Term Frequency-Inverse Document Frequency algorithm (TF-IDF). For example, a word like *the* is very common and appears in many different contexts. It is unlikely that there is a lot of signal we can extract from it. On the other hand, a word like *epilepsy* will be much more rare and specific to a given task, and we would like to raise its importance. This has the net effect of allowing us to find good representations for larger word sequences. To address the second point, we will give a brief introduction into Deep Learning (DL) and the extremely powerful concept of *embeddings*: one that is not only relevant in NLP, but in the world of artificial intelligence in general.

## 13.2 Deep Learning

Deep neural networks (DNNs) have revolutionized the field of NLP, along with many other fields. NLP has seen three main architectures emerge over time: fully connected neural networks (FCNN), recurrent neural networks (RNNs), and Transformers.

### 13.2.1 Fully Connected Neural Networks

FCNNs are the simplest form of neural networks and are characterized by their feedforward structure, where the input is mapped to one or more output nodes, and with an adjustable number of hidden layers in between. Each node is connected to every other node in the previous and following layer, via a linear transformation (i.e. a matrix multiplication) followed by a non-linear activation function (e.g. a sigmoid). The addition of a non-linear activation function allows for the capture of non-linear relationships between the input and output; without it, the transformation could be rewritten as just a single matrix

**TABLE 13.1**
Common loss functions used for various machine learning tasks. Mean squared error is used for regression tasks, binary cross entropy for binary classification, and cross entropy for multi-class classification.

| Loss name | Function |
|---|---|
| Mean Squared Error | $\frac{1}{N}\sum_{i=1}^{N} \lvert\hat{y}_i - y_i\rvert^2$ |
| Binary Cross Entropy | $-\frac{1}{N}\sum_{i=1}^{N}(y_i \cdot log(\hat{y}_i) + (1-y_i)\cdot log(1-\hat{y}_i))$ |
| Cross Entropy | $-\frac{1}{N}\sum_{i=1}^{N} y_i \cdot log(\hat{y}_i)$ |

multiplication. The key advantage of DNNs is their ability to automatically learn complex representations of the input data using multiple hidden layers, allowing for the capture of high-level features that could not be easily hand-engineered.

While glossing over some details, training any type of DNN can summarized in the following steps:

1. Prepare data pairs $(x_i, y_i)$, where $x_i$ is an input sample, and $y_i$ is the desired output.
2. Determine a function $f$, such that $f(\theta, x_i) = \hat{y}_i \approx y_i$, where $\theta$ are model parameters and $f$ is the model architecture.
3. Define a loss function $L(\theta) = \sum_i L(\hat{y}_i, y_i)$ that measures how close the model's output is to the desired output.
4. Optimize $\theta$ to minimize $L(\theta)$.

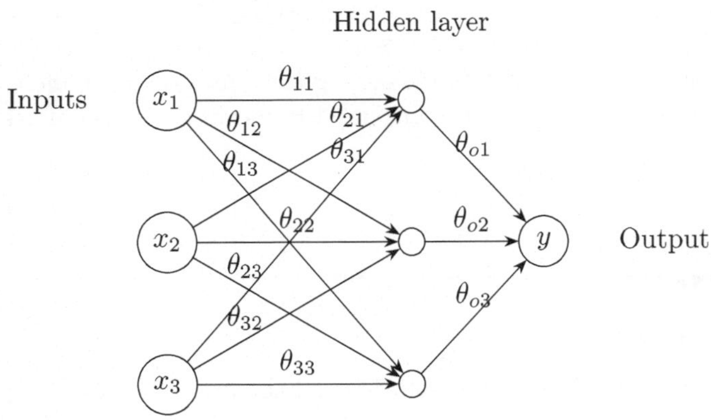


**FIGURE 13.1**
Generic architecture of a fully connected neural network. The input is mapped to the output via a series of linear transformations and non-linear activation functions. The number of hidden layers and the number of nodes in each layer are hyperparameters that can be tuned.

Here, the loss function can take on many forms, depending on the training task. We summarize some of the most common ones in Table 13.1. Training is then formulated as the task of finding the parameter configuration that minimizes the loss function. We visualize the loss function of just a single parameter in Figure 13.2. In order to move toward the global minimum, we need to update the parameters in the direction of the steepest descent, which can be calculated by taking the derivative of the loss function with respect to the

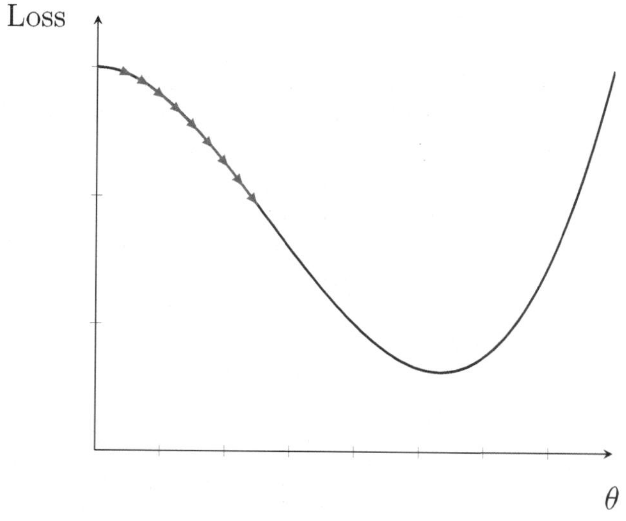


**FIGURE 13.2**
To minimize the loss function, we adjust the parameter $\theta$ in the direction of the steepest descent, which can be calculated by taking the derivative of the loss function with respect to $\theta$. (Color version available in electronic supplement.)

parameter. Parameters in the last layer are then updated according to the following rule until convergence:

$$\theta \to \theta - \alpha \frac{\partial L}{\partial \theta}, \tag{13.1}$$

where $\alpha$ is called the *learning rate* and determines the step size, the partial derivative of the loss function with respect to the parameters is called the *gradient*. Consequently the algorithm is called *gradient descent* and is the workhorse of all modern deep learning. The algorithm trivially extends to the case of multiple parameters in the last layer. A similar rule applies to parameters in the hidden layers. Once the gradients of the subsequent layer have been computed we can apply the chain rule from calculus to compute the gradients of the parameters in the current layer – this is called *backpropagation*.

Simple FCNNs have several limitations in NLP. For example, it is difficult to capture the sequential structure of text data, and they do not scale well to large vocabularies. Remember that, in order to represent a word in a FCNN, we need to have a one-hot vector of size $|V|$. To represent a sentence of length $n$, we need to have $n$ vectors of size $|V|$, which entails a lot of parameters.

### 13.2.2 Recurrent Neural Networks

To overcome this, RNNs were introduced. RNNs are a type of neural network that have loops in their structure, allowing information to flow both forward and backward through the network. The idea is that we can use the output of the previous step as input to the current step, and the output of the current step as input to the next step, and so on. To encode the meaning of a sentence or paragraph, the model reads the tokens one by one, updating the representation in the hidden state, which can then be used for subsequent predictions. This allows us to reuse a large part of the parameters, which is crucial for efficient training. It also means that this architecture is suitable to varying length inputs, as we can stop reading the input once we reach the end of the sentence. This is in contrast to FCNNs, where we have to define the maximum length of the input in advance. However, this comes at a cost.

For the purpose of training this architecture, think of unrolling the network into a sequence of layers, where each layer is a single step in the sequence. This quickly leads to very deep neural networks, which tend to be difficult to train because the training signal has to flow through each layer. This is related to a common problem in DL that is known as *vanishing gradients*. It occurs when the gradients used to update the network's parameters become extremely small, a consequence of the backpropagation algorithm where gradients are multiplied by the derivative of the activation function of the subsequent layer. In the case of a *sigmoid*, its derivative is smaller than one, so that this factor decays exponentially in the number of layers. This means that the maximum sequence length that can be learned is strongly limited. There are some workarounds, such as using different activation functions (e.g., *tanh*, *ReLU*) or gating mechanisms (e.g., Long Short-Term Memory or Gated Recurrent Units) to allow the information to propagate more freely through the network. But even then, the maximum achievable sequence length is limited to about 100 tokens before the network "forgets" what happens at the beginning.

Lastly, RNNs are inherently sequential because the output of a step depends on the output of the previous step, and vice versa during backpropagation. We can not parallelize this process making parameter updates, and therefore scaling to large datasets, as well as inference, is very slow.

**Attention:** One way to address the vanishing gradient problem is to use a so-called attention mechanism [3]. The intuition behind the attention mechanism is to assign a weight to each part of the input sequence, indicating the importance of that part for the current task. These weights are computed dynamically for each step in the processing of the input sequence and allow the model to focus on the most relevant parts of the sequence. They are implemented as additional layers in the model that calculate the attention weights using a set of learnable parameters and use these weights to weight the hidden states of the RNN at each step in the processing of the input sequence. The weighted hidden states are then combined and passed through a feedforward neural network to produce the final output.

There are several different types of attention mechanisms, including additive attention, multiplicative attention, and self-attention. Each of these mechanisms has its own strengths and weaknesses, and the choice of mechanism to use depends on the specific requirements of the task and the nature of the input data.

### 13.2.3 Transformers

The development of attention mechanisms in RNNs laid the foundation for the development of the Transformer architecture, which is now the state-of-the-art in many natural language processing tasks.

The main drawback of attention mechanisms in RNNs is that they require sequential processing of the input sequence, which can be slow and inefficient for long sequences, and does not scale to large datasets. The Transformer architecture was introduced as a solution, as it uses self-attention mechanisms to allow for parallel processing of the entire sequence.

Self-attention works by first embedding the input sequence into a continuous vector space. Then, for each position in the input sequence, the model calculates a set of attention scores, which indicate the degree of dependence between that position and all other positions in the sequence. These attention scores are used to compute a weighted sum of the input representations, which is then used as the input to the next layer of the model. It is called self-attention because the model is able to put the representations of each token into context of all surrounding tokens.

Each token is assigned an embedding which is multiplied with three trainable weight matrices to obtain three vectors, called Queries, Keys, and Values. The model first computes the dot product of the Query vector with each of the Key vectors, and then applies a softmax function to the resulting vector to obtain attention scores that are between 0 and 1 and sum to 1, where the softmax function is defined as:

$$\text{softmax}(x_i) = \frac{e^{x_i}}{\sum_{j=1}^{n} e^{x_j}}. \tag{13.2}$$

Finally, the resulting vector of attention scores for each token is multiplied with the Value vectors to obtain the representation for this token. The outputs of the self-attention mechanism are then passed through a feedforward neural network to produce the output of a so called *encoder block*. Many such encoder blocks are stacked on top of each other to form the encoder of the Transformer architecture. In some architectures one wants to generate new text, for which we need a *decoder*. It has a very similar structure, but we will defer that discussion here. For more details on the Transformer architecture, we refer the reader to other sources [1, 19].

**Pre-training and Fine-tuning:** The state of the art in NLP is currently dominated by Transformer-based models, which are trained using a two-stage process called *pre-training* and *fine-tuning*. Starting with a model pre-trained on a broad set of topics significantly reduces the amount of task-specific training data required to achieve great performance.

Pre-training refers to the process of training a model on a large corpus*[7] of text, sometimes in multiple languages, or on domain-specific datasets. For more information on domain-specific models in medicine, see Section 13.3.2. The model is trained to predict masked tokens in a sequence, or to reconstruct the input sequence itself, using only the context information provided by surrounding tokens. This process enables the model to learn general language patterns and relationships between words and concepts, and can be compared to a human learning a new language. Just as a human needs to understand the basic rules and patterns of a language before they can use it to apply it effectively, a model needs to do the same. Pre-trained Transformer models are freely available for download† and can be used as a starting point for many NLP tasks. They are able to produce robust sentence embeddings with a fine-grained understanding of syntactic structure, semantics, and general knowledge of the world. One can also pre-train one's own model from scratch, but this requires a lot of data, time, and money and is rarely worth the investment.

Fine-tuning, on the other hand, refers to the process of adapting the pre-trained model on a much smaller dataset to a specific task, such as classification, sentiment analysis, question answering, or machine translation. This can be compared to a human adapting their language skills to a specific context. For example, a person who has learned a new language may need to modify their language skills to fit a particular situation, such as a formal business setting or a casual conversation with friends. During fine-tuning, a task-specific layer is added on the on top of the pre-trained model and either only that layer or the entire network is trained end-to-end on the task-specific data.

### 13.2.4 Practical Considerations

In contemporary architectures, there are millions to hundreds of billions of parameters, and updating them efficiently is crucial.

*BooksCorpus (800M words, Wikipedia 2,500M words)

†Huggingface

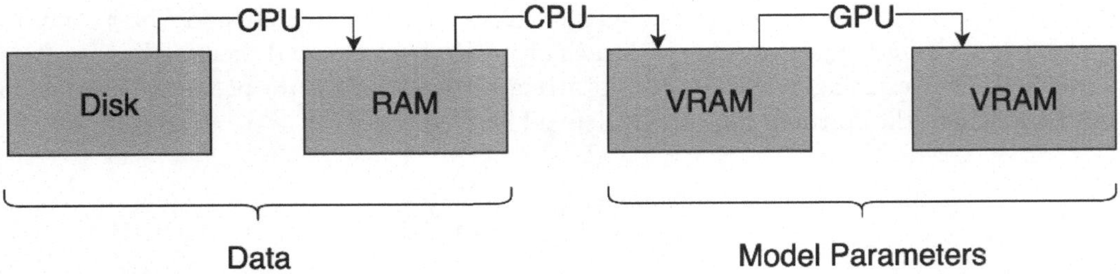


**FIGURE 13.3**
Data needs to be moved from disk to random access memory (RAM) to video random access memory (VRAM) so that it can be used to update the model parameters. CPU, central processing unit; GPU, graphics processing unit. (Color version available in electronic supplement.)

**Feeding Data to the Model:** Model parameters are stored in Graphics Processing Unit (GPU) memory, also known as Video Random Access Memory (VRAM); in order to update them, the GPU needs to process data from the training set. After downloading the data from cloud storage, it resides on local disk, from where it needs to be moved to RAM and finally VRAM (Figure 13.3). Loading data into the model needs to be fast, or we run the risk of starving the GPU, meaning the GPU processes each batch of data faster than the CPU can deliver the next one, leading to low resource utilization and slow training. We use PyTorch's `DataLoader` class to parallelize this process across multiple CPU workers. A `DataLoader` takes as argument a `Dataset` and provides a stream of batches of data. The *batch size* is an important parameter that needs to be tuned on a case by case basis, as we will explain in the next section.

**Mini-Batch Gradient Descent:** To optimize the parameters as outlined in Eq. 13.1, we need to evaluate the gradient of the loss function given the data $(x_i, y_i)$. To compute the optimal update step, we need to sum over all samples in the dataset, compute and store all the gradients, update the parameters once, and repeat the process until convergence. This, however is not practical, given the size of typical datasets and the number of model parameters – each step would be very computationally expensive and the training slow.

On the other end of the spectrum, we could use only a single sample to compute approximations of the optimal gradients, and they will take us close to the global minimum. This method is called *stochastic gradient descent* and generally works well, but it comes with some tradeoffs:

- Loading single samples from the dataset is slow, due to Central Processing Unit (CPU), RAM and bus overhead when copying data to VRAM;
- There is overhead in the GPU related to scheduling of compute operations; and
- The gradients are much more noisy than the optimal ones, and the model will learn more slowly.

There is a happy middle ground called *mini-batch gradient descent* which is a combination of stochastic gradient descent with mini-batches. Using mini-batches allows for a more accurate estimate of the gradient, and reduces the overhead per sample, as we can take advantage of hardware accelerated vectorized compute operations in CPUs and GPUs. In practice, we will choose a batch size that is much smaller than the number of samples in the dataset, and as big as possible without running out of VRAM, where the latter condition is typically the more relevant constraint.

Many optimization algorithms exist that aim to minimize the objective loss function that represents a deep learning model. Stochastic gradient descent is often a good first choice for this optimization. It requires tuning the *learning rate* parameter, which controls how much the parameters will adjust on each step of the iteration after calculating the relative error of the model with respect to each of these parameters. A large learning rate will often get stuck in local optima because it is unable to find the minimum in a complex multi-dimensional optimization space, whereas a smaller learning rate might take too long to train. Learning rate schedules are often used that aim to get the best of both worlds. One schedule that is often used is to begin with a higher learning rate and to slowly decay it as training proceeds. This often allows for faster overall training but still converging to a lower final loss. Another technique that is used in practice is to cycle learning rates between high and low numbers, as this allows the loss functions to escape from local optima and finely explore other parts of the decision space.

As mentioned, mini-batch gradient descent is not the only loss function available to us. Most deep learning libraries support many others that automatically compute these partial derivatives for each parameter and adjust them on every backpropagation pass. Some incorporate weighted averages to establish a momentum term to smooth out the jumpiness of the loss value. Others have learning rates that exist for each separate parameter and not a single global learning rate. The Adam optimizer is a good first choice that combines these techniques and works out of the box quite well for a variety of NLP problems.

**Regularization:** A common problem in machine learning is the balance between over- and underfitting. Underfitting can happen when the model is too simple, i.e., it is not able to capture the underlying function (rarely a problem in deep learning). Overfitting happens when the model is too complex or has too many degrees of freedom, such that it can fit the training data well, but does not capture the essence of the true data generating process, leading to poor generalization performance when applied to new data.

An easy way to detect these issues is by observing training and validation metrics as a function of training steps or epochs, called learning curves. We want to see that both training and validation metrics continue to improve as training progresses until they both taper off at a certain point. Note that it is normal to see a difference in the absolute value and rate of change between the training and validation metrics. This is called the generalization error and is nothing to be too concerned about; ultimately, only the validation and test metrics are relevant. What *is* problematic is if we observe that the validation metrics start to get worse, while the training metrics continue to improve – this is a clear sign of overfitting, and we should stop the training early (Figure 13.4). To address underfitting, the easiest remedy is to increase the complexity of the model (e.g. add more layers) or to increase the number of training steps. We can also try to add more features to the dataset, such as adding more words to the vocabulary. When dealing with overfitting in deep learning, we usually don't want to reduce the model complexity, but instead add *regularization* and more data. Regularization is a technique that restricts the freedom of the model, for example by introducing a penalty on the magnitude of the model parameters. For this, the loss functions in Table 13.1 are modified as:

$$\tilde{L}(\theta) = L(\theta) + \frac{1}{2}\sum_i |\theta_i|^2, \tag{13.3}$$

where $L$ is the loss function and $\theta$ is the model parameters.

Another common technique is to add *dropout*, where a fraction of neurons in the network is randomly turned off for each training step. This ensures that each neuron has a unique

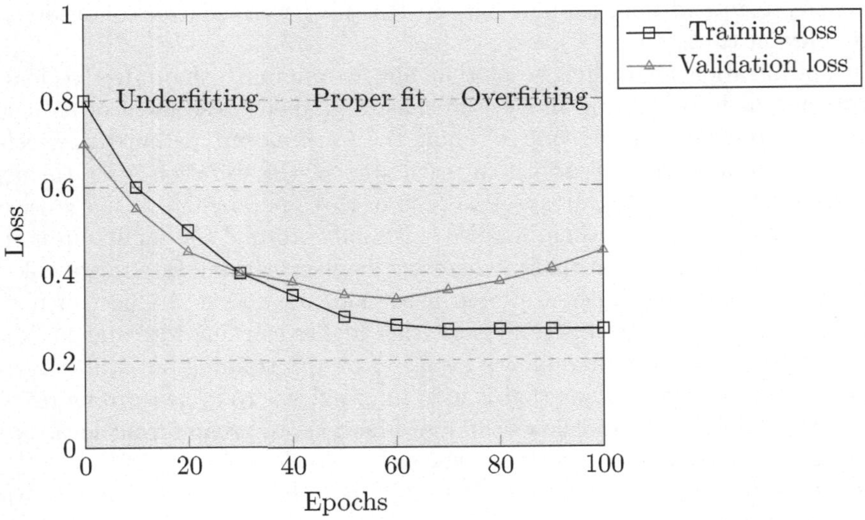


**FIGURE 13.4**
Learning curves, the training and validation loss are plotted as a function of the number of training steps/epochs. The training loss continues to improve, while the validation loss worsens after a certain point, indicating overfitting.

purpose and learns to detect a specific set of features in the data, without co-adapting to the output of other neurons. Another interpretation of dropout is that it can be seen as an approximation to a bagging technique, where the outputs of different models at each iteration are averaged, leading to an overall reduction in errors if they are uncorrelated. This tends to reduce generalization error, prevent the model from fitting to irrelevant details, and make it more robust to noise.

There are many other regularization techniques that are used in practice. They are all designed to reduce generalization error, and not training error. Often they come in the flavor of the additional terms added to the objective function, as exemplified in Eq. 2.3, or as model restrictions, such as dropout. Another common technique is on the dataset level, wherein practitioners will directly augment datasets. This happens often in image classification tasks, where a dataset will create random copies of samples that are rotated and stretched in different directions to make the model robust to such invariance. Direct injection of noise, randomly generated numbers, also occurs on both the inputs as well as labels.

## 13.3 Embeddings

An embedding is a representation of a vector space that captures the similarity between the entities we are encoding, where entities can be words, images, e-commerce products, movies, houses, and many other data modalities. Scientific progress in the field of machine learning is often directly about finding algorithms that can learn high-quality robust embeddings in an efficient and scalable way. The final performance of a given architecture is often largely determined by the quality of the embeddings it learns.

To illustrate this concept, we will discuss briefly one of the earliest algorithms that has been used to learn embeddings for words: *word2vec*, a technique pioneered by a team led by

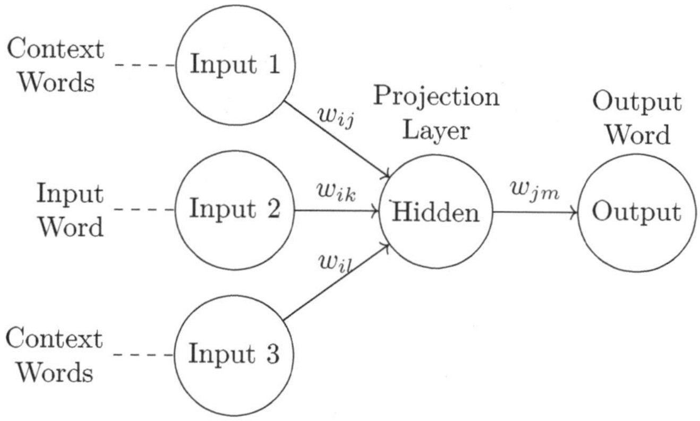


**FIGURE 13.5**
Illustration of the continuous bag of words (CBOW) approach to the word2vec model. The model takes a window of surrounding (context) words as input, and the goal is to predict the input word. The context words are first projected onto a hidden layer, and the input word is predicted based on the activations in the hidden layer. The weights are learned through training.

Thomas Mikolov [11]. The idea behind *word2vec* is to set a word into context with the words surrounding it. As it turns out, the idea that similar words appear in similar contexts, is an extremely powerful signal for achieving quality word embeddings. In NLP, the study of techniques that determine the probability of a given sequence of words is known as language modeling.

For example, the word *epilepsy* may appear in the context of words like *symptom*, *medication*, or *episode* and vice versa. However, we would not expect that *epilepsy* would appear in the context of words like *potato*. We then translate this idea into a training task: Given the sum of the one-hot encoded word vectors of the words surrounding the target word, map it to the one-hot encoded vector of the target word.

This is a task that can be solved by a neural network with the following setup: Add a layer $l_1$ that maps from the input dimension (of size $|V|$) to an intermediate dimension of size $h$, and then another layer $l_2$ that maps from the intermediate dimension to the output dimension (of size $|V|$). Here $h$, is what is called the embedding dimension and $h << |V|$.

While $h$ is generally a hyperparameter that can be optimized at a later stage, a reasonable choice is to use a value according to the rule of thumb:

$$h \approx 4\sqrt[4]{|V|} \tag{13.4}$$

For a vocabulary size $|V| = 30,000$, this comes to a value of $h$ of about 50. During training, the network will learn to encode the original sparse indicator vectors in a way that preserves the maximum amount of information necessary to predict the target word, while being forced to squeeze the information through the low dimensional bottleneck. An interesting side effect of this approach is that we can use part of the network to encode a given word in $V$ by using for example the inverse of $l_2$ as a lookup table. The vectors that we obtain from this lookup table are called word embeddings and they have some very useful properties:

- Similar words tend to be close together (e.g. in terms of Euclidean distance).
- Averaging word embeddings of a sentence will give us a more robust representation than our naive approach.

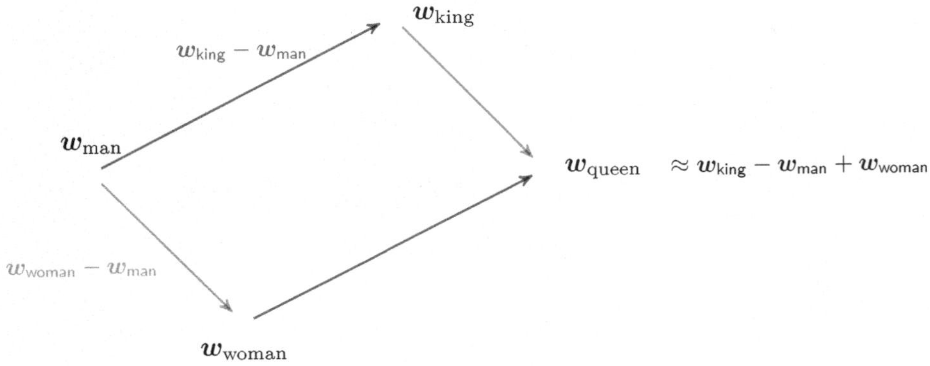


**FIGURE 13.6**
Geometric illustration of word2vec performing vector arithmetic using word embeddings. If we take the representation of "king," subtract away the representation of "man," and add the representation of "woman," the vector representation closest to the result in our vocabulary table is the vector of the word "queen."

- We can perform some arithmetic, such as adding and subtracting the embedding vectors to traverse the space.

These properties also imply that the represenstions for two sentences will be close together if they are semantically similar, which will make the job of, say, a downstream classifier much more straightforward – it only has to slice the embedding space. The hard part of understanding the meaning of the sentence is already done. Since the training data can be generated from just raw text, it is sufficient to train the embeddings once on a very large corpus and then reuse them, in effect giving us a headstart when building task-specific models [14]. Instead of also having to learn what words mean, and some of the syntactic rules behind written language, we can get a head start on this and focus our computational resources on adapting this knowledge to a specific task.

Using these pre-trained text representations is often critical. Without doing so, the majority of what a machine learns is the basic syntax and semantics of language. By using these pre-trained word embeddings, we allow our models to learn to focus more on the downstream task. By simplifying the learning task with these pre-trained embeddings, we need to use far fewer labeled examples than we would training from scratch.

This underlying assumption that similar neighboring words share a semantic similarity to center words is powerful, and at the heart of many modern training objectives for embeddings that are used in many downstream machine learning systems. We do not inherently inject a great deal of model bias, but rather rely on having a large enough training set that the word vectors will become meaningful representations with respect to one another. A corpus such as Common Crawl,which contains roughly 840 billion tokens of over two million unique words, provides such scale. There are other corpora used in these unsupervised processes, one such common candidate being a collection of all Wikipedia articles.

In practice, one training objective can be to use the distributed representation of a set of context words to guess a center word. This is known as the continuous bag of words (CBOW) model and is illustrated in Figure 13.5.

Consider a training document describing patients with epilepsy, where we are attempting to train a model with a predefined vocabulary $V$ of the top $|V|$ most common words in

English to learn. The document being chosen in this training iteration may contain the following excerpt:

```
... recommended administering Lamictal to treat their focal
seizures, the patient continued experiencing symptoms though
reported a 50% reduction in ...
```

In training our word embeddings, we will randomly mask one of the words, in this case *patient*. Our model makes use of an additional parameter, a context window size $c$, that helps to provide necessary context. If we choose $c = 8$, our training sample would become

```
... lamictal to treat their focal seizures, the [MASK] continued
experiencing symptoms though reported a 50% ...
```

For a given center word at index $i$, we consider previous words at indexes $i-1$, $i-2$, ..., $i-c$, and all subsequent words at indexes $i+1$, $i+2$, ..., $i+c$. In our word sequence $S$, we may then choose to sum the word vectors of each of these context words. Our context input can be written as:

$$\sum_{\substack{j=-c \\ j\neq 0}}^{c} w_{i+j}. \tag{13.5}$$

Our task is then to predict a probability distribution over the size of our vocabulary $|V|$, where the target is a vector of all 0's with a 1 at the index in the vocabulary for the word *patient*. There are a few additional takeaways from this example, many of which will be addressed in the sections to follow:

- The training process will likely consider this text many times, and mask out different words in each iteration.
- Our processed sentence is slightly modified from our original input. Notice that the number and percent symbol are split, and that Lamictal is lowercased.
- The word *patient* can also be an adjective. Our *patient* embedding will also capture this meaning in our model, dependent upon how often it is used with that meaning.
- If our context window is too small, we lose information. If it is too large, our signal becomes fuzzy as we converge to the global mean vector.

What if we choose to use only a center word, and have our model predict all of the surrounding context words? This is a common training technique for embeddings as well and is known as the Skip-Gram model.

**Example 13.3.1.** (Spacy example of word embeddings).

```
import spacy

sample_words = ["epilepsy", "seizure",
                "patient", "language"]

nlp = spacy.load("en_core_web_md")
docs = [nlp(sample) for sample in sample_words]

#Spacy's Medium English Model Stores Words As
# Vectors of Dimension 300
#Note each word has this vector size
for doc in docs:
```

```
    assert doc.vector.shape[0] == 300

#The cosine distance, ranging from [0,1], of
# the vectors tells us how similar the words are
print(docs[0].similarity(docs[1]))
#epilepsy and seizure -> 0.9999
print(docs[0].similarity(docs[2]))
#epilepsy and patient -> 0.4434
print(docs[0].similarity(docs[3]))
#epilepsy and language -> 0.1273
```

### 13.3.1 Character and Subword Embeddings

In Example 13.1.1, we covered the issue of missing vocabulary that is frequently encountered when using word-level tokenization. However, there are other strategies that are commonly used that help to avoid this issue. One such simple way around out-of-vocabulary tokens is to use character-level tokenization. Instead of having a vocabulary that is tens of thousands of words long, the vocabulary only contains the characters in that specific language , with the addition of punctuation, digits, and a few special tokens for sentence and word marking. As long as the tokenizer is able to mark which characters start a word and which characters are continuations of a word, then the original sequence of words can always be recovered.

Unfortunately, the tradeoff for a small vocabulary size with no unknown word entries is that the length of tokens to represent a sentence is clearly much larger. Empirically, these models do not perform as well, partially because of this sequence length but also because of the loss of information that is represented in word vectors.

In practice, the best models are often somewhere in the middle, in what is known as word-piece, or subword, vocabularies. These tokenizers and vocabularies contain a rich set of common words but also have subword units that can be used to piece together out-of-vocabulary words. These subword units behave like normal word vectors and can store semantic and syntactic information.

**Example 13.3.2.** (Wordpiece tokenizers).

```
from transformers import BertTokenizer

sample = "After a temporal lobe resection, the " \
         "atonic and clonic seizure frequency " \
         "fell by 50%."

bert_tokenizer = BertTokenizer.from_pretrained(
    'bert-base-uncased'
)

ids = bert_tokenizer.encode(sample)
tokens = bert_tokenizer.convert_ids_to_tokens(
    encoded_ids
)

for token, id  in zip(tokens, ids):
    print("{}: {}".format(token,id))

#output:
# [CLS] 101
# after: 2044
# a: 1037
# temporal: 15850
# lobe: 21833
# res: 24501
```

```
# ##ection: 18491
# ... (output continues)
#   %: 1003
# .: 1012
# [SEP]: 102
```

In the tokenizer output in Example 13.3.1 above, note the following:

1. The text is silently preprocessed to be lowercased. Other functions, such as whitespace trimming, are common.
2. The output token sequence includes the specialized tokens (CLS), and (SEP), that not only help to mark the beginning and end of a sequence but aid in downstream classification in the model.
3. The word "resection" is split into two tokens, with a special marker for the continuation of a word that was split.

### 13.3.2 Domain-Specific Medical Embeddings

Many of the datasets and models that are available online are trained on general text, and not specific to any particular domain. Unsurprisingly, vocabularies that include medical terminology are used in practice, as are the models that have been trained to represent these vectors in NLP tasks specific to areas in medicine. Using these models is a common practice and often yields better results than a general-purpose approach. Because data collection is an expensive process, the better the pre-trained embeddings that are available, the more quickly we can produce high-quality models for specialized tasks.

Predictive models from electronic health records have been used to train transformer-based models, and `Med-Bert`[15] is an example of one such model giving a boost to prediction accuracy with respect to the number of training examples required by a specialized model. The `BioBERT`[9] and `Bio_ClinicalBERT`[2] models can be loaded as drop-in replacements for a BERT model from the Huggingface library to achieve better results in clinical tasks. Many other such models exist, and it is recommended to keep an eye out for advancements in this area when using pre-trained models for tasks in epilepsy as well as other domains.

## 13.4 Natural Language Processing Tasks in Epilepsy

Armed with an understanding of some basics of computational representations of language data, let us now consider some modern use cases for NLP that may be pertinent to epileptologists or researchers working with epilepsy data.

### 13.4.1 Unstructured Text from the Electronic Health Record

In the electronic health record, there are many sources of unstructured text that are primarily aimed as a either a communication channel between specialists, or a way to convey information about patients that is not captured in a structured format. History & physicals, progress notes, operative notes, surgery conference notes, discharge summaries, and pathology reports: all of these sources carry information, but traditionally require experts in the field to extract it. If we can teach systems to read through this unstructured text and perform respectably close to these experts, we can perform large-scale clinical retrospective research much faster and at a much lower cost.

Because pre-trained language models can draw upon information from so many domains and have a sound understanding of language, they need relatively few labeled examples to begin to perform tasks such as classifying text. All they have to learn is the task at hand, not the nuances of languages. If a team of experts is able to identify a set of labels in which they are interested, they can label this data in a single shot. The next step is to fine-tune a pre-trained language model, often by just attaching a logistic regression layer to the outputs of the language model, to recognize each of these labels.

Rather than requiring time and expense from experts to perform large-scale retrospective research on unstructured text, fine-tuned pre-trained language models can perform admirably on text classification with, in many cases, only a few hundred labeled examples. The trained model can then read through and extract targeted text with much reduced cost and human time investment. For example, this strategy has been used for three pretrained neural language models, `Bio_ClinicalBERT`, to extract seizure frequency from epilepsy clinical notes [22].

### 13.4.2 Unstructured Text from Surveys

Another source of unstructured text in epilepsy research is acquired from surveys. While often surveys call for responses on numeric scales, such as the Likert scale or multiple choice responses, many offer unstructured text as a method for patients to freely communicate their responses. Allowing for free-form responses allows for researchers to avoid constraining the respondent to pre-defined response categories, but it can be difficult to parse responses at scale without modern natural language processing techniques.

Sentiment analysis, the task of extracting and studying subjective sentiment in text and speech data, is yet another field of NLP that has greatly benefited from the widespread adoption of transformer architectures, particularly in specialized domains. Sentiment analysis can identify freeform responses as positive or negative, or sometimes into more granular sentiments, using machine learning methods. It is worth noting that naive methods on sentiment tend to capture some cases well. The words *love* and *hate* are strong signals, but even their simple negation becomes a diluted signal with possible interpretations of sarcasm that become subjective. Add in the many colorful ways that people write, and we start to see why rule-based text-mining systems for sentiment are so difficult. Sentiment analysis models using transformer architectures such as RoBERTa aim to project the large-dimensional output vector of the textinto a basic sentiment of two classes: positive or negative. Often a third class may also be used to represent neutral sentiment. This method should be used when analyzing free-form responses in patient surveys using NLP models trained on sentiment. While a model trained on epilepsy-specific or medical data would ideal, it is quite impressive how well a model trained on movie reviews will transfer over to other sentiment tasks.

The same methods for analyzing basic sentiment can be used to label tones, more granular emotional classifications, or other task-specific points of interest. It is important to have domain experts label these targeted semantic expressions of patients. Once a model is trained with a set of positive examples of these targets, it can be used on any text response.

### 13.4.3 Named Entity Recognition and Personally Identifiable Information

Named Entity Recognition (NER) is a subtask of information extraction that classifies unstructured text into personal names, locations, time indications, organizations, and other tags. NER is an important task in medicine due to the ability to mask out Personally Identifiable Information (PII). Although some PII text is easy to catch with rule-based approaches and regular expressions, such as credit card numbers, other information requires contextual understanding and an machine learning solution to achieve the necessary performance. If a model, such as a transformer architecture, is able to identify text as a first name, a home address, or a credit card number, then we can anonymize this information to mask PII-specific text.

Spacy, NLTK, and Stanford NLP all provide out-of-the-box NER models that perform well on unstructured text. Example 13.4.3 shows how to implement a simple PII anonymizer in Python.

**Example 13.4.1.** (Simple anonymizer for masking personally identifiable information).

```
import spacy

sample = "The patient, John Smith, began feeling " \
         "symptoms at his home in Seattle, and was " \
         "taken to Virginia Mason Medical Center " \
         "for treatment"
nlp = spacy.load("en_core_web_md")

doc = nlp(sample)

for word in doc.ents:
    sample = sample.replace(word.text, word.label_)

print(sample)
# The patient, PERSON, began feeling symptoms at his
# home in GPE, and was taken to ORG for treatment
```

### 13.4.4 Clinical Trial Matching and Surgical Candidacy

There has been an emergence of NLP technologies aimed at matching patients against eligibility criteria, such as clinical trial matching, which is the process of matching different patient characteristics against eligibility criteria of available trials, or in the identification of candidates for epilepsy surgery. While sometimes the data on patient characteristics and eligiblity criteria exists in a structured form, oftentimes they are composed of free-form responses with critical information. The NLP algorithms discussed in this chapter can help to create features on this type of text for these tasks. For example, Criteria2Query [23] is a hybrid system that uses NLP methods to transform text into eligibility criteria features that can be extracted with structured queries. The Clinical Trial Parser and accompanying dataset of 3,314 trials [18], made publicly available from Meta Research, is a system with a similar goal that combines a number of information extraction techniques from NLP to determine trial level eligibility. NLP approaches have also been used to identify candidates for epilepsy surgery using clinical notes [20].

These examples provide a broad introduction into some of the ways that the field of epilepsy may continue to incorporate computational linguistics into research in coming years. As a general rule, when evaluating the potential candidacy of an NLP model for a specific task, the following questions may be informative:

1. Is there text data in this task that provides signal toward a targeted classification that typically requires human involvement?
2. Have others in the medical field tried using NLP models on a similar task?

3. Does the task require either a substantial amount of time, money, or scarce resources of domain expertise?
4. Is there a dataset I can use that is in good shape and does my group have full permissions to work with it on the required hardware?

If the answer is yes to any of these questions, it may be worth trying an NLP technique for the task at hand.

## 13.5 Example: Parsing Surveys on Quality of Life in Epilepsy

Next, we demonstrate how the techniques discussed in Sections 13.3–13.3.2 may be applied to a practical example in the field of epilepsy: analysis of unstructured or semi-structured text data from survey responses. Full code is available at the repository accompanying this book and `https://github.com/chris-boson/epilepsy`.

### 13.5.1 Problem Definition

For this example, we will consider a set of deidentified free-text responses derived from a survey about quality of life collected by SeizureTracker.com™ as part of the *It's Not Just Seizures*™ initiative [5]. We focus our example on responses from 178 respondents to one specific survey question:

*What comments do you have about the financial impact of epilepsy?*

Let us focus on a binary task. We will analyze the 178 responses and label each response as to whether or not the respondent expressed that the individual with epilepsy and/or their family was experiencing difficulty obtaining or maintaining employment. We choose this label in this example because it is moderately difficult to annotate, and therefore would may be tedious and costly to annotate at scale. A positive example to this survey question, in which the respondent expressed difficulty obtaining or maintaining employment, might be something like:

*We have found that employers are far less likely to want to hire our son because of his condition.*

A negative example to this survey question, in which the respondent did not express a sentiment related to obtaining or maintaining employment, might be:

*The medication costs are through the roof and it is simply too much for us to be able to handle.*

The dataset used in this example is small enough to illustrate the NLP concepts discussed in this chapter, but the techniques discussed here scale well into the order of millions (or even billions) of samples. In general, if we can train an NLP model to identify this type of employment burden with few training examples, this gives us confidence that these types of survey responses can be summarized by machine learning models at large scale. The fewer training samples needed, the less time required by skilled professionals to to perform such an analysis.

### 13.5.2 Walkthrough: Few-Shot Learning with Folds

First, let us load the dataframe and examine the label distribution.

```
import evaluate
import numpy as np
import pandas as pd
from datasets import Dataset
from transformers import (AutoModelForSequenceClassification, AutoTokenizer,
    Trainer, TrainingArguments, pipeline,
)
df = pd.read_csv("~/financial_surgery.csv", header = 0)
df = df[["financial_impact", "employment_burden"]]
df["label"] = df["employment_burden"].astype("int32")
print(df["label"].value_counts())
df = df.sample(frac=1, random_state = 123456).reset_index(drop = True)

#Value Counts are:
# 0 (negative) - 106
# 1 (positive) - 71
```

If we run the above code, we see that there are 71 positives and 106 negatives. This means 71 people surveyed expressed a financial burden with respect to their ability to obtain or maintain employment.

Rather than tuning a model from scratch, we will fine-tune one of the Transformer-based architectures. Our goal will be to provide some examples of positive and negative expressions of a financial burden, fine-tune a transformer-based architecture, and evaluate how it performs on the 178 samples in our dataset. Due to small sample size, we will split the dataset into five folds, training on four of the folds and testing on the hold-out fold. We will do this for all five folds, and stitch together the results in order to get an accurate representation of our learner.

Let us load our transformer model and tokenizer from HuggingFace [21], a state-of-the-art library for Transformer models. The following code downloads and prepares the RoBERTa [10] model from HuggingFace, a model that was trained by Facebook AI in 2019.

```
tokenizer = AutoTokenizer.from_pretrained("roberta-base")

# Create vanilla fine-tuner
model = AutoModelForSequenceClassification.from_pretrained("roberta-base",
    num_labels = 2)
training_args = TrainingArguments(output_dir = "financial_impact_trainer",
    save_total_limit = 2)
```

We will also need to estimate several binary machine learning performance metrics, as discussed in Chapter 12; let us load those as well.

```
metric_functions = {"precision": evaluate.load("precision"), "recall": evaluate.
    load("recall"), "f1": evaluate.load("f1"), "accuracy": evaluate.load("accuracy
    ")}

def compute_metrics(eval_pred):
    logits, labels = eval_pred
    predictions = np.argmax(logits, axis=-1)

    metrics = {}
    for metric_name, metric_fn in metric_functions.items():
        metrics[metric_name] = metric_fn.compute(predictions = predictions,
    references = labels)[metric_name]
    return metrics
```

The *compute_metrics* function will be passed to our *Trainer* class so that it can run the metrics whenever we are done with a training epoch. We now need to take our dataset and pass it to the tokenizer in order to prepare our inputs. We will make use of HuggingFace's Dataset and pass our dataset to the tokenizer that we created.

```
N_FOLDS = 5
dfs = np.array_split(df, 5)
train_df = pd.concat([dfs[idx] for idx in range(N_FOLDS-1)])
test_df = dfs[N_FOLDS-1]

train_df = train_df.reset_index(drop=True)
test_df = test_df.reset_index(drop=True)

train_dataset = Dataset.from_pandas(train_df)
test_dataset = Dataset.from_pandas(test_df)

train_dataset = train_dataset.map(tokenize_function, batched=True)
test_dataset = test_dataset.map(tokenize_function, batched=True)
```

Our dataset is now ready to train. If we create a *Trainer* class, we will be able to pass our train and test datasets, as well as our metrics function, and get outputs as the model trains. Let us define those now, and start training.

```
# Fine-tune
training_args = TrainingArguments(output_dir = f"financial_impact_trainer",
    evaluation_strategy = "epoch", num_train_epochs = 2)

trainer = Trainer(model = model, args = training_args, train_dataset =
    train_dataset, eval_dataset = test_dataset, compute_metrics = compute_metrics
    ,)
trainer.train()
trainer.save()
```

We have now successfully loaded a dataframe, loaded a pre-trained transformer model, fine-tuned it to a specific task of our choosing, and reported performance metrics on the dataset we created. The last step is to take our final code and put it into a loop that runs a trainer for each separate *k*-fold. Table 13.2 shows the estimated performance of the transformer model for identifying responses indicating job insecurity:

**TABLE 13.2**
Five-fold cross validation performance of transformer model for identifying job insecurity from quality of life dataset.

| Fold | Precision | Recall | F1 score | Accuracy |
|---|---|---|---|---|
| Fold 1 | 0.824 | 1.0 | 0.903 | 0.916 |
| Fold 2 | 0.714 | 0.833 | 0.769 | 0.833 |
| Fold 3 | 0.938 | 1.0 | 0.968 | 0.971 |
| Fold 4 | 1.0 | 1.0 | 1.0 | 1.0 |
| Fold 5 | 1.0 | 1.0 | 1.0 | 1.0 |
| Total | 0.876 | 0.986 | 0.927 | 0.938 |

Using five-fold cross-validation, we see that the transformer model obtains quite good performance with an accuracy of 0.94, precision of 0.88 and recall of 0.99, with an $F_1$ score of 0.93.

## 13.6 Generative Artificial Intelligence and Large Language Models

A recent trend, one that has gained notoriety in circles far outside of machine learning, is the usage of generative artificial intelligence (AI), or Large Language Models, for both machine learning and non-machine learning applications. These are largely unsupervised, or sometimes semi-supervised, algorithms that generate content from analyzing existing content. This content is often text, such as in ChatGPT, but in recent multi-modal models such as OpenAI's GPT-4 [12], can include non-text modalities such as imagess, or even a combination thereof.

Large Language Models have gained traction specifically because they have arguably reached human-level performance, and according to some even surpassed it, on various tasks of generating text. The word "large" here is an understatement, as these models have billions upon billions of parameters, and rely on neural architectures that stack transformers and other large computational operations across many GPUs. They are trained on massive amounts of text, sometimes on the order of trillions of tokens [17].

What makes these newer language models such as OpenAI's ChatGPT, Meta AI's Llama [17], or Google's Bard so special is their ability to generalize to new tasks *without any fine-tuning or training.* What this means is that we can simply provide an instruction (also called a *prompt*) to the model, and it will generate text that is consistent with it. Moreover, these models exhibit remarkable emergent abilities, meaning things they were never explicitly trained on. These include common-sense reasoning, the ability to use tools (e.g., to search, calculate, write and execute code, invoke APIs), and even theory of mind (e.g., understanding that other agents have their own beliefs, desires, and intentions) [4, 12].

As it turns out, the key to unlocking these abilities lies in an elaborate fine-tuning process after extensive pre-training on a large corpus of text. In the case of ChatGPT, this was done in a novel way using a method called Reinforcement Learning with Human Feedback (RLHF) to align the model on human preferences, specifically rewarding high-quality content and penalizing toxic content [13]. Because these models are trained on text across the internet, which, unsurprisingly, included troves of nonsense and hate speech, these models must be pushed away from purely unchecked generation of content, as this can be dangerous. While the possibility of generating this text can never be fully eliminated, or can be circumvented with the right prompts, it remains true that this can be controlled as we add more human feedback.

One great remaining challenge in Large Language Models is to control the tendency of these models to hallucinate, or make up facts that are not true or not provided in the context, while sounding very confident and authoritative. It is important never to trust the output of a Large Language Model unchecked, especially when providing medical advice or making other critical decisions. Nevertheless, Large Language Models can still be very useful if used with caution and in the right context, yielding potentially enormous savings in time and effort.

### 13.6.1 Instruction Tuning

"Instruction tuning" refers to fine-tuning a language model of NLP tasks described with instructions, often with the aim of having the model perform admirably on tasks on which it was never trained. Let us take a look at an example.

Consider the Google FLAN model [6]. This model was provided not only wih a variety of datasets, but tuned with a variety of different tasks. Instructions were provided for the model to reason through many types of question answering but also text generation tasks, common-sense reasoning tasks, and even tasks related to program execution. Researchers found that by fine-tuning a variety of instruction sets in this manner, models were able to generalize to not only these types of tasks but other tasks as well. This is a powerful step in the field of Artificial Intelligence. A model receiving instructions on common-sense reasoning tasks and generalizing these instructions to performing tasks like arithmetic is a step toward generalized intelligence in AI systems. If enough of these types of prompts are instruction sets related to medical tasks, would a model be able to generalize to other types of information in the field?

### 13.6.2 Large Language Models for Medical Decision-Making

Large language models, while extremely powerful, should never solely be relied upon for medical advice. The examples in this text, as well as the models that are referenced, are used solely for educational purposes. These models are growing at rapid pace, a trend which will very likely continue in the coming years. As generative language become more powerful, there will inevitably be questions as to how they can or should be used in medicine. As these questions arise, it is important to remember that this AI is trained on reading the text on the internet, a haven for misinformation; this by itself should be all you need to know that this AI should never be used to make a decision about a patient. What might be more dangerous than this misinformation is the tendency for these types of models to *hallucinate*, a term that refers to these models generating sequences that are inconsistent with their training data. What makes this particularly dangerous is that these hallucinated sequences are often confident responses.

That being said, that does not mean that large language models are not useful. Consider the task in Section 13.5, where we used a large language model to identify whether or not respondents were experiencing difficulty in attaining or maintaining employment. This is an example of the sort of task that Large Language Models can also help with. All we have to do is design a prompt that lets the Large Language Model know what we are trying to model and provide the text sample.

### 13.6.3 Privacy Concerns

There has been a great deal of interest in exploring Large Language Models in clinical areas of medicine. One question that has arisen is whether it is acceptable to simply send patient data, or even survey responses, to a Large Language Model such as ChatGPT and ask for results?

Of course not. ChatGPT is a model owned by OpenAI, and sensitive patient data including identified or deidentified data should not be sent over an API, especially in the absence of secure and compliant solutions. However, there are Large Language Models with weights that can be downloaded and used on a local machine, or within the compute plane of a healthcare organization. There are likely to be more Large Language Models to come in the near future that will be specialized to medicine and that may be of use. If you download one of these models, it is no different than using any other machine learning model. It is worth noting that, at the time of this book's publication, there are active efforts toward developing institutional, state, and national regulations surrounding the ethical use of AI models, particularly Large Language Models, with respect to user data, and that as these regulations develop it will be critical to ensure compliance.

### 13.6.4 Prompt Engineering

Consider the following example output from a state-of-the-art unnamed Large Language Model that targets the task from Section 13.5. First, let us try the sample positive:

> **Prompt:** Does the following quote express a person's financial difficulties in their ability to maintain or attain employment: "We have found that employers are far less likely to want to hire our son because of his condition."
>
> **Large Language Model Response:** Yes, the quote suggests that the parents of a child with a disability are saying that employers are less likely to want to hire their son due to his condition. This could have a significant financial impact on the person's ability to attain or maintain employment.

It looks like the Large Language Model got this example correct. And now we can try the sample negative:

> **Prompt:** Does the following quote express a person's financial difficulties in their ability to maintain or attain employment: "The medication costs are through the roof and it is simply too much for us to be able to handle."
>
> **Large Language Model Response:** Yes, the quote suggests that the person is struggling to afford the cost of their epilepsy medication. This could have a significant financial impact on their ability to maintain or attain employment.

Notice that this example is incorrect, though the reasoning is sound. This illustrates an important point in the usage of Large Language Models, and that is Prompt Design.

Prompt design is key to the success of Large Language Models. In the above example, the model believes that the cost of epilepsy medication itself may lead to a difficulty in maintaining or attaining employment. While this might be true, the target was a direct expression of this difficulty. If we modify the query to express this directly, we get the kind of result we were looking for, at least in this case:

> **Prompt:** Does the following quote discuss the difficulty in maintaining or attaining employment: "The medication costs are through the roof and it is simply too much for us to be able to handle."
>
> **Large Language Model Response:** No, the statement you provided does not specifically discuss the difficulty in maintaining or attaining employment. It focuses on the high cost of medication and how it's difficult for the person making the statement to handle it.

When working with Large Language Models, it is important to remember that iterating on your prompts is a valuable use of time. You should work to clearly express what you are trying to solve. Some of these models have larger context lengths than others. What this means is that they can handle more input tokens, such as a longer set of instructions, or in our case a longer quote. In general, try to use a model that can fit the entire context of the task at hand.

### 13.6.5 Fine-Tuning

It is very likely that Large Language Models will soon be fine-tuned to the medical domain. What this means is that they will tradeoff accuracy in their abilities to answer general prompts, for increased accuracy in their ability to answer prompts related to a target. In the same way that a transformer model like RoBERTa was fine-tuned to our task in Section 13.5, a Large Language Model can have its weights fine-tuned. Currently, Large Language Model fine-tuning to specific tasks comes at prohibitive costs. However, LoRA optimization techniques are the method most often used to combat these costs [8]. These techniques inject trainable decomposed matrices into the transformer architectures that are easier to train than the entire model, which may be extremely large. Although this is beyond the scope of the current chapter, these tools will soon become commonplace, and it is not beyond the realm of possibility for a Large Language Model to be fine-tuned specifically to deal with epilepsy.

## 13.7 Summary

The development of natural language processing and Large Language Models will continue in the years to come. At the time of this book's publication, artificial intelligence with respect to NLP is growing as fast as it ever has, and the general public is becoming increasingly aware of its abilities. In the future, it is likely that we will be able to fine-tune Large Language Models on data such as the electronic health record for a series of questions relating to retrospective research. Until then, we recommend the reader monitor the regulations around Large Language Models as well as the tools and frameworks created by researchers and engineers in the field. Above all else, we must remain vigilant with respect to privacy concerns, bad actors, and the understanding that these models should not be used for medical advice.

## Bibliography

[1] Jay Alammar. The illustrated transformer.

[2] Emily Alsentzer, John R. Murphy, Willie Boag, Wei-Hung Weng, Di Jin, Tristan Naumann, and Matthew B. A. McDermott. Publicly available clinical BERT embeddings. arXiv preprint arXiv:1904.03323, 2019.

[3] Dzmitry Bahdanau, Kyunghyun Cho, and Yoshua Bengio. Neural machine translation by jointly learning to align and translate. arXiv preprint arXiv:1409.0473, 2014.

[4] Sébastien Bubeck, Varun Chandrasekaran, Ronen Eldan, Johannes Gehrke, Eric Horvitz, Ece Kamar, Peter Lee, Yin Tat Lee, Yuanzhi Li, Scott Lundberg, Harsha Nori, Hamid Palangi, Marco Tulio Ribeiro, and Yi Zhang. Sparks of artificial general intelligence: Early experiments with GPT-4. arXiv preprint arXiv:2303.12712, 2023.

[5] Sharon Chiang, Robert Moss, John M Stern, Inna Hughes, S Andrew Josephson, Jennifer R Pearce, Brandon E Kopald, Anup D Patel, and Vikram R Rao. Development of a core outcome set for quality of life for adults with drug-resistant epilepsy: A multistakeholder Delphi consensus study. *Epilepsia*, 64(1):170–183, 2023.

[6] Hyung Won Chung, Le Hou, Shayne Longpre, Barret Zoph, Yi Tay, William Fedus, Yunxuan Li, Xuezhi Wang, Mostafa Dehghani, Siddhartha Brahma, Albert Webson,

Shixiang Shane Gu, Zhuyun Dai, Mirac Suzgun, Xinyun Chen, Aakanksha Chowdhery, Alex Castro-Ros, Marie Pellat, Kevin Robinson, Dasha Valter, Sharan Narang, Gaurav Mishra, Adams Yu, Vincent Zhao, Yanping Huang, Andrew Dai, Hongkun Yu, Slav Petrov, Ed H. Chi, Jeff Dean, Jacob Devlin, Adam Roberts, Denny Zhou, Quoc V. Le, and Jason Wei. Scaling instruction-finetuned language models, 2022.

[7] Jacob Devlin, Ming-Wei Chang, Kenton Lee, and Kristina Toutanova. BERT: Pretraining of deep bidirectional transformers for language understanding. arXiv preprint arXiv:1810.04805, 2018.

[8] Edward J. Hu, Yelong Shen, Phillip Wallis, Zeyuan Allen-Zhu, Yuanzhi Li, Shean Wang, Lu Wang, and Weizhu Chen. LoRA: Low-rank adaptation of large language models. arXiv preprint arXiv:2106.09685, 2021.

[9] Jinhyuk Lee, Wonjin Yoon, Sungdong Kim, Donghyeon Kim, Sunkyu Kim, Chan Ho So, and Jaewoo Kang. BioBERT: A pre-trained biomedical language representation model for biomedical text mining. Bioinformatics 36(4), 1234-1240, 2020.

[10] Yinhan Liu, Myle Ott, Naman Goyal, Jingfei Du, Mandar Joshi, Danqi Chen, Omer Levy, Mike Lewis, Luke Zettlemoyer, and Veselin Stoyanov. RoBERTa: A robustly optimized BERT pretraining approach. arXiv preprint arXiv:1907.11692, 2019.

[11] Tomas Mikolov, Kai Chen, Greg Corrado, and Jeffrey Dean. Efficient estimation of word representations in vector space. arXiv preprint arXiv:1301.3781, 2013.

[12] OpenAI. GPT-4 technical report, 2023.

[13] Long Ouyang, Jeff Wu, Xu Jiang, Diogo Almeida, Carroll L. Wainwright, Pamela Mishkin, Chong Zhang, Sandhini Agarwal, Katarina Slama, Alex Ray, John Schulman, Jacob Hilton, Fraser Kelton, Luke Miller, Maddie Simens, Amanda Askell, Peter Welinder, Paul Christiano, Jan Leike, and Ryan Lowe. Training language models to follow instructions with human feedback. Advances in Neural Information Processing Systems 35:27730-27744, 2022.

[14] Jeffrey Pennington, Richard Socher, and Christopher Manning. GloVe: Global vectors for word representation. In *Proceedings of the 2014 Conference on Empirical Methods in Natural Language Processing (EMNLP)*, pages 1532–1543, Doha, Qatar, October 2014. Association for Computational Linguistics.

[15] Laila Rasmy, Yang Xiang, Ziqian Xie, Cui Tao, and Degui Zhi. Med-BERT: Pretrained contextualized embeddings on large-scale structured electronic health records for disease prediction. NPJ Digital Medicine 4(1): 86, 2021.

[16] Claude E. Shannon. A mathematical theory of communication. *The Bell System Technical Journal*, 27(3):379–423, 1948.

[17] Hugo Touvron, Thibaut Lavril, Gautier Izacard, Xavier Martinet, Marie-Anne Lachaux, Timothée Lacroix, Baptiste Rozière, Naman Goyal, Eric Hambro, Faisal Azhar, Aurelien Rodriguez, Armand Joulin, Edouard Grave, and Guillaume Lample. Llama Open and efficient foundation language models. arXiv preprint arXiv:2302.13971, 2023.

[18] Yitong Tseo, M. I. Salkola, Ahmed Mohamed, Anuj Kumar, and Freddy Abnousi. Information extraction of clinical trial eligibility criteria. arXi preprint arXiv:2006.07296, 2020.

[19] Ashish Vaswani, Noam Shazeer, Niki Parmar, Jakob Uszkoreit, Llion Jones, Aidan N. Gomez, Lukasz Kaiser, and Illia Polosukhin. Attention is all you need. Advances in neural information processing systems, 30, 2017.

[20] Benjamin D. Wissel, Hansel M Greiner, Tracy A. Glauser, Katherine D Holland-Bouley, Francesco T. Mangano, Daniel Santel, Robert Faist, Nanhua Zhang, John P. Pestian, Rhonda D. Szczesniak, and Judith W. Dexheimer. Prospective validation of a machine learning model that uses provider notes to identify candidates for resective epilepsy surgery. *Epilepsia*, 61:39–48, 2019.

[21] Thomas Wolf, Lysandre Debut, Victor Sanh, Julien Chaumond, Clement Delangue, Anthony Moi, Pierric Cistac, Tim Rault, Rémi Louf, Morgan Funtowicz, Joe Davison, Sam Shleifer, Patrick von Platen, Clara Ma, Yacine Jernite, Julien Plu, Canwen Xu, Teven Le Scao, Sylvain Gugger, Mariama Drame, Quentin Lhoest, and Alexander M. Rush. Huggingface's transformers: State-of-the-art natural language processing. arXiv preprint arXiv:1910.03771, 2019.

[22] Kevin Xie, Ryan S Gallagher, Erin C Conrad, Chadric O Garrick, Steven N Baldassano, John M Bernabei, Peter D Galer, Nina J Ghosn, Adam S Greenblatt, Tara Jennings, Alana Kornspun, Catherine V Kulick-Soper, Jal M Panchal, Akash R Pattnaik, Brittany H Scheid, Danmeng Wei, Micah Weitzman, Ramya Muthukrishnan, Joongwon Kim, Brian Litt, Colin A Ellis, and Dan Roth. Extracting seizure frequency from epilepsy clinic notes: A machine reading approach to natural language processing. *Journal of the American Medical Informatics Association*, 29(5):873–881, 2022.

[23] Chi Yuan, Patrick B Ryan, Casey Ta, Yixuan Guo, Ziran Li, Jill Hardin, Rupa Makadia, Peng Jin, Ning Shang, Tian Kang, and Chunhua Weng. Criteria2Query: A natural language interface to clinical databases for cohort definition. *Journal of the American Medical Informatics Association*, 26(4):294–305, 2019.

# Part IV

# Clinical Studies

# 14

# *Prospective Observational Study Design and Analysis*

**Carrie Brown**

*The Emmes Company (USA)*

**Kimford J. Meador**

*Department of Neurology, Stanford University (USA)*

**Page B. Pennell**

*Department of Neurology, University of Pittsburgh (USA)*

**Abigail G. Matthews**

*The Emmes Company (USA)*

## CONTENTS



Observational prospective studies are required for investigating epilepsy-related issues when a randomized clinical trial would not be ethical or practical. This chapter reviews critical aspects of prospective study design and analysis pertinent to epilepsy populations. Observational studies for epilepsy face unique trial design issues related to population heterogeneity and the collection and analysis of seizure data. Study design considerations discussed include the selection of appropriate outcome measures, selection of the study

DOI: 10.1201/9781003254515-14

population to balance homogeneity with generalizability, common sources of bias in epilepsy studies, and considerations for calculating power and sample size. This chapter also discusses effective approaches for determining and collecting data on potential confounders, mediators, effect modifiers, and risk factors of interest; methods for prospective collection of seizure data including the use of mobile health applications and considerations when collecting anti-seizure medication dose and blood level concentrations. Analysis methods commonly employed in observational data are highlighted with specific attention to variable selection, multiple regression, and multiple imputation for missing data. Throughout this chapter, we highlight lessons learned from the Neurodevelopmental Effects of Antiepileptic Drugs (NEAD) and Maternal Outcomes and Neurodevelopmental Effects of Antiepileptic Drugs (MONEAD) prospective observational studies.

## 14.1 Introduction

Prospective observational studies have been a powerful tool in epilepsy research for decades. As with any clinical indication, there may be research topics which cannot, or should not, be addressed using the rigorous randomized controlled trial (RCT). Examples include scenarios where randomization is not possible or ethical, where independent variables of interest cannot be controlled, where there is a lack of equipoise and, similarly, where participants or clinical staff may not accept randomization. Further, research areas for which prospective observational studies may be ideal include big data/health sciences research, genetic/genomic studies, implementation studies and certain pragmatic trials.

Two examples of an epilepsy study where randomization is not ethical, practical or accepted by participants/clinicians are the NEAD and MONEAD studies [24, 25], which will be highlighted throughout this chapter as examples of prospective observational studies in epilepsy. These studies enrolled pregnant women with epilepsy and followed them and their offspring to assess the neurodevelopmental effects of antiseizure medication (ASM) exposure in utero and via breastmilk, as well as neonatal and maternal outcomes in the MONEAD study. In order to have conducted an RCT, women with epilepsy would have to have been (1) enrolled prior to getting pregnant, (2) willing to have their ASM randomly assigned by the study for their future pregnancy and postpartum, and (3) treated by a clinician willing to change their ASM or be willing to change providers. The first criterion would have greatly restricted generalizability since it would only have applied to women who actively tried and succeeded in getting pregnant and delivering an infant who was subsequently followed for neurodevelopmental outcomes (i.e., not a miscarriage or spontaneous abortion). Requiring women to be willing to change their ASM or provider in order to be randomized for an RCT would also hinder generalizability. Beyond generalizability, such a study would be highly impractical and even questionable ethically.

Other studies where prospective observational studies are advantageous and pragmatic are effectiveness studies where the real world environment is of interest, as well as using existing data sources, such as electronic medical records (EMR) or existing control or comparator groups of interest. Quality improvement studies often fit into this category and can rely on EMR data, such as interventions that involve updating the EMR system itself [13, 19]. For example, both of these studies involved updating the EMR and a pre-/post-comparison of data collected via EMR and participant self-report to evaluate any changes in patient perceptions or communications. Comparative effectiveness studies where interest lies in assessing differences, or lack thereof, between two active treatment groups can be conducted via RCT; however, in order to adhere to the spirit of the real world nature of comparative effectiveness, the limited generalizability of an RCT could impede achievement of study goals. In general, real world evidence and real world data, which can be collected via a prospective observational study design, are a focus amongst clinical decision makers and even the U.S. Food and Drug Administration (https://www.fda.gov/science-research/science-and-research-special-topics/real-world-evidence). Another research area within epilepsy where prospective observational studies are valuable is with respect to developing predictive models for seizure frequency when the predictors of interest cannot be controlled, such as intelligence quotients, genetic biomarkers, or sociodemographic factors (e.g., socioeconomic status, rurality and insurance status). In this chapter, we focus on the issues of trial design, data collection, and methods for statistical analysis with respect to epilepsy research studies using a prospective observational approach.

## 14.2 Study Design

First, we start by reviewing critical aspects of prospective study design.

### 14.2.1 Selection of Outcome Measures and How to Best Collect the Data

For many studies in epilepsy, the outcome of interest is related to seizure occurrence or seizure frequency [11]. Some seizure-related metrics commonly used as study outcomes include the change in seizure frequency compared to the individual's baseline, achieving greater than 50% seizure reduction (or other percentages) within a pre-specified time frame, number of seizure-free days within a pre-specified time frame, rate of seizure freedom, and time-to-event measures such as rate of relapse or time to first seizure recurrence (see Chapter 6) [2]. Understanding the research question and analysis population is critical for determining the appropriate outcome for a given study. Factors that should be considered include study design considerations, such as the planned length of follow-up time, as well factors related to the study population, such as understanding of the seizure pathology studied and whether seizure events in the study population are expected to be rare or more frequent. Safety outcomes and outcomes related to quality of life and development of co-morbidities are also often included in epilepsy research.

While seizure outcomes are common in epilepsy research and often the most clinically relevant outcome, reliable measurement and collection of seizure data are quite challenging. This is one of the biggest challenges for prospective studies in epilepsy. While the most common approach for collecting seizure data continues to be through patient self-report via online or paper diaries, it is known that these approaches may be inaccurate and underreporting of seizures is common [5, 6]. Despite these limitations, there are presently few viable or cost-effective alternatives, and patient report continues to be the most common approach for the collection of seizure data. However, due to the known limitations in patient report, development of alternate methods is rapidly evolving and new approaches such as scalp implants, wearable scalp devices, and other wearable devices that measure movements or other bodily changes are being developed and tested [6, 9, 21]. Additional details regarding methods for seizure collection are provided in Section 14.3.3; however, it is essential that the method of seizure data collection is considered during the initial phase of trial design, as well as how the limitations of the selected approach may impact the study outcomes. It is also important to note that most studies of epilepsy are limited to seizures which are observable (e.g., focal aware seizures with motor components). Collection of seizure information for non-observable seizures can be complex and resource intensive.

Seizure type is another important variable that must be considered when defining study outcomes. There is a large amount of heterogeneity across seizure and epilepsy types, and patients may experience more than one type of seizure [11, 31]. Depending on the research question and study population, it may be desirable to limit outcomes only to specific seizure types. How the study plans to incorporate seizure types in the outcome will also impact the methods for collecting seizure data. For example, some types of wearable seizure recording devices are only sensitive to specific seizure types, most commonly tonic-clonic seizures, and may not apply to the study if other seizure types are intended to be included. If using seizure diaries, collection of information on seizure type and duration may be necessary. Many patients with epilepsy may not be aware of when all of their seizures occur, what types of seizures they experience, or the standard terminology used to describe these seizure types [10]. Participant education may be necessary to ensure accurate reporting within seizure diaries.

### 14.2.2 Selection of Study Population

In observational studies, there are a variety of issues to consider when selecting the study population and developing recruitment and retention plans, some of which are particularly relevant in epilepsy research. As noted in the introduction to this chapter, prospective observational studies can offer greater generalizability of results than RCTs. When the study population selected is highly heterogeneous and truly reflects the source population, then generalizability will be maximized. The flip side to the heterogeneity coin is that such large variability across study participants can mask group differences/effects and thus decrease power and necessitate a larger sample size. When selecting the relevant study population to target for an epilepsy study following participants through time, there must be a balance between an achievable sample size and maximizing generalizability of results. In 2013, Friedman & French discussed several challenges encountered in developing effective ASMs [11]. Those authors noted that even the diagnosis of epilepsy can be uncertain and require extensive clinical history, electroencephalography (EEG) and/or imaging to be definitive in determining epilepsy. They further note that underserved communities with low-resource health care systems may not have the resources available to patients for proper epilepsy evaluation and monitoring. This phenomenon may result in the lack of representation in clinical research for such patients, which impacts generalizability and may pose ethical quandaries.

Recruitment is not the only factor that can impact generalizability of results. The study procedures themselves must be feasible for all enrolled participants so as to ensure data collection is as complete as possible for all those in the study. For example, if one is seeking to evaluate a novel medication for treating Dravet syndrome and collecting parent-reported seizures via a smartphone app, it will be important to ensure that all parents have similar access to the app so that under-resourced communities, or rural communities with limited cellular and wireless internet access, can contribute to the research. One potential solution is the provision of telephone cards with relevant data plans or hotspots to ensure parents can report seizures in real time, regardless of their financial resources, thus maximizing the generalizability of the results to patients with Dravet syndrome from various backgrounds.

One potential design solution to the heterogeneity in diagnosis noted by Elger & Hoppe [9] would be to require rigorous diagnostic testing when determining eligibility. However, requiring more rigorous diagnostic testing to determine eligibility may lead to more restrictions and reduced generalizability. Not all potential participants may be willing, for example, to undergo EEG and MRI testing to confirm a proper diagnosis of epilepsy. Those individuals who are unwilling or unable to undergo such rigorous testing may be systematically different with respect to seizure frequency, quality of life, and cognitive function, for example. Thus the eligibility criteria, and the assessment of those criteria, must match the targeted goals of the study, including the appropriate level of generalizability, while also ensuring that a sufficient number of people will be eligible and willing to participate in the study. If the eligibility criteria or study procedures are too restrictive, researchers may not be able to achieve their recruitment goals or may enroll a sample that is unrepresentative of the intended source population. In general, there is always a need to balance the feasibility of study implementation with the desire for rigorous designs. Some observational study designs for epilepsy studies may not be possible for sites to implement successfully, and if the study cannot be implemented as designed, then interpretation of results may be viewed with skepticism when disseminated.

The comparator groups used in prospective observational studies should also be carefully chosen. For example, given the potential heterogeneity in epilepsy diagnosis, control participants may be challenging to identify. In order to maximize power, differences between the control and comparator groups must be minimized (i.e., groups should be balanced across demographics and baseline covariates), and heterogeneity in either group may mask differences. These challenges in selecting a control group or specifying control group eligibility criteria must be thought through during the design stage, and care must be taken to ensure that inclusion of controls will facilitate research and not further muddy the waters. Matching can be a very powerful tool for selecting control and comparator patients for recruitment. A common approach to matching involves matching recruitment across all groups for basic demographics (e.g., age and sex); however, additional criteria may be warranted for epilepsy research. For example, one criterion that may be appropriate to consider is seizure type (e.g., generalized versus focal), though even such a designation may not be simple since some people with epilepsy experience both types of seizures. Section 14.3 provides additional discussion of methods of collection for epilepsy and seizure types. Yet another matching criterion for consideration is matching on type of ASM or whether one's epilepsy is treatment-resistant. Despite these challenges, if selection of the control group is completed and implemented appropriately, then use of such groups can greatly add to the rigor of prospective observational studies.

### 14.2.3 Bias and Confounding

The main advantages of randomizing participants in clinical research is that it creates, but does not guarantee, balance with respect to potential confounders and minimizes bias. Observational research requires *a priori* planning during the design phase to reduce the impact of confounding and utilize approaches to prevent bias to the greatest extent possible.

With respect to confounding, it is vital to collect information on as many confounders as possible so that they can be adjusted for in analyses. Consultation with clinicians and research investigators, as well as literature searches, can be used to generate such a list of potential confounders. While completeness is imperative, it must be balanced with resourcing. Even in the ideal situation where all potential confounders are known and can be collected during the study, it may not be logistically possible or affordable to do so. Consider a scenario where eliciting data from participants at baseline on all identified confounders would require a five-hour visit with the research team. This would be very burdensome for the participant and could have several negative impacts: (1) only highly motivated individuals or those who are not employed and do not have children may agree to participate, which hinders generalizability; (2) participants may not complete all of the data collection, and confounders would end up being incompletely measured; and (3) participants may become frustrated with the repeated burden of these assessments after baseline and withdraw from the study completely. All of these potential consequences can result in bias and residual confounding.

The main three types of bias that arise with observational prospective studies are: (1) selection bias, (2) recall bias, and (3) information bias. *Selection bias* occurs when the enrolled sample systematically differs from the target source population. In the previous example of a medication study in patients with Dravet syndrome, selection bias could occur if children in rural communities were not enrolled because of challenges with completing seizure frequency assessment via a smartphone app. Another example of selection bias that is particular to studies in young children relates to the motivation of the parent. Perhaps, in a study of Dravet syndrome, parents of children with extensive development delay by age three would be more likely to agree to participate than parents of children whose developmental delay is more mild. In such a case, the results of the study cannot be said to reflect Dravet syndrome as a whole, but rather only those for whom there is extensive developmental delay by age three. *Recall bias* is another type of systematic error that occurs when participants may not remember and/or report events accurately. For example, different types of seizures differentially impact cognitive function and recall; therefore, if a study allows for such variability in seizure type, then more objective outcome measures than participant self-report may be warranted to reduce recall bias. *Information bias*, also known as *measurement bias*, is a third type of systematic error where the association metric is distorted by inaccurate measurement or reporting of key study variables (e.g., outcomes, potential confounders, medication exposure). This type of bias is also important to address during the design phase, and particularly when developing the data collection plan and selecting assessments and metrics of interest.

### 14.2.4 Power and Sample Size

Calculating power and necessary sample size can be challenging for any observational study. Consideration generally needs to be paid to the primary analytic model, missing data, and potential covariate imbalance. In some circumstances, power calculations can be simplified and standard software used; however, simulation-based calculations can offer improvements.

Observational studies tend to have numerous secondary, and occasionally tertiary, outcomes. The large number of outcomes must be considered when interpreting results since it is not possible to power a study for that many statistical tests and maintain the appropriate overall type I error rate. With limits on resources and feasible sample sizes, it is common to power the study for 80% and consider only the primary outcome.

In addition, the need to consider covariate imbalance can complicate sample size calculations. Methods exist for incorporating propensity scoring into power computations [3, 20]; however, these are not currently available in existing standard software packages. With respect to confounding, statistical approaches to power calculations have been developed that incorporate information on confounding [14, 23, 41].

Last, missing outcome data is a common problem in prospective observational studies and must be considered in power calculations. Based on prior knowledge, assumptions should be made about the mechanism of missing data, as well as the anticipated rates and patterns of missingness. These can be used to adjust the target sample size such that the study will be sufficiently powered for the outcome of interest even if not all outcome data is available for analysis.

## 14.3 Data Collection

We now turn our attention to aspects of data collection.

### 14.3.1 Covariates

A key design factor of prospective observational studies is that the study groups of interest are not randomly assigned. In RCTs, randomization helps to create balance across other variables that may be associated with the outcome of interest to help isolate the effect of interest. The comparative lack of randomization in observational studies may introduce systematic bias into the analysis since the study groups may not be balanced across other factors associated with the effect of interest. Without the advantage of randomization to create balance, other methods must be employed to reduce this source of bias. These imbalances may lead to biased estimates and incorrect conclusions.

There are a variety of analytical methods that can be employed to account for these imbalances and reduce bias. When building analytical models, it is important to understand the types of variables that may impact the association between your exposure and outcome of interest. Variables that need to be considered include mediators, moderators, and confounders. *Mediators* include intermediate variables on the causal pathway between the exposure and the outcomes. These are often not adjusted for in the analysis, but may be analyzed in a path analysis to estimate the magnitude and significance of potential mediators. *Confounders* are variables that are related to both the exposure or study group assignment and the outcome but are not on the causal pathway. *Moderators* are variables in which the causal relationship between the exposure or study group of interest and outcome is heterogeneous across levels of the moderating variable.

In order to ensure accurate inference and estimation of causal effects, it is essential to consider the presence of potential confounders, effect modifiers, and mediators when identifying the appropriate analytical model to use. While confounders and effect modifiers should be incorporated as variables in the model, inclusion of mediators could obscure the effect of the exposure on the outcome and should not be included in the analytical model. While mediators should not be included in the model, collection of potential explanatory variables may help to elucidate the underlying pathways in the treatment effect. Directed acyclic graphs can be a useful tool in identifying these potential confounders, mediators, and modifiers as well as hypothesizing the causal relationships between the variables. Understanding the causal framework can help both in trial design, as well as in the model building phase of the analysis. There are other tools, such as statistical model building, also referred to as empirical variable selection [30]. These methods include forward, backward, and stepwise selection procedures, as well as regularized methods such as the least absolute shrinkage and selection operator (LASSO). All are valid approaches to handling confounding. When using these statistical approaches for model building, it is important to consider both potential confounders as well as covariates independently associated with the outcome for inclusion in the regression model.

Since data is collected prospectively, all potential confounders, mediators, and effect modifiers must be identified during the trial design phase, so they may be collected throughout the study. This step is critical during the trial design phase since if potential confounders and modifiers are not collected, they will not be available for inclusion in the analysis model, potentially leading to biased estimates and faulty conclusions.

Determination of potential confounders and moderators involves close collaboration with study investigators and subject matter experts to determine variables that may be associated with the exposure or study group assignment and variables that may be associated with the outcome of interest. As many prospective studies include multiple outcomes, it is important to consider confounders and modifiers for all outcomes of interest, not solely the primary outcome. Literature reviews of similar analyses can also help to identify any confounders and modifiers that have been observed in previous research. Literature review can also provide examples of how similar studies have measured and accounted for these variables. Using similar methods to previous research can help increase homogeneity in the research field and make it easier for future meta-analyses to combine or compare findings across multiple studies. When determining the final list of covariates to collect, it is also important to consider participant burden. While from a statistical perspective it may be ideal to collect as many potential confounders or effect modifiers as possible [12], this may not be practical due to study budget constraints as well as undue burden on study participants. Therefore, is it critical to consider which variables are most important to include in study design.

Observational research in epilepsy populations must all consider, comorbidities as a potential confounder. Previous studies have found that between 26.8% and 84% of epilepsy patients had at least one comorbid medical condition, and psychiatric conditions were particularly prevalent [33]. Given these high rates of comorbidities, it is essential that they be measured and accounted for in the analysis, especially for studies which compare outcomes with non-epilepsy populations, to ensure that any observed effect can be attributed to the exposure of interest and not to one of these underlying conditions. Comorbidities may be collected by participant self-report or through medical records. For the collection of psychiatric conditions such as measures of depression and anxiety, assessments that provide a continuous measure of those conditions may be considered, which may provide additional power to detect an impact on that analysis.

### 14.3.2 Epilepsy and Seizure Types

Any epilepsy-related clinical trial, including observational studies, will require the collection of epilepsy and seizure types. There is considerable heterogeneity among participants who experience different seizure types and epilepsy syndromes. Additionally, different epilepsy syndromes are strongly correlated with specific intellectual, psychiatric, and other comorbidities or the absence of various morbidities [42]. Due to this heterogeneity, studies may elect to restrict the analysis population to a subset of seizure or epilepsy types. To do so, seizure or epilepsy type needs to be specified as part of the inclusion and exclusion criteria for the study and requires accurate assessment during screening. Studies not restricted to specific seizure types will still need to collect seizure and epilepsy types to use as potential risk factors, confounders, or effect modifiers in analysis. Misclassification or inconsistent classification of seizure types in a study can introduce bias or additional variability. Additionally, consistent classification of seizure and epilepsy types across studies is vital for the reproducibility of study findings [36].

In 2017, the International League Against Epilepsy (ILAE) released updated guidelines for the classification of seizure type, epilepsy type, and epilepsy syndrome [31]. While primarily proposed to assist with diagnosing patients, this classification system also provides a systematic framework for epilepsy research. A thorough review of this classification system and additional literature for updates to these guidelines is essential during the protocol development phase and should inform the selection of the study population and assessment required during screening. For observational studies with longer follow-up periods, sufficient information regarding the history of seizure types should be collected. Additionally, studies may want to consider specifying how they will handle changes in seizure classification guidelines regarding seizure type or diagnosis at the participant level after enrollment in the study.

A systematic process for the collection of seizure history and classification of seizure types is essential and should be clearly outlined in the study protocol. For studies that involve multiple sites or centers, training across sites is critical to ensure high inter-rater reliability for seizure classification. Additionally, studies may consider using a central review board for adjudication of seizure and epilepsy types to ensure accurate classification. The application of data standards such as the National Institute of Neurological Disorders and

Stroke (NINDS) Epilepsy Common Data Elements is also recommended to ensure accurate classification.

### 14.3.3 Seizure Frequency

Outcomes related to seizure frequency are critical in observational studies in epilepsy and accurate capture of seizure occurrences is essential for unbiased inference. Seizure data is often collected through the use of seizure diaries. These can be paper-based; however, paper-based diaries have more commonly been replaced with electronic diaries that can be installed on smartphones or accessed online.

While seizure diaries remain the most common way to measure seizure frequency, studies have found that seizure reports from patients and caregivers generally undercount or in some cases may serve as an unreliable proxy for electrographic seizures. One study comparing patient-reported seizures to video-EEG monitoring showed a discrepancy of more than 50% between patient-reported and electrographic seizures [5]. It has also been shown that under-reporting of self-reported seizures can be associated with seizure type and exhibit within-subject variability over time [9]. This may impact observation study outcomes such as change in seizure frequency, in which a seizure frequency at a later time point is compared with an earlier baseline assessment.

A key issue with self-reported seizures is that patients may be partially or fully amnestic during or after seizures, and unable to provide accurate self-report [6]. A study in which patients wore wearable monitoring found that only 26% were always aware of all their seizures, and 30% were never aware [5]. Seizure type and vigilance state have also been shown to impact seizure self-reporting. In a study of adults with focal epilepsy comparing patient self-report with video EEG monitoring, patients failed to report 73.2% of complex partial (focal impaired aware) seizures compared with 26.2% of simple partial (focal aware) seizures and 41.7% of secondarily generalized (focal to bilateral) tonic-clonic seizures. Additionally, 85.8% of all seizures during sleeping went unreported, compared with 32.0% of seizures during the awake state [17]. Studies with children have also shown that 40–50% of seizures in the pediatric population go unreported [9], suggesting that it is not just due to the patient being unable to recall. Underreporting of seizures can reduce statistical power in clinical trials and variability in seizure reporting can introduce heterogeneity and lead to biased estimates.

To overcome limitations of seizure reporting, various technologies are being developed, such as wearable sensing devices including wrist accelerometers, non-invasive surface electromyography (EMG) wearables, and multimodal devices employing measures such as accelerometry and heart rate. Many of these technologies are still in development and testing phases, and validated devices are currently only available for specific seizure types (i.e., convulsions), which creates a challenge to employ these devices in studies including participants with a broader range of seizure types. A working group evaluated currently available devices and concluded that there was only a sufficient level of evidence for the accuracy of automated detection of generalized tonic-clonic seizures (GTC) and focal-to-bilateral tonic-clonic seizures (FTBTC) [4]. The use of devices was not recommended for any other seizure type for use in clinical studies. In addition to accuracy in seizure counts, there are additional challenges when employing such technologies for observational prospective studies, which may aim to study a larger number of participants over longer time frames. Data from the Responsive Neurostimulation (RNS®) System, for example, is routinely transferred by patients to a secure online databank, Patient Data Management System (PDMS), from where it can be reviewed by clinicians [18, 26]. Concerns about data processing and security can make these sensing devices challenging to employ on a larger scale [6].

It is commonly thought that the use of traditional seizure diaries is a cost-effective way to collect seizure data compared with some of these newer technologies. However, since larger sample sizes may be required when using diaries to account for potential inaccuracy in reporting, this may override potential cost-savings in the overall cost of the trial. As more research is performed to develop and validate these new technologies, the use of devices such as shake watches and implantable devices will likely become standard in clinical trials.

Despite limitations in self-report, seizure diaries remain one of the most common approaches to assist in the collection of prospective seizure data. In the prospective study MONEAD, we employed an approach that combined self-reported seizure data collected via an eDiary application which could be used on a smartphone or iPod with information about seizure occurrence collected at each study visit, occurring about every three months across a two-year period. In our approach, we sought to not only classify days with seizures but also seizure-free days using these sources. Data on seizure type and duration were also collected.

Participants were instructed to use the eDiary daily to record seizure activity. Not all women complied with this instruction, and approximately 50% of the participant study days were able to be classified as seizure-free or with seizures based on the eDiary daily reports. Several strategies were employed to minimize the amount of missing data. When the eDiary application was opened, if the participant had not entered data for the previous day, a pop-up question asking "Did you have a seizure yesterday?" was displayed before the participant could continue to use the application. If the answer was yes, the user was prompted to enter seizure details. An additional 22% of the seizure days analyzed were attributed to the eDiary pop-up question (43, 242 seizure-free days, 636 seizure days). Data from the eDiary was further supplemented by questions asked during each study visit, in which research coordinators were instructed to review the eDiary with the participant to assess compliance. The Visit Documentation case report form included the question "Has the subject experienced any seizures since the last visit?" and if 'Yes' included a follow-up question to confirm whether all seizures were entered in eDiary. If the participant reported that seizures were missing from the eDiary, the study coordinator could enter them into a Seizure Log case report form during the study visit. If the case report form indicated that either the subject had no seizure since the last visit, or all seizures were entered into the eDiary or Seizure Log, then any days that were missing from the eDiary that couldn't be classified were then imputed as seizure-free days. Seizure day classification from the visit documentation questions and seizure log case report form accounted for about 16% of all days, including about 250 additional reports of seizures captured in the Seizure Log that had been missed in the eDiary. This combined approach allowed us to classify 89% of all study days as being seizure-free or seizure days, and also collect information on the type and number of seizures occurring on seizure days [25].

From a data management perspective, several challenges needed to be addressed throughout the study to enable the combination of data across multiple sources. Since seizure data were collected at the level of seizure type, nightly data quality reports were run to check that all seizure types reported within the eDiary had a link to the participants' data collected through the case report forms. Any discrepancies were flagged, and queries were sent to the site for review and correction. This process helped to minimize data quality issues in the analysis phase, which often occurred years after the seizure report.

An additional advantage of collecting data using this approach is we were able to create a seizure database that captured for each day in the study whether or not the participant had a seizure, and if so, the number of each seizure type for that day. This has enabled us to easily calculate seizure frequencies for any timeframe within the study (i.e., all pregnancy, postpartum, or by trimester) and across several seizure types and epilepsy types.

The MONEAD approach for collecting seizure data provided a cost-efficient and scalable approach for collecting seizure data in pregnant and non-pregnant women for a moderately sized observational study across multiple years and including a wide range of epilepsy types. While we sought to minimize missing data and underreporting of seizures through a multimodal approach, it still relied entirely on self-report, which would not be immune to the challenges of this collection method discussed earlier in this section. This may not be the optimal approach for all prospective studies. Studies with shorter duration, smaller sample size, or more homogenous study populations may wish to take advantage of newer wearable methods that may provide more accurate seizure assessments for certain seizure types of interest. Additionally, newer seizure detection technologies are continually being developed and tested. When designing a study, a review of the current literature is recommended to assess which method may best meet the needs of that particular study within limitations of size, budget, and scope. Understanding the limitations of the seizure collection method that is employed is essential for interpreting results and should be clearly explained in any presentation of findings from the study.

### 14.3.4 Anti-Seizure Medication Dose, Blood Concentrations, and Compliance

Depending on the research questions of interest, prospective collection of ASM dosages, ASM blood concentration levels, and medication compliance may be of importance for collection. Additionally, depending on study outcomes, data collection on non-ASM medications may also be of interest.

One challenge in prospective trials is that it is difficult to collect accurate data on the above quantities when dosages change frequently, such as in pregnancy and in the early postpartum period. Use of a daily diary is critical to capture the details of each dose change. Dosage information can also be collected via case report forms at each study visit; such forms should collect information on the dosage, formulation, and medication regimen for each ASM. Dosage information can be collected from a variety of other sources, including participant self-report, prescriptions, or health records. For longitudinal studies, it is essential to collect dosage information at each visit to monitor dose or drug changes. Data quality checks should be put in place to check the correct entry of start and stop dates, and any overlapping dates or unexpected gaps should be queried throughout the study.

Medication adherence is a common issue in observational studies. Compliance with medication has been shown to be associated with changes in seizure frequency or breakthrough seizures [35], so it is of particular importance to track in prospective studies in epilepsy. Medication adherence can be measured by several methods, including patient self-report, therapeutic drug monitoring (TDM), electronic devices, and pick-up/refill rates.

Subjective methods such as patient self-report are generally the most cost-effective approach to monitor medication adherence. Methods for collecting patient-reported medication adherence measures can include questionnaires administered at study visits or through daily electronic diaries. The use of electronic diaries to collect medication information may be useful for epilepsy studies already employing diaries for seizure monitoring. However, self-report is subject to bias and patient recall. Additionally, medication adherence may itself be correlated with self-report accuracy, which may serve as an additional source of bias in the study.

If more accurate estimates of medication compliance are critical to the study, other non-subjective methods may be employed to complement self-report. Pill counts are an approach that is commonly used in randomized trials, but can also be employed in observational research. In this approach, participants provide evidence of how many doses were taken between visits, and this is compared with how many doses were provided to calculate compliance. However, this method cannot prove that the participant actually ingested the missing doses. Electronic medication monitoring, such as inclusion of a computer chip in a bottle cap that records the date and time the pill bottle is open, or review of electronic databases such as records that the drugs were picked up from the pharmacy, are additional methods that can assess compliance [1]. These methods may be more accurate than patient self-report; however, they are more expensive and may be difficult or impractical to implement for large prospective studies with long follow-up times, and may still not accurately assess medication adherence. The advantages and disadvantages of each approach, as well as factors regarding cost and implementation, should be considered during the study design phase.

ASM blood concentration levels are another method to assess ASM exposure that does not rely on patient self-report. Aside from providing a proxy for medication compliance, collection of ASM blood levels may be necessary for studies where the dose is not expected to be a good approximation for concentration, such as in pregnant women [40]. However, since ASM blood levels only reflect medication levels at a single time point, they may not be reflective of the levels across the entire study. Frequency of collection should be considered when designing the study, and may be a limitation in the analysis. When collecting ASM blood levels, it is also essential to collect information on the time of the last dose prior to blood draw and the dosage amount. For details on the collection and analysis of ASM concentration data, see Chapter 16.

For analyses involving ASM dose or blood levels, if the study includes more than one ASM, it may be necessary to standardize the dosage amounts so that they are comparable across the different drugs. One approach is to use internal standardization, that is, standardization using the collected data. Within each drug, the dosage is standardized to a mean of zero and standard deviation of one, as shown in the formula below:

$$\text{Standardized dose} = \frac{\text{Prescribed daily dose} - \text{Average daily dose for ASM}}{\text{Standard deviation of daily dose for ASM}}.$$

This yields standardized dosages which are now on the same scale across drugs and can be used within the same model. This approach works well when working with a large population with a sufficient number of subjects within each dose group. A second requirement of this approach is that the mean dose for each dose group should be similar to the mean dose for the population to which each dose group is intended to generalize.

A second approach is to use external standardization, that is, standardization using externally collected data. Dosages can be standardized using the World Health Organization (WHO) Defined Daily Dose values. A ratio Defined Daily Dose (DDD) can be calculated by dividing the participant prescribed daily dose by the WHO DDD available on the WHO website (`https://www.whocc.no/atc_ddd_index/`). For participants on more than one ASM, a total ratio Defined Daily Dose can be derived by summing across the ratio Defined Daily Dose values for all prescribed ASMs:

$$\text{Ratio DDD per ASM} = \frac{\text{Prescribed daily dosage}}{\text{WHO DDD}}$$

$$\text{Ratio DDD across prescribed ASMs} = \sum \text{Ratio DDD per ASM}.$$

A similar approach can be used for blood concentrations. A ratio ASM concentration value can be calculated by dividing the ASM concentration by the upper limit of published therapeutic ranges:

$$\text{Ratio ASM concentration per ASM} = \frac{\text{Measured ASM concentration}}{\text{WHO upper limit therapeutic range}}$$

$$\text{Ratio ASM concentration across prescribed ASMs} = \sum \text{Ratio ASM concentration per ASM}.$$

Therapeutic ranges for common ASMs can be found in published references [34]; however, therapeutic ranges may not be available for all ASMs in the study. For both ASM dose and blood levels, within-ASM sub-analyses should be performed to assess if any observed trends across ASMs apply within single ASM groups.

## 14.4 Analysis

We conclude with an overview of analytical methods commonly encountered in prospective trials of epilepsy populations.

### 14.4.1 Modeling Considerations

For observational studies in general, it is rarely appropriate to perform a simple unadjusted statistical analysis. As discussed previously, there are quite often potential confounding factors that need to be adjusted for and this is accomplished via modeling. The selection of the appropriate model depends on many factors, including the type of outcome measure and the research question of interest. Frequently, observational studies of epilepsy focus on comparing two interventions with respect to the relationship with a seizure-related outcome measure.

If assessing seizure frequency, the operational definition of the outcome measure can impact the selection of the appropriate model. For example, if looking at the number of seizures in a specified timeframe, then it is possible to implement a Poisson regression model or related model if there is overdispersion (e.g., zero-inflated Poisson, Beta-Binomial). Alternatively, one may be simply interested in whether seizures occurred at all in the specified timeframe, in which case a logistic regression would be appropriate. Pennell et al. (2020) [25] took another approach, using as a primary outcome measure the change in seizure frequency categorized as an increase, decrease, and no-change, by comparing the seizure frequency during the time period of interest to the individual's baseline seizure frequency. Survival analysis methods could also be used for outcomes such as time to seizure control.

The independent variables in the model can be potential confounders, and risk factors to aid in prediction precision. Measures that are deemed to be colliders (i.e., variables independently caused by both the outcome and another independent variable) should not be included as independent variables in any modeling, and care should be taken to avoid including collinear variables in the model. These scenarios can negatively impact model fit/convergence and interpretation.

In some prospective observational studies, performing mediator analyses may be of interest. For example, in a study comparing two ASMs, one may be interested whether the treatment difference is a function of adherence to the medication. Wang et al. (2022), for example, performed a mediation analysis to evaluate whether certain variables mediated the relationship between ASMs and health-related quality of life amongst people with epilepsy [39]. A review of mediation analysis methods and review of literature is available in Rijnhart et al. (2021) [27].

Yet another analytic method important in observational studies is moderation analysis, where interest lies in evaluating whether the relationship between the dependent and independent variable varies across different levels of another independent variable. Typically, this is handled by including an interaction term in the regression model between the two relevant independent variables. A recent study of seizures and epilepsy in COVID-19 patients, for example, included a moderator analysis for age group [38]. These analyses are akin to subgroup analyses, where interest lies in identifying particular patient subgroups for which a treatment effect differs.

One of the key challenges with observational studies is bias due to imbalance in baseline or other variables also related to the study outcome. Randomization in RCT studies can help to provide balance across known and unknown potential confounders. However, in prospective observational studies, the lack of randomization may introduce bias when assessing the effect of exposure on the outcome. When interpreting model results, one must ensure that any observed associations (or lack of associations) are not the result of other variables that may be associated with the exposure and outcome.

Multiple regression is a common analytical method to statistically control for confounders and to isolate the association with the outcome for the particular exposure of interest. Prior to estimating a multiple regression model, the list of covariates to include must be identified. Determining which variables are likely to be confounders and should be included in the regression model can be based on background knowledge, collaboration with subject matter experts, and estimation of directed acyclic graphs to elucidate the relationships among those variables. For some research questions, this may be sufficient for selecting a succinct list of appropriate confounders to include in the regression model. However, often in observational research, the number of potential confounders is quite large and there may be insufficient degrees of freedom to estimate all main effects and interactions if all covariates are included in the regression model. Additionally, there may be strong collinearity among two or more potential covariates. Common approaches for handling this situation include variable selection procedures to reduce the number of variables included in the final regression model and the use of a propensity score matching to reduce the dimensionality of a collection of covariates into a single value. Dimension reduction methods are discussed in detail in Chapter 12.

### 14.4.2 Variable Selection Methods

Empirical variable selection procedures use an algorithmic approach to either add or eliminate variables from the statistical model using a pre-defined selection criterion. Here we limit our discussion to several simple variable selection procedures, including forward selection, backward selection, stepwise selection, and best subsets selection (Table 14.1). Regularized linear regression is covered in Chapter 13.

Using significance levels (i.e., p-values or model $R^2$) is a common approach for selecting or excluding individual variables from the model in stepwise selection. Information criteria, such as the Akaike information criterion (AIC) and Bayesian information criterion (BIC) can also be used to compare model goodness-of-fit and select the best fit model. Both AIC and BIC involve a goodness of fit term plus a penalty to reduce overfitting and can be used to compare two models even if they are not hierarchically nested. Therefore, these statistics can be used when selecting the best fit model among the collection of models with all possible combinations of covariates. For AIC and BIC, lower values indicate better fit.

AIC is calculated as:

$$AIC = -2LL + 2k,$$

where $LL$ is the log-likelihood and $k$ is the number of estimated parameters in the model. AIC tries to select the best fit model with the fewest possible independent variables. BIC is very similar to AIC and is defined as:

$$BIC = -2LL + k\log(n)$$

where $k$ is the number of estimated parameters in the model and $n$ is the sample size. Compared to AIC, BIC is more stringent and places a stronger penalty on the number of parameters, therefore tending to select simpler models compared with AIC [8]. Additionally,

**TABLE 14.1**
Comparison of stepwise and best subsets variable selection procedures.

| Procedure | Description | Advantages/Disadvantages |
|---|---|---|
| Forward Selection | 1. Specify an $\alpha$ level of significance for covariate entry.<br>2. Start with an empty model (or model including only *a priori* variables) and add each potential variable separately to the model.<br>3. Select the covariate with the best model fit, or with the smallest p-value.<br>4. Repeat until no remaining variables have a p-value below the pre-specified $\alpha$ level for covariate entry. | Can include a large number of starting covariates.<br>Once a variable enters the model, it is not able to be selected out even if no longer necessary in presence of other variables. |
| Backward Selection | 1. Specify an elimination $\alpha$ level of significance.<br>2. Start with a model with all potential variables and identify the variable with the largest p-value. If the p-value is greater than the predetermined threshold, then drop the variable.<br>3. Repeat until no further variables have p-value greater than the pre-specified $\alpha$ level for elimination. | If larger number of covariates, may not be able to run initial model.<br>Once a variable exits the model, it is not able to be selected in. |
| Stepwise Selection | 1. Pre-set significance levels $\alpha$ for entry and elimination.<br>2. Specify either Forward or Backward regression.<br>3. With forward selection, if variables selected in previous steps drop below the elimination $\alpha$ level, may be removed from model.<br>4. With backwards selection, variables eliminated from the model are assessed again at subsequent step.<br>5. Repeat until all covariates in the model have p-value below the $\alpha$ level for covariate entry, and all variables excluded have p-values above the elimination $\alpha$ level. | Can include a large number of starting covariates.<br>Variables can enter and exit the model throughout the variable selection process |
| Best Subsets Regression | Estimate all possible combinations of covariates and select the model with the best fit according to pre-specified model criterion (e.g., AIC, BIC, DIC, Mallow's Cp, $R^2$). | If the set of potential covariates is large (e.g., $> 30$) may require substantial computational time. |

BIC assumes that there is a true model, and that model is included in the model selection. If this assumption holds, then selection using BIC will converge to the true model [16]. In practice, the assumption of a true model being included amongst all models may not be practical and AIC may be a more appropriate information criterion.

Stepwise variable selection algorithms are available in most statistical analysis packages. If using `SAS`, all the variable selection algorithms discussed above can be implemented using

`PROC GLMSelect`. For `R` users, the `stepAIC()` function in the `MASS` package can be used to perform stepwise variable selection using the AIC.

### 14.4.3 Matching

Matching is another approach to control for confounding in cohort studies, by ensuring equal distribution of the confounding variable across the exposed and control populations. *Frequency matching* is matching at the population level. Control subjects are selected so that the distribution of the confounding variables in the control population is equivalent to the exposed population. For example, if the exposed population is 30% female and sex is a known confounder for the research question of interest, a subset of controls may be selected from the cohort that is also 30% female, so that the distribution of sex in the control population is equivalent to the exposed population. For cohort studies, no additional statistical methods are necessarily applied to account for the matching. *Individual matching* is when each subject within the exposed population is matched to one or more controls on one or more confounders. In the final analysis population, matched variables should have an equal distribution among both groups, removing or reducing the confounding effect, and isolating the exposure of interest.

Individual matching is rarely used during the primary data collection phase in most prospective trials due to practical challenges in collection, and since data is often collected with a number of research questions in mind requiring different exposures and sets of confounders. However, individual matching can be applied in secondary use of existing cohort data. Analyses with matching on the exposure in cohort studies can be analyzed using the same methods as unmatched studies and do not require additional methods in the analysis phase to account for the matching.

### 14.4.4 Propensity Scores

Another method that can be used for matching as well as other analytical approaches to account for the imbalance in covariates is *propensity score matching*. The propensity score was first defined by Rosenbaum and Rubin as the probability of being in the treatment group conditioned on a set of observed baseline covariates

$$e(x) = P[z = 1|x], \tag{14.1}$$

where $z = 1$ for subjects in the treatment group and $z = 0$ for subjects in the control or comparison group [28].

For observational studies, Eq. (14.1) has been extended to include the conditional probability of being in the exposed or study group of interest. The derivation of propensity scores reduces the dimensionality of the set of baseline covariates into a single number. In theory, participants with similar propensity scores come from a similar distribution of the baseline covariates. Propensity scores can be used for matching using similar methods described above or for stratification, or as a covariate in a regression model.

For observational studies with two groups of interest, propensity scores can be derived using logistic regression. The dependent variable in the logistic regression model is the group assignment, and the independent variables are the set of baseline covariates. The propensity scores are then equal to the predicted probability from the logistic regression model.

$$\log\frac{e(x)}{1 - e(x)} = \alpha + \beta^T x_i,$$

where $e(x) = P[z = 1|x]$ and $x$ denotes the covariates.

Covariates included in the logistic regression model should include only baseline covariates. Measurement of these variables should precede group membership. Additionally, propensity scores cannot be derived if covariate values are missing, so this may not be practical if there is a large amount of missing data. When selecting the variables to include in a propensity score model, variables associated with the outcome in the final analysis model are the most important and should always be included. Variables associated with treatment should also be considered for inclusion, although these are generally less important if not associated with the outcome [32].

One important consideration with the use of propensity scores in epilepsy research is that the conceptual framework of propensity scores is best applied with a well-defined intervention or treatment. Applications of the propensity score to underlying disease state, since disease state is not modifiable, would not fit within this framework. Therefore, propensity scores may not be applicable to observational studies when comparing participants with epilepsy to those without, or between various types of epilepsy, and would be better suited for studies in which the analysis groups of interest are based on things like specific interventions or treatments among patients with epilepsy. While the statistical theory underlying these methods does not prohibit them from being applied in condition states, additional care must be taken when selecting the covariates included in the model [32].

Common applications of propensity scores include stratification, matching, and model adjustment. For stratification, strata are derived based on percentiles of the propensity scores. Diagnostic tests are then run to assess balance across covariates within each stratum. Once balance has been achieved, the analytic model comparing the treatment groups is assessed within strata. When using propensity scores for matching, balance within the exposed group is achieved by matching each exposed with an unexposed subject with the closest propensity score. Diagnostic tests are run to assess balance; the matched pairs analysis is used to assess the effect of interest. This approach is only applicable when the set of unexposed participants is large enough to provide sufficient matched samples.

Derivations of propensity scores can be easily implemented in most statistical software packages using a logistic regression model. The `R` package `MatchIt` provides functions for both estimating propensity scores and also matching participants using the derived propensity score, as well as other approaches to matching. The `SAS` procedure `PROC PSMATCH` can also be used for calculating propensity scores, matching or stratifying participants using the derived propensity scores, and running a number of diagnostics to assess balance across the model covariates.

### 14.4.5 Missing Data

Missing data is a common problem in observational prospective studies, and studies of epilepsy populations are no exception. Missing data can be the results of missed or incomplete visits, treatment non-adherence, participant dropout, or loss to follow-up. While is it essential to try to ensure maximum participant retention and compliance with the study protocol, some non-compliance issues are inevitable, and missing data must be addressed and accounted for during the analysis phase.

From a statistical perspective, missing data is typically classified into three different categories: *missing completely at random (MCAR)*, *missing at random (MAR)*, and *missing not at random (MNAR)*. For data that is MCAR, the missingness is completely independent of the observed and unobserved data. A common example would be data that is missing due to machine malfunction which would be expected to affect all missing samples equally. Excluding data that is MCAR would not introduce bias; however, exclusion may reduce statistical power depending on the amount of missingness. MAR occurs when the missing values are associated with, or systematically related to, the observed data, not the unobserved data. For example, in an analysis examining scores on a depression assessment, if younger participants are less likely to complete the assessment, and age is fully observed in the study, then the data may be classified as MAR. Missing data is considered MNAR when the missing value is related to unobserved data, often the missing data itself. For example, if subjects who are more depressed are more likely to miss the study visit and depression assessment, the missing data on that assessment would be associated with the score and classified as MNAR. The various methods for handling missing data and whether they produce unbiased or approximately unbiased estimates depends on the type of missingness, so it is important to consider the mechanism when employing these methods.

*Complete case analysis* or *listwise deletion* is one approach for treating missing data, where records with missing data are excluded from the analysis. This approach may be appropriate if the amount of missing data is very small, or missing data is assumed to be MCAR. However, MCAR is generally regarded as a strong and often unrealistic assumption. If the amount of missingness is non-trivial, additional approaches should be considered.

Another approach for handling missing data is to use *single-point imputation*, in which the missing data are replaced with a single value prior to analysis. There are various approaches for which value to use for imputation. A common approach for longitudinal studies is to use the last observation carried forward (LOCF), where the subject's last observation prior to the missing values is imputed for subsequent missing values. Similar approaches include best or worst observation carried forward. A summary statistic of available data such as the median or mean can also be used in single value imputation. These approaches may introduce bias even if the missingness is MCAR [37]. However, they may be useful for sensitivity analyses and assessing the robustness of results obtained from other approaches such as multiple imputation.

A more sophisticated approach to handling missing is multiple imputation, which uses the distribution of the observed data to estimate multiple possible values for each missing value, generating multiple complete analysis datasets. During the analysis phase, the statistical model is run on each dataset and the resulting estimates from each dataset are pooled to derive approximately unbiased point estimates for data that are MAR. The additional uncertainty around the missing values is incorporated into the standard errors for inference.

The most common approach for pooling parameter estimates across multiple imputed datasets is using Rubin's rule [29]. An example of Rubin's rule for a single parameter of interest $Q$, such as a regression coefficient, is shown below. The multiply imputed point estimate for $Q$ is:

$$\bar{Q} = \frac{1}{m}\sum_{i=1}^{m}\hat{Q}_i$$

where $m$ is the number of imputed datasets and $Q_i$ is the point estimate of the parameter from each imputed data. The total variance for the overall multiply imputed estimate is:

$$T = \bar{U} + (1 + \frac{1}{m})B,$$

where $\bar{U} = \frac{1}{m}\sum_{i=1}^{m} U_i$ is the estimated imputation variance and $B = \frac{1}{m-1}\sum_{i=1}^{m}(\hat{Q}_i - \bar{Q})^2$ is the between-imputation variance.

While multiple imputation requires additional steps, most statistical packages offer methods for both generating the imputed datasets and also combining parameter estimates across the multiply imputed datasets for the final model. Methods such as

PROC MI/PROC MIANLYZE in SAS or using the mice package in R. Here is some sample syntax for performing multiple imputation by chained equations using the R mice package:

```
# Imputation step: Specify number of imputed datasets as m and the imputation
    method using the meth argument
IMPDat <- mice(data, m = 5, maxit = 50, meth = 'pmm', seed = 500)
summary(IMPDat)

# Run linear regression on each imputed dataset
modelFit1 <- with(IMPDat, lm(Outcome ~ Var1 + Var2 + Var3))

# Pool parameter estimates across the missing value samples in order to obtain a
    single point estimate.
summary(pool(modelFit1))
```

In general, the imputation model should include all variables that will be used in the analysis. Variables that are not used in the analysis but are highly correlated with responses or explanatory variables, as well as variables that are associated with the pattern of missing data, should also be included. However, it has been shown that inclusion of too many variables, and particularly variables with low correlation with the imputed variable, can decrease precision and lead to a downward bias of the estimate [15]. Therefore, auxiliary variables should be reviewed prior to inclusion in the imputation model.

Standard multiple imputation models as described above assume that the data is MAR and that all variables have been measured and included in the imputation model. A challenge in handling missing data is that since the pattern of missingness depends on unseen data, in many cases, the observed data cannot be used to verify if the data is MAR versus MNAR. Therefore, sensitivity analyses that assess departures from MAR are necessary to examine the robustness of this assumption. Common MNAR imputation techniques include pattern-mixture models and tipping-point analyses. A common pattern-mixture model is reference-based imputation, where, depending on the type of missing data, subjects in one group would be imputed as if in the control group or reference group [7]. Another approach would be to add a delta value to the imputed values within each imputed data set [22]. In a tipping-point analysis, the multiple imputation model is run using a range of delta values added to the imputed values to determine the minimum delta value needed to change the conclusion from the initial model (i.e. until the statistical test being used yields a $p$-value $> 0.05$) [22].

## 14.5 Summary

In this chapter, we have presented some of the experimental design and statistical issues relevant for observational studies of persons with epilepsy. An elucidation of all issues that may arise with such studies is out of the scope of this chapter; however, the topics discussed here represent the authors' experience in the design, implementation, and data analyses as investigators in the NEAD and MONEAD studies. In general, the statistical challenges and methodologies encountered in prospective trial analysis are similar to observational studies, with this chapter highlighting a few topics specific to epilepsy. Specifically, there are unique issues with heterogeneity in phenotype, such as the numerous different types of seizures. In addition, studies of epilepsy also need to consider measurement issues particularly as they relate to data collection regarding seizures and the numerous covariates needed to address potential confounding.

## Bibliography

[1] Laura Alexandra Anghel, Andreea Maria Farcas, and Radu Nicolae Oprean. An overview of the common methods used to measure treatment adherence. *Medicine and Pharmacy Reports*, 92(2):117, April 2019.

[2] A Arzimanoglou, L Kalilani, MA Anamoo, M Cooney, A Golembesky, C Taeter, A Bozorg, A Tofighy, and J Wheless. Role of observational studies in supporting extrapolation of efficacy data from adults to children with epilepsy—A systematic review of the literature using lacosamide as an example. *European Journal of Paediatric Neurology*, 23(4):589–603, July 2019.

[3] Peter C. Austin. Informing power and sample size calculations when using inverse probability weighting using the propensity score. *Statistics in Medicine*, 40(27):6150–6163, November 2021.

[4] Sándor Beniczky, Samuel Wiebe, Jesper Jeppesen, William O. Tatum, Milan Brazdil, Yuping Wang, Susan T. Herman, and Philippe Ryvlin. Automated seizure detection using wearable devices: A clinical practice guideline of the International League Against Epilepsy and the International Federation of Clinical Neurophysiology. *Clinical Neurophysiology*, 132(5):1173–1184, May 2021.

[5] DE Blum, J Eskola, JJ Bortz, and RS Fisher. Patient awareness of seizures. *Neurology*, 47(1):260–264, July 1996.

[6] Benjamin H. Brinkmann, Philippa J. Karoly, Ewan S. Nurse, Sonya B. Dumanis, Mona Nasseri, Pedro F. Viana, Andreas Schulze-Bonhage, Dean R. Freestone, Greg Worrell, Mark P. Richardson, and Mark J. Cook. Seizure diaries and forecasting with wearables: Epilepsy monitoring outside the clinic. *Frontiers in Neurology*, 12, 2021.

[7] James R. Carpenter, James H. Roger, and Michael G. Kenward. Analysis of longitudinal trials with protocol deviation: A framework for relevant, accessible assumptions, and inference via multiple imputation. *Journal of Biopharmaceutical Statistics*, 23(6):1352–1371, 2013.

[8] John J. Dziak et al. Sensitivity and specificity of information criteria. *Briefings in Bioinformatics*, 21(2):553–565, 2020.

[9] Christian E. Elger and Christian Hoppe. Diagnostic challenges in epilepsy: Seizure under-reporting and seizure detection. *The Lancet. Neurology*, 17(3):279–288, 2018.

[10] Robert S. Fisher, J. Helen Cross, Jacqueline A. French, Norimichi Higurashi, Edouard Hirsch, Floor E. Jansen, Lieven Lagae, Solomon L. Moshé, Jukka Peltola, Eliane Roulet Perez, Ingrid E. Scheffer, and Sameer M. Zuberi. Operational classification of seizure types by the International League Against Epilepsy: Position paper of the ILAE commission for classification and terminology. *Epilepsia*, 58(4):522–530, 2017.

[11] Daniel Friedman and Jacqueline A. French. Designing better trials for epilepsy medications: The challenge of heterogeneity. *Clinical Investigation*, 3(10):927–934, October 2013.

[12] Thomas A. Glass, Steven N. Goodman, Miguel A. Hernán, and Jonathan M. Samet. Causal inference in public health. *Annual Review of Public Health*, 34:61, 2013.

[13] Randall W. Grout, Jeffrey Buchhalter, Anup D. Patel, Amy Brin, Ann A. Clark, Mary Holmay, Tyler J. Story, and Stephen M. Downs. Improving patient-centered communication about sudden unexpected death in epilepsy through computerized clinical decision support. *Applied Clinical Informatics*, 12(01):090–099, 2021.

[14] Sebastien Haneuse, Jonathan Schildcrout, and Daniel Gillen. A two-stage strategy to accommodate general patterns of confounding in the design of observational studies. *Biostatistics*, 13(2):274–288, April 2012.

[15] Jochen Hardt, Max Herke, and Rainer Leonhart. Auxiliary variables in multiple imputation in regression with missing x: A warning against including too many in small sample research. *BMC Medical Research Methodology*, 12:1–13, 2012.

[16] Georg Heinze, Christine Wallisch, and Daniela Dunkler. Variable selection–A review and recommendations for the practicing statistician. *Biometrical Journal*, 60(3):431–449, 2018.

[17] Christian Hoppe, Annkathrin Poepel, and Christian E. Elger. Epilepsy: Accuracy of patient seizure counts. *Archives of Neurology*, 64(11):1595–1599, 2007.

[18] Beata Jarosiewicz and Martha Morrell. The RNS system: Brain-responsive neurostimulation for the treatment of epilepsy. *Expert Review of Medical Devices*, 18(2):129–138, 2021.

[19] Felipe J. S. Jones, Jason R. Smith, Neishay Ayub, Susan T. Herman, Jeffrey R. Buchhalter, Brandy E. Fureman, Sydney S. Cash, Daniel B. Hoch, and Lidia M. V. R. Moura. Implementing standardized provider documentation in a tertiary epilepsy clinic. *Neurology*, 95(2):e213–e223, 2020.

[20] Sin-Ho Jung, Shein-Chung Chow, and Eric M. Chi. A note on sample size calculation based on propensity analysis in nonrandomized trials. *Journal of Biopharmaceutical Statistics*, 17(1):35–41; discussion 43, 2007.

[21] Abhinav V. Kurada et al. Seizure detection devices for use in antiseizure medication clinical trials: A systematic review. *Seizure*, 66:61–69, 2019.

[22] Katherine J. Lee et al. Framework for the treatment and reporting of missing data in observational studies: The treatment and reporting of missing data in observational studies framework. *Journal of Clinical Epidemiology*, 134:79–88, 2021.

[23] K. J. Lui. Sample size determination under an exponential model in the presence of a confounder and type I censoring. *Controlled Clinical Trials*, 13(6):446–458, 1992.

[24] Kimford J. Meador, Gus A. Baker, Nancy Browning, Morris J. Cohen, Rebecca L. Bromley, Jill Clayton-Smith, Laura A. Kalayjian, Andres Kanner, Joyce D. Liporace, Page B. Pennell, et al. Fetal antiepileptic drug exposure and cognitive outcomes at age 6 years (NEAD study): A prospective observational study. *The Lancet Neurology*, 12(3):244–252, 2013.

[25] Page B. Pennell, Jacqueline A. French, Ryan C. May, Elizabeth Gerard, Laura Kalayjian, Patricia Penovich, Evan Gedzelman, Jennifer Cavitt, Sean Hwang, Alison M. Pack, et al. Changes in seizure frequency and antiepileptic therapy during pregnancy. *New England Journal of Medicine*, 383(26):2547–2556, 2020.

[26] Vikram R. Rao. Chronic electroencephalography in epilepsy with a responsive neurostimulation device: Current status and future prospects. *Expert Review of Medical Devices*, 18(11):1093–1105, 2021.

[27] Judith J. M. Rijnhart, Sophia J. Lamp, Matthew J. Valente, David P. MacKinnon, Jos W. R. Twisk, and Martijn W. Heymans. Mediation analysis methods used in observational research: A scoping review and recommendations. *BMC Medical Research Methodology*, 21:226, 2021.

[28] Paul R. Rosenbaum and Donald B. Rubin. The central role of the propensity score in observational studies for causal effects. *Biometrika*, 70(1): 41–45, 1983.

[29] Donald B. Rubin. *Multiple Imputation for Nonresponse in Surveys*, volume 81. John Wiley & Sons, 2004.

[30] Brian Sauer, M. Alan Brookhart, Jason A Roy, and Tyler J. VanderWeele. *Chapter 7: Covariate Selection.* Agency for Healthcare Research and Quality, 2013.

[31] Ingrid E. Scheffer et al. ILAE classification of the epilepsies: Position paper of the ILAE commission for classification and terminology. *Epilepsia*, 58(4):512–521, 2017.

[32] Phillip J. Schulte, and Edward J. Mascha. Propensity score methods: Theory and practice for anesthesia research. *Anesthesia & Analgesia*, 127(4):1074–1084, October 2018.

[33] Michael Seidenberg, Dalin T. Pulsipher, and Bruce Hermann. Association of epilepsy and comorbid conditions. *Future Neurology*, 4(5):663–668, 2009.

[34] Erik K St. Louis. Monitoring antiepileptic drugs: A level-headed approach. *Current Neuropharmacology*, 7(2):115–119, 2009.

[35] L Stanaway, DG Lambie, and RH Johnson. Non-compliance with anticonvulsant therapy as a cause of seizures. *The New Zealand Medical Journal*, 98(774):150–152, 1985.

[36] Claude Steriade, Michael R. Sperling, Bree DiVentura, Meryl Lozano, Renée A. Shellhaas, Sudha Kilaru Kessler, Dennis Dlugos, and Jacqueline French. Proposal for an updated seizure classification framework in clinical trials. *Epilepsia*, 63(3):565–572, 2022.

[37] Jonathan A. C. Sterne, Ian R. White, John B. Carlin, Michael Spratt, Patrick Royston, Michael G. Kenward, Angela M. Wood, and James R. Carpenter. Multiple imputation for missing data in epidemiological and clinical research: Potential and pitfalls. *BMJ*, 338:b2393, 2009.

[38] Maxime Taquet, Orrin Devinsky, J. Helen Cross, Paul J. Harrison, and Arjune Sen. Incidence of epilepsy and seizures over the first six months after a COVID-19 diagnosis: A retrospective cohort study. *Neurology*, 100(8):e790–e799, 2023.

[39] Meng Wang, Kevin Perera, Colin B. Josephson, Mubasiru Lamidi, Oluwaseyi A. Lawal, Oluwagbohunmi Awosoga, Pamela Roach, Scott B. Patten, Samuel Wiebe, and Tolulope T. Sajobi. Association between antiseizure medications and quality of life in epilepsy: A mediation analysis. *Epilepsia*, 63(2):440–450, 2022.

[40] Andreas Austgulen Westin, Karl Otto Nakken, Svein I. Johannessen, Arne Reimers, Kari Mette Lillestølen, and Eylert Brodtkorb. Serum concentration/dose ratio of topiramate during pregnancy. *Epilepsia*, 50(3):480–485, 2009.

[41] J Andrew Wilson et al. The reporting of studies using routinely collected health data was often insufficient. *Journal of Clinical Epidemiology*, 119:21–31, 2020.

[42] Elaine Wirrell, Paolo Tinuper, Emilio Perucca, and Solomon L. Moshé. Introduction to the epilepsy syndrome papers, 2022 (see the journal and volume information here: https://pubmed.ncbi.nlm.nih.gov/35503711/).

# 15

# *Pharmacokinetic and Pharmacodynamic Modeling*

**Ashwin Karanam**

*Pfizer, Inc. (USA)*

**Yuhan Long**

*Department of Experimental & Clinical Pharmacology, University of Minnesota (USA)*

**Angela Birnbaum**

*Department of Experimental & Clinical Pharmacology, University of Minnesota (USA)*

## CONTENTS



Neurologists and clinical pharmacologists have been measuring and analyzing antiseizure medication concentrations for decades as instrumentation has become available and sensitivity sufficient. Measurement of drug concentrations can provide a surrogate for overall drug exposure in an individual patient. Establishment of the optimal concentration for an individual such that seizure control and adverse events are balanced allows for evaluation of medication adherence and assessment of changes in seizure control. Therapeutic drug monitoring is regularly employed in patients with epilepsy with the premise that the concentration in the blood is correlated to concentration of drug at the active site; in the case of antiseizure medications, the site of action is the central nervous system, specifically the brain. Knowledge of mechanism and compartmentalization of drug in the body is important when developing pharmacostatistical models in order to incorporate valid assumptions and

DOI: 10.1201/9781003254515-15

create meaningful models. A suite of analyses and model types are available, and the choice of method used can depend on study design and the availability of intensive data versus sparse data sampling in an individual.

## 15.1 Pharmacokinetic Parameters

Pharmacokinetics involves the movement of drug through the body from entry to exit. In order to characterize the pharmacokinetics of a medication, particular parameters are used to describe the processes involved. The parameters most often reported in literature are included in Table 15.1.

**TABLE 15.1**
Commonly reported pharmacokinetic parameters.

| Parameter shorthand | Parameter name |
|---|---|
| $D$ | Dose |
| $C_{max}$ | Maximum concentration, peak concentration |
| $T_{max}$ | Time to maximum concentration |
| $C_{min}$ | Minimum concentration |
| $AUC$, $AUC_a^b$ | Area under the concentration-time curve |
| $F$ | Bioavailability |
| $CL$, $Cl$ | Clearance |
| $V_d$ | Volume of Distribution |
| $k_e$, $k_{el}$ | Elimination rate constant |
| $k_a$ | Absorption rate constant |
| $t_{1/2}$ | Half-life |

$C_{max}$ and $T_{max}$ refer to the highest concentration and when it occurs after a dose, respectively. These parameters help define the fluctuation of the overall concentrations during a dosing interval. $AUC$ is the area under the concentration time curve and is typically used as a measure for overall drug exposure. $F$ or bioavailability indicates the amount of drug from a dose that reaches systemic circulation and is then available at the site of action. Bioavailability is defined by both the rate and extent of absorption.

Clearance ($CL$) and volume of distribution ($V_d$) are two independent parameters that form the basis for most pharmacokinetic models. Clearance describes how fast the drug leaves the body and is expressed in units of volume per time to signify the volume of plasma cleared of drug over a specific amount of time. Volume of distribution is a representation of how drug distributes throughout the body. Volume of distribution, expressed with units of volume, is driven by the lipophilicity of a compound and indicates if a drug remains mostly in the plasma or whether it passes out of plasma into tissue compartments. Because drug does not evenly distribute in the body, volume of distribution is theoretical and dependent on the model. This can lead to situations where volumes can be higher than the total volume of body water (approximately 42 liters in humans). Both clearance and volume of distribution help define the half-life, $t_{1/2}$, of a drug by the following equation:

$$t_{1/2} = \frac{log(2)V_d}{CL}.$$

Depending on the model used, there may be further parameters included, such as additional rate constants that dictate transfer between "compartments." A common addition is the absorption rate constant ($k_a$) for non-intravenous drug administration. The choice of parameters to be estimated depends on the data collected, including the number and timing of concentration measurements during a dosing interval. Therefore, sample collection and study design are important determinants of which parameters can or should be estimated from a model.

## 15.2 Concepts of Pharmacokinetic Processes

In order to create valid pharmacokinetic models, it is critical to understand the mechanisms that describe how the drug travels through the body from delivery of a formulation to excretion. Pharmacokinetics is divided into four main processes: absorption, distribution, metabolism, and elimination [12, 16]. These processes are reflected in the equations used during model building. Models often use a simple exponential growth/decay equation for approximation, though more complex models can be developed that incorporate unique aspects of physiology and drugs; however, models are often limited by the lack of data collected that can address a particular process or parameter leading to overparameterization and nonconvergence of the overall model. Foundational concepts of the processes most often included in pharmacokinetic models will be discussed further in this section.

Pharmacokinetics can also be classified into linear and nonlinear processes. When clearance is constant over time in the central compartment (see Section 15.4.2 for details on compartments), pharmacokinetics is considered linear, which can be modeled with exponential growth/decay. If clearance varies over time within individuals, we observe nonlinear pharmacokinetics resulting in dose increases that do not exhibit a proportional increase in concentration. There are examples of antiseizure medications that show a lower than proportional increase in concentrations due to autoinduction of metabolizing enzymes (e.g., carbamazepine) and higher than proportional increase due to the inhibition of metabolizing enzymes at clinical doses (e.g., phenytoin). It should be noted that the terms linear and nonlinear are used to refer to different aspects of pharmacokinetics and care should be taken with respect to context. A later topic of population pharmacokinetics will involve discussion of "nonlinear mixed effects modeling," where the nonlinear term refers to the statistical method rather than the pharmacokinetic process.

### 15.2.1 Absorption

The pharmacokinetic model parameters most often associated with absorption are the absorption rate constant ($k_a$) and bioavailability ($F$). Absorption refers to the processes involved in systemic absorption of the drug from the site of administration. Several physiological, chemical, and physiochemical factors (e.g., pH of the solution, membrane permeability, transporters) modulate the gradient of influx of the drug into systemic circulation. For orally administered drugs, potential sites of absorption in the gastrointestinal tract include the oral mucosa, stomach, duodenum, and intestinal tract. Absorption in the gastrointestinal tract is usually driven by surface area, pH, blood flow, and permeability. For almost all orally administered drugs, the absorption from small intestine is the fastest owing to the large surface area of microvilli and large blood flow. Other routes of administration, such as lungs and skin, have their own absorption characteristics. Since antiseizure medications are mostly administered orally, oral administration will be our focus. There are situations where drug is administered intravenously such as for acute seizure control. The ability to administer a medication by the intravenous route is usually limited by absence of appropriate formulations.

As mentioned above, the term bioavailability is used to describe the extent and rate of systemic absorption of a drug administered by an extravascular route relative to intravenous dose. As 100% of a drug given intravenously is delivered to the systemic circulation, $F$ will be 1.0 for intravenously delivered products. Thus, intravenous administration is used as the reference formulation for determination of absolute bioavailability. When the pharmacokinetics following an intravenous dose is known, $F$ of an orally administered drug can be computed by the following equation:

$$F = \frac{AUC_{po}/D_{po}}{AUC_{iv}/D_{iv}},$$

where $AUC$ is the area under the concentration time curve and $D$ is dose. The subscript $po$ refers to oral administration and $iv$ to intravenous administration. For an orally administered drug, the bioavailability is usually less than one. Physiologically, the vasculature from the gastrointestinal tract drains into the portal vein and then to the liver. As drug concentration data may not be available from intravenous administration due to lack of a suitable formulation or more complicated sample collection (i.e., need for higher level staff to place an indwelling catheter), relative bioavailability is more practical to report. For relative bioavailability the comparison would be made between two nonparental formulations, such as comparison between the immediate and extended release formulations.

There are several processes involved in the passage of drug from the site of administration to the systemic circulation that can reduce drug absorption, thereby reducing bioavailability. First, drug may be lost by degradation in the lumen. The remaining fraction ($F_a$) of drug may be subject to enzymatic metabolism (e.g., CYP3A4) in the gut. The fraction escaping gut metabolism ($F_g$) is further metabolized by the liver via the portal vein. Finally, the fraction remaining after liver extraction ($F_h$) would be the fraction available systemically. The metabolism in the gastrointestinal tract and liver prior to systemic circulation is referred to as first pass metabolism. First pass metabolism is defined as the metabolism that occurs to the drug before it reaches systemic circulation, so first pass metabolism from non-oral administration can involve metabolism from other sources. A drug that exhibits a high first pass metabolism usually results in a low oral bioavailability. The measure of oral bioavailability is determined by:

$$F = F_a \times F_g \times F_h.$$

Other processes such as dissolution of a capsule or tablet take place, but information for this parameter is typically not available in clinically obtained data. Factors such as dosage form, gastrointestinal motility, and food administered with a dose can also modulate the absorption process. Being familiar with factors that may affect absorption can aid in determining the variables to include when designing a pharmacokinetic study.

### 15.2.2 Distribution

Distribution describes the passage of drug through the body, such as from an oral formulation after ingestion to systemic circulation and then to site of action. Movement of drug usually occurs either through the cell (transcellular) or between the cells (paracellular). Most drugs bind to plasma proteins and tissue components to some extent. Only unbound drug is capable of moving through membranes. Hence, in this section, drug transport refers to movement of unbound drug. Changes in protein binding can lead to changes in unbound drug. Some ASMs are more highly bound to proteins than others and unbound concentrations are considered more relevant than total drug concentrations in drugs that exhibit high protein binding (> 85%).

Diffusion is one of the main processes by which drugs move through membranes. Passive diffusion is guided by permeability, the available surface area for transport, and most importantly the concentration gradient between the membranes. Permeability across a membrane is also affected by drug properties such as lipophilicity, molecular size, and the ionization of the molecule. The influence of lipophilicity across membranes is most clearly seen in the transport of molecules across barriers such as the blood brain barrier.

### 15.2.3 Metabolism and Elimination

Both metabolism and excretion contribute to overall drug elimination from the body. Metabolism is predominantly mediated by the liver, with a small fraction mediated by gastrointestinal wall, blood, lungs, and kidneys. Excretion, on the other hand, is almost entirely mediated by the kidneys via renal elimination.

Metabolic reactions are chemical alteration of medications carried out by enzymes so that they can be more easily eliminated from the body. Typically, this involves increasing the polarity of the drug, thereby increasing its water solubility. These include oxidation, reduction, hydrolysis, and conjugation reactions. Conjugation reactions in particular add polar moieties (such as glucuronic acid, acetate, or sulfate) to the drug. Depending on the drug and metabolite properties, metabolism can also be sequential with one metabolite leading to further metabolism (e.g., oxidation followed by conjugation). Enzymes that mediate these reactions are most highly concentrated in the liver, but metabolic enzymes can be found in almost every organ.

Oxidation reactions, previously referred to as Phase I metabolism, are mediated predominantly by the cytochrome P450 (CYP450) system. The CYP450 system is subdivided into 5 subfamilies from A through E. CYP3A is the largest by abundance in the liver and is found in the gastrointestinal wall as well. Relative abundance does not necessarily reflect the contribution to metabolism. For example, CYP2D6 is the major metabolizing enzyme for approximately one fourth of all prescribed drugs, but only accounts for 2% of liver CYP450 enzymes (see Figure 15.1 for relative CYP450 abundance in the liver). Conjugation reactions, previously referred to as Phase II metabolism, are mediated by several superfamilies of which the most well characterized is the UDP-glucuronosyltransferase (UGT) superfamily. Glucuronidation increases polarity of molecules by forming glucuronides, which are usually excreted by the kidneys.

Renal excretion is a combined result of filtration, secretion, and reabsorption at the nephron. Filtration and secretion work to remove the drug from the body whereas reabsorption works to move drug back into the systemic circulation. Filtration clears approximately 10% of the volume of blood that passes through the glomerulus and works through pressure exerted by arterial blood, clearing the unbound drug in blood. The glomerular filtration rate (GFR) is a metric used to quantify the rate at which plasma is filtered. Creatinine is an endogenous compound which is used to calculate creatinine clearance, a surrogate method of estimating GFR. Creatinine does not bind to plasma proteins, nor is it secreted which makes it ideal for calculating estimated GFR (eGFR).

Secretion is active transport of drug from blood to lumen. Active secretion occurs on the apical and basolateral membranes of the proximal tubule. Reabsorption is the last factor mediating renal elimination occurring throughout the nephron. Active reabsorption occurs for many endogenous molecules such as glucose and amino acids. Due to the nature of membranes, lipophilic molecules are well reabsorbed and polar water-soluble molecules are not. Most of the water filtered at the glomeruli is reabsorbed, which concentrates drug and metabolites in urine.

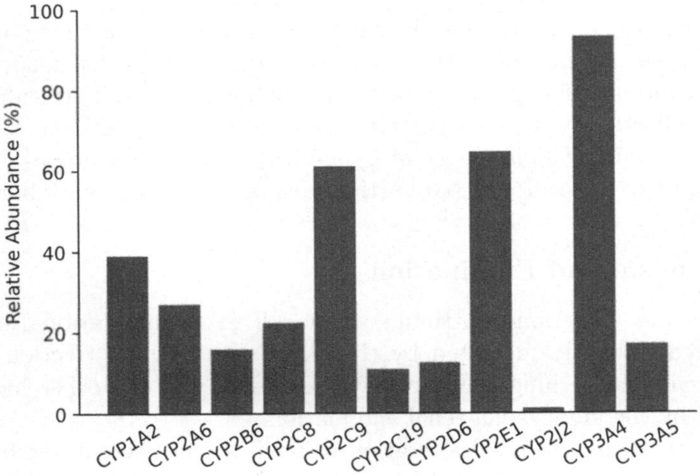


**FIGURE 15.1**
CYP450 abundances in the liver for notable drug metabolizing CYP450s [1]. The bar heights represent enzyme concentrations as a percentage relative to CYP3A4 (100%).

The clearance of a drug can be computed as the summation of clearance of drug by multiple organs. For example, if the liver and kidneys are the only two clearance mechanisms for a drug then:

$$CL = CL_R + CL_H,$$

where $CL$ is the total clearance, $CL_R$ is the renal clearance, and $CL_H$ is the hepatic clearance.

## 15.3 Pharmacokinetic Study Design

To incorporate pharmacokinetics into a study, a method of measuring drug movement is necessary. For these pharmacokinetic studies, the main parameter of interest is drug concentration in the blood. Blood samples are relatively straightforward to collect via venipuncture, though the type of sample collected can depend on characteristics of the drug(s) of interest. Drug concentrations from tissues can be used to provide data that will allow more extensive pharmacokinetic analyses; however, these are not usually readily available and collection can be more difficult, or even impossible. How a sample is collected is important to ensure that concentration measurements will reflect the patient sample and not an artifact of the collection process. Time of last dose and time of sample collection should be recorded for every biological sample collected. Date and time of collection should be included for all collected variables, so that the timing of measures can be correlated to drug concentration data. For example, if a cognitive test is being preformed in a pharmacokinetic study, it is important to record the timing of both the drug concentration measurement and when the cognitive test was performed in order to adequately characterize the concentration-response relationship.

When designing the protocol, the timing of each test should be considered to optimize the effect and control for variability within and across individuals [8]. A goal of pharmacokinetic modeling is to explain variability in pharmacokinetic parameters to determine potentially significant influences of covariates. Potential sources of variability should be recorded to minimize unexplained variability. For instance, if samples are being shipped and are not in control of study personnel, then assurances of stability and recording of storage conditions should be implemented. The use of a central laboratory can allow samples to be batched and analyzed by the same technique on the same day, thereby decreasing both inter-day and inter-run variability of concentration measurements.

Where data points are collected in relation to time after dose can determine how well parameters can be estimated in your analysis. For instance, early time points will capture information concerning absorption, whereas later time points will aid in estimation of volume of distribution. Potential problems with estimation of parameters can be introduced when collection of data is limited. To help alleviate these risks, alternative study designs and data analysis methods have been developed to optimize the information that can be collected from sparse sampling designs (e.g., optimal sampling) [17].

### 15.3.1 Intensive Sampling

The pharmacokinetics of drugs are typically represented by parameters that characterize processes in the body, such as clearance to represent elimination. For the most part these processes are best characterized through intensively sampled protocols that provide the most information at all key times after the administration of a dose. For example, intensive sampling protocols can include up to fifteen time points within a dosing interval. As one would expect, collection of more data points allows for better characterization of the concentration-time profile and increases the chance that particular pharmacokinetic parameters will be estimated adequately. However, intensive designs can be impractical or ethically challenging in certain populations of patients or subjects, such as infants and pregnant women. For example, collecting fifteen blood samples per participant for intensive pharmacokinetic design is not possible in infants.

### 15.3.2 Sparse Sampling

Although having an extensive amount of data collected over a dosing interval gives the most complete characterization of most pharmacokinetic profiles, it is not always practical or possible. In addition, data collected during regular clinical practice is usually very sparse in nature. Samples can also be difficult to collect due to the need for participants to be available for a large amount of time. Sparse sampling involves taking a small number of samples from many individuals as opposed to a large number of samples from few individuals. These sampling methods are especially useful in studies of neonates and children as well as adult patient populations including pregnant patients and older adults. While sparse sampling is useful for population analysis, it can fail to capture pharmacokinetics peculiarities in an individual.

## 15.4 Pharmacokinetic Analysis Methods

Two types of basic analysis methods are usually employed in pharmacokinetic analyses: non-compartmental and compartmental [6, 9].

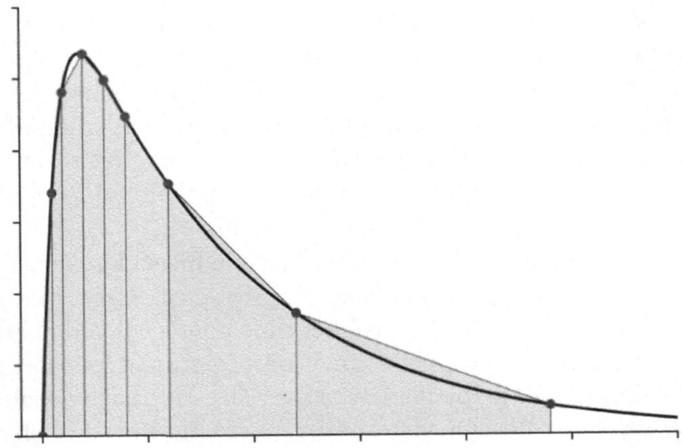

**FIGURE 15.2**
Trapezoid rule for calculate AUC for a pharmacokinetic model. The solid line shows the pharmacokinetic profile, while black circles show sampled concentrations.

### 15.4.1 Non-Compartmental Analysis

Non-compartmental analyses (NCA) are computed directly from concentration-time data and do not depend on a pharmacokinetic model [11]. These analyses are most often used when intensive sampling is available.

For non-compartmental analysis, $AUC$ is the base pharmacokinetic parameter used to calculate other parameters. Trapezoidal approximations for area are calculated from consecutive pairs of measured concentrations (see Figure 15.2). These areas are then summed together to determine the area-under-the-concentration-time-curve ($AUC_0^\infty$) which represents overall drug exposure. As the concentration at the last time point measured in a dosing interval is often not zero, the last trapezoid is extrapolated from the curve based on the last measurable time point to approximate $AUC_{last}^\infty$. Although the example given is for a single dose to illustrate the basic concept, it should be noted that antiseizure medications are typically taken daily to maintain a steady-state concentration. In this case, the $AUC$ is calculated using a single dosing interval for the non-compartmental analysis as drug will always be present in the system. Although there will be a contribution from the previous dose, there will be a similar corresponding contribution of the current peak to the next dose. At steady-dose dosing, assuming equal dosing per interval, the contributions will essentially cancel each other and the $AUC$ of a single dosing interval gives a good approximation of the $AUC$, irrespective of previous and subsequent doses. Calculation of pharmacokinetic parameters for antiseizure medications at steady state dosing use standard pharmacokinetic equations for multiple dosing and can be simplified as:

$$CL = \frac{F \times D \times \tau}{AUC} \text{ or } CL = \frac{F \times D \times \tau}{t \times C_{p,ss}},$$

where $t$ is time of data collection and $\tau$ is dosing interval. The steady-state concentration ($C_{p,ss}$) can be substituted for $AUC$ signifying that the absorption rate will equal the elimination rate. Timing of the blood sample collection can be important to signify if concentrations represent peak versus trough (i.e., the time before the next dose) or single (e.g., medications given for rescue therapy) versus steady-state concentrations. Drugs with short half-lives will have more fluctuation in concentrations than longer half-life drugs. Peak and trough concentrations will be more similar when longer half-life medications are given at similar dosing regimens as doses become more superimposed on each other than medications with shorter half-lives. Therefore, a concentration of a drug with a long half-life will be similar no matter when it is measured; whereas a shorter half-life drug will result in more varying concentrations depending on its proximity in time to when the dose was given.

Half-life is calculated based on the elimination portion of the curve – those points after $C_{max}$ and the absorption phase. In order to estimate half-life with good accuracy, sampling time points need to be spread over 3–5 half-lives to capture a majority of exposure (97%). As some antiseizure medications have long half-lives, it can add significant time to a protocol to include time points that capture information for 5 half-lives. For example, a drug with a half-life of 20 hours will require approximately 5 days of sample collection. Adding multiple days and blood collection time points to a protocol will need to be balanced with any issues such as noncompletion of the protocol and what data is needed to estimate the relevant parameters of interest. One advantage of non-compartmental analysis is that it uses direct calculations and does not require model assumptions as needed in compartmental analysis.

### 15.4.2 Compartmental Modeling

The compartmental approach divides the whole body into one or more compartments by assuming that the drug is uniformly distributed within hypothetical compartments where drug can be sampled. A compartment is not necessarily physiological and can consist of partial, single, or multiple organs. The number of compartments used to describe the drug in the body can depend on how much and what kind of data you have. For instance, the most basic compartment representation of a drug would be intravenous administration of a medication directly into the blood (i.e., central compartment). Each compartment has its own associated volume of distribution, which is typically not a true volume. With the additional consideration of bioavailability, these volumes are often called apparent volume of distribution.

For a one-compartment model (Figure 15.3), the term $A$ signifies the amount, or mass, of drug in the body and can be related to the dose given. As this is an intravenous administration, 100% of the dose would reach the systemic circulation (i.e., blood). The volume of distribution ($V_d$) will usually be determined as liters. Therefore, the concentration can be calculated as $A/V_d$, resulting in mg/L, the units of blood concentration measurements. Rate of elimination ($k_{el}$) is usually a first order process where the rate at any one time is dependent on the concentration of drug present at that instance. For most drugs the active, or parent, total drug (both unbound and bound drug) is measured in the blood as that is a convenient and obtainable biospecimen. For this one-compartment

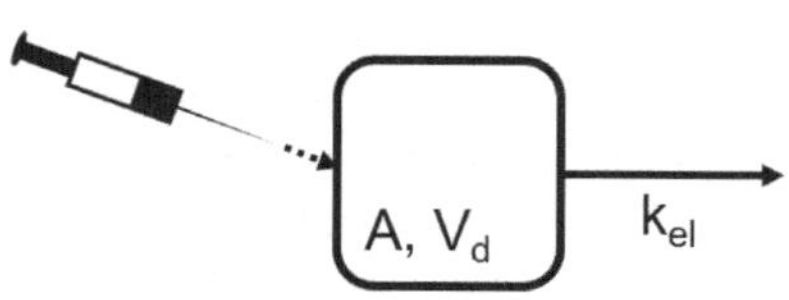


**FIGURE 15.3**
A one-compartment model with intravenous bolus administration. The drug injected into the body is approximated by a single instant, so the only rate constant will be due to exiting the compartment.

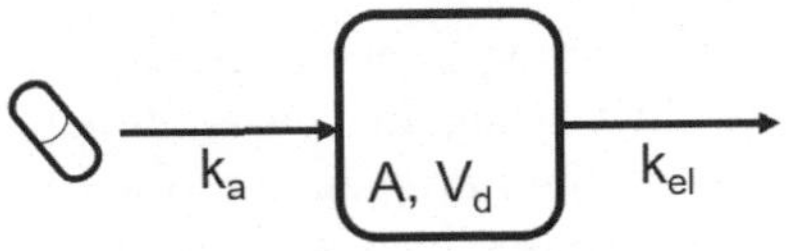


**FIGURE 15.4**
A one-compartment model with oral administration. After a patient takes the drug, it will remain in the gastrointestinal tract and be absorbed over time into the compartment, hence the additional absorption rate constant compared to intravenous administration.

intravenous model, the rate expression derived from mass balances would be represented by the differential equation:

$$\frac{dA}{dt} = -k_{el}A.$$

Therefore, the amount of drug eliminated from the body over a time interval depends on the elimination rate constant and the amount in the body at any given time. Solving this differential equation with initial condition $A_0$ equivalent to the dose, $D$, gives us our typical exponential decay formula:

$$A = D\exp(-k_{el}t).$$

Dividing both sides by $V_d$ and substituting $k_{el} = \frac{CL}{V_d}$, we get the following equation for concentration, $C_p$, as a function of time.

$$C_p = \frac{D}{V_d}exp(-\frac{CL}{V_d}t),$$

which can be linearized by taking the natural log of both sides to:

$$log(C_p) = log(\frac{D}{V_d}) - \frac{CL}{V_d}t$$

In practice, most antiseizure medications are given orally and thus we need to account for absorption from the gut. An absorption rate constant, $k_a$, is added to represent the time of transfer from the gut to the central (i.e., blood) compartment (Figure 15.4).

Similar to the intravenous model, we derive a differential equation from mass balances. In this case, we have an extra term $G$ representing the amount of drug remaining in the gastrointestinal tract during absorption.

$$\frac{dA}{dt} = k_aG - k_{el}A.$$

Compartmental analyses require assumptions to be made and the analyst needs to determine if these assumptions are valid given the data that is available for analysis. Assumptions in a one-compartment model would be that the drug follows linear pharmacokinetics and is instantaneously distributed throughout the body. This assumption allows the whole body to be treated as one unit and is known as the well-mixed assumption. Although few drugs may distribute instantaneously or have minimal distribution, a one-compartment model may be adequate for approximation of pharmacokinetic parameters. There are also situations where data are lacking and there is only enough information for a one-compartment model, even when previous studies show more complex pharmacokinetics.

Another common compartmental model is the two-compartment model (Figure 15.5), which attempts to capture distribution of the drug to peripheral compartments. Usually, clinical data does not contain enough information to describe two-compartments and a one-compartment model would be used. However, intensive sampling protocols may contain

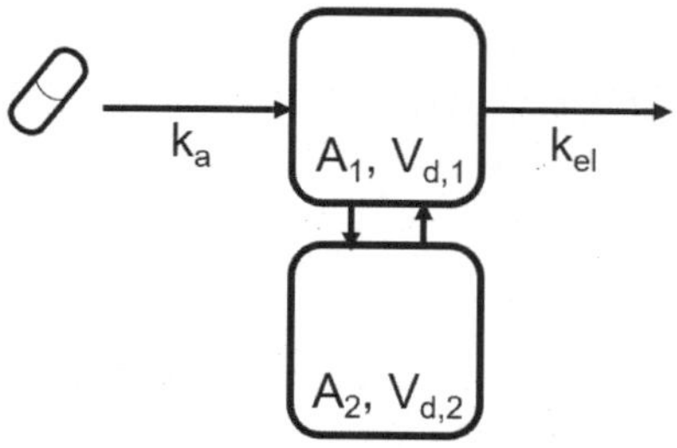


**FIGURE 15.5**
A two-compartment model with oral administration. The difference between a one-compartment and two-compartment is the addition of an extra theoretical area where the drug distributes to. Note that the amount of drug and the volume of distribution are not necessarily the same between the compartments.

enough blood samples collected between the absorption and elimination phases of the curve to justify a two-compartment model. Assumptions for a two-compartment model can include instantaneous mixing within each compartment, the drug travels in and out via the central compartment, and distribution of drug between compartments is slow relative to within compartments. Additional compartments can be added to represent organs or other measured compounds such as metabolites. Furthermore, multiple-compartment models can be modified, such as with partition coefficients, to predict theoretical concentrations such as the amount of drug concentrations in specific tissue. These models form the basis of physiologically based pharmacokinetic (PBPK) modeling. More complex PBPK models can include absorption through different gastrointestinal segments, metabolism and elimination due to different organs.

In summary, whether we use a one- or multiple-compartment model depends on our drug as well as our data as we may not have the data to observe the distribution phase. Typically, we want to choose the simplest model that adequately characterizes the data to avoid model overparameterization.

### 15.4.3 Population Pharmacokinetic Modeling

Population pharmacokinetic (popPK) modeling is a pharmacostatistical approach that seeks to characterize the time course of drug exposure in a patient through estimation of pharmacokinetic parameters and account for variability both within and among individuals [7, 10, 13]. The models use concentration-time data for the drug of interest and can be expanded to include pharmacodynamic modeling (Section 15.5). The popPK approach allows evaluation of the sources for both intrinsic (e.g., renal impairment or genetic polymorphism) and extrinsic (e.g., food effect, measurement error) factors in populations of interest. These models can estimate pharmacokinetic parameters with few sparse samples across multiple individuals as opposed to intensive sampling within each individual. Thus, a population focused analysis is especially useful in special populations such as in pediatrics and older adults where investigators are limited to sparse sampling due to ethical and logistic considerations, and in studies with routine clinical data and samples used in therapeutic drug monitoring.

Nonlinear mixed effects modeling is a common method used to estimate pharmacokinetic parameters in population analyses. This method is particularly well suited for studies with unbalanced designs, which is typical in clinical data where each patient can have a different number of observations. Specialized software such as NONMEM (ICON Development

Solutions, Ellicott City, MD) and Phoenix NLME (Certara, Princeton, NJ) are commonly used, but those will not be described in detail here. NONMEM is especially prevalent and literature often uses terminology that originated from it [4, 5]. Pharmacokinetic nonlinear mixed effects models consist of two parts: a structural model and an error model. The structural models describes the pharmacokinetics of the drug (e.g., one- versus two-compartments) along with covariance structures. To construct the structural model, factors that are known to influence the pharmacokinetics of the compound should first be incorporated into the base compartmental model. In NONMEM, once the base model is determined, covariates can be added to the model and tested for significance based on a decrease in objective function value. Covariates are included/excluded using a forward-backward variable selection procedure. That is, they are added and tested one at a time based on the objective function (forward inclusion). Then, added covariates are removed one at a time (backward exclusion) based on the objective function to confirm significance. More stringent criteria are usually employed with backward exclusion to reduce Type 1 statistical error. An alternative strategy is to begin with all covariates included and then remove them one at a time (backward selection). Attention must be taken to identify collinearities among covariates. Testing is based on a $\chi^2$ distribution to approximate p-values and it is assumed that covariates are nested.

A popPK model uses two levels of error to describe parameter variability. Error placed at the individual level, which captures the variability in predicted drug concentrations, can be described by the following equation:

$$Y_{ij} = f\left(x_{ij}, \Theta_i\right) + \varepsilon_{ij},$$

where $Y_{ij}$ is a particular observation ($j$th observation) in an individual ($i$th individual), and $f$ refers to the structural model function according to independent variables such as time and dose ($x_ij$). $\Theta_i$ represents parameter estimates for subjects and $\varepsilon_{ij}$ represents the residual error (residual unexplained variability) in an individual subject. The first level of the random error is signified by $\varepsilon_{ij} \sim \mathcal{N}(0, \sigma^2)$. $\varepsilon_{ij}$ represents "unexplained" variability including model misspecification, measurement error, analytical error, intraindividual variability, and other unaccounted randomness.

Error is also added at the population level to capture the variability due to variation of structural parameters between the individuals, called BSV for between subject variability, which can generally be written as:

$$\Theta_i = g\left(V_i, \theta\right) + \eta_i,$$

where $g$ is a function defining the covariate model of the parameters with $V_i$ representing the vector of covariates for an individual; $\theta$ is a typical value for a parameter and represents the fixed effects. Error is added through inclusion of $\eta_i \sim \mathcal{N}(0, \Omega)$, where $\Omega = Cov(\theta)$, to represent the between subject variability of the parameters for an individual.

Estimation for nonlinear mixed effects models use maximum likelihood methods. Due to nonlinearity of pharmacokinetic models, a linearization approximation is used to compute the likelihood function. The first order (FO) method approximates the likelihood function based on a first-order Taylor series expansion with both random error models set to zero. The first-order conditional estimation (FOCE) method is an advancement of the FO estimation method, which uses first-order Taylor series expansion about individual's empirical Bayes estimates of interindividual random effect ($\eta_i$) instead of zero. Interaction can also be included with FOCE estimation, resulting in the first-order conditional estimation with interaction method (FOCE-I). The conditional estimation methods require more computational power, though modern advances in computer hardware have led to this to no longer be of significant concern.

Models are only as good as the data used for their development, and care must be taken to ensure that data are representative of the population and the question being asked. For instance, data should be checked for inconsistencies and accuracy. Different approaches can be employed to clean data, with one of the main goals being to determine whether outliers exist. No data should be removed without a plausible reason for removal. Valid reasons for not including a data point can be impossible concentration/dose or known data entry errors. Tracking which sites contributed particular data can aid in detection of site recording inconsistencies with the overall protocol. As drug concentration is the main dependent variable, it is particularly important to consider particular aspects of the protocol, including the analytical assay, in order to decrease residual error. For instance, unusually high concentrations may have been measured after dilution of samples adding another source of possible error to the measurement. Knowledge of the lower end of an assay (e.g., lower limit of quantification, LLOQ) can also be important. It is not unusual for a laboratory to report a value at or below the lower limit of quantification value. Different methods are available for handling of concentrations that are below the limit of quantification as using a value of zero will give an artificially lower than true value and using the limit of quantification of the assay will be artificially higher value. An assay with a high lower limit of quantification relative to values expected from study design can also introduce problems. For example, if the values over the dosing interval are much higher with few values at the lower limit of quantification then the overall $AUC$ will not be affected as much compared to dosing intervals with a low $C_{max}$ and many observations below the lower limit of quantification. Even when data is collected perfectly, there can be hidden correlation due to the population. For example, therapeutic drug monitoring is common with antiseizure medications and involves adjustment of doses to achieve desired concentrations. This inherently correlates clearance and dose, so dose should not be used as a covariate [2]. Therefore, population pharmacokinetic analysis within this patient population can show pharmacokinetic nonlinearity with clearance, even if the medication follows linear pharmacokinetics in actuality.

### 15.4.4 Model Evaluation

Once models are developed, they must be evaluated to determine the robustness of the model and its ability to provide relevant and accurate estimates of parameters [15]. Several methods are used including goodness-of-fit plots. Goodness-of-fit plots such as population predicted concentrations versus observed concentrations, individual predicted concentrations versus observed concentrations, and residual plots are used for model diagnostics. One example of an evaluation plot is the visual predictive check (VPC), which typically involves plotting of the original dataset with the population model and confidence intervals [14]. Predicted concentrations of a VPC can be normalized to obtain the prediction-corrected visual predictive check (pcVPC). These visual evaluations are the most standard method for model evaluation. Model evaluation can also be performed using bootstrapping to calculate nonparametric parameter precision. Due to the complexity of nonlinear models, bootstrapping is a common way to obtain confidence and prediction intervals.

## 15.5 Pharmacodynamics

We are often interested in the response or outcome to drug exposure. While pharmacokinetic modeling connects dose to concentrations, pharmacodynamic modeling

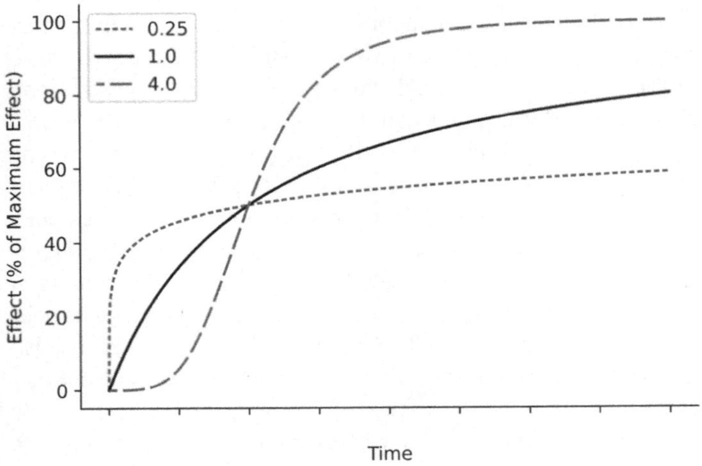


**FIGURE 15.6**
Illustration of how the effect ($y$-axis) as a percentage of maximum effect ($E_{max}$) varies with different values of $\gamma$ (lines). Note that when $\gamma = 1$, we have the Michaelis-Menton model.

connects concentration to outcomes. Pharmacodynamic (PD) models vary depending on the application. Models can include characterization of variables such as enzyme kinetics or seizure frequency. The most common pharmacodynamic model is the sigmoidal $E_{max}$ model, which is based on the Hill function and is represented by following equation:

$$E = E_0 + \frac{E_{max} \times [C]^\gamma}{[EC_{50}]^\gamma + [C]^\gamma},$$

where $E$ is the effect, $E_0$ and $E_{max}$ are the minimal and maximal effects respectively, $C$ is the drug concentration, $EC_{50}$ is the concentration at which the effect is at 50%, and $\gamma$ is a coefficient that defines the shape of the curve, also known as the Hill coefficient. A specific case of the $E_{max}$ model appears when $\gamma = 1$ as seen in the following equation:

$$v = \frac{V_{max} \times [C]}{K_M + [C]},$$

where $v$ is the velocity, $V_{max}$ is the maximal velocity, and $K_M$ is the Michaelis constant. This equation is the Michaelis-Menton equation, which can be used for pharmacodynamic modeling when appropriate.

In Figure 15.6, we can see how the $E_{max}$ model plateaus, which reflects how pharmacodynamic processes can be saturable, leading to diminishing returns as concentrations increase. The nonlinear features of the $E_{max}$ model increase the complexity when balancing pharmacological and toxicological effects, which can also be modeled with pharmacodynamic models such as $E_{max}$.

Other common models include, but are not limited to, threshold and linear models. For threshold models, the drug is assumed to take effect when the systemic concentration reaches a certain threshold. Linear models assume systemic concentration is directly proportional with effect. Pharmacodynamic models can be much more varied as they typically depend on the pharmacological mechanism. Pharmacodynamic models can also be based on physiology, similar to physiologically based pharmacokinetic models. These include quantitative systems pharmacology (QSP) models, which use systems biology to build interactions between the drug and the body. We can combine pharmacokinetic and pharmacodynamic models, allowing us to determine response to a drug after dosing. Linking pharmacokinetics and pharmacodynamics can be done directly using concentration. This assumes no time delay and response occurs instantly with variations in concentration. Though this can lead to an adequate model, sometimes we will see a delay between concentration and response. This can be accounted for with the addition of a pharmacodynamic compartment that holds an insignificant volume. By adjusting the rate between the pharmacokinetic compartment and pharmacodynamic compartment, a time delay for response can be incorporated into the model. These pharmacokinetic-pharmacodynamic (PKPD) [18] models can be developed sequentially where the pharmacokinetic parameters are estimated first and then pharmacodynamic measures, or simultaneously where both are modeled together. The sequential approach is typically less computationally expensive as the pharmacokinetic model and pharmacodynamic models are developed separately. This method comes with the assumption that the pharmacokinetic and pharmacodynamic models are independent of each other. On the other hand, the simultaneous PKPD model treats the pharmacokinetic and pharmacodynamic models as one unit with potential interaction between the two. While this model does not necessarily require drug concentration data, it is still beneficial to obtain drug concentrations to boost the robustness of the model.

## 15.6 Case Study: Population Pharmacokinetic Model Simulation

In this section, we present a popPK model which is typically used to quantify pharmacokinetic parameters, variability, and the effect of various covariates on drug disposition. The popPK model presented here is for a hypothetical drug with a few covariate effects. The model is developed for the `R` package `mrgsolve` [3]—the associated model code and simulation specifics are also presented here.

### 15.6.1 Model Specifications

In this exercise, a simulation will be performed for a hypothetical drug with known pharmacokinetic parameters in younger adults and covariate effects to illustrate how a popPK model works. The pharmacokinetic parameters of this drug are presented in Table 15.2.

This drug follows first order absorption, mono-exponential (one-compartment) elimination behavior. Assume that the drug is given orally at 500 mg twice a day. The oral bioavailability is 90%, with an apparent volume of distribution ($V/F$) of 90 L and a rapid apparent clearance ($CL/F$) of 2.15 L/hr. Both apparent volume and clearance are hypothesized to have a 30% between subject variability. In addition, there are two covariate effects that will be identified. The first covariate is sex on apparent volume of distribution. Males have 1.45-times higher $V/F$ compared to females. Second, a single nucleotide polymorphism (SNP) in a metabolic enzyme gene increases $CL/F$ by 1.65-fold compared to wild type.

The covariate effects are modeled using a power function as follows:

$$TV\theta_i = TV\theta \times \theta COV^{\ COV},$$

**TABLE 15.2**
Model parameters.

| Parameter (Unit) | Value | Between-subject Variability (%) |
|---|---|---|
| **Preconception Parameters** | | |
| $F$: Oral Bioavailability (%) | 90 | - |
| $k_a$: Absorption Rate Constant ($h^{-1}$) | 3.17 | - |
| $V/F$: Apparent Volume of Distribution (L) | 90 | 30 |
| $CL/F$: Apparent Clearance (L/hr) | 2.15 | 30 |
| **Covariate Effects** | | |
| Male Sex on $V/F$ | 1.45 | - |
| SNP on $CL/F$ | 1.65 | - |
| Residual Unexplained Variability (%) | 15 | |

where $TV\theta_i$ is the typical parameter estimate for the $i$th individual, $TV\theta$ is the typical value of the parameter in the population, $\theta COV$ is the parameter for effect of covariate on the pharmacokinetic parameter and $COV$ is an indicator variable (0 or 1).

The parameters are modeled log-normally as follows:

$$\theta_i = TV\theta_i \times e^{-\eta^{\theta i}},$$

where $\theta_i$ is the parameter estimate for the $i$th individual, $TV\theta_i$ is the parameter estimate for the $i$th individual, $\eta_i^\theta \sim \mathcal{N}(0, \Omega)$ are individual-specific random effects for the $i$th individual.

Lastly, the residual variability is modeled as a proportional error model as follows:

$$C_{ij} = \hat{C}_{ij} \times (1 + \varepsilon_{ij,PROP}),$$

where $C_{ij}$ is the $j$th observed concentration of the $i$th individual, $\hat{C}_{ij}$ is the $j$th model predicted concentration based on the individual parameters for $i$th individual. $\varepsilon_{ij,PROP} \sim \mathcal{N}(0, \sigma^2)$ is the proportional error, for the $j$th measurement in the $i$ individual.

These parameters are specified in a .cpp file, as shown below. While this is written in the C language, significant knowledge of C is not required. Note that, in C, "//" indicates a comment. This model specification file for `mrgsolve` is similar to that of NONMEM. The model file is split into blocks which each specify specific components. Other blocks may be specified for different analyses, such as parameter estimation. As there are software-specific model files, it is best to refer to the software documentation and tutorials for detailed information. Some information to help parse this specific model file is provided below and in comments.

- $PROB is the problem statement and the text following is a free text comment.
- $PARAM is the parameter specification for known parameters. These are typically constants or individual specific values that are known beforehand.
- $CMT specifies the compartment variables; here, DEPOT is a depot compartment for absorption and CENT is the central compartment for the one compartment model. These also specify what the program is looking for.
- $MAIN is where the relationship between the models and parameters is specified for population pharmacokinetic analysis.

- $THETA specify the parameter means, for this case volume and clearance for a one compartment model. These are estimated parameters and subject to variability. These can be matched with the equations mentioned previously in this section.
- $OMEGA, $SIGMA specify between-subject variability and within-subject random effects, respectively. These represent the covariance matrices, and can be specified as such. When covariance is zero, the diagonal variances can be specified alone, as with this case.
- $ODE specifices the differential equations that model the pharmacokinetics (see Section 15.4.2).

```
1cmt_sex_SNP.cpp

$PROB
1 cmt model - Simulation with sex on volume, genetics on clearance

$PARAM
KA = 3.17, //First order rate of absorption
SEX = 0, //0 = Female; 1 = Male
SNP = 0, //0 = Wild Type; 1 = Mutated
SEX_EFF = 1.45, //Effect of male sex on volume
SNP_EFF = 1.75 //Effect of SNP on clearance

$CMT DEPOT CENT //One compartment model plus depot for oral dosing

$GLOBAL
#define Cp (CENT/V) //Define central concentration (ug/mL)

$MAIN
F_DEPOT = 0.9; //Oral bioavailability

double TVV = THETA1 * pow(SEX_EFF,SEX); //Typical volume
double TVCL = THETA2 * pow(SNP_EFF,SNP) ; //Typical clearance

double V = TVV*exp(ETA(1)); //Population volume
double CL = TVCL*exp(ETA(2)); //Population clearance

$THETA
90 //Volume
2.15 //Clearance

$OMEGA
0.09 //BSV on V
0.09 //BSV on CL

$SIGMA
0.0225

$ODE
dxdt_DEPOT = -KA*DEPOT; //Absorption compartment
dxdt_CENT = KA*DEPOT - CL*Cp; //Central compartment

$CAPTURE
Cp, V, CL, SEX, SNP //Capture variables you want to report
```

### 15.6.2 Simulation Specifications and Results

The population simulation here assumes a sample size of 500 individuals, all receiving a 500 mg twice a day dosing regimen a steady state. In this sample size, assume a 40% male demographic and SNP allelic frequency of 20%. A 24-hour steady-state time and concentration profile is simulated with the R code provided.

```
1cmt simulations.R

# Load required libraries ====
library(mrgsolve)
library(dplyr)
library(ggplot2)
library(gridExtra)

# Simulation ====
set.seed(15)

# Compile .cpp model with mrgsolve
modpop2 <- mread("1cmt_sex_SNP.cpp")

# Generate input data file for simulation
# Simulation of 500 individuals,
#   40% males and 20% population having the SNP mutation
input_data <- data.frame(ID=c(1:500), SEX = rbinom(500,1,0.4), SNP = rbinom
   (500,1,0.2))

#Assume a dosing regimen of 500 mg given twice a day at steady state
dosing <- ev(amt=500,ss=1,ii=12, addl=1)

# Generate simulation
out <- modpop2 %>%
  Req(Cp,V,CL,SEX,SNP)%>% #Request variables in simulation output
  obsonly() %>%
  idata_set(input_data)%>%
  mrgsim(events=dosing,end=24,delta=1,obsonly=TRUE) %>%
  as.data.frame()

# Add names to the indicator covariate variables
sim.out <- out %>%
  mutate(SEX_Name = if_else(SEX ==0,"FEMALE","MALE"), SNP_Name = if_else(SNP
  ==0,"WILD TYPE","MUTATED"))

# Generate summary data (used for plots)
sim.summ_sex <- sim.out %>%
  group_by(SEX_Name,time) %>%
  summarise(LOW_CI = quantile(Cp,0.05),
            HI_CI = quantile(Cp,0.95))

sim.summ_snp <- sim.out %>%
  group_by(SNP_Name,time) %>%
  summarise(LOW_CI = quantile(Cp,0.05),
            HI_CI = quantile(Cp,0.95))

sim.param <- sim.out %>%
  distinct(ID,.keep_all = T)
```

Let us look at the simulation results. Figure 15.7 presents the median concentrations and 90% CIs for the wild type and the SNP groups. This illustration represents how a 65% higher clearance for the SNP ("mutated") group results in a nearly 1-fold lower steady-state concentration, which could have severe repercussions clinically depending on the outcomes and side effect profile of the drug. The faster clearance and lower concentrations may lead to

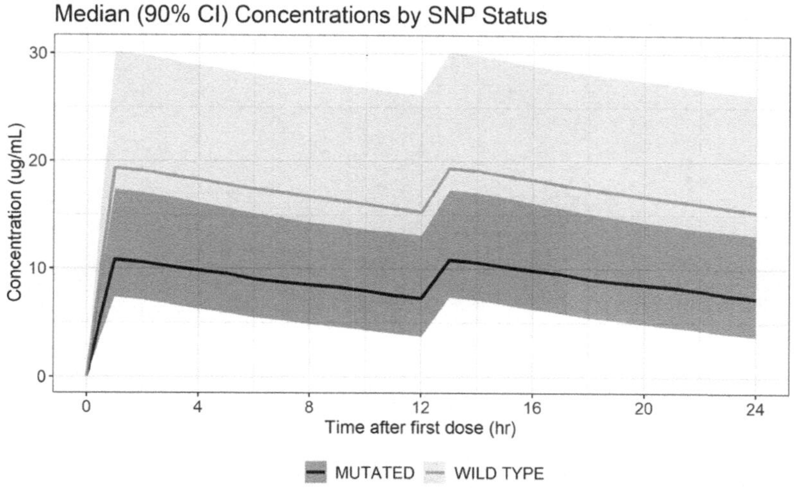


**FIGURE 15.7**
Median concentrations and 90% confidence intervals for the wild type and SNP groups.

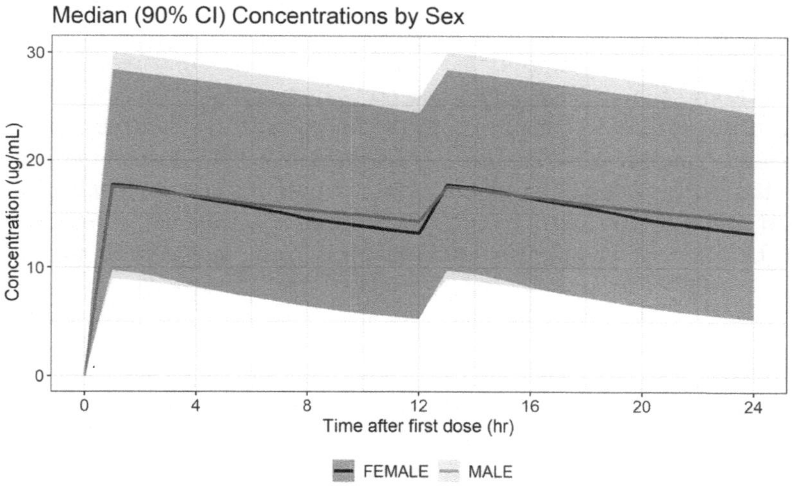


**FIGURE 15.8**
Median concentrations and 90% confidence intervals for the two sexes.

subtherapeutic concentrations for the individuals with the SNP necessitating dose changes for clinical efficacy.

Figure 15.8 presents the median concentrations and 90% CIs for the two sexes. In contrast to clearance, though males have 45% higher volume of distribution, there is minimal difference in concentrations compared to females at steady-state. The higher volume would not require any changes to dosing.

The differences in parameters by the covariates can be presented with the use of boxplots. It is easy to see the effect of sex on volume and SNP on clearance in Figure 15.9. However, the clinical implication of these statistically significant covariate effects is dependent on how they affect steady-state concentrations and clinical outcomes in relation to the therapeutic window for an individual.

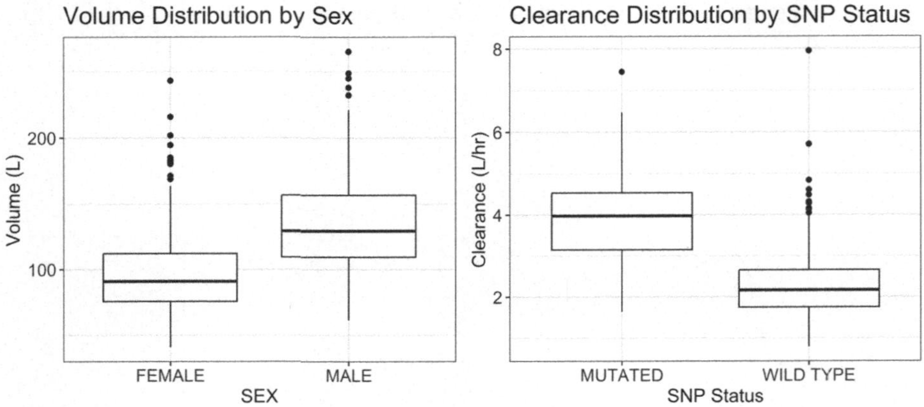


**FIGURE 15.9**
Boxplots showing the effect of sex on volume and SNP on clearance.

## 15.7 Summary

Measurement of drug concentrations have enabled clinicians and researchers to see more of the drug in body. How the drug and the body interact is essential for individuals with epilepsy that utilize antiseizure medications to manage seizures. Knowledge of physiological mechanisms and compartmentalization of drugs help in the development of meaningful pharmacostatistical models that can be useful for populations and individuals. Here, we have reviewed common pharmacokinetic and pharmacodynamic models and analyses, which provide insight into the connection between antiseizure medication dosage and seizure control.

## Bibliography

[1] Brahim Achour, Jill Barber, and Amin Rostami-Hodjegan. Expression of hepatic drug-metabolizing cytochrome p450 enzymes and their intercorrelations: A meta-analysis. *Drug Metabolism and Disposition*, 42(8):1349–1356, 2014.

[2] Jae Eun Ahn, Angela K. Birnbaum, and Richard C. Brundage. Inherent correlation between dose and clearance in therapeutic drug monitoring settings: Possible misinterpretation in population pharmacokinetic analyses. *Journal of Pharmacokinetics and Pharmacodynamics*, 32(5-6):703–718, 2005.

[3] Kyle T. Baron. *mrgsolve: Simulate from ODE-Based Models*, 2023. R package version 1.0.9.

[4] Robert J. Bauer. NONMEM tutorial part I: Description of commands and options, with simple examples of population analysis. *CPT: Pharmacometrics and Systems Pharmacology*, 8(8):525–537, 2019.

[5] Robert J. Bauer. NONMEM tutorial part II: Estimation methods and advanced examples. *CPT: Pharmacometrics and Systems Pharmacology*, 8(8):538–556, 2019.

[6] Peter L. Bonate. *Pharmacokinetic and Pharmacodynamic Modeling and Simulation*. Springer, second edition, 2011.

[7] W Byon, MK Smith, P Chan, MA Tortorici, S Riley, H Dai, J Dong, A Ruiz-Garcia, K Sweeney, and C Cronenberger. Establishing best practices and guidance in population modeling: An experience with an internal population pharmacokinetic analysis guidance. *CPT: Pharmacometrics and Systems Pharmacology*, 2(7):e51, 2013.

[8] Ann-Cathrine Dalgård Dunvald, Ditte Bork Iversen, Andreas Ludvig Ohm Svendsen, Katrine Agergaard, Ida Berglund Kuhlmann, Christina Mortensen, Nanna Elman Andersen, Erkka Järvinen, and Tore Bjerregaard Stage Tutorial: Statistical analysis and reporting of clinical pharmacokinetic studies. *Clinical and Translational Science*, 15(8):1856–1866, 2022.

[9] Ene I. Ette and Paul J. Williams, editors. *Pharmacometrics: The Science of Quantitative Pharmacology*. John Wiley & Sons, 2007.

[10] Food and Drug Administration. Population pharmacokinetics. *Guidance for Industry*, 2022.

[11] Johan Gabrielsson and Daniel Weiner. Non-compartmental analysis. *Methods in Molecular Biology*, 929:377–389, 2012.

[12] Milo Gibaldi and Donald Perrier. *Pharmacokinetics*. Informa Healthcare, second edition, 1982.

[13] Tony K. L. Kiang, Catherine M. T. Sherwin, Michael G. Spigarelli, and Mary H. H. Ensom. Fundamentals of population pharmacokinetic modelling: Modelling and software. *Clinical Pharmacokinetics*, 51(9):573–590, 2012.

[14] Anne Kümmel, Peter L Bonate, Jasper Dingemanse, and Andreas Krause. Confidence and prediction intervals for pharmacometric models. *CPT: Pharmacometrics and Systems Pharmacology*, 7(6):360–373, 2018.

[15] THT Nguyen, M Mouksassi, N Holford, N Al-Huniti, I Freedman, AC Hooker, J John, MO Karlsson, DR Mould, JJ Perez Ruixo, EL Plan, R Savic, JGC van Hassalt, B Weber, C Zhou, E Comets, and F Mentré. Model evaluation of continuous data pharamcometric models: Metrics and graphics. *CPT: Pharmacometrics and Systems Pharmacology*, 6(2):87–109, 2017.

[16] Malcolm Rowland and Thomas N. Tozer. *Clinical Pharmacokinetics and Pharmacodynamics: Concepts and Applications*. Lippincott, William & Wilkins, fourth edition, 2010.

[17] C Stockmann, JS Barrett, JK Roberts, and CMT Sherwin. Use of modeling and simulation in the design and conduct of pediatric clinical trials and the optimization of individualized dosing regimens. *CPT: Pharmacometrics and Systems Pharmacology*, 4(11):630–640, 2015.

[18] Huixi Zou, Parikshit Banerjee, Sharon Shui Yee Leung, and Xiaoyu Yan. Application of pharmacokinetic-pharmacodynamic modeling in drug delivery: Development and challenges. *Frontiers in Pharmacology*, 11:997, 2020.

# 16

# *Randomized Clinical Trial Analysis*

**Joseph E. Sullivan**

*Department of Neurology, University of California, San Francisco (USA)*

**Michael Lock**

*UCB Biosciences, Inc. (USA)*

## CONTENTS



The development of anti-seizure medications for use in the clinical environment requires a rigorous process to demonstrate efficacy in the targeted patient population. For patients with epilepsy, this has historically been done with a randomized, double-blind, placebo-controlled trial design, where the new treatment of interest is added to standard baseline therapy, and overall reduction in seizures compared to placebo is analyzed at the end of a pre-defined treatment period. In this chapter, we discuss many of the statistical challenges that should be considered when designing a clinical trial for patients with epilepsy, with illustrative examples provided in the R programming language. These include controlling Type 1 error rates when there are multiple clinical endpoints of interest, and determining the length of the baseline period needed to obtain a reliable estimate of seizure reduction. We also present several methods for analyzing highly skewed seizure reduction data, illustrated with data from clinical trial of patients with Dravet syndrome. Finally, we discuss a time-to-event clinical trial design that may allow for shortened placebo exposures – an important safety consideration to minimize the overall risk of ongoing seizures when receiving placebo as part of a clinical trial.

DOI: 10.1201/9781003254515-16

## 16.1 Epilepsy Clinical Trials

Clinical trials in epilepsy have largely focused on studying the efficacy, safety and tolerability of new investigational compounds that satisfy both regulatory requirements for approval but also meet the needs of clinicians who will be prescribing these new medications in everyday practice. The gold-standard study design that has been utilized for the last two decades has been a double blind, randomized, placebo-controlled trial where the new compound is added as adjunctive therapy to a stable baseline of one or more anti-seizure medications (ASMs). This study design allows patients to receive standard treatment while also having the opportunity to add a novel therapy with the goal of improved seizure control. There are several limitations to this type of study design, particularly with a disorder such as epilepsy, where seizure frequency is highly variable from patient to patient and some seizure types may be difficult to count. For these reasons, some seizure types are not included in the determination of the primary endpoint. Furthermore, due to the non-normal distribution of seizure frequency across patients, special statistical considerations need to be employed. In epilepsy trials there is also a higher risk of sudden unexpected death in epilepsy patients (SUDEP) in placebo recipients than in patients receiving the novel therapy [11] Philippe Ryvlin, et al, 2011. This raises additional ethical and statistical questions about the standard RCT design. In this chapter, we review critical statistical considerations when designing these types of trials. We also explore an alternative study design that may offer some advantages in specific epilepsy diagnoses where seizure frequency is very high, and, therefore, there is a strong interest in minimizing the duration of placebo exposure. We also review the importance of secondary outcomes that are increasingly more focused on patient-oriented outcomes and how these can best be measured.

### 16.1.1 Patient Demographics

Epilepsy is a common condition affecting over 3 million persons in the United States. Approximately 70% of these patients will become seizure free with currently available ASMs [6] Linda Kalilani, et al, 2018. It would be unwise and perhaps unethical to enroll patients in trials of new medications until they have first been treated with other, approved ASMs. This would usually exclude enrolling patients with newly diagnosed epilepsy. Instead, trials of new epilepsy drugs are studied as adjunctive therapy and include patients who are resistant to current ASMs yet continue to have seizures on a monthly basis.

Determining the number of seizures that are necessary for patient inclusion also has practical considerations especially since insufficient seizure frequency has been identified as potentially the most common reason for exclusion from medication-resistant epilepsy trials [8], Wesley T. Kerr, Hai Chen, et al, 2023. On one hand, a patient who has one seizure per month is considered to have drug-resistant epilepsy. However, in order to detect a statistically significant improvement in seizures with a novel therapy, a longer maintenance/observation phase would be necessary compared to a patient who is having 4 or more seizures per month. The longer maintenance/observation period would expose placebo patients to a longer period of time, when changes to their treatment regimen are not allowed. It is these competing interests of meeting a predetermined primary endpoint while simultaneously minimizing placebo exposure that are important practical and clinical factors that must be considered when deciding on inclusion criteria and overall study duration in clinical trial trial design.

### 16.1.2 General Considerations for Epilepsy Clinical Trials

As mentioned above, the gold standard in Phase 3 epilepsy trials has been the randomized, double-blind, placebo-controlled clinical trial. As such, the basic design of a Phase 3 trial in epilepsy patients is similar to other confirmatory trials. Nevertheless, it is worth a short discussion of each of the descriptors of the clinical trial – randomized, double-blind, and placebo-controlled – in the context of a new epilepsy treatment.

- *Randomized*: One aspect of clinical trial design is choosing the randomization ratio, i.e., the proportion of patients who are randomly assigned the active treatment compared to the proportion assigned placebo. While not a requirement, regulators and investigators often prefer to assign an equal number of patients to each group. This avoids the presumption that patients assigned treatment will necessarily benefit more than placebo recipients. In addition, equal-sized treatment groups make it easier to compare the groups on the rate of adverse events and other safety signals.

- *Double-blind*: Maintaining blinding over the course of a clinical trial requires a sizeable amount of logistical effort. For a new drug, the placebo needs to match the novel drug in appearance and route of administration. Oral treatments must also match in taste and smell. Unblinded personnel must be available throughout the trial to ensure that the correct treatment or placebo is delivered to each patient, to review and deliver unblinded data to the safety monitoring committee, and to break the blind if necessary for patient safety. Other treatments such as devices or surgical interventions are subject to similar blinding requirements.

- *Placebo-controlled*: As noted above, the term "placebo-controlled" in an epilepsy trial means adding either a placebo or a novel treatment to each patient's stable baseline of one or more ASMs. This ensures that all patients in the trial receive standard treatment while simultaneously evaluating whether the new treatment improves seizure control. Patients should be encouraged to maintain the baseline regimen throughout the trial, since any changes would make it more difficult to ascribe improvement or worsening to the novel treatment.

### 16.1.3 Multiple Comparisons

This chapter is focused mostly on clinical trials where the primary endpoint is a reduction in seizures. Of course, investigators are rarely interested in only a single endpoint and typically have an extensive list of other endpoints, meaningful to both investigators and patients, worth examining. For example, in a disorder with infrequent seizures, an investigator may believe that a significant improvement in a quality-of-life endpoint such as Clinical Global Improvement (CGI) is as important or perhaps even more important than seizure reduction. Patients and caregivers can also play an important role in identifying which endpoints matter the most to them.

Dealing with more than one important endpoint brings up the well-known problems inherent to multiple comparisons (Chapter 4). These problems are far from insurmountable, but their solutions require careful attention to the objectives of the trial. In the situation above, the investigator may consider that the new treatment is useful if it can satisfy either endpoint; i.e., the trial would be a success if the patients experienced either a significant reduction in seizure frequency or a significant improvement in CGI score. Testing both endpoints at the $\alpha = 0.05$ level leads to an increase in the probability of a Type 1 error, or the probability of concluding that a difference is significant when it occurred merely by chance. A simple technique for avoiding an increase in Type 1 error is to "split the alpha" across the two comparisons, also known as the Bonferroni correction. Specifically, treatment would be compared to placebo on the reduction in seizures at the $\alpha = 0.025$ level and independently on the change in CGI at the $\alpha = 0.025$ level. If either comparison is significant, then the new treatment can be claimed to be successful at the overall $\alpha = 0.05$ level.

While simple to implement, splitting $\alpha$ makes it harder to attain significance within each of the multiple comparisons. Thus, sample size should be increased to maintain overall power. Adding more comparisons would require splitting the overall $\alpha$ level of 0.05 into smaller and smaller portions, leading to either less overall power or a greater increase in sample size. Thus, other approaches are often used for larger numbers of comparisons.

Consider a trial where there are two treatment dose levels and, again, two important endpoints – seizure reduction and improvement in CGI. This setup yields four comparisons of treatment to placebo. If the investigator is willing to rank each of the comparisons in order of importance, then a "gatekeeper" strategy can be implemented to maintain Type 1 error. For example, say the investigator decides that the following list of endpoints and comparisons corresponds to the most important objectives of the trial:

1. Reduction in seizures: High dose treatment vs. placebo
2. Improvement in CGI: High dose treatment vs. placebo
3. Reduction in seizures: Low dose treatment vs. placebo
4. Improvement in CGI: Low dose treatment vs. placebo

The gatekeeper strategy performs comparisons in the order specified in the list above. If the high dose of treatment is superior to placebo at the $\alpha = 0.05$ level, then that comparison is considered statistically significant and testing moves on to the next comparison on the list. If any comparison in the list is not significant at the $\alpha = 0.05$ level, then that comparison, and any other comparison lower on the list, are considered not statistically significant.

The gatekeeper is an excellent approach for trials where it is difficult to increase sample size to accommodate multiple comparisons, but it does require a hierarchy of endpoints to be specified in advance. Other, more general approaches, such as the Simes method, allow more flexibility in assessing multiple comparisons [12] R.J. Simes, et al, 1996. In general, such methods attempt to maximize the number of comparisons that can be considered significant by ranking them according to $p$-value. Comparisons with the lowest $p$-values are the most likely to be considered significant. See [5] for more details on theory and implementation.

## 16.2 Significance and Magnitude of Treatment Effects

The remainder of this chapter will reference a recently completed Phase 3 randomized, double-blind, placebo-controlled trial in a cohort of children with Dravet syndrome to illustrate many of the statistical and methodologic issues that should be considered when designing a study of a new ASM that balances patient safety and reaching the primary outcome measure for the purposes of regulatory approval and later use in clinics [9] Lieven Lagae, et al, 2019.

### 16.2.1 Analysis Challenges

One of the biggest challenges in analyzing clinical trial seizure data is handling the variability among patients in the number of seizures they experience. This number is usually expressed as a frequency, for example the number of seizures per month, where a month is defined as 28 days. Depending on the disorder under study, seizure frequencies could range from just a few per month in some patients up to several hundred per month in others. Statistical methods used to assess the efficacy of a new treatment need to take into account the background seizure frequency of the patients involved to avoid having the results dominated by the subjects with the most seizures. This, in turn, requires having a good estimate of a patient's background seizure frequency. While such an estimate could be obtained from the patients themselves or from their caregivers, many of whom keep personal seizure diaries, the most rigorous approach entails measuring seizure frequency over the course of a baseline period prior to the first administration of study treatment in the trial. The baseline period must be long enough to obtain a reasonably solid estimate of the patient's background seizure frequency. Determining the length of the period is discussed further in Section 16.3. Using seizure data collected in a diary over the course of the baseline period, a background or baseline seizure frequency, $SF^B$, can be readily calculated.

Following the baseline period, patients enter a blinded treatment period, where subjects receive either an active treatment or a matching placebo, typically in addition to standard of care therapy. Again, using a seizure diary, the seizure frequency per 28 days during the treatment period, $SF^T$, is calculated. Comparing the seizure frequency during treatment to the frequency during baseline affords a test of the efficacy of the new treatment.

It is helpful to use real world data from the Dravet syndrome trial mentioned above to illustrate seizure frequency and methods for analysis. This was a randomized, double-blind, placebo-controlled clinical trial with the monthly frequency of convulsive seizures as the primary endpoint. It entailed a 6-week observation period to establish baseline monthly (28 days) convulsive seizure frequency followed by a 14-week treatment period where patients were randomly assigned in a 1:1:1 ratio to placebo or fenfluramine 0.2 or 0.7 mg/kg/day (maximun daily dose 26 mg) added to existing ASMs. (Patients taking concomitant stiripentol were excluded.) For simplicity, we consider only the placebo (n=40) and higher dose fenfluramine (n=40) groups here.

Figure 16.1 shows histograms of convulsive seizure frequency of fenfluramine-treated subjects during the baseline and treatment periods of the trial. Both histograms depict high variability and highly skewed distributions with most patients having fewer than 30 convulsive seizures per month but a handful experiencing many more. The skewness is more pronounced during the treatment period shown in the histogram at right due to the efficacy of treatment with fenfluramine: twice as many patients experienced 10 or fewer seizures per month during treatment than during baseline. High variability and skewness engender analysis challenges; methods to overcome some of the challenges are presented below.

### 16.2.2 Percentage Change from Baseline

A common statistical approach to reducing variability is to adjust for baseline. That is, it is reasonable to posit that patients who have the highest baseline seizure frequencies will likely also have the highest frequency following treatment. Adjusting for baseline takes advantage of that relationship, if present, to yield a statistic with lower variability while often enhancing interpretability. The simplest way to adjust for background seizure frequency is to calculate the arithmetic difference from baseline, $SF^T - SF^B$. A more popular adjustment, though, is the percent change from baseline, $SF^{\Delta\%} = \frac{(SF^T - SF^B)}{SF^B} \times 100$. Other methods for baseline adjustment are discussed later in this section.

One of the main advantages of using the percent change from baseline is that it is familiar and readily interpretable. It has also been used in many epilepsy trials and so affords a means to compare treatment efficacy across numerous trials. However, although

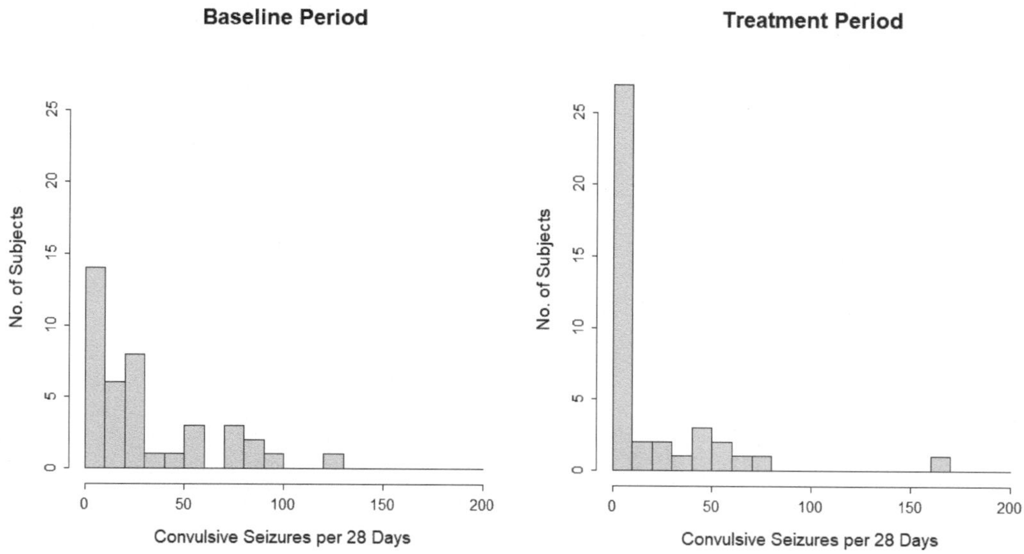


**FIGURE 16.1**
Histograms of convulsive seizure frequency during the baseline (left panel) and treatment (right panel) periods for patients treated with 0.7 mg/kg/day fenfluramine in the Dravet syndrome trial.

percentage change does adjust for baseline differences in seizure frequency across patients, it does so in a rigid manner. For example, it assumes that a decrease of four seizures per month in a patient with a background monthly frequency of 8 seizures per month – i.e., a 50% reduction – is equivalent to a decrease of 40 seizures in a patient with a background frequency of 80. In addition, the distribution of the percent change from baseline creates some difficult challenges for analysis methods. As can be seen in the histogram at left in Figure 16.2, the distribution is highly skewed to the right in the treatment group since most subjects had large reductions in convulsive seizure frequency during the treatment period. The asymmetry of the distribution is inherent to percent change statistics; specifically, any reduction from baseline must be between −100% and 0%. Conversely, increases from baseline can extend well past +100% and could theoretically go to infinity. A final problem with percent change is that it highly dependent on the denominator, the baseline seizure frequency, especially when the denominator is small.

### 16.2.3 Wilcoxon Rank-Sum Test

The skewness of the percent change statistic precludes analysis by standard, normal-based methods like $t$-tests and ANOVA, all of which require at least some degree of symmetry to yield powerful, accurate comparisons. In particular, the median and interquartile range offer more reliable summaries of the percent change from baseline than do the mean and standard deviation, both of which can be inflated greatly by large increases in seizure frequency in only a small number of patients. The Wilcoxon rank-sum test affords an excellent, robust alternative to the $t$-test for comparing the change from baseline measured in the treatment and placebo groups. Since the Wilcoxon test relies on ranks, it doesn't matter whether the most extreme increase in seizure frequency is 500% or 1000%. The biggest increase in a sample of $N$ data points is simply assigned the rank of $N$.

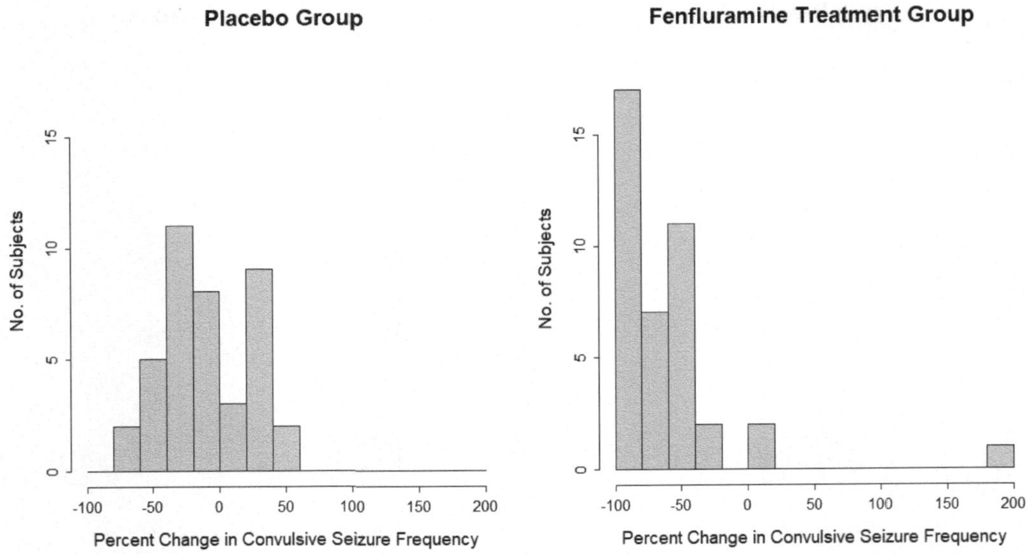


**FIGURE 16.2**
Histograms of the percent change from baseline in convulsive seizure frequency per 28 days for the placebo (left panel) and treatment (right panel) groups in the Dravet syndrome trial.

Below is some sample `R` code that uses a Wilcoxon rank-sum test to compare the fenfluramine treatment group to the placebo group in the Dravet syndrome trial introduced earlier. The data frame `Szr.Data` includes a column, `SF.PChg`, that contains the percentage change between the treatment and baseline periods in monthly convulsive seizure frequency for each of the 80 patients in the trial. The variable `Grp` indicates which treatment group each subject is in. To implement the Wilcoxon test, we run:

```
wilcox.test(SF.PChg ~ Grp, data = Szr.Data)
```

Here is the output from the call:

```
 Wilcoxon rank sum test with continuity correction

data:  SF.PChg by Grp
W = 186, p-value = 3.558e-09
alternative hypothesis: true location shift is not equal to 0
```

$W$ is the Wilcoxon test statistic, which is not particularly useful, at least in this situation. The $p$-value though is much less than 0.0001, indicating a statistically significant difference between treatment and placebo.

While the Wilcoxon rank-sum test affords a reliable means to assess the significance of a comparison, it does not yield an estimate of the numerical size of the treatment effect. That is, the Wilcoxon can tell us whether treatment is significantly superior to placebo, but does not provide an interpretable estimate of the size of the treatment's advantage. The treatment estimate could be estimated by simply subtracting the median percent change in the placebo group from the analogous statistic calculated from the treatment group. The bootstrap method can be used to provide a 95% confidence interval for difference in medians. An alternative to calculating the difference between medians is the Hodges-Lehmann (HL) estimator. It estimates the difference between the two groups using ranked data, like the

Wilcoxon test, and also provides a confidence interval for the difference. The HL estimator can be implemented in R by adding a single argument to the call for the Wilcoxon test:

```
wilcox.test(SF.PChg ~ Grp, data = Szr.Data, conf.int = TRUE)
```

This call generates the following output:

```
    Wilcoxon rank sum test with continuity correction

data:  SF.PChg by Grp
W = 186, p-value = 3.558e-09
alternative hypothesis: true location shift is not equal to 0
95 percent confidence interval:
 -71.24753 -41.02023
sample estimates:
difference in location
     -56.90791
```

This means that in the Dravet syndrome trial, the Hodges-Lehmann estimate of the percentage difference in seizure reduction between treatment and placebo is 56.9 percentage points with a 95% confidence interval of $(-71.2, -41.0)$ percentage points. (The HL estimate can also be obtained by calling the R function `HodgesLehmann()`.)

### 16.2.4 Rank ANCOVA

Incorporating explanatory variables such as age or sex into the comparison between treatment and placebo requires a different method than the Wilcoxon test. One such method that maintains much of the advantages of the Wilcoxon test, while allowing for the inclusion of potentially explanatory factors, is a rank-based analysis of covariance, or ANCOVA. ANCOVA and the analysis of variance, ANOVA, are very similar statistical models. The primary difference between the two is that all explanatory factors in an ANOVA must be categorical, like sex, while the ANCOVA can handle a mixture of continuous and categorical factors like age and sex. A rank ANCOVA is identical to an ordinary ANCOVA except that the response variable is the rank of the original data point. The ranked data are then analyzed using the same methods used to analyze an ordinary ANCOVA including testing for the influence of other potentially explanatory factors.

Consider again the example of Dravet syndrome, which may evolve as children grow, leading to the possibility that age could have an impact on treatment efficacy. Assume that, like above, the clinical trial has a single active treatment group comprised of $n_1$ patients and a placebo group comprised of $n_2$ patients, all of whom have been diagnosed with Dravet syndrome. The percent change from baseline in seizure frequency is calculated for each patient and the resulting percentages are then lumped into a single group of $N = n_1 + n_2$ patients and ranked from smallest to largest. Using the previous Dravet syndrome trial example, the R code for adding a new variable to hold the rank percent change from baseline, `SF.PChg.Rank`, to the `Szr.Data` data frame, is as follows:

```
Szr.Data$SF.PChg.Rank <- rank(Szr.Data$SF.PChg)
```

Given the concern about the impact of patient age on the course of Dravet syndrome, it is prudent to include age as a factor in the analysis. (Additionally, enrollment in this trial was stratified to maintain balance between treatment and placebo within two age groups: $< 6$ years, $\geq 6$ years.) Here age is a continuous variable running from two to 18 years. The general form of the rank ANCOVA may then be written as:

$$rank\left(SF_{ij}^{\Delta\%}\right) = \alpha + \beta_1 A_{ij} + T_i + \varepsilon_{ij}, i = 1, 2; j = 1, \ldots, n_i \tag{16.1}$$

where $SF_{ij}^{\Delta\%}$ is the percent change in seizure frequency for the $j^{th}$ patient in the $i^{th}$ treatment group, $\alpha$ is an overall mean, $A_{ij}$ is the patient's age, $\beta_1$ is a coefficient modulating the effect of age, $T_i$ is the effect of the treatment (i.e., $T_1$ is the effect of the active treatment and $T_2$ is the effect of placebo), and $\varepsilon_{ij}$ is a randomly distributed error term specific to each patient. The following code and output illustrate how this model can be implemented in R:

```
Rank.ANCOVA <- lm(SF.PChg.Rank ~ Grp + Age, data = Szr.Data)
> anova(Rank.ANCOVA)

Analysis of Variance Table

Response: SF.PChg.Rank

    Df  Sum Sq  Mean Sq F value Pr(>F)
Grp     1   18849.8    18849.8    60.9708    2.377e-11
Age   1   2.8        2.8        0.0091  0.9244
Residuals 77  23805.4    309.2
```

Like the Wilcoxon test, the rank ANCOVA yields a test of whether there is a significant difference between treatment groups but here the significance level is assessed while taking the potential effect of age into account. The $p$-value corresponding to the difference between treatments is found at the end of the line labeled `Grp` in the analysis of variance table and is highly significant ($p = 2.377 \times 10^{-11}$). The rank ANCOVA also yields a significance test of the effect of age that is far from significant ($p = 0.9244$). However, like the Wilcoxon test, the rank ANCOVA does not produce an interpretable estimate of the treatment effect or its confidence interval.

### 16.2.5 Log-Transformed ANCOVA

As mentioned above, there are other ways to adjust for baseline seizure frequency that do not rely on the percent change from baseline. Another potentially more powerful method is to include baseline seizure frequency as a covariate in an ANCOVA. The basic form of the model is similar to the rank ANCOVA except that no ranking is involved and a factor is added to adjust for baseline seizure frequency:

$$SF_{ij}^{T} = \propto + \beta_1 A_{ij} + \beta_2 SF_{ij}^{B} + T_i + \varepsilon_{ij}, \tag{16.2}$$

for $i = 1, 2$ and $j = 1, \ldots, n_i$, where $SF_{ij}^{B}$ and $SF_{ij}^{T}$ are the seizure frequencies for the $j^{th}$ patient in the $i^{th}$ treatment group during the baseline and treatment period, respectively; and $\beta_2$ is a coefficient modulating the effect of baseline seizure frequency. The other terms are the same as for the rank ANCOVA. Note that the percent change from baseline does not appear in the model.

This model, though, is unlikely to satisfy the assumptions needed to assess significance in an ANCOVA due to skewness of the distribution of the seizure frequency data. Log transformations are frequently used in data analysis to handle skewed data and can be profitably applied here as well. Here is the model where the seizure frequency from both the baseline and treatment periods have been log-transformed:

$$\log\left(SF_{ij}^{T}\right) = \propto + \beta_1 A_{ij} + \beta_2 \log\left(SF_{ij}^{B}\right) + T_i + \varepsilon_{ij}, i = 1, 2; j = 1, \ldots, n_i. \tag{16.3}$$

A standard ANCOVA assumes that the error term, $\varepsilon$, is normally distributed, although the analysis is still likely to yield valid results as a long as the sample size is not terribly small and the distribution of $\varepsilon$ is roughly symmetrical.

The ANCOVA using log-transformed seizure data can be analyzed using standard techniques except that estimates of effect size will be on a log scale. Estimated marginal means (EMMs, also known as least squares means or LSMs) can be used to estimate the baseline-adjusted effect of the active treatment on a log scale. For example, the EMM of the log-transformed seizure frequency of the active group during the treatment period is

$$\hat{\alpha} + \hat{\beta}_1\overline{A} + \hat{\beta}_2\overline{\log\left(SF^B\right)} + \hat{T}_1 \tag{16.4}$$

where $\overline{A}$ is the mean age of all subjects, $\overline{\log\left(SF^B\right)}$ is the mean over all subjects of the log-transformed seizure frequency during baseline, and $\hat{\alpha}, \hat{\beta}_1, \hat{\beta}_2$, and $\hat{T}_1$.are estimated parameters from the ANCOVA. The estimate can be back-transformed to the original data scale by exponentiation:

$$\exp\left(\hat{\alpha} + \hat{\beta}_1\overline{A} + \hat{\beta}_2\overline{\log\left(SF^B\right)} + \hat{T}_1\right). \tag{16.5}$$

EMMs can be calculated straightforwardly in `R` using the `emmeans` package by calling the `emmeans()` function. The `R` package also returns a confidence interval for the estimate. Exponentiating the endpoints of the confidence interval transforms the interval back to the original scale of the data.

The overall treatment effect, i.e., the estimated difference between treatment and placebo, can also be calculated for the log-transformed data using EMMs:

$$\begin{aligned}\left\{\hat{\alpha} + \hat{\beta}_1\overline{A} + \hat{\beta}_2\overline{\log\left(SF^B\right)} + \hat{T}_1\right\} - \left\{\hat{\alpha} + \hat{\beta}_1\overline{A} + \hat{\beta}_2\overline{\log\left(SF^B\right)} + \hat{T}_2\right\} \\ = \hat{T}_1 - \hat{T}_2.\end{aligned} \tag{16.6}$$

The resulting difference between treatment groups is on the log scale, but like above, it can be exponentiated to produce a more interpretable result. Exponentiating a difference yields a ratio:

$$\exp\left(\hat{T}_1 - \hat{T}_2\right) = \frac{\exp\left(\hat{T}_1\right)}{\exp\left(\hat{T}_2\right)}. \tag{16.7}$$

Here a ratio of 1 indicates no difference between groups, while a ratio $< 1$ indicates an advantage to the active treatment. The ratio is a meaningful quantification of the treatment effect. That is, a ratio of 0.25 indicates a greater reduction in seizure frequency than a ratio of 0.50. The endpoints of the confidence interval for the difference on the log scale can be exponentiated to provide a confidence interval for the ratio.

One further algebraic manipulation can produce a result that may be even easier to interpret. Specifically, the ratio of treatment to placebo can be turned into a percent difference from placebo as follows:

$$\left\{1 - \frac{\exp\left(\hat{T}_1\right)}{\exp\left(\hat{T}_2\right)}\right\} \times 100. \tag{16.8}$$

This manipulation transforms a ratio of 0.25 into a $-75\%$ change from placebo. Or in another words, the active treatment yielded a 75% greater reduction than placebo in baseline-adjusted seizure frequency. The same algebraic manipulation may be applied to the confidence interval endpoints to yield a confidence interval for the percent change from placebo.

### 16.2.6 Negative Binomial Model

In recent years, another approach to analyzing seizure data has become popular: negative binomial regression [14] Joseph J. Tharayil, et al, 2017. This type of analysis does not require calculating seizure frequencies or a data transformation prior to analysis, but the analysis model itself is more complex than those described so far, and some care must be taken to extract the estimates of interest from analysis software packages such as R.

Several variations of negative binomial regression have been proposed and studied; here we explore the mixed-effects repeated measures (MMRM) negative binomial model. The "repeated" part of the MMRM refers to using seizure measurements from two nonoverlapping time periods – the baseline and treatment periods – as outcome measures in the model. That is, the model includes two outcomes per subject: the number of seizures experienced during the baseline period and the number of seizures experienced during the treatment period. The two outcomes are typically arranged vertically in the dataset and denoted by one of two values (1, 2) of an indicator variable, $P$, for time period.

The "mixed" part of the MMRM indicates that the model includes both fixed factors and random effects. To ensure that the model takes baseline into account, the fixed effects include treatment, period, and the interaction between treatment and period. The fixed effects can also include other factors such as age group. One random effect is included – a random intercept that is allowed to vary for each subject.

The model also requires a smooth link function to linearize the relationship among the explanatory factors. A log link function is used here. It fills the same need as the log transformation used above but does so in a different manner. Optionally, an "offset parameter" can be incorporated into the model to help adjust for discrepancies among subjects in the amount of time spent in the treatment period. The offset parameter essentially changes the outcome variable from a seizure count into a seizure frequency and is helpful if, for example, many subjects discontinue treatment early and end up with much shorter treatment times than subjects who completed the trial. Finally, seizures are assumed to follow a negative binomial distribution conditional on the other components of the model.

The fixed effects part of the basic negative binomial model takes the following form:

$$\log (S_{ijk}) = \propto + T_i + P_j + (TP)_{ij} + \varepsilon_{ijk}, i = 1, 2; j = 1, 2; k = 1, \ldots, n_j \tag{16.9}$$

where $P_j$ indicates the $j^{th}$ time period, either baseline or the treatment period; $(TP)_{ij}$ is the interaction between the $i^{th}$ treatment and the $j^{th}$ time period; and $S_{ijk}$ is the number of seizures experienced by the $k^{th}$ patient in the $i^{th}$ treatment group in the $j^{th}$ time period.

This type of model can be evaluated using the R function `glmer.nb()` using the following call:

```
NB1 <- glmer.nb(S ~ T + P + T*P) + (1|SubjID))
```

The last part of the call, `(1|SubjID)`, where `SubjID` is a unique identifier for each subject, fits a random intercept for each subject. The results of the model are stored in a data structure called `NB1`. The R function, `emmeans()`, can again be used to obtain an estimate of the difference between treatments and its confidence interval:

```
NB1.emm <- emmeans(NB1.model, specs = ~T * P, type = "response")
confint(contrast(NB1.emm, interaction = "pairwise", adjust = "none"))
```

Since a log link function was implicitly used in `glmer.nb`, the resulting estimate of the treatment effect and its confidence interval are on the log scale. But as with the log-transformed model described above, the estimated difference can be exponentiated to yield a ratio of treatment to placebo. Other factors such as age group can be readily added to the model.

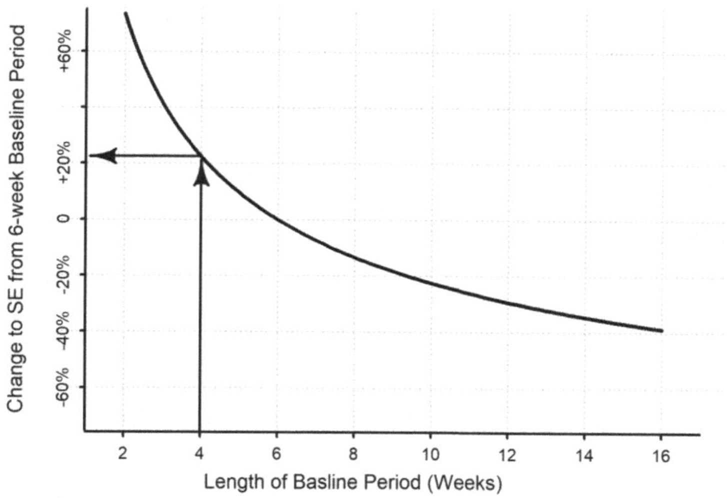


**FIGURE 16.3**
Simplified curve showing how the standard error of the estimated baseline seizure changes as the length of the baseline period is shortened or lengthened from an oft-used duration of four weeks.

## 16.3 Trial Duration

Last, we discuss considerations in epilepsy in determining the length of a clinical trial.

### 16.3.1 Length of Baseline Period and Overall Length of Trial

Statistically, seizure frequency is a sample mean. For any given patient, it is calculated as the number of seizures experienced over a specified time period divided by the length of the time period. Under the simplifying, if a bit unrealistic, assumption that seizure frequency measured within each time period is independent of every other period, the standard error (SE) of seizure frequency decreases in direct proportion to the square root of the length of the period.

The decrease in the SE of seizure frequency is illustrated by the square root curve in Figure 16.3. The $x$-axis represents the number of weeks over which patients are followed in the baseline period of a hypothetical trial. The height of the curve depicts how much the SE of the baseline seizure frequency of a single patient would change if the baseline period differed from the six weeks specified in the Dravet syndrome trial. For example, if the baseline period were shortened from six weeks to four, the SE of the baseline seizure frequency for any single subject would be expected to increase by about 22%. Increasing the baseline period to eight weeks would decrease the SE by about 13%.

The curve in Figure 16.3 shows that there are diminishing returns to extending the length of the baseline period but also shows that shortening the period too much would lead to high variability in the estimate of baseline seizure frequency. For example, Kerr, et al. (2023) describe a patient in an ongoing trial who had 15 seizures in the first four weeks of the baseline period and only four seizures in the subsequent four weeks of baseline [11]

Philippe Ryvlin, et al, 2011. The estimate of that patient's baseline seizure frequency would vary greatly depending on how baseline was defined. High baseline variability would, in turn, increase the variability of the estimate of change from baseline leading to a decrease in the overall power of the trial. It is difficult, however, to quantify exactly how much the length of the baseline period might impact the outcome of a trial. The curve in Figure 16.3 is a simplified idealization, and baseline seizure frequency factors into the efficacy in a variety of different, nonlinear ways.

One approach to estimating the impact of the length of the baseline period is to reanalyze the Dravet syndrome trial using seizure data from only the last four weeks of the actual 6-week baseline period. Using a 4-week baseline period led to only minor changes in the descriptive statistics of the baseline seizure frequency in the trial. Among fenfluramine-treated patients, the mean (SD) seizure frequency using the full six weeks of baseline data was 31.4 (30.6) seizures per month compared to 30.2 (28.8) when using only four weeks of baseline data. Among the placebo recipients the mean (SD) baseline frequency was 45.2 (40.2) seizures per month using the 6-week baseline period compared to 45.5 (39.8) using the 4-week baseline period.

The real test of the shortened baseline period is whether it added enough variability to have a significant impact on the power of the efficacy comparison between treatment and placebo. Here, the treatment groups are compared using the ANCOVA model with log-transformed data described in Section 16.2.5. That model includes baseline seizure frequency as a covariate. Using the original 6-week baseline period, the model estimated that the reduction in monthly seizure frequency was 61.0% (95% CI: 45.4%, 72.2%) greater in the treatment group than in the placebo group. The reduction estimated using the 4-week baseline period was 59.7% (95% CI: 43.4%, 71.2%). The shorter baseline period was expected to lead to greater variability in the overall efficacy comparison and this turned out to be true – but just barely. Specifically, the confidence interval for the estimated reduction in seizure frequency based on the 4-week baseline was one percentage point wider than the analogous CI when all 6 weeks of baseline data was used. The difference is small enough in this case to be considered negligible.

This example suggests that a 4-week baseline period may be used in trials of Dravet syndrome or other disorders with relatively high seizure counts at baseline. However, other study designs for those with high seizure counts, such as time-to-event, may provide a better approach. One possible explanation for why the shorter baseline period had such little impact may be related to the way baseline seizure frequency was used in the efficacy analysis (i.e., as a factor in a model modulated by a coefficient). A shorter baseline period may have had a larger impact on the comparison if, for example, percentage change from baseline were used as the outcome variable. This is because the baseline seizure frequency appears in the denominator of the percentage change from baseline, and small changes in the denominator may result in outsized effects on the overall statistic. The relatively high seizure frequency often seen in Dravet syndrome also likely mitigated the impact of shortening the baseline period. A short baseline period might be unworkable for disorders with infrequent seizures, since some patients may have zero seizures during the baseline period if it is too short.

### 16.3.2 Time-to-Event Trials in Epilepsy

Patients who are recruited to participate in epilepsy clinical trials by definition have medically refractory epilepsy and these patients have a well-defined risk of SUDEP [11]. Even more concerning is that, in a meta-analysis of 112 published placebo-controlled add-on studies, the rate of SUDEP was higher among placebo-treated participants (6.9 per 1,000 patient years) compared to those who received active add-on treatment (0.9 per

1,000 patient years). Therefore, it is critical to minimize the duration of placebo exposure without negatively impacting the ability to detect a treatment difference between treatment groups. This becomes increasingly important in more severe epilepsy conditions, such as the developmental and epileptic encephalopathies, where it is not uncommon for patients to experience multiple seizures per day. A time-to-event study design is one possible alternative approach to minimizing the duration of placebo exposure in such studies.

Time-to-event (TTE) analyses, discussed in depth in Chapter 6, have several advantages for epilepsy clinical trials. TTE models are readily available in statistical software, are relatively simple to fit, and output from the models is easy to interpret [7], Wesley T. Kerr, Stephane Auvin, et al, 2023. There are several potential choices for which kind of event would be most appropriate for a particular trial [7]. For example, the time to first or second seizure after initiation of treatment could be appropriate for patients who experience only infrequent seizures, while time to remission could also be useful [10] ILAE Commission on Antiepilepic Drugs, 1998.

A more general endpoint is the time to the $N^{th}$ seizure following the initiation of treatment, where $N$ can be specifically chosen for each patient [1, 4]. This approach is described below and applied to the data from the Dravet syndrome trial discussed earlier. In this example, $N_i$ is determined individually for each patient in the trial and is set to the number of convulsive seizures the subject experienced during the 6-week baseline period of the trial. This can be considered a time to treatment failure. A short time to the $N_i^{th}$ seizure indicates a poor treatment, a time of six weeks to the $N_i^{th}$ seizure indicates no benefit to treatment, and a time longer than six weeks is a sign of treatment efficacy. Once a suitable event has been identified, TTE data from epilepsy clinical trials can be analyzed using survival analysis methods such as Kaplan-Meier curves, log-rank tests, and Cox proportional hazards models (Chapter 6).

In a retrospective analysis of the Dravet syndrome trial, the event of interest for the $i^{th}$ subject was defined as the number of seizures, $N_i$, experienced during the 6-week baseline period [13] Joseph Sullivan, et al, 2021. The TTE endpoint for the $i^{th}$ subject was defined as the elapsed time from randomization to when the subject experienced their $N_i^{th}$ seizure during the 14-week treatment period. If a patient experienced fewer than $N_i$ seizures during the treatment period – i.e., never had as many seizures during the treatment period as during baseline – that patient was considered right-censored at their last observed time, $T_i^+$, during or at the end of the treatment period.

A Kaplan-Meier curve from the TTE analysis of the Dravet syndrome study is shown in Figure 16.4. The graph shows that 56% of fenfluramine-treated subjects never experienced as many seizures through the entire 14-week treatment period as they had in the 6-week baseline period. The analogous percentage in the treatment group was only 5%. The log-rank test affords a way to test whether there is a difference between the treatment groups at any time point in the treatment period [2]. The $p$-value from the log-rank test in this example was $< 0.001$. Like the Wilcoxon test discussed earlier, the log-rank test does not yield an estimate of the size of the treatment effect, and it does not take into account other potential explanatory factors such age, sex, or baseline seizure frequency. These limitations can be overcome by using a Cox proportional hazards model to analyze the TTE data.

It is useful in this example, though, to compare the Kaplan-Meier curves at earlier time points than the planned end of treatment. For example, at Week 7 – the halfway point through the planned treatment period – the curves from the treatment and placebo groups had already diverged greatly. In particular, by Week 7, 58% of placebo subjects had either discontinued or had already experienced as many or more seizures than they had during baseline. If the design of the trial considered those subjects as treatment failures, they could have discontinued treatment and simply continued their original treatment or switched to unblinded fenfluramine treatment. Either option would be preferable to continuing with

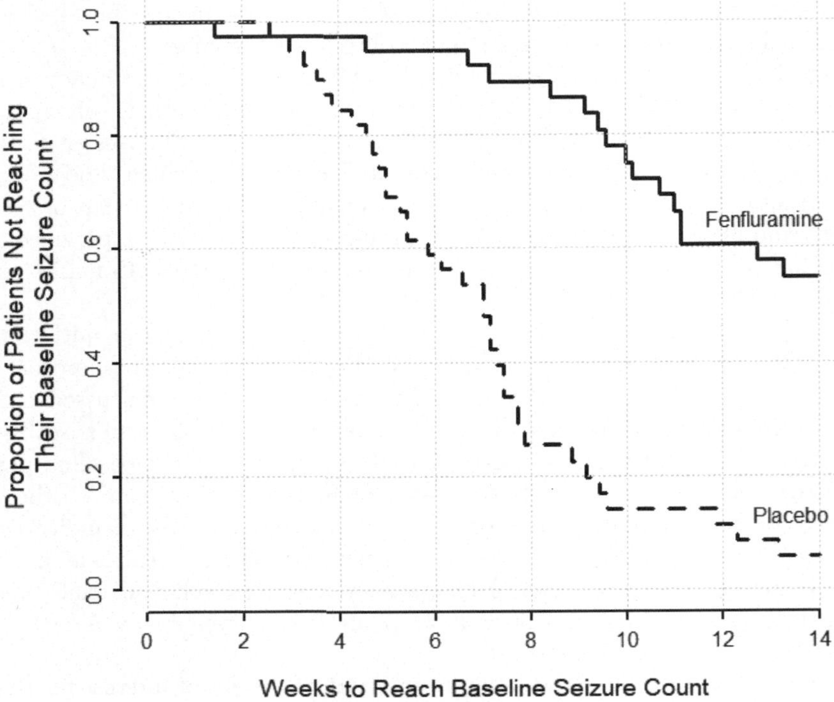


**FIGURE 16.4**
Kaplan-Meier curves comparing fenfluramine-treated patients (n = 40) to placebo recipients (n = 40) using the time after treatment each patients takes to reach their baseline seizure count. Patients who never reach their baseline seizure count during treatment are right-censored.

placebo. At Week 10, 87% of subjects in the placebo group could be considered treatment failures. With the right design, it is likely that the trial could have been stopped early at this point saving four weeks of additional treatment on placebo when the superiority of an alternative could already be clearly established.

## 16.4 Summary

In summary, clinical trials are necessary to investigate the efficacy and safety of novel treatments for epilepsy patients; however, the study design must take into consideration many clinical variables that are unique to individuals with epilepsy. By taking these variables into account for the various different types of epilepsy, innovative trial designs and statistical methods may optimize the overall sample size and trial duration while still gaining the necessary data for regulatory approval and subsequent use in clinical practice.

## Bibliography

[1] Stéphane Auvin, Jacqueline French, Denis Dlugos, Kelly G. Knupp, Emilio Perucca, Alexis Arzimanoglou, Ed Whalen, and Renée A. Shellhaas. Novel study design to assess the efficacy and tolerability of antiseizure medications for focal-onset seizures in infants and young children: A consensus document from the regulatory task force and the pediatric commission of the international league against epilepsy (ILAE), in collaboration with the pediatric epilepsy research consortium (PERC). *Epilepsia Open*, 4(4):537–543, September 2019.

[2] J. Martin Bland and Douglas G. Altman. The logrank test. *BMJ*, 328(7447):1073, April 2004.

[3] Laura J. Bonnett, Jane L. Hutton, and Anthony G. Marson. Modelling seizure rates rather than time to an event within clinical trials of antiepileptic drugs. *BMC Medical Research Methodology*, 20(1), April 2020.

[4] J.A. French, A. Gil-Nagel, S. Malerba, L. Kramer, D. Kumar, and E. Bagiella. Time to prerandomization monthly seizure count in perampanel trials: A novel epilepsy endpoint. *Neurology*, 84(20):2014–2020, April 2015.

[5] Jason Hsu. *Multiple Comparisons.* Chapman and Hall/CRC, February 1996.

[6] Linda Kalilani, Xuezheng Sun, Barbara Pelgrims, Matthias Noack-Rink, and Vicente Villanueva. The epidemiology of drug-resistant epilepsy: A systematic review and meta-analysis. Epilepsia, 59(12):2179–2193, December 2018.

[7] Wesley T. Kerr, Stephane Auvin, Serge Van der Geyten, Christopher Kenney, Gerald Novak, Nathan B. Fountain, Caitlin Grzeskowiak, and Jacqueline A. French. Time-to-event clinical trial designs: Existing evidence and remaining concerns. Epilepsia, 00:1–10, 2023.

[8] Wesley T. Kerr, Hai Chen, Mariana Figuera Losada, Christopher Cheng, Tiffany Liu, and Jaqueline French. Reasons for ineligibility for clinical trials of patients with medication-resistant epilepsy. Epilepsia, 64(5):e56–e60, 2023.

[9] Lieven Lagae, Joseph Sullivan, Kelly Knupp, Linda Laux, Tilman Polster, Marina Nikanorova, Orrin Devinsky, J. Helen Cross, Renzo Guerrini, Dinesh Talwar, Ian Miller, Gail Farfel, Bradley S. Galer, Arnold Gammaitoni, Arun Mistry, Glenn Morrison, Michael Lock, Anupam Agarwal, Wyman W. Lai, and Berten Ceulemans. Fenfluramine hydrochloride for the treatment of seizures in dravet syndrome: a randomised, double-blind, placebo-controlled trial. *The Lancet*, 394(10216):2243–2254, December 2019.

[10] ILAE Commission on Antiepileptic Drugs. Considerations on designing clinical trials to evaluate the place of new antiepileptic drugs in the treatment of newly diagnosed and chronic patients with epilepsy. *Epilepsia*, 39(7):799–803, July 1998.

[11] Philippe Ryvlin, Michel Cucherat, and Sylvain Rheims. Risk of sudden unexpected death in epilepsy in patients given adjunctive antiepileptic treatment for refractory seizures: a meta-analysis of placebo-controlled randomised trials. *The Lancet Neurology*, 10(11):961–968, November 2011.

[12] R.J. Simes. An improved Bonferroni procedure for multiple tests of significance. *Biometrika*, 73(3):751–754, 1986.

[13] Joseph Sullivan, Nicola Specchio, Orrin Devinsky, Stéphane Auvin, M. Scott Perry, Adam Strzelczyk, Antonio Gil-Nagel, David Dai, Bradley S. Galer, and Arnold R. Gammaitoni. Fenfluramine significantly reduces day-to-day seizure burden by increasing number of seizure-free days and time between seizures in patients with dravet syndrome: A time-to-event analysis. *Epilepsia*, 63(1):130–138, October 2021.

[14] Joseph J. Tharayil, Sharon Chiang, Robert Moss, John M. Stern, William H. Theodore, and Daniel M. Goldenholz. A big data approach to the development of mixed-effects models for seizure count data. *Epilepsia*, 58(5):835–844, March 2017.

# *Index*

**T**